TAPPAN'S HANDBOOK OF HEALING MASSAGE TECHNIQUES

Classic, Holistic, and Emerging Methods

Fourth Edition

Patricia J. Benjamin, PhD
Licensed Massage Therapist, Illinois
Chicago, Illinois

Frances M. Tappan, PT, EdD
Formerly of the University of Connecticut
Storrs, Connecticut

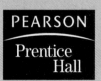

PEARSON
Prentice
Hall

Upper Saddle River, New Jersey

Library of Congress Cataloging-in-Publication Data

Tappan, Frances M.
    Tappan's handbook of healing massage techniques / Frances M. Tappan,
        Patricia J. Benjamin.—4th ed.
        p. ; cm.
    Includes bibliographical references and index.
    ISBN 0-13-098715-8
    1. Massage therapy. 2. Acupressure.
    [DNLM: 1. Massage—methods. WB 537 T174ha 2005] I. Title: Handbook
of healing massage techniques. II. Benjamin, Patricia J. III. Title.

    RM721.T2178 2005
    615.8'22—dc22
                                                            2004006732

Publisher: Julie Levin Alexander
Publisher's Assistant: Regina Bruno
Senior Acquisitions Editor: Mark Cohen
Associate Editor: Melissa Kerian
Editorial Assistant: Jaquay Felix
Director of Manufacturing and Production: Bruce Johnson
Managing Editor for Production: Patrick Walsh
Production Liaison: Cathy O'Connell
Production Editor: Bruce Hobart/Pine Tree
    Composition, Inc.
Manufacturing Manager: Ilene Sanford
Manufacturing Buyer: Pat Brown
Creative Director: Cheryl Asherman
Senior Design Coordinator: Christopher Weigand
Cover Designer: Mary Siener
Director of Marketing/Marketing Manager: Karen Allman
Channel Marketing Manager: Rachele Strober
Marketing Coordinator: Janet Ryerson
Media Editor: John Jordan
Media Production Manager: Amy Peltier
Media Project Manager: Stephen Hartner
Composition: Pine Tree Composition, Inc.
Printing and Binding: Courier/Westford
Cover Printer: Phoenix Color Corp.

NOTICE

The authors and the publisher of this volume
have taken care that the information and
technical recommendations contained herein
are based on research and expert consultation,
and are accurate and compatible with the
standards generally accepted at the time of
publication. Nevertheless, as new information
becomes available, changes in clinical and
technical practices become necessary. The
reader is advised to carefully consult manufacturers' instructions and information material
for all supplies and equipment before use, and
to consult with a healthcare professional as
necessary. This advice is especially important
when using new supplies or equipment for
clinical purposes. The authors and publisher
disclaim all responsibility for any liability, loss,
injury, or damage incurred as a consequence,
directly or indirectly, of the use and application of any of the contents of this volume.

Inside Front Cover and Facing Page: Muscles of the Human Body
Inside Back Cover and Facing Page: Energy Channels of Traditional Asian Medicine

Pearson Education, Ltd., *London*
Pearson Education Australia Pty. Limited, *Sydney*
Pearson Education Singapore, Pte. Ltd.
Pearson Education North Asia Ltd., *Hong Kong*
Pearson Education Canada, Ltd., *Toronto*

Pearson Education de Mexico, S.A. de C.V.
Pearson Education—Japan, *Tokyo*
Pearson Education Malaysia, Pte. Ltd.
Pearson Education, Upper Saddle River, *New Jersey*

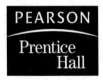

10 9 8 7 6 5 4 3 2 1
ISBN 0-13-098715-8

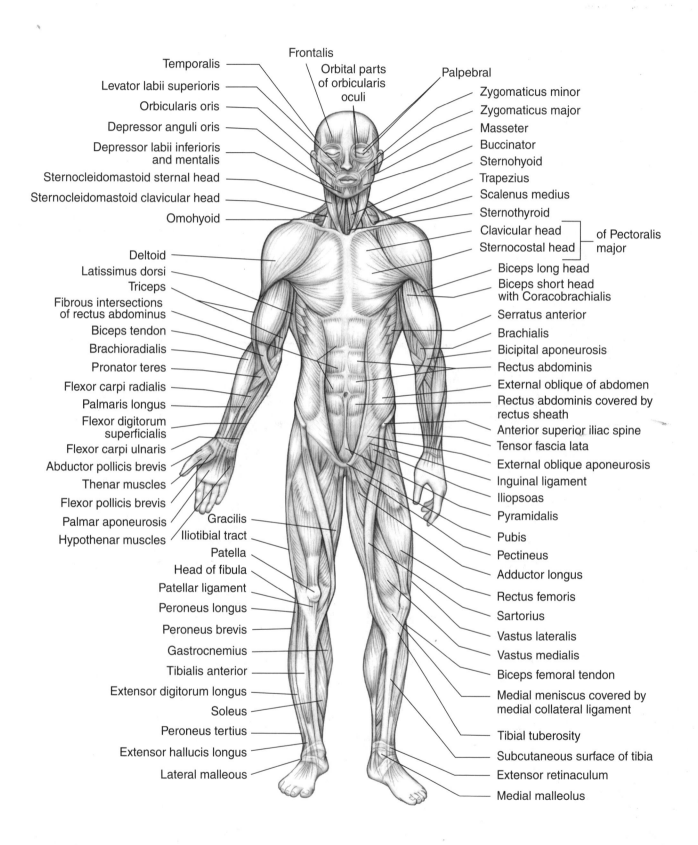

Temporalis

Levator labii superioris

Orbicularis oris

Depressor anguli oris

Depressor labii inferioris
and mentalis

Sternocleidomastoid sternal head

Sternocleidomastoid clavicular head

Omohyoid

Deltoid

Latissimus dorsi

Triceps

Fibrous intersections
of rectus abdominus

Biceps tendon

Brachioradialis

Pronator teres

Flexor carpi radialis

Palmaris longus

Flexor digitorum
superficialis

Flexor carpi ulnaris

Abductor pollicis brevis

Thenar muscles

Flexor pollicis brevis

Palmar aponeurosis

Hypothenar muscles

Gracilis

Iliotibial tract

Patella

Head of fibula

Patellar ligament

Peroneus longus

Peroneus brevis

Gastrocnemius

Tibialis anterior

Extensor digitorum longus

Soleus

Peroneus tertius

Extensor hallucis longus

Lateral malleous

Frontalis

Orbital parts
of orbicularis
oculi

Palpebral

Zygomaticus minor

Zygomaticus major

Masseter

Buccinator

Sternohyoid

Trapezius

Scalenus medius

Sternothyroid

Clavicular head

Sternocostal head

of Pectoralis
major

Biceps long head

Biceps short head
with Coracobrachialis

Serratus anterior

Brachialis

Bicipital aponeurosis

Rectus abdominis

External oblique of abdomen

Rectus abdominis covered by
rectus sheath

Anterior superior iliac spine

Tensor fascia lata

External oblique aponeurosis

Inguinal ligament

Iliopsoas

Pyramidalis

Pubis

Pectineus

Adductor longus

Rectus femoris

Sartorius

Vastus lateralis

Vastus medialis

Biceps femoral tendon

Medial meniscus covered by
medial collateral ligament

Tibial tuberosity

Subcutaneous surface of tibia

Extensor retinaculum

Medial malleolus

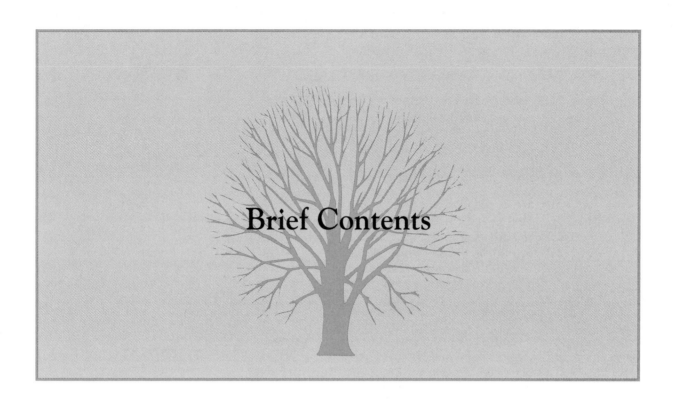

Brief Contents

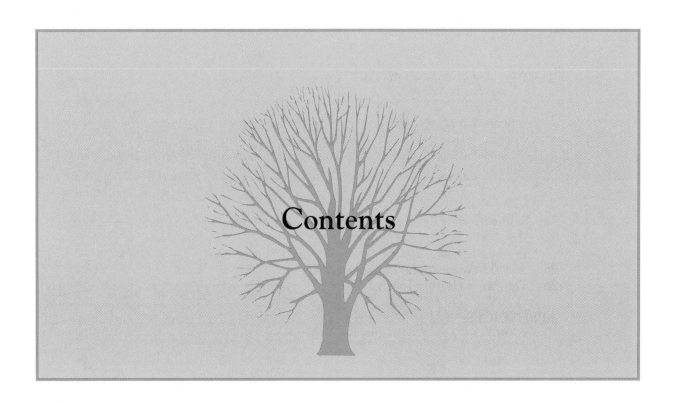

Contents

x   Contents

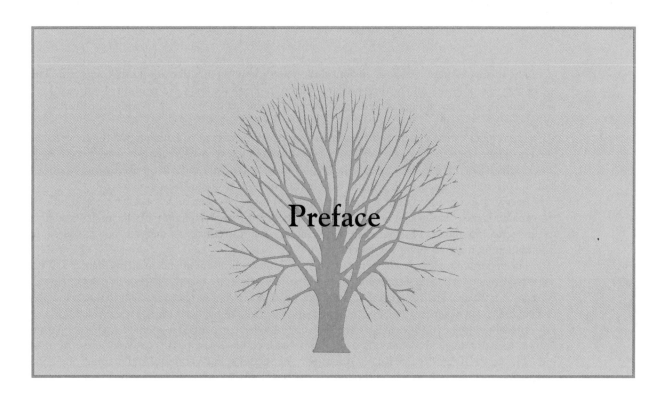

Preface

Tappan's Handbook of Healing Massage Techniques has been updated and revised to reflect the changes in massage therapy and its use in the health professions over the past several years. Massage continues to be a mainstay of the spa and salon, health club, and private practice scenes, while being integrated into an increasing number of heath care settings.

The number of states in the United States that license massage therapists has grown from 24 in 1998, when the third edition was published, to 31 in 2004. A massage therapy research database sponsored by the AMTA Foundation is now available on the Internet. The Canadian Touch Research Centre is holding its second International Symposium on the Science of Touch in Montreal in May 2004.

As the massage universe expands, and massage therapy enjoys increasing recognition within the health professions, the expectations for massage therapy education also grow. Massage therapy training programs must educate their students for the future by giving them a firm foundation to build on.

Tappan's Handbook of Healing Massage Techniques has been redesigned, with several learning aids to help students and teachers in their studies. These include a detailed Table of Contents formatted as chapter outlines, and a complete list of figures and tables for easy location. Each chapter contains learning outcomes, key terms and concepts, and references including books, videos and Web sites. Chapter study guides include suggestions for studying key terms and concepts, as well as study questions for information recall, and suggested activities for a deeper understanding of important topics.

A CD-ROM video that demonstrates basic Western and contemporary massage techniques, as well as applications for special populations, is included with the text. Use of this modern technology helps make up for the limited ability of words and still pictures to depict satisfactorily what is essentially a performance-based art and science.

Frances Tappan's original vision for the textbook remains intact. Dr. Tappan wanted students of massage to have descriptions of massage techniques and approaches from all over the globe. The inside front and back covers showing the muscular system from Western anatomy, and energy channels from Traditional Asian Medicine, reflect her interest in the worldwide reach of massage.

Part I: Foundations provides the theoretical underpinning and context for later chapters on massage techniques. Chapter 1, Healing Massage—A Wellness Perspective, discusses massage as a natural healing art found all over the world. The relationship between massage and Western medicine in the context of integrative health care is explored. The concept of *wellness* is discussed at greater length, and a new paradigm called the Wellness Massage Pyramid offers a fresh image of massage in its broad scope.

The history of massage as an ancient and modern healing practice is told in Chapter 2. The use of massage for health and healing predates current professions, and its universality for humankind is evident. A section on more recent developments in the health professions brings this history up to date.

The science of the effects and benefits of massage is examined in Chapter 3. This chapter has been rearranged to be more compatible with human anatomy texts used in many massage programs. It looks at the effects of massage at the tissue, organ system, and organism levels, as well as its physiological and psychological effects. A holistic view of the effects of massage is also presented.

A new chapter called Clinical Applications of Massage has been added as Chapter 4. It reflects the expanding use of massage in health care and in the treatment of different pathologies. It also points to the increasing number of research studies being done on the efficacy of massage, and to sources of information on massage therapy research.

The important topics of endangerment sites and contraindications are taken up in Chapter 5. With a greater diversity of people seeking massage for a variety of reasons, massage therapists need to be well versed in how to avoid harm. The information on contraindications has been rearranged into principles as a guide to good judgment, and a section on cautions related to medications has been added.

Guidelines for giving massage in Chapter 6 have also been expanded to include more information on how to maintain good therapeutic relationships with clients, some pitfalls to avoid, and ethical issues. The new HIPAA Privacy Rule is discussed. The sections on positioning and draping, and good body mechanics, are enriched by still photos from the CD-ROM video of massage techniques.

Part II is devoted entirely to Western Massage, which forms the basis for most therapeutic massage applications found in physiotherapy, in natural healing, and for wellness in Europe and North America. Chapter 7, Western Massage Techniques, and Chapter 8, Joint Movements, describe basic techniques in detail. Chapter 9, Full-Body Western Massage, offers a massage routine to illustrate a one-hour wellness-focused session and practice sequence. Chapter 10, Regional Applications, looks at massage techniques for each body region and includes the meaning of the region in human terms, its anatomy, and more detailed massage treatment descriptions. Chapter 11, Hydrotherapy/Thermal Therapies is an addition to *Tappan's Handbook of Healing Massage Techniques* that focuses on applications of water, and hot and cold modalities typically associated with massage therapy. It does not cover the full range of physical agents found in physical therapy texts. It does offer valuable descriptions of modalities to use with massage, and summary tables of useful information.

Part III Contemporary Massage and Bodywork explores five systems of massage and bodywork theory and techniques that can be used in conjunction with basic Western massage. Three are grounded in Western science and are concerned with specific body tissues or systems, i.e., myofascial massage, neuromuscular therapy, and lymphatic drainage massage. Two involve alternative ways of understanding the human body. Foot reflexology is based on the theory of zone therapy and involves compression massage of the feet. Polarity therapy considers the body's theoretical energy fields and methods of balancing that energy for better health and disease prevention.

Asian massage and bodywork traditions based on Chinese medicine are covered in Part IV. Chapter 17 is a treatise on the theory of Traditional Asian Medicine (TAM). Just as Western anatomy and physiology forms the theoretical basis of Western massage, TAM underpins Asian Bodywork Therapy (ABT). This new chapter contains a more thorough explanation of the theoretical basis of Asian bodywork including yin/yang, concepts of qi, five elements, energy assessment, and acupoints. Chapters 18–20 look at different forms of ABT including Amma: Traditional Japanese Massage, Zen Shiatsu (a modern Japanese bodywork form), and Jin Shin Do®, a contemporary derivative.

Applications of massage are covered in Part V. Massage for special populations such as athletes, pregnant women, infants, the elderly, and the terminally ill are described. Seated massage is explained in the context of providing massage in the workplace.

These chapters have been updated and enhanced with still photos from the CD-ROM, which has a section on each population treated in the text.

Dr. Tappan's essay on The Art of Healing Touch appears as Chapter 26. It offers her insight into the role of the massage practitioner, the nature of health and disease, and the power of healing touch.

Rounding out the content of the book is reference material, including a Bibliography and listing of useful Web sites mentioned in the text, and an updated glossary. Appendix A is new, and contains concise information on 25 popular massage and bodywork systems. The list of important organizations and publications in Appendix B has been expanded and updated, as has the list of states which license massage therapists in Appendix C. Appendix D provides an evaluation tool for massage therapy students and teachers, and Appendix E contains sample health history forms for planning safe and effective massage sessions.

My hope continues to be that those of you who read and study from this book not only value the basic information presented, but also sense the wonder and potential of hands-on healing for the simplest of intentions—to help fellow human beings in their quest for good health and optimum wellbeing.

Patricia J. Benjamin, PhD

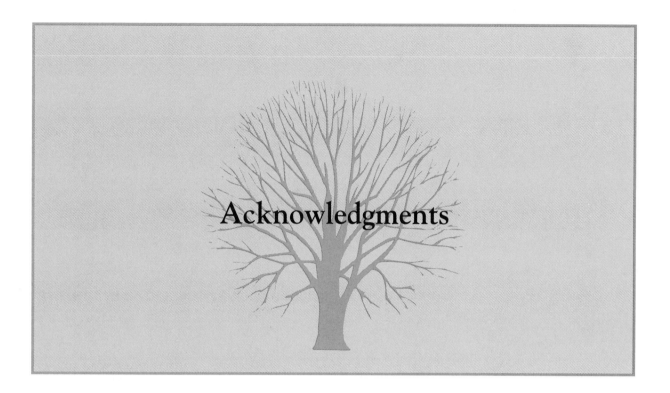

Acknowledgments

Writing and producing a text like *Tappan's Handbook of Healing Massage Techniques* involves the contributions of many people both known and unknown to the author. They all deserve thanks. A few who stand out will be acknowledged here.

Gratitude is extended to the many people who gave of their knowledge and experience in the production of the first three editions of *Tappan's Handbook of Healing Massage Techniques*. They laid the foundation for this current edition. Many thanks are reserved for the colleagues and friends of Frances Tappan at the School of Physical Therapy at the University of Connecticut in Storrs who assisted with the first two editions.

Thanks also to Steve Kitts and Beverly Schoenberger, founders of the Connecticut Center for Massage Therapy, for their consultations and writing in earlier editions. The faculty and staff at CCMT offered encouragement and support during production of the 3rd edition, reviewed drafts and served as models for many of the drawings. Special recognition goes to Victoria Carmona and Lee Stang for their help with photography from which technique drawings were made.

I am grateful to all those who reviewed drafts of the current manuscript and made suggestions for improvement from correcting grammar to refining the details of content. The process was anonymous, but you know who you are, and you have my thanks. I'd like to acknowledge Christopher Alvarado and Lisa Holk for their reviews of key chapters, ideas, and videos. Other faculty and staff of the Chicago School of Massage Therapy lent their ideas and suggestions. It is a better book for their input.

Appreciation also goes to the contributing authors who offer their expertise in special areas of study including Gary Bernard — Amma, Pauline Sasaki — Zen Shiatsu, Beverly Schoenberger — Polarity Therapy, Jasmine Wolf and Iona Teeguarden — Jin Shin Do®. Special welcome is extended to Barbara Esher and John Johnston who are new contributing authors to the Asian Bodywork Therapy section.

Thanks to the staff at Prentice Hall Health who put it all together. Melissa Kerian, Assistant Editor, and Mark Cohen, Senior Editor of Health Professions guided the project throughout. Jody Small was producer of the CD-ROM video, and Hector Grillone its director. Massage therapists who performed for the cameras were Lisa Barnacz, Elyce Cooper, Caleb Edmond, and Harry Purcell. Thank you for your cooperation, patience, and skill in demonstrating massage.

Of course, a project like this is a culmination of the life experiences, study, and work of a number of people. Acknowledgement goes to all of the teachers and students who have used the book and made valuable suggestions, to all of my friends and colleagues, to clients who have taught me so much, and to massage practitioners from various professions who practice healing massage in their work.

Special appreciation is reserved for Martha Fourt who offered encouragement throughout the writing of the 4th edition. Her patience and support, and that of my family and friends were invaluable.

Patricia J. Benjamin, Ph.D.

Frances M. Tappan Remembered
1917–1999

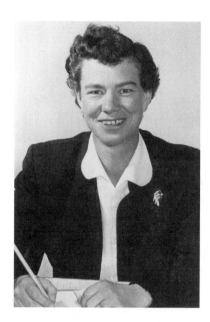

Frances M. Tappan at the University of Connecticut c. 1960.

Frances M. Tappan passed away on August 17, 1999. Her spirit endures in the memories of the many people she touched throughout her full life. Fran was an adventurous soul with a big heart. She was an inspiration to her family, friends, and colleagues—and to two professions dear to her heart, physical therapy and massage therapy.

Dr. Tappan organized the physical therapy program at the University of Connecticut in Storrs in 1950, and served as its leader for the next 25 years. She was active in the American Physical Therapy Association. After she officially retired, Fran continued her work, helping the founders of the Connecticut Center for Massage Therapy in Newington in the early 1980s. She received the American Massage Therapy Association, Council of Schools Award for Excellence in Education in 1989.

Although her other professional accomplishments are many, she will be remembered here for love of massage therapy. Fran believed in massage and its healing capabilities. In the 1940s, she began her study of the different massage techniques used at the time in the developing field of physical therapy. Her first book on massage was called *Massage Techniques: A Case Method Approach* (1961).

Fran traveled to Germany to study Bindegewebsmassage at the Elizabeth Dicke School in Überlingen. In 1975, she went to Taiwan to learn about Chinese medicine and how finger pressure to acupoints can be used to enhance healing. The first edition of *Tappan's Handbook of Healing Massage Techniques* was published in 1980 and reflected her interest in massage techniques practiced worldwide. It was called *Healing Massage Techniques: A Study of Eastern and Western Methods*.

Chapter 26, "The Art of Healing Touch," appeared as "Creating Positive Attitudes towards Healing" in that first edition. It is recommended reading for anyone wanting a sense of Dr. Tappan's personal belief in the healing power of touch.

The next editions of *Tappan's Handbook of Healing Massage Techniques* included even more forms of massage and bodywork, some with alternative ways of understanding human health, disease, and healing. The book's subtitle changed to *Classic, Holistic, and Emerging Methods*.

Tappan's Handbook of Healing Massage Techniques, including this latest edition, is a product of Dr. Tappan's vision. She set the scope, the tone, and the basic philosophy that continues in the work that she began so many years ago. It is a tribute to her dedication and love of hands-on healing.

May Frances M. Tappan be remembered as the curious, open, and kind-hearted spirit that she truly was.

Patricia J. Benjamin

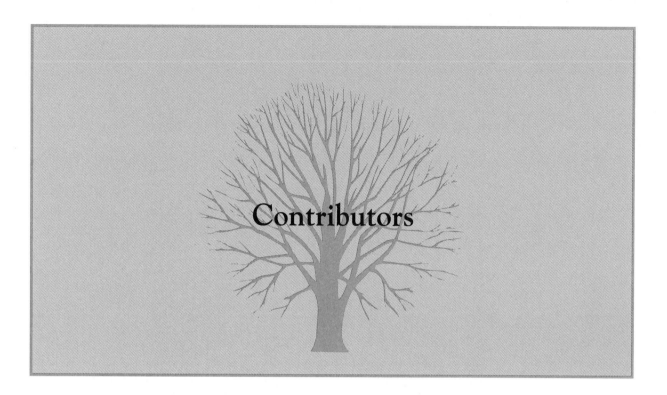

Contributors

Gary Bernard
Owner, Touch Wellness: Chair Massage
for the Workplace
San Francisco, California
Amma Instructor, Milberry Fitness and
Recreation Center
University of California at San Francisco

**Barbara Esher, Dipl. Ac. & ABT
(NCCAOM)**
Senior Instructor and Curriculum Coordi-
nator for the Shiatsu Program and Asian
Bodywork Program at the Baltimore
School of Massage
Baltimore, Maryland

John Johnston
Shiatsu Instructor at the Baltimore
School of Massage
and Anne Arundel Community College
Baltimore, Maryland

Pauline Sasaki
Quantum Shiatsu Instructor
Certified Practitioner and Instructor,
AOBTA
Teacher throughout the United States
and Europe
Westport, Connecticut

Beverly Schoenberger, RPT
Co-founder, Connecticut Center for Massage
Therapy
Licensed Psychotherapist and Physical
Therapist
Newington, Connecticut

**Iona Marsaa Teeguarden, MA, Executive
Director**
Jin Shin Do® Foundation for Bodymind
Acupressure
Author of *A Complete Guide to Acupressure—
Jin Shin Do*®
Idyllwild, California

Jasmine Ellen Wolf, BA
Authorized Jin Shin Do instructor
Jin Shin Do teacher throughout New England
Coventry, Connecticut

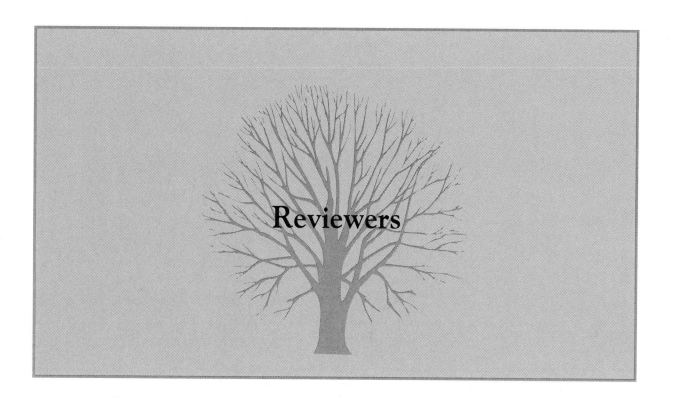

Reviewers

Melodie A. Adinolfi, LMT
Founder
The Alternative Conjunction Clinic
and School of Massage Therapy
Lemoyne, Pennsylvania

Linda Aldridge, LMT, MA
Instructor
McKinnon Institute of Massage
Oakland, California

Michael Avenoso, M.T.I.
Co-owner and Instructor
White River School of Massage
Fayetteville, Arkansas

Nancy W. Dail, LMT, NCTMB
Director
Downeast School of Massage
Waldoboro, Maine

Patricia M. Donohue, LMT
Professor
New York College for Health Professions
Syosset, New York

Marty Downey, RN, MSN, HNC
Associate Professor
Department of Nursing
Boise State University
Boise, Idaho

Randy Ellingson, FLCSP(Phys)
President
Wellington College of Remedial Massage
Therapies
Winnipeg, Manitoba
Canada

Western College of Remedial Therapies
Regina, Saskatchewan
Canada

Patrick Goff, Ed.D
Professor of Health Psychology and Wellness
Institute for Therapeutic Massage
and Wellness
Davenport, Iowa

Lisa Mertz, PhD, LMT
Massage Therapy Program
Queensborough Community College
Bayside, Queens

Maureen Rattensperger, PT, OCS, MS
Associate Professor and Director
Physical Therapy Assistant Program
Missouri Western State College
St. Joseph, Missouri

John P. Sanko, PT, Ph.D.
Associate Professor
Physical Therapy Department
University of Scranton
Scranton, Pennsylvania

Cheryl L. Siniakin-Baum, Ph.D
Associate Professor and Director
Massage Therapy Program
Community College of Allegheny County
Pittsburgh, Pennsylvania

Ann Vendrely, PT, MS, OCS
Professor
Physical Therapy Program
Governors State University
University Park, Illinois

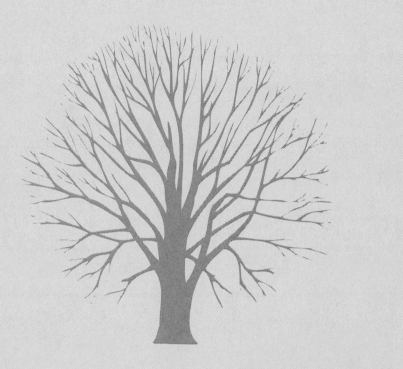

I

Foundations

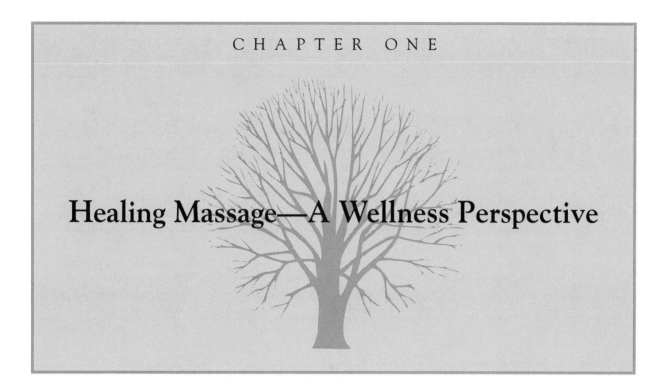

CHAPTER ONE

Healing Massage—A Wellness Perspective

LEARNING OUTCOMES

After studying this chapter, the student will have information to:

1. Explain massage as a natural healing art, and as manual therapy.
2. Identify important tenets of the natural healing philosophy.
3. Define the meaning of healing, and contrast it to curing.
4. Define holistic, and discuss the idea of the whole person.
5. Define massage, and analyze the nature of massage techniques, including action and intention.
6. Describe four major world traditions of massage and bodywork.
7. Identify the seven major categories of Western massage techniques.
8. Analyze the relationship of massage to Western medicine as a CAM therapy, and within a system of integrative health care.
9. Use Travis' Illness/Wellness Continuum to compare the wellness and treatment models.
10. Use the Wellness Massage Pyramid to describe the broad scope of massage, and its contributions to achieving high level wellness.
11. Discuss the scope of different health professions using the Wellness Massage Pyramid.
12. Use the language of wellness and treatment appropriately.

 MEDIALINK

A companion CD-ROM, included free with each new copy of this book, supplements the techniques presented in this chapter. Insert the CD-ROM to watch video clips of massage techniques being demonstrated. This multimedia feature is designed to help you add a new dimension to your learning.

KEY TERMS/CONCEPTS

Alternative therapy
Asian bodywork therapy
   tradition
Ayurvedic massage tradition
CAM therapy
Clients, guests, patients
Complementary therapy
Contemporary massage and
   bodywork
Eclectic practitioner
Effleurage
Folk and native traditions
Friction
Giver
Healing

High level wellness
Holistic
Illness/wellness continuum
Integrative healthcare
Intention
Joint movements
Manual therapy
Massage
Massage and bodywork
Massage technique
Medical spa
Natural healing arts
Natural healing philosophy
Petrissage
Practitioner

Receiver, recipient
Session
Tapotement
Therapist
Touch without movement
Traditions of massage and
   bodywork
Treatment model
Treatment, procedure
Vibration
Wellness Massage Pyramid
Wellness model
Western massage technique
   categories
Western massage tradition

INTRODUCTION

In this first decade of the 21st century, massage is available around the globe—on the streets of China, in the spas of Europe, in the temples of Thailand, in tribal villages in Africa and Australia, and in health clubs and day spas in the United States. Soft tissue manipulation is used by traditional healers such as Hispanic curanderas, and is an integral part of medical systems such as Traditional Chinese Medicine, and Ayurveda in India. It is also being reclaimed as a valuable therapy within modern Western medicine. Its many benefits for preventing illness, healing, and optimizing well-being are being rediscovered by a growing number of people worldwide.

NATURAL HEALING ART

Massage is one of the traditional **natural healing arts.** It has been used for centuries to promote and restore health along with other gifts of nature such as nutritious food, herbs, healing waters, exercise, relaxation, fresh air and sunshine. Massage is a **manual therapy,** i.e., performed by hand. Simple hand tools and electric devices are sometimes used in conjunction with massage by hand. But it is the person-to-person touch that defines massage, and gives massage its unique healing potential.

Many of the tenets of the **natural healing philosophy** formalized in late 19th century are still adhered to by many massage practitioners. These include preference for natural methods of healing, a belief in the existence of an innate healing force, and a holistic view of human life. The wellness perspective described later in this chapter is a modern adaptation of the natural healing philosophy.

The term **healing** has many shades of meaning. Healing in its broader sense means to make healthy, whole, or sound. The word healing also means enhancing health and well-being, as well as the process of regaining health or optimal functioning after an injury, disease, or other debilitating condition. Modern science is confirming the efficacy of massage and other natural methods for maintaining health and for healing.

Healing, especially natural healing, may be contrasted to the concept of *curing*. The connotation of the term *cure* is of something coming from the outside, and given to a passive recipient. Healing, on the other hand, implies the existence of a force at work from within, with the recipient as an active participant in their own recovery. In this text, massage is presented as a method for enhancing the innate healing force already at work as living beings continuously repair themselves and try to maintain an integrated wholeness.

Holistic refers to those approaches to health and healing that take into account the wholeness of human beings, including body, mind, emotions, and spirit. In the holistic paradigm, massage is applied to the physical body, yet it affects all other aspects of the whole person. Although the term holistic is relatively new in the health professions, the concept is of ancient origin and is a basic tenet of the natural healing philosophy. It is also a fundamental principle of the wellness perspective discussed later in the chapter.

MASSAGE DEFINITION

Massage is the intentional and systematic manipulation of the soft tissues of the body to enhance health and healing. Joint movements and stretching are commonly performed as part of massage. The primary characteristics of massage are touch and movement.

The actions and intentions of the practitioner constitute the **massage technique.** Massage techniques are generally described in active terms such as gliding or sliding, percussion, compression, broadening, kneading, friction, vibrating, stretching, and holding. Through the medium of touch, the massage practitioner's actions cause movement in the soft tissues of the recipient. Different massage techniques have different effects. Techniques are chosen by the practitioner and applied in such a way to accomplish the goals of each massage session.

Intention is the aim that guides the action, that is, what the practitioner hopes to accomplish. The intent might be to enhance a biophysical process such as relaxation or circulation, or to balance energy, or to evoke a positive emotional state. It might also be expressed in a more functional way, such as to recover from an athletic competition, to improve posture, or to diminish pain. Intention helps determine choice of techniques and guides the action in subtle ways. Intention is an essential part of the effective application of massage.

Massage falls into the more general category of **massage and bodywork.** The term *bodywork* was coined in the latter 20th century to encompass a wide variety of manual therapies including systems of soft tissue manipulation, movement integration, structural integration, energy balancing, and other approaches to health and healing that involve touch and movement. The terms *massage* and *bodywork* are often used together to describe the broad scope of the occupational field of massage therapy, for example, as in National Certification for Therapeutic Massage and Bodywork. The types of massage described in this text fall into the broad category of massage and bodywork. Some of the more popular systems of massage and bodywork are described in Appendix A. (The book to read for a survey of massage and bodywork systems is *Discovering the Body's Wisdom*, by Mirka Knaster.)

MASSAGE AND BODYWORK TRADITIONS

A *tradition* implies some element of culture that is passed down from generation to generation within a group of people. A tradition is typically defined as originating from an ethnic group, geographic location, or civilization.

Occasionally a tradition of one group is adopted by other groups of people. This has happened time and again throughout history, for example in music, art, games, writing, and health and healing practices. Tradition is not an immutable concept; some say that a tradition is established after only two generations. However, tradition is a useful concept for identifying the origin, and categorizing the many different systems of massage and bodywork.

There are four traditions that encompass most of the systems of massage and bodywork used widely today. These are folk and native traditions, Ayurvedic massage, Asian bodywork therapies (ABT), and Western massage and bodywork. The map in Figure 1–1 shows the origin of these world traditions of massage. Information about the history of these traditions may be found in Chapter 2 and in Part IV.

Folk and native traditions of massage and bodywork are characterized by being specific to a small or narrowly defined group of people, and passed down by apprenticeship either through families, or from tribal or village healers. They include both general health and healing goals. Folk and native healing practices are based on how things have been done in the past, and on experience about what brings are about the desired results. These practices are most often performed in a larger context that includes herbal remedies, rituals, and religious beliefs. These traditions often served as the foundations for the more formal and larger traditions that evolved over time. Examples are rubbing techniques of

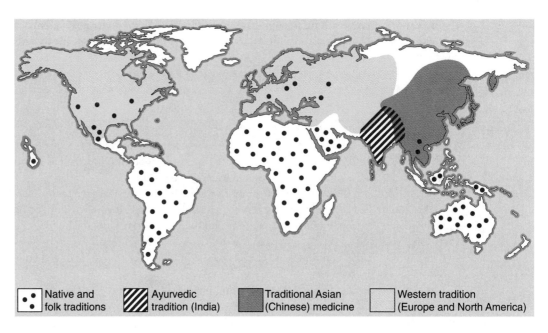

Native and folk traditions   Ayurvedic tradition (India)   Traditional Asian (Chinese) medicine   Western tradition (Europe and North America)

FIGURE 1–1. Map of World Traditions of Massage and Bodywork.

the tribal healers in Africa; lomi-lomi of the Hawaiians; and soft tissue techniques of traditional Hispanic healers, called curanderas.

The **Ayurvedic massage tradition** originated in India, and is based on a comprehensive system of beliefs about health and disease. Its theory can be traced to an ancient text called the Vedas written in the 5th century BCE. Massage is considered essential in Ayurvedic practices to circulate "vayu" (or wind) in vessels called "siras" to promote healthy body functioning. The oil used in massage is chosen carefully according to the recipient's body type, the atmosphere, and the season. Different types of bodywork are also used to balance energy in centers called chakras. Related practices include hatha yoga, breathing exercises, cleansing and vegetarianism. (The book to read is *Ayurvedic Massage*, by Harish Johari.)

The **Asian bodywork therapy (ABT) tradition** includes systems of massage and bodywork with roots in Chinese medicine. These are characterized by reference to energy (chi, ki) channels or meridians, and points along the channels called acupoints. Pressing and rubbing techniques stimulate the movement of energy through the channels to promote balance and harmony. Examples of ABT are tuina or medical massage from China, amma and shiatsu from Japan, and a contemporary system called Jin Shin Do®. Related practices include tai chi, qigong, and acupuncture.

The **Western massage tradition** can be traced to ancient Greek and Roman practices as developed over the centuries in Europe and North America. The Western tradition encompasses massage as a heath practice, for beauty and pleasure, as well as for healing. Its foundation is Western science including anatomy, physiology, and pathology. Scientific research about the efficacy of massage for healing has increased dramatically in the past few decades, and is providing a solid grounding for the use of massage in treatment of certain pathologies, as defined by Western medicine.

Modern Western massage is a system of soft tissue manipulation that evolved out of the work of Pehr Ling and Johann Mezger at the end of the 19th century. Five classic massage technique categories are *effleurage, petrissage, friction, tapotement,* and *vibration*. The classic terminology is common to Swedish massage, and massage as taught in most physical therapy programs. Some schools today use their English equivalents, i.e., sliding/gliding, kneading/compression, friction, percussion, vibration. Touch without movement and joint movements are also incorporated into Western massage. These seven **Western massage technique categories** are simple, adaptable, and useful for describing a variety of healing massage techniques.

Effleurage techniques slide or glide over the skin with a smooth continuous motion. **Petrissage** techniques lift, wring, or squeeze soft tissues in a kneading motion, or press or roll tissues under the hands. **Friction** is performed by rubbing one surface over another repeatedly. **Tapotement** consists of rapid percussive movements performed in a rhythmic manner. **Vibration** may be described as an oscillating, quivering, or trembling motion, or movement back and forth or up and down performed quickly and repeatedly. **Touch without movement** includes passive touch, holding, or laying the hands on the body. **Joint movements** within the scope of Western massage include mobilizing techniques within normal range of motion, and stretching. Figure 1–2 illustrates the basic Western massage techniques.

Contemporary massage and bodywork systems that go beyond the basic Western techniques were developed in the 20th century. Some—like lymphatic massage, trigger points, and myofascial massage—are based in Western anatomy, while others—like polarity therapy and reflexology—rely on alternative health perspectives. In recent years there has been an explosion of interest in many different forms of massage and bodywork as consumers have rediscovered their many benefits for promoting optimal health and healing. Part III describes five systems of contemporary massage and bodywork.

Many practitioners grounded in Western massage incorporate elements of theory and technique from other systems or traditions for an eclectic approach. For example, an **eclectic practitioner** might combine basic Western techniques with contemporary approaches like myofascial or trigger point techniques, and perhaps some reflexology or shiatsu. Part of the art of massage is in choosing the appropriate techniques to accomplish the goals of a session.

MASSAGE AND WESTERN MEDICINE

Massage and bodywork therapies are sometimes called alternative or complementary in relation to Western medicine. This is a curious concept, since massage has been used in Western medicine since ancient Greek times. The reason for this contradiction can be traced to the mid-20th century when massage lost favor within regular medicine, and was largely dropped from mainstream health care. Renewed interest in massage in the late 20th century happened largely within the natural healing tradition during the counterculture of the 1960–1970s. Since the revival occurred outside of what was considered conventional medicine at the time, and included approaches to healing at the fringes or outside of Western science, massage therapy was then considered to be alternative.

This attitude has gradually changed as more scientific research about massage is conducted within mainstream medical institutions. For example, research studies about massage are conducted by the Touch Research Institute at the University of Miami (www.miami.edu/touch-research), and can be found in the AMTA Foundation database (www.amtafoundation.org).

When massage is called an **alternative therapy,** it is generally meant as an *either/or* option outside of mainstream medicine. When it is seen as a **complementary therapy,** it is considered secondary to the treatments of mainstream medicine, but contributing to the patient's recovery.

CAM is an acronym for Complementary and Alternative Medicine. CAM is a broad concept that includes therapies like biofeedback, herbal remedies, homeopathic remedies, acupuncture, Ayurveda, naturopathic medicine, environmental medicine, and various forms of massage and bodywork. Wide use of CAM therapies by consumers prompted the establishment of the National Center for Complementary and Alternative Medicine (NCCAM) within the National Institutes of Health (NIH) in 1998. (www.nccam.nih.gov).

The White House Commission on CAM Policy (2002) cites therapeutic massage, bodywork, and somatic movement therapies as a major CAM domain. Other domains include alternative healthcare systems (e.g., Traditional Chinese Medicine, Ayurveda, chiropractic and naturopathic medicine), mind-body interventions (e.g., meditation and hypnosis), biological-based therapies (e.g., herbal remedies and special diets), energy therapies (e.g., qigong and Reiki), and bioelectromagnetics (e.g., magnet therapy). (www.whccamp.hhs.gov).

A more progressive viewpoint considers massage and bodywork as a choice within an **integrative health care** system offering many options for healing. In integrative health care systems, different therapies exist on equal status, and are chosen for a particular case based on the greatest benefit for the patient. Manual therapies like massage are being integrated into an increasing number of medical settings today.

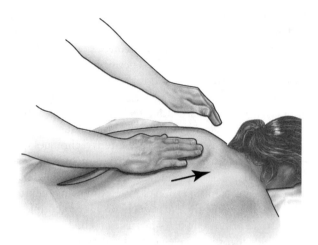

Effleurage—sliding and gliding techniques.

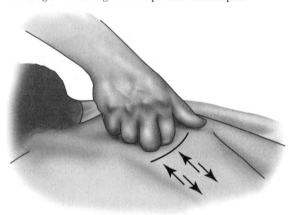

Petrissage—kneading and compression techniques.

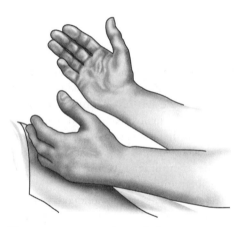

Tapotement—percussion techniques.

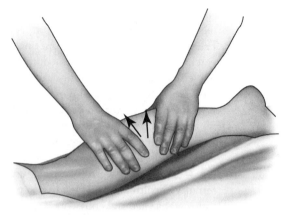

Friction—rubbing techniques.

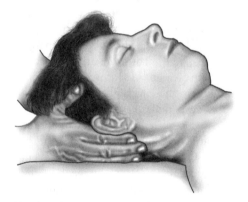

Touch without movement—holding and touching techniques.

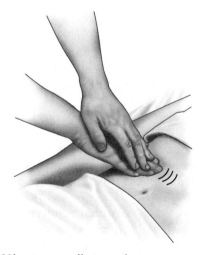

Vibration—oscillating techniques.

FIGURE 1–2. Seven Basic Western Massage Techniques.

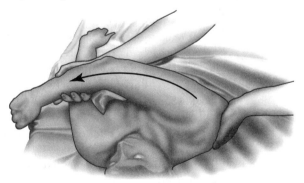

Joint movements—mobilizing and stretching techniques.

In a parallel trend, some North American spas are providing conventional as well as complimentary therapies to patrons who come to them for health and healing services. An integrative approach has been common in European spas for years. The International Spa Association (ISPA) includes "medical spa" as one of the seven categories of spas. A **medical spa** is one that provides "comprehensive medical and wellness care in an environment which integrates spa services, as well as conventional and complementary therapies and treatments" (www.experienceispa.com).

WELLNESS PERSPECTIVE

A wellness perspective goes beyond the old idea of health as the mere absence of disease to the goal of achieving a vibrant, meaningful life. In this paradigm, the individual takes personal responsibility for forming life habits to achieve optimal wellbeing in many areas of their lives. "Wellness" is a concept that took form in the 1970s United States and has been adopted in professions devoted to physical education and fitness, health, recreation and leisure, and health care.

Illness/Wellness Continuum

The diagram of the **illness/wellness continuum**, shown in Figure 1–3, is a useful illustration of the concept of wellness, and of the wellness and treatment models. It was developed by John Travis, MD, a pioneer of the wellness movement, who founded the Wellness Resource Center in Mill Valley, California in 1975. Wellness Associates, a nonprofit educational foundation, continues Travis' work today (www.thewellspring.com).

Travis's **wellness model** spans the entire illness/wellness continuum, from premature death to high level wellness. It includes treatment for disability and the signs and symptoms of disease, as well as movement towards greater awareness, education, and growth to achieve high level wellness. In this diagram the **treatment model** is shown separately and corresponds to the half of the wellness model to the left of "neutral."

High Level Wellness

In its broadest sense, **high level wellness** is a condition of optimal physical, emotional, intellectual, spiritual, social, and vocational wellbeing. It is holistic at its core. The components of wellness and a healthy lifestyle are explained in practical terms in Table 1–1. Achieving optimal wellness in each of these arenas is a lifetime process.

There are many aspects of living that contribute to high level wellness. They include things like good nutrition, adequate exercise, rest, recreation, satisfying and healthy relationships, seeking counsel for handling problems, spending time in nature, and finding meaningful work.

Many have found massage to be an effective method to enhance wellness in a number of ways. Looking at the components of wellness in Figure 1–4, several potential ways come to mind. Massage helps keep soft tissues in healthy condition, improves sleep, and promotes relaxation. It can help one cope with stress, reduce anxiety, and find inner peace. It supports participation in exercise and sports.

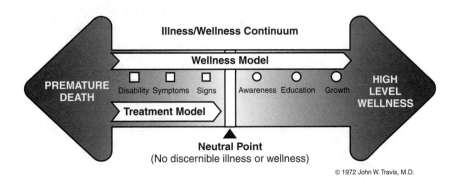

FIGURE 1–3. The illness/wellness continuum. (*Reprinted with permission, Wellness Workbook, Travis & Ryan, Ten Speed Press, Berkeley, CA. © 2000 John W. Travis, MD*)

Table 1–1 COMPONENTS OF WELLNESS AND A HEALTHY LIFESTYLE

Physical wellbeing involves being physically fit; eating nutritiously; being free from chemical dependency and other harmful behaviors; being aware of early signs of illness; getting adequate sleep and rest; preventing accidents.

Emotional wellbeing involves balance in emotions; expressing emotions appropriately and comfortably; showing respect and affection for others; coping successfully with stress and personal problems; seeking counsel when needed.

Intellectual wellbeing includes clear thinking and problem solving; processing information; questioning and evaluating; learning from life experiences; being flexible, creative, and open to new ideas.

Social wellbeing means having satisfying relationships and interacting well with others; having a network of family, friends, and others who can help you in time of need; establishing a sense of belonging within your community.

Spiritual wellbeing is whatever brings meaning and purpose in your life; knowing your purpose in life and being more comfortable expressing love, joy, peace, and fulfillment; feeling connected to your inner self, significant others, and the universe; having hope after setbacks; appreciating nature.

Vocational wellbeing includes school and job satisfaction; working in harmony with others to accomplish something worthwhile.

Source: Seiger, L., Vanderpool, K., & Barnes, D. (1995). *Fitness and wellness strategies.* Madison, WI: Brown & Benchmark (pp. 5–6).

It can provide an avenue for learning more about the body, mind and emotions. It helps develop body awareness and sense of connectedness to the inner self. It can relieve isolation, and help establish a sense of connectedness to others. It offers caring touch in a safe environment. Because each person is an interconnected whole, improving any one of these aspects can help improve others. Each person benefits from massage for their own unique reasons.

WELLNESS MASSAGE PYRAMID

While the illness/wellness continuum is useful, it leaves the impression of a dichotomy between the wellness and treatment models. This is problematic when trying to express one broad scope for massage therapy. This dichotomy in thinking is evident in how the terms are commonly used, that is, with the word

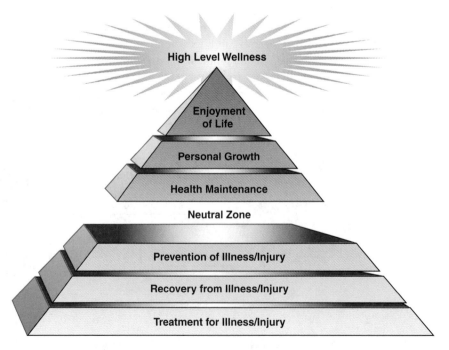

FIGURE 1–4. Wellness massage pyramid.

treatment reserved for massage therapy left of the neutral point (i.e., disability, symptoms, signs), and *wellness* practices reserved for the neutral point to high level wellness (i.e., awareness, education, growth). A different illustration is needed to capture a concept of wellness that includes the entire range of wellness related to massage therapy.

The **Wellness Massage Pyramid** (WMP) in Figure 1–4 tries to capture the inclusive nature of a wellness perspective for massage therapy. The WMP uses some concepts from the illness/wellness continuum, but adds others specific to the potential contributions of massage to high level wellness.

Each level on the WMP represents a major contribution massage can make on a journey to high level wellness, and each level serves as the platform for the next level. The pyramid includes from the base to the top: treatment and recovery from illness and injury, prevention of illness and injury, a neutral zone (absence from illness and injury), and on to health maintenance, personal growth and the enjoyment of life. A three-dimensional view of the pyramid would reveal each of these levels for body, mind, emotions, and spirit.

Using a pyramid to depict a hierarchy of levels for achieving a specific goal is borrowed from Maslow's Hierarchy of Needs in psychology. At the base of the pyramid in Maslow's theory of human motivation are *deficiency needs* that have to be satisfied before *growth needs* may be addressed. Maslow's deficiency needs are physiological, safety, love, and esteem. Once these are met, then growth needs, such as understanding and aesthetic needs, may be addressed, finally allowing for self-actualization and transcendence (Huitt 2002). Maslow's theory is meant to explain human motivation, but the general idea of a pyramid also works well to illustrate needs to be met on the road to high level wellness.

At the base of the WMP is treatment for, recovery from, and prevention of illness or injury. If successful at these levels, i.e., eliminating deficiencies, one gets to a neutral point. Beyond the neutral point, growth toward high level wellness proceeds to the maintenance of good health. This provides a base for physical, psycho-emotional, and spiritual growth, and enjoyment of life. Theoretically, the foundation would be laid on each level to enable a person to proceed to the next level, but it is important not to take this hierarchy too literally.

There is significant gray area between levels. Throughout a lifetime, levels would be revisited periodically to repair any weaknesses from the wear and tear of living, and to address challenges faced in different life stages. And given the multidimensional nature of wellness, you could be addressing different levels simultaneously. For example, from a wellness perspective, people with chronic illnesses might always be in treatment, but may also be maintaining health in other areas, working on personal growth (e.g., spiritual development), and progressing to high level wellness in other dimensions of their lives. The pyramid is simply a tool for understanding the possible contributions of massage therapy on the journey to high level wellness.

The pyramid can be used to explain the many different reasons people seek massage. The treatment and recovery level is perhaps the easiest to understand. A client comes in with a complaint of pain or dysfunction, and massage is used to diminish pain and help in the healing process. Once an acute phase is past, the slow rebuilding of a healthy state begins. It is in the recovery phase that massage is often used to complement a primary treatment.

At the level of prevention, a client may be aware that their stress level is getting too high and may use massage as a strategy to reduce their stress and prevent illness. Or a client may feel their muscles tightening up from repetitive motion and seek massage to prevent damaging strain. These are subclinical situations that would eventually lead to illness or injury if left to progress.

The neutral zone indicates the absence of deficiencies, i.e., signs and symptoms of disease and injury. It is characterized by absence of pain, tolerable stress level, and function for daily living activities. This was the goal in old theories of health. In the WMP, it is a plateau on the way to high level wellness.

At the level of health maintenance, a client might receive regular massage as part of a healthful lifestyle. At this point they are moving past the neutral zone on their way to high level wellness. Massage can help keep the body and mind functioning well both as a kind of pre-prevention strategy, as well as a foundation for being able to participate in personal growth activities and to enjoy life to its fullest.

Beyond health maintenance are the reasons people seek massage as a life enhancement. These might include the healthful pleasure of caring touch, developing greater awareness of our inner selves, feeling integrated in body and mind, or improving physical condition for recreation activities.

The wellness massage pyramid can be used to describe the goals of a massage session. The goals might fall within one or more levels, depending on the client/patient needs at the time and the setting.

A session may be focused primarily at the base of the pyramid in the treatment arena, or on treatment and prevention, or on health maintenance and personal growth, or at several levels simultaneously. Any one massage session could be described as having a certain percentage of time or focus at a particular level of the pyramid.

WELLNESS AND THE HEALTH PROFESSIONS

Several health professions include massage in their scope of practice, e.g., massage therapists, physical therapists, nurses, athletic trainers, chiropractors, and naturopaths. Depending on the profession, massage may be called massage therapy, bodywork, manual therapy, physiotherapy, or simply a modality.

In the context of a profession that utilizes several different modalities, or methods of treating pathology, massage may play a minor role overall. It may be in the same category of modalities as ice packs, hot packs, ultrasound, or whirlpool baths. This is true of most health professions listed above.

In the massage therapy profession, massage and bodywork is the main "modality." Massage therapists are specialists in soft tissue applications, and are called upon to perform massage within the full range of the wellness massage pyramid. Massage therapists themselves sometimes call different systems of massage and bodywork "modalities." This is discouraged, since it does not reflect the complexity of these approaches to healing. *Systems, approaches,* and *forms* are suggested instead of the term modality.

Massage practitioners commonly specialize in one or two aspects of the wellness massage pyramid. For example, most physical therapists concentrate on treatment, recovery and prevention, while many massage therapists focus on health maintenance and personal growth. However, some physical therapists help clients reach personal goals such as improving athletic performance, and a growing number of massage therapists specialize in rehabilitation and in treatment of patients with pathology. Nurses may include massage as part of palliative care for patients in hospitals or nursing homes. Most health professions include at least some aspects of the broad scope of wellness, although individual practitioners may choose to practice within a narrower range of client goals.

Health practitioners in states with occupational licensing generally have their scope of practice defined by law, although that scope may change over time. For example, many jurisdictions now include treatment in the scope of practice of massage therapists, although they are legally prohibited from diagnosing medical conditions in most states.

Massage is used somewhat differently in different health professions according to their scope and theoretical bases, but these professions share a common bond, that is, the massage techniques themselves. The heart of this book is the description of massage techniques and their applications for enhancing health and healing.

CLARIFYING TERMINOLOGY

Terminology used within different health professions and in different settings varies. For example, some health professionals will say they have **clients** or **guests,** while others use the term **patients.** Some call themselves technicians or **practitioners,** while others prefer **therapists.** Some refer to what they do as **treatments** or **procedures,** while others use the term **sessions.**

The word *treatment* has become particularly problematic for massage therapists in their interface with mainstream medicine. Historically, the term *treatment* has been used for a number of different services in settings like spas. For example, a facial, mud bath, or massage might be called a treatment even though its aim is health, beauty, or pleasure.

This becomes confusing for practitioners in health care professions where *treatment* specifically means a method of healing a medical condition. Because many massage therapists are working in mainstream medical settings, and it is important to be clear about scope of practice, it may be time to limit the use of the term *treatment.* It should be reserved for when massage and bodywork is used for treatment of or recovery from a specific medical condition.

The chart in Table 1–2 contains suggestions for terminology to distinguish more clearly when massage is being used in the medical model. The column on the left lists terms more appropriate for more general wellness situations, and the column on the right is more treatment oriented language. Using

Table 1–2 WELLNESS/TREATMENT TERMINOLOGY CHART

The terminology listed below can be used to distinguish more clearly between the broad scope of wellness, and specific treatment applications of massage. Wellness terminology is appropriate in a wide variety of settings, while the treatment terminology is used more in clinical or medical settings.

Note: The intent of massage from a wellness perspective is high level wellness in many dimensions of life, and in treatment applications is the alleviation of a specific diagnosed medical condition.

Wellness Terminology	Treatment Terminology
• Client	• Patient, case
• Client history, health history	• Medical history, case history
• Session, appointment	• Treatment
• Assessment, evaluation	• Assessment, diagnosis
• Benefit	• Indication
• Contraindication	• Contraindication
• Problem solving skills, session organizing skills	• Clinical reasoning skills
• Client management	• Case management
• Session plan, session strategy	• Treatment plan, protocol
• Therapeutic approach	• Intervention
• Therapeutic	• Therapy, rehabilitation
• Health profession	• Health care profession
• Practice environment	• Medical environment, health care environment
• Practitioner, massage therapist, bodyworker	• Therapist

the word *treatment* and related terms only in the context of addressing a medical condition would help clarify the intention of a specific massage application.

The terminology used throughout this text is deliberately more inclusive. The one who performs massage will be called the **giver** or practitioner, while the one receiving massage will be called the **receiver** or **recipient.** The word *practitioner* specifically refers to someone trained in massage techniques, and who uses massage in the practice of his or her profession. Session will refer to the period of time in which massage is performed. The term treatment will be reserved for descriptions of medical applications.

SUMMARY

Massage is one of the traditional natural healing arts. It is a manual therapy, i.e., performed by hand, and it is the person-to-person touch that defines massage and gives it a unique healing potential. Many massage practitioners adhere to the tenets of a natural healing philosophy, including a preference for natural methods of healing, the belief in an innate healing force, and a holistic view of human life.

Healing means to make healthy, whole, or sound. It also means to enhance health and wellbeing, and the process of regaining health or optimal functioning after an illness or injury. Healing comes from the inside, and recipients are active participants in their own recovery. In contrast, the connotation of the word *curing* is something coming from the outside, and given to a passive recipient. Massage is presented in this text as a method for enhancing the innate healing force already at work as living beings continuously repair themselves and try to maintain an integrated wholeness.

Holistic refers to approaches to health and healing that take into account the wholeness of human beings including body, mind, emotions, and spirit. In the holistic paradigm, massage is applied to the physical body, yet it affects all other aspects of the whole person.

Massage is the intentional and systematic manipulation of the soft tissues of the body to enhance health and healing. Its primary characteristics are touch and movement. The actions and intentions of the practitioner constitute the massage technique. Through the medium of touch, the practitioner's actions (e.g., sliding, kneading, or stretching) cause movement in the soft tissues. Intention is the aim that guides the action, and is an essential part of the effective application of massage. Massage falls into the general category of massage and bodywork.

Traditions are elements of culture passed down from generation to generation. There are four traditions that encompass most of the systems of massage and bodywork used widely today. These are folk and native traditions, the Ayurvedic massage tradition of India, Asian bodywork tradition based in Chinese medicine, and the Western massage tradition from Europe and North America.

Modern Western massage is a system of soft tissue manipulation first developed in 19th century Europe. The seven Western massage technique categories are effleurage (sliding and gliding), petrissage (kneading and compression), tapotement (percussion), friction, vibration, touch without movement (holding and touching), and joint movements (mobilizing and stretching techniques). Contemporary massage and bodywork systems developed in the 20th century include lymphatic massage, trigger points, myofascial massage, polarity therapy, and reflexology. Eclectic practitioners combine Western massage techniques with techniques from other systems or traditions to accomplish the goals of a massage session.

Massage and bodywork are sometimes called alternative or complementary to Western medicine. Although renewed interest in massage occurred outside of conventional Western medicine in the late 20th century, a growing number of scientific studies are currently conducted within mainstream medical institutions. When massage is referred to as alternative, it is looked upon as an either-or option outside of mainstream medicine. When it is called complementary, it is considered secondary to a conventional treatment but as contributing to a patient's recovery. CAM is the acronym for complementary and alternative medicine. The United States government considers therapeutic massage, bodywork, and somatic movement therapies a major CAM domain.

In an integrative health care system, massage is considered of status equal to other conventional and CAM therapies. Massage is being integrated into many medical settings today, as well as in spas that offer comprehensive medical and wellness care.

The illness/wellness continuum extends from premature death to high level wellness. The wellness model spans the entire length of the continuum with the aim of high level wellness, while the treatment model spans the continuum to the neutral point. High level wellness is a condition of optimal physical, emotional, intellectual, spiritual, social, and vocational wellbeing. Massage can help individuals achieve high level wellness in a number of ways.

The wellness massage pyramid (WMP) combines concepts from the illness/wellness continuum and Maslow's hierarchy of needs to illustrate the many contributions massage can make toward achieving high level wellness. Moving up from the base of the WMP, levels of contribution are treatment of, recovery from, and prevention of illness and injury, the neutral zone, and then health maintenance, personal growth, and enjoyment of life. The WMP can be used to explain reasons people seek massage, as well as describe the goals of a massage session.

Several health professions include massage in their scope of practice. In many health professions, massage is just one modality among others for treatment of a medical condition. For massage therapists, massage is their specialty and is used for the full range of the wellness goals. Although massage is used somewhat differently in different professions, they share a common bond, that is, the massage techniques themselves.

Various health professions use terminology related to massage differently. The terminology used in this text is deliberately inclusive. The one who performs massage will be called the *giver* or *practitioner*, while the one receiving massage will be called the *receiver* or *recipient*. *Session* will refer to the time period in which massage is performed. *Treatment* will be reserved for medical applications.

A look ahead . . .

Our current understanding and practice of massage therapy has evolved over many centuries. In Chapter 2 we will take a closer look at the history of massage to get a sense of its ancient origin, and its development into a valued health and healing practice for the 21st century.

REFERENCES

Huitt, W. G. (2002) Maslow's hierarchy of needs. Retrieved: March 2003 (*http://chiron.valdosta.edu/whuitt/col/regsys/maslow.html*).

Johari, H. (1996) *Ayurvedic massage: Traditional Indian techniques for balancing body and mind.* Rochester, VT: Healing Arts Press.

Knaster, M. (1996) *Discovering the body's wisdom: A comprehensive guide to more than fifty mind-body practices.* New York: Bantam Books.

Seiger, L., Vanderpool, K., & Barnes, D. (1995). *Fitness and wellness strategies.* Madison, WI: Brown & Benchmark.

Travis, J. W., & Ryan, R. S. (2000). *Wellness Workbook.* 2nd edition. Berkeley, CA: Ten Speed Press.

White House Commission on Complementary and Alternative Medicine Policy (2002). *Final Report.* Department of Health and Human Services. (*www.whccamp.hhs.gov*).

WEB SITES

www.amtafoundation.org AMTA Foundation—Research Database

www.experienceispa.com International Spa Association

www.miami.edu/touch-research Touch Research Institute at the University of Miami

www.nccam.nih.gov National Center of Complementary and Alternative Medicine at the National Institutes of Health, Washington, DC.

www.thewellspring.com Wellness Associates

www.whccamp.hhs.gov White House Commission on CAM Policy Report

S T U D Y   G U I D E

LEARNING OUTCOMES

Use the learning outcomes at the beginning of the chapter as a guide to your studies. Perform the task given in each outcome, either in writing or verbally into a tape recorder or to a study partner. This may start as an "open book" exercise, and then later from memory.

KEY TERMS/CONCEPTS

To study key words and concepts listed at the beginning of this chapter, choose one or more of the following exercises. Writing or talking about ideas helps you remember them better, and explaining them to someone else helps deepen your understanding.

1. Write a one or two sentence explanation of each key word and concept.

2. Make study cards by writing the explanation from problem 1 on one side of a 3 × 5 card, and the key word or concept on the other. Shuffle the cards and read one side, trying to recite either the explanation or word on the other side.

3. Pick out two or three key words or concepts and explain how they are related.

4. With a study partner, take turns explaining key words and concepts verbally.

5. Make up sentences using one or more key words or concepts.

6. Read your sentences from problem 5 to a study partner, who will ask you to clarify your meaning.

STUDY OUTLINE

The following questions test your memory of the main concepts in this chapter. Locate the answers in the text using the page number given for each question.

Natural Healing Art

1. Along with other therapies that use the healing gifts of nature, massage is considered a _____. (p. 4)

2. The natural healing philosophy includes these tenets: (1) _____, (2) _____, (3) _____. (p. 4)

3. Massage is considered manual therapy because it is performed _____. (p. 4)

4. The term *healing* means _____ _____. (p. 4)

5. In contrast to the term *healing*, the term *curing* implies _____. (p. 4)

6. The term *holistic* includes a person's (1) _____, (2) _____, (3) _____, and (4) _____ (p. 4)

Massage Definition

1. *Massage* is the _____ and _____ manipulation of the _____ of the body to enhance health and healing. (p. 5)

2. The _____ and _____ of the practitioner constitute the massage technique. (p. 5)

3. The aim that guides the action is called its _____. (p. 5)

4. The words _____ and _____ are often used together to describe the broad scope of the occupational field of massage therapy. (p. 5)

Massage and Bodywork Traditions

1. A *tradition* is an element of culture that is passed down from _____. (p. 5)

2. Four major world traditions of massage and bodywork are (1) _____, (2) _____, (3) _____, (4) _____. (p. 5)

3. The system of soft tissue manipulation that evolved out of the work of Ling and Mezger in the 19th century is known as _____. (p. 6)

4. Match the classic Western massage techniques listed below with the descriptions on the right: (p. 7)

   _____ effleurage   a. percussion

   _____ petrissage   b. rubbing surfaces together

   _____ tapotement   c. sliding or gliding

   _____ friction   d. oscillating

   _____ vibration   e. kneading or pressing

5. Two additional techniques commonly performed in Western massage are _____ and _____. (p. 7)

6. Lymphatic massage, trigger points, and reflexology are categorized as _____ Western massage and bodywork systems. (p. 7)

7. Practitioners who incorporate techniques from two or more traditions or systems of massage and bodywork are said to be _____. (p. 7)

Massage and Western Medicine

1. When massage is considered an either/or option outside of mainstream medicine, it is referred to as _____. (p. 7)

2. When massage is used to contribute to a patient's recovery, but as secondary to a treatment by mainstream medicine, it is referred to as _____. (p. 7).

3. CAM is an acronym for C _____ & A _____ M _____. (p. 7)

4. In _____ health care systems, different therapies exist on an equal footing and are chosen for the greatest benefit of the patient. (p. 7)

Wellness Perspective

1. A wellness perspective goes beyond the old idea of health as the absence of disease to one of achieving _____. (p. 9)

2. The diagram by Travis that shows the scope of the wellness model from premature death to high level wellness is called the _____. (p. 9)

3. The goal of treatment is to bring a person to the _____ point on the illness/wellness continuum. (p. 9)

4. Since it addresses many different aspects of a person's life, the idea of high level wellness is _____ _____ at its core. (p. 9)

5. The wellness massage pyramid is a tool for understanding the _____ _____ on the journey to high level wellness. (p. 11)

6. The levels of the wellness massage pyramid from the foundation up to high level wellness are (1) _____, (2) _____, (3) _____, (4) neutral zone, (5) _____, (6) _____, and (7) _____ (Figure 1–4)

7. Which of the following statements are true according to a wellness perspective? (pp. 9–12)

_____ a. Treatment for a medical condition is an aspect of wellness.

_____ b. A person with a chronic illness cannot achieve high level wellness.

_____ c. Health care professionals are responsible for their patients achieving high level wellness.

_____ d. Freedom from illness or injury is a neutral point in terms of wellness.

_____ e. Once high level wellness is achieved, it remains for life.

Wellness and the Health Professions

1. The professions that include massage in their scope of practice are _____ _____. (p. 12)

2. A method of treating a pathology is called a _____. (p. 12)

3. Rather than calling systems of massage bodywork *modalities*, it is recommended that they be called _____ or _____. (p. 12)

4. True or False. Physical therapists only perform treatment applications of massage and other therapeutic modalities. Explain. (p. 12)

5. True or False. Massage therapists only perform massage for personal growth and pleasure. Explain. (p. 12)

4. Nurses sometimes include massage as part of _____ care of patients in hospitals and nursing homes. (p. 12)

5. Although different health professions use massage somewhat differently, they share a common bond, that is, the _____ themselves. (p. 12)

Clarifying Terminology

1. Someone trained in massage and who uses massage in the practice of his or her profession is called a _____. (p. 13)

2. A _____ refers to the period of time in which massage is performed. (p. 13)

3. The word _____ is reserved for descriptions of medical applications of massage. (pp. 12–13)

FOR GREATER UNDERSTANDING

The following exercises are designed to take you from the realm of theory into the real world. They will help give you a deeper understanding of the subjects covered in this chapter. Action words are *underlined* to emphasize the variety of activities presented to address different learning styles, and to encourage deeper thinking.

1. Visit two or more places where massage is offered, for example, a spa, health club, rehabilitation clinic, or integrative medicine facility. Compare and contrast the settings, clientele, and types of massage offered. Get a massage at one or more places for a more personal experience.

2. Interview someone who receives regular massage to find out how they think massage has benefited them over a period of time. Ask them to be specific. Analyze their responses using the wellness massage pyramid.

3. Interview two or more people as in problem 2, and compare their responses.

4. Receive a massage from a trained practitioner. After the massage, interview the practitioner about their choice of techniques and their intention(s) in applying the techniques during the session. Write a report of your experience.

5. Interview someone who performs massage in his or her occupation and analyze their work according to the wellness massage perspective. Note their

occupational field or profession, the setting, clientele, goals of massage sessions, and types of massage and bodywork provided.

6. Think about how you might use massage for your own health and healing, looking at benefits for body, mind, emotions, and spirit. Discuss your thoughts in class or a study group, and compare with others.

7. Using Table 1–2, write a short story about a client or patient using wellness or treatment terminology as appropriate. For example: (Wellness) Jane went to the spa for a massage session after planting her vegetable garden and experiencing sore and stiff back and legs. The massage therapist took a health history, assessed the situation, developed a session strategy, and performed Western massage focusing on circulation and muscle relaxation in the back and legs. (Treatment) John's doctor referred him for massage to help in recovery from a repetitive strain injury in the shoulder.

The therapist took a medical history, noting that John was taking muscle relaxants and pain medication. Using clinical reasoning skills, the therapist developed a treatment plan, and performed Western massage with trigger point therapy on the affected region.

8. Look through a massage and bodywork magazine or journal, and make a list of the types of massage and bodywork written about or advertised. Categorize the types into the four world traditions. Explain your decisions.

9. Read the White House Commission Report on Complementary and Alternative Medicine Policy, and in class or with a study group, discuss the implications of the report for the future of massage therapy. (*www.whccamp.hhs.gov*).

10. Visit the Web sites listed throughout this chapter for further information about a particular topic.

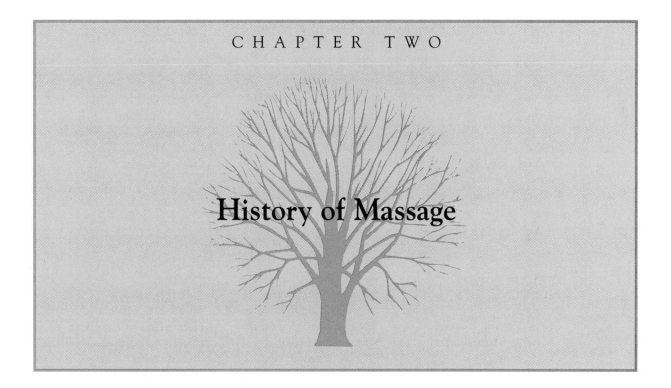

CHAPTER TWO

History of Massage

LEARNING OUTCOMES

After studying this chapter, the student will have information to:

1. Appreciate massage as an ancient and global practice.
2. Discuss massage as part of daily life in different native and folk cultures.
3. Describe evidence of massage in the ancient civilizations of Sumer, China and Japan, India, Greece and Rome.
4. Explain how the practice of massage was preserved during Medieval and Renaissance Europe.
5. Describe the beginning of modern Western massage, including the roles of P. H. Ling and J. Mezger.
6. Discuss the uses of massage within conventional medicine from simple medical rubbing to its use in nursing and physical therapy.
7. Discuss the natural healing movement of the early 20th century, including the contributions of J. Harvey Kellogg and Bernarr Macfadden.
8. Describe Swedish massage in its heyday from 1920 to 1950.
9. Trace the development of massage for sports and fitness.
10. Explain the significance of Esalen massage in the 1970s.
11. Identify milestones in the advancement of massage therapy at the turn of the 21st century.

MEDIALINK

A companion CD-ROM, included free with each new copy of this book, supplements the techniques presented in this chapter. Insert the CD-ROM to watch video clips of massage techniques being demonstrated. This multimedia feature is designed to help you add a new dimension to your learning.

KEY HISTORICAL PEOPLE

Avicenna	Ling, Pehr Henrik	Namikoshi, Torujiro
Celsus	Lucas-Champoinnière, Marie	Pare, Ambrose
Curanderas	Marcellin	Reconstruction Aides
Galen	Macfadden, Bernarr	Roth, M.
Graham, Douglas	McMillan, Mary	Taylor, George
Hippocrates	Mennell, James	
Kellogg, J. Harvey	Mezger, Johann Georg	

KEY TERMS/CONCEPTS

Amma	Massage parlor	Rubdown
AMTA Foundation	Medical rubbing	Shiatsu
Anatriptic art	National Certification	Swedish massage
Ayurveda	Examination for Therapeutic	Swedish movement cure
Commission on Massage	Massage and Bodywork	Touch Research Institute
Therapy Accreditation	National Center for	Traditional Chinese Medicine
Counterculture	Complementary and	Turkish bath
Esalen massage	Alternative Medicine	Wellness movement
Greek gymnasium	Natural Healing Movement	Yellow Emperor's Classic of
Hawaiian lomi-lomi	Roman Baths	Internal Medicine
Human potential movement	Royal Institute of Gymnastics	

ANCIENT AND GLOBAL HERITAGE

The history of massage is both ancient and global. Its origin is before recorded history, and it is found in some form in every known culture in the world. Isolated peoples developed their own unique forms of massage and bodywork, which were transformed when their cultures came into contact with each other. Travel, war, trade, immigration, international study, and modern forms of communication have all facilitated the exchange of ideas, and the evolution of the practice of massage on a global scale. Access to the Internet with its vast potential as a reservoir of information is a major advancement for sharing knowledge and transforming the practice of massage today.

The Western massage tradition currently forms the foundation of massage therapy in North America. However, Asian bodywork therapies and Ayurvedic massage are also gaining popularity here. Diverse ethnic populations bring their traditions to the mix.

Knowing about the history of these various traditions helps massage practitioners develop a sense of the vast heritage of which they are a part. (The book to read is *The History of Massage* by Robert N. Calvert, 2002.) Some interesting facts about the uses of massage at various times and in a variety of places will be presented in this chapter. Some of the major forces that shaped massage therapy in North America in the latter part of the 20th century will also be identified.

It will become evident that forms of massage from different time periods, and from all over the world, span the broad scope of the wellness perspective. You will find massage for medical applications, health and fitness, sports massage, and for personal and spiritual development. Some of these forms of massage and bodywork are both historical *and* contemporary to the extent that they continue to be performed in their traditional ways.

As is the custom in many history texts, the more universal designation of dates will be used. The abbreviation "BCE" will be used to denote *before the common era,* often referred to as "BC." The abbreviation "CE" is used to mean *in the common era,* referred to as AD in the Roman calendar.

NATIVE AND FOLK TRADITIONS

In cultures without written records, historical evidence of health practices like massage is difficult to find. The knowledge and skills were handed down in families and in communities through the generations from person to person, and many of these oral traditions have been lost. However, we can learn some things from explorers who first came in contact with indigenous peoples of the world and who described their daily lives in written records. In addition, some ancient forms are still performed by groups who continue to practice their honored traditions. Massage by the South Sea Islanders before their contact with Western civilization and by the curanderas of the southwest United States are examples of native and folk traditions for which we have some reliable information.

South Sea Islands

Descriptions from European and American adventurers offer glimpses of massage as practiced in the South Sea Islands in the 1800s. It was reported that the Maoris of New Zealand called their version of massage *romi-romi*, and the natives of Tonga Island performed *toogi-toogi* for relief of sleeplessness and fatigue. "Melee denotes rubbing with the palm, and fota kneading with the thumb and fingers" (Kellogg, 1923, p. 12). In 1874, Nordhoff described a wellness massage called **Hawaiian lomi-lomi** performed by the natives of the Sandwich Islands:

> To be lomi-lomied you lie down upon a mat, or undress for the night, if you prefer. The less clothing you have on the more perfectly the operation can be performed. To you thereupon comes a stout native with soft fleshy hands, but a strong grip, and beginning with your head and working down slowly over the whole body, seizes and squeezes with indefatigable patience, until in half an hour, whereas you were weary and worn out, you find yourself fresh, all soreness and weariness absolutely and entirely gone, and mind and body soothed to a healthful and refreshing sleep (Murrell, 1890, p. 10).

The Maori of New Zealand are reported to have treated clubfoot in infants with massage. In his study of the genetics of clubfoot, Beals tells of the practice of continuous massage of the clubfoot by the older women of the family, which he said had surprisingly good results. It was a practice passed down from generation to generation, but which virtually disappeared with the advent of European medicine in New Zealand (Beals, 1978).

Curanderas

Today in the Southwestern United States, Hispanic healers called **curanderas** continue folk traditions from Spain and Mexico that are combined with Native American remedies. Their roots can be traced to the Moors of 8th century Spain, then to the Spaniards who came to the Americas in the 15th century, and also to Native Americans, particularly the Aztecs of ancient Mexico (Torres).

Curanderas are female healers called upon when a family's chief caregiver needs assistance. Curanderas totals are those who practice all the various healing specialties, including herbs, midwifery, massage, and ritual. Curanderas totals have a strong spiritual dimension to their methods and are described as using "ritualism and symbolism in their art and are able to move in and out of dimensions not bound to earth." It is believed that curanderas inherit their power to heal, although some families with no heritage of healing may be given the *don*, translated as "gift," or more loosely as the "heart."

Sobardoras are curanderas who specialize in massage and may also use herbal remedies in their work. They perform soft tissue manipulations as well as "bonesetting" types of joint manipulations. Sobardoras learn their art by apprenticeship (Perrone, Stockel, & Krueger, 1989).

ANCIENT CIVILIZATIONS

Written and pictorial records from the ancient civilizations of Sumer, China and Japan, India, Greece, and Rome contain descriptions of massage and exercise. Many of the forms of massage and bodywork found today trace their roots to these ancient practices.

Sumer

A clay tablet from Sumer dating from 2100 BCE describes a remedy that uses an herbal mixture and "rubbing" and "frictions."

> Pass through a sieve and then knead together turtle shells, naga-si plant, salt, and mustard. Then wash the diseased part with beer of good quality and hot water, and rub with the mixture. Then friction and rub again with oil, and put on a poultice of pounded pine (Time-Life Books, 1987, p. 41).

China and Japan

Since Chapters 17–20 each contains information on the history of Asian bodywork therapy, we will simply mention some of the highlights in this chapter.

The **Yellow Emperor's Classic of Internal Medicine** (c. 500 BCE), is often cited as the first book on Chinese medicine. It became the foundation for **traditional medicine** practiced in the Asian countries of China, Japan, and Korea (Monte, 1993, p. 20). Essential concepts in Chinese medicine include yin and yang, life energy called *qi* or *chi,* which moves in patterns defined by energy channels, and the five element (fire, wood, water, metal, earth) theory. Ancient health practices and therapies from China include acupuncture with needles, acupressure using finger pressure on acupuncture points, a form of massage called tuina, and forms of exercise called chi kung and tai chi. The basic theory of Chinese medicine is explained more thoroughly in Chapter 17.

Massage and bodywork was not confined to medicine in China. In the 1700s, Chinese barbers offered a form of massage to seated patrons in addition to other personal services like cutting hair and cleaning ears. Figure 2–1 is a drawing from an actual street scene in China in the 1790s. It appears to be a form of percussion (Benjamin 2002).

Anma, or **amma,** is a form of Japanese massage that was brought from China via the Korean peninsula in the sixth century CE. At that time, the Japanese assimilated the Chinese medical philosophies that came to Japan as kampo, i.e., "the Chinese way." Amma became an accepted Japanese healing practice, as described in more detail in Chapter 18.

Shiatsu is a modern form of Japanese bodywork developed in the 1940s by **Torujiro Namikoshi.** Shiatsu incorporates many of the ideas from Western science with traditional Japanese amma. Shiatsu was introduced into the United States in the 1950s by Torujiro's son, Toru Namikoshi. See Chapter 19 for more detailed information about the history of shiatsu.

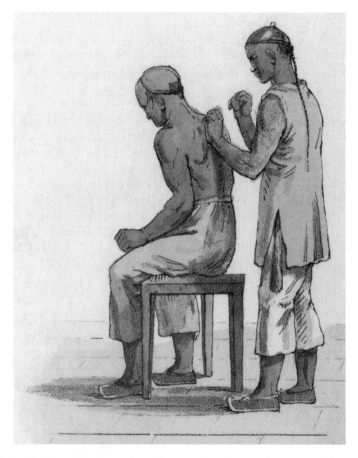

FIGURE 2–1. Chinese barber performing a form of percussion on a seated patron in China in the 1790s. From *Picturesque Representations of the Dress and Manners of the Chinese* by Thomas M'Lean, published 1814.

India

Ayurveda, "knowledge of long life" and the traditional medicine of India, is said to have been given to a Hindu seer by the god Indra. The Ayurvedic system goes back to at least the fifth century BCE and is based on the Vedas, the ancient philosophical and spiritual writings of India (Monte, 1993, p. 30).

Ayurvedic health practices include guidelines for vegetarian eating, forms of cleansing, movements and postures (hatha yoga), breathing exercises, meditation, and massage. Essential concepts in Ayurvedic theory include a life force called *prana*, energy centers called *chakras*, the five great elements (earth, water, fire, air, ether), and the three *doshas* (*vata, pita, kapha*). The ancient wisdom of Ayurveda continues to be practiced today and has been popularized in the West in the writings of Deepak Chopra (Chopra, 1991).

The recent revival of infant massage in the United States has been patterned in part on the ancient practice of baby massage in India. Leboyer's popular book, *Loving Hands: The Traditional Indian Art of Baby Massage* (1982), shows Shantala, an Indian woman, massaging her baby as she learned from her mother, who learned from her mother, and so on back in time.

Greece

In ancient Greece, the uses of massage for healing, health, and sports were well advanced. **Hippocrates** (450–377 BCE) wrote of the utility of friction after sprains and reduced dislocations and recommended abdominal kneading and chest clapping (Kleen, 1921, p. 2). Aristotle (384–322 BCE), a Greek philosopher and tutor of Alexander the Great, is said to have recommended rubbing with oil and water as a remedy against weariness. Alexander the Great (356–323 BCE), who conquered a vast empire from Egypt to India, reportedly had a personal *triptai* (massage specialist) named Athenophanes, "whose business it was to rub the great emperor and to prepare his bath" (Kleen, 1921, p. 2).

The **Greek gymnasia** in ancient Athens and Sparta were centers run by the state for free men and youths, which contained facilities for exercises, frictions, and baths. The exercises included wrestling, boxing, running, jumping, throwing the quoit and spear, and some ball games. Massage with oil was used to prepare the young men before their exercises and to refresh them after their exercises and after their baths (Johnson, 1866, pp. 15–16).

A description of massage performed in the Greek gymnasia is offered by **Galen** (c. 130–200 CE). Galen was a respected Greek doctor who early in his career was physician to the gladiators, and who later went to Rome and served several emperors. Galen's writings preserve knowledge of the Greek traditions and contain valuable descriptions of how massage was performed in ancient times. Galen describes the effects of massage before exercises (*tripsis paraskeuastike*) and after exercises (*apotherapeia*):

> Rubbing which prepares for gymnastic exercises, and that which follows the same, is subservient to the exercises. The former heats and moderately opens the pores, and liquifies the excretions retained in the flesh, and softens the solid parts, and this is termed preparatory or paraskeuastic rubbing. But the other is termed after-administering (apotherapeutic); and as it is applied with a larger amount of oil, it at the same time moistens by means of the grease, and softens the solid parts, and carries off what is contained in the pores (Johnson, 1866, pp. 19–20).

Rome

The Roman Empire dates from approximately 27 BCE to 476 CE. At the height of its power, the Roman Empire extended from present-day Turkey and Asia Minor in the east to the British Isles in the west and included the territories of southern Europe and northern Africa. The Romans adopted much of Greek culture and spread it throughout their empire.

Aulus Cornelius **Celsus** (25 BCE–50 CE), a Roman physician, is credited with compiling a text called *De Medicina,* a series of eight books covering all of the medical knowledge of his time. In the text, he describes the use of exercises, frictions, inunctions (i.e., applying oil or ointment), rubbing, brushing, ligatures, and dry cupping to prevent and treat certain diseases. Active movements prescribed include walking, running, swimming, riding on horseback, and playing at ball (Georgii, 1880, p. 3).

The Romans borrowed many of the features of the Greek gymnasia to create the **Roman Baths.** The ruins of a famous Roman Bath may still be toured in the former Roman city of Aquae Sulis, now the city of Bath, England. Also at this site is a temple to the Roman goddess of wisdom, Minerva. The Aquae Sulis baths were in operation from approximately 60 to 410 CE. The baths themselves consisted of a space for undressing (*apodyterium*), an exercise court, a warm room (*tepidarium*), a type of steam-room (*caldarium*), and a cold pool (*frigidarium*). At Aquae Sulis, there was also a great swimming pool and immersion baths where one could sit up to the neck in hot curative waters. Both men and women came to these baths.

The Roman writer Seneca (4 BCE–65 CE) left a vivid description of the noise of the Roman bath above which he was trying to study. The passage included complaints about the noise of people exercising and the following passage about massage:

> Or perhaps I notice some lazy fellow, content with a cheap rub-down, and hear the crack of the pummelling hand on his shoulder varying in sound according as the hand is laid on flat or hollow (Cunliffe, 1978, p. 16).

Turkey

After the fall of the Roman Empire in 476 CE, the idea of the Roman Bath was preserved in Turkey and brought back into Western civilization as the **Turkish bath** during the Renaissance. In Turkey it was customary for women, as well as men, to go to the baths as part of their health regimen. The Turkish bath became very popular in the big cities of Europe and the United States in the 19th century.

After partaking of the various forms of hot and cold waters at the *hammam* or Turkish baths, a patron would receive a rather rigorous form of bodywork. The following is a description of a bodywork session given at the *hammam* in Constantinople in the mid-19th century:

> The tellack (two, if the operation is properly performed) kneels at your side, and bending over, grips and presses your chest, arms, legs, passing from part to part like a bird shifting its place on a perch. He brings his whole weight on you with a jerk; follows the line of muscle with an anatomical thumb . . . draws the open hand strongly over the surface, particularly round the shoulder, turning you half up in doing so . . . You are now turned on your face; and . . . he works his elbow round the edges of your shoulder-blades, and with the heel, hard, the ankle of the neck . . . You are then raised for a moment to a sitting posture, and a contortion given to the small of the back with the knee, and a jerk to the neck by the two hands holding the temples (Johnson, 1866, pp. 29–30).

Turkish baths can still be found in some of the major cities of the world. It is noteworthy that the tradition of the Greek gymnasia, the Roman baths, and the Turkish baths is still with us in the form of the modern health club. The basic format of exercise space, swimming pool, showers, steamroom, sauna, whirlpool, and massage room, continue this ancient tradition.

MIDDLE AGES AND RENAISSANCE EUROPE

The Middle Ages in Europe extended roughly from 500 to 1300 CE. This is often considered a period of backwardness in Europe, where the Roman Empire collapsed with the invasion of "barbarian" tribes like the Celts and Saxons. The classical Greek and Roman medical writings, including those about the medical use of friction and rubbing, were lost for a time, and not brought back to Europe until the Renaissance (1300–1600 CE). The Arabs in Turkey and the Near East, as well the monks in Ireland, preserved the writings of Hippocrates, Galen, and others. Some of the information concerning rubbing and frictions was also preserved at this time in the folk healing traditions in Europe.

The Middle Ages were not all darkness, however. A book translated from Arabic into Latin in the 11th century called the *Tacuinum Sanitatis* expounded on the six things that are necessary for everyone in the daily preservation of health. These were listed as the treatment of air, right use of foods and drink, correct use of movements and rest, proper sleep, correct use of elimination and retention of humors, and the regulating of the person by moderating joy, anger, fear, and distress. It notes that "the secret of the preservation of health, in fact, will be in the proper balance of all these elements, since it is the disturbance of this balance that causes illnesses" (Arano, 1976, p. 6).

The *Tacuinum Sanitatis* is evidence of the rich knowledge about healthy living that was known in the Middle Ages and of an early holistic philosophy of health and disease in Europe. It contains the seeds of the philosophy and practices of natural health and healing, which were in full swing by the late 19th century. Natural healing is one of the major traditions of which massage is a significant part.

It should be noted that the Arabic physician **Avicenna** (980–1037 CE) wrote about massage in his famed medical texts. Avicenna said: "the object of massage is to disperse the effete matters formed in the muscles and not expelled by exercise. It causes the effete matter to disperse and so remove fatigue" (Wood & Becker, 1981).

The classical writings of the Greeks and Romans were reintroduced into Europe during the Renaissance. These included writings about the use of frictions and rubbing in the treatment of disease and injuries. This no doubt renewed interest in massage as a medical treatment in the great learning centers of Europe, particularly in France, England, Germany, Russia, and Sweden.

One of the founders of modern surgery, **Ambrose Pare** (1517–1590) of France, wrote about the use of frictions for joint stiffness and wound healing. Pare described different types of frictions simply as gentle, medium, and vigorous.

WESTERN MASSAGE

Two figures loom large in the history of massage in the 19th and early 20th centuries: Pehr Henrik Ling of Sweden and Johann Georg Mezger of Amsterdam. Their pupils have taken their systems of active and passive movements, combined and expanded upon them, and spread them throughout the world. Western massage is a synthesis of techniques developed by these two men.

Ling

Pehr Henrik Ling (1776–1839) was a fencing master, poet, playwright, and educator. He believed that movements of the body had the power to protect, educate, express, and heal. Ling developed four different systems of movement: military, educational, aesthetic, and medical. He described them in his treatise *The General Principles of Gymnastics,* published one year after his death in 1840 (Ling, 1840a). In the late 19th and early 20th centuries, Ling's educational gymnastics were taught in the public schools of the United States as Swedish gymnastics, and his system of medical gymnastics was known popularly as the **Swedish movement cure.** The movement cure consisted of passive and active movements used to treat chronic disease conditions.

Ling is eulogized as having put medical gymnastics on scientific ground. However, a reading of his treatise in the original Swedish reveals the more metaphorical thinking of a poet. He believed that human beings are made up of mechanical, chemical, and dynamic forces. The mechanical force is roughly equivalent to movements of the muscles, and the chemical force has to do with processes like digestion, elimination, and the secretions of glands. The dynamic force is an interesting mix of mental, emotional, and spiritual aspects. Balance in these three forces is necessary to maintain health, while imbalance results in disease. The mechanical force, the realm of passive and active movements, is sometimes used to reestablish balance and, therefore, health, in the human organism (Roth, 1851, pp. 25–32).

Ling's medical gymnastics included both active and passive movements. In his *Notations to the General Principles,* Ling identified the passive movements with descriptive terms like shaking, hacking, pressing, stroking, pinching and squeezing, kneading, clapping, vibrations, and rolling. He instructed that oil may be used to decrease skin friction, but that "this hinders the manipulation of the inner abdominal organs" (Ling, 1840b).

The types of diseases treated by medical gymnastics in the 19th century included a variety of ailments such as congestion of the head, humming in the ears, asthma, emphysema, gastritis, constipation, incontinence, and hernia. Nervous conditions such as epilepsy, neuralgic pain, and paralysis were also treated. Explorations into the treatment of mental diseases by movements were also conducted (Roth, 1851).

Ling believed that practitioners of his work need a thorough grounding in anatomy and physiology. However, in the *Means or Vehicles of Gymnastics,* he cautioned his pupils against a mechanistic view of the human body with these words:

> May anatomy—that holy genesis, which reveals the great work of the Creator to the eye of man, and teaches him at one and the same time how small and yet how great he is—be the gymnast's most treasured fundamental principle; but let him contemplate these forms—not as if they were lifeless ones— but . . . as though they were living, not as constituting an inert mass, but the instrument of the soul, animated with the latter throughout (Ling, 1840c).

Ling established the **Royal Institute of Gymnastics** in Stockholm in 1813 to teach his systems of gymnastics. His pupils took educational and medical gymnastics to major cities all over the world, and by the late 19th century, people interested in natural health and healing were traveling to the Royal Institute to learn Ling's systems from those who carried on his work.

Ling's major legacy to the practice of massage lies in his belief that active and passive movements skillfully applied can help maintain and restore health and balance in the human organism. His holistic view of human beings has persisted, and his work was part of the evolution of the modern concepts of holistic health and wellness. The exercises of Ling's educational gymnastics were the forerunners of modern forms of calisthenics and physical fitness. In addition, the Swedish movements were carried on in the early practice of physical therapy.

Mezger

Johann Georg Mezger (1838–1909), a physician in Amsterdam, also believed that passive movements had the power to heal. Although he never published a detailed description of his work, his pupils von Mosengeil and Helleday did write articles about Mezger's massage. Mezger categorized the methods of soft tissue manipulation into four broad technique categories using the French terms *effleurage* (stroking), *petrissage* (kneading), *friction* (rubbing), and *tapotement* (tapping).

The popularity of Mezger's work was instrumental in reviving the interest in massage in medical settings (Nissen, 1920, pp. 7–8). The general categories of movements he defined have proved very useful and form the basis of Western massage. Vibration was added later as a fifth category as it gained popularity in the late 1800s.

Swedish Movement Cure in the United States

Ling's medical gymnastics, or movement cure as it was known in English-speaking countries, was well established in England and in the United States by the late 1800s. **Dr. M. Roth** studied at the Royal Institute and wrote the first book in English on Ling's system in 1851, *The Prevention and Cure of Many Chronic Diseases by Movements*. Figure 2–2 shows two drawings from Roth's book. One drawing depicts superficial friction being performed for respiratory congestion, and the other shows passive rotation of the foot used to increase circulation in the lower limbs to affect circulation in the head and chest. Note that the patient (recipient) and the operator (practitioner) are in various positions to best facilitate the

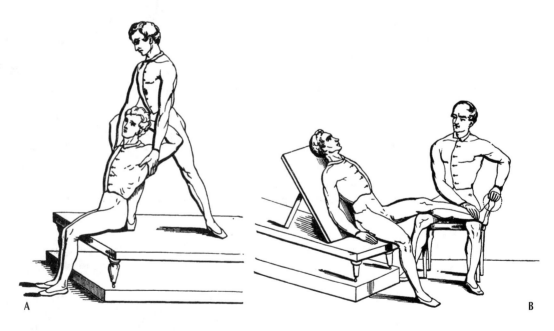

FIGURE 2–2. Drawings from Dr. Roth's book, *The Prevention and Cure of Many Chronic Diseases by Movements*, published in 1851. A. Superficial friction on the sides of the chest for respiratory congestion. B. Passive rotation of the foot to increase circulation.

movements being performed. The convention of lying on a table during the entire session was a later development adopted after the popularization of full-body massage.

The Swedish movement cure was first brought to the United States in 1854 by **Dr. George Taylor** of New York. Other prominent names in the early history of the movement cure in the United States are Hartvig Nissen in Washington, DC (1889), Baron Nils Posse in Boston (1894), Kurre Ostrom in Philadelphia (1905), and Axel Grafstrom in New York (1904).

By the early 20th century, Mezger's massage was adopted by practitioners of the Swedish movement cure, and you begin to see the two terms used together. For example, they are both used in the title of Ostrom's book, *Massage and the Original Swedish Movements* (1905). Figure 2–3 shows drawings of massage of the the neck and shoulders from Ostrom's book.

CONVENTIONAL AND NATURAL HEALING

Various forms of soft tissue manipulation and passive movements continued to be developed as methods for promoting health and healing into the 1900s. The most popular forms continued to be massage and the Swedish movements, later combined into what was called Swedish massage.

Massage in Conventional Medicine

The use of massage in conventional medicine (as opposed to folk remedies, natural healing, and other "alternative" practices) can be found in the medical literature of Europe and the United States dating from the 1700s. It was generally called frictions, rubbing, or **medical rubbing.** In 1866 Walter Johnson wrote a history of medical massage with the lengthy title, *The **Anatripic Art:** A history of the art termed anatripsis by Hypocrates, tripsis by Galen, friction by Celsus, manipulation by Beveridge, and medical rubbing in ordinary language, from the earliest times to the present day.*

Marie Marcellin Lucas-Championnière (circa 1880) claimed that in fractures, the soft tissue union as well as the bony union should be considered from the start. Sir William Bennett of England was impressed with Lucas-Championnière's idea and started a revolutionary treatment with the use of massage at St. George's Hospital in circa 1899. Albert J. Hoffa published his book, *Technik der Massage,* in Germany in 1900. This book is still a good basic text on massage, giving clear descriptions of how to execute the techniques and advocating the procedures that underlie all modern techniques. The book by Max Bohm, *Massage: Its Principles and Techniques,* written in 1913, includes interpretations of Hoffa's techniques. In 1902, **Douglas Graham** published *A Treatise on Massage, Its History, Mode of Application and Effects.* This text finally aroused the interest of the medical profession in the United States in massage and its therapeutic effects.

Sir Robert Jones, a leading orthopedic surgeon in England, was an enthusiast of the Lucas-Championnière treatment of fractures. Jones was to have an influence on two of the great figures of

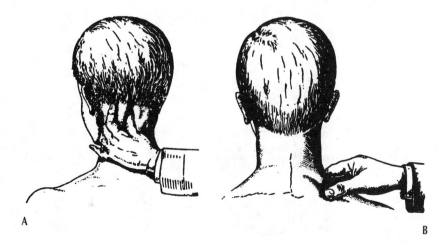

A   B

FIGURE 2–3. Drawings of kneading the neck muscles from Ostrom's book, *Massage and the Original Swedish Movements,* published in 1905. A. Kneading the posterior neck muscles. B. Kneading the upper trapezius.

physical therapy in the United States. Mary McMillan was associated with Jones's clinic at Southern Hospital in Liverpool, England, from 1911 to 1915, and **James B. Mennell** worked with Jones at the Special Military Surgical Hospital, Shepherd's Bush, England. Mennell (1880–1957) wrote his text, *Physical Treatment by Movement, Manipulation and Massage*, in 1917 during World War I. Mennell's text was a compilation of the manual therapeutics that he saw in various European countries, and he considered his book to be a rationale of massage treatment. He endeavored to show the importance of care and gentleness in giving massage. Mennell was a medical officer and lecturer on massage at the Training School of St. Thomas' Hospital in London, England, from 1912 to 1935. He was very influential in shaping the practice of physical therapy in its early years.

During World War I, E. G. Bracket and Joel Goldthwait became interested in the reconstruction (i.e., rehabilitation) work that was being done among the Allied nations. They initiated the Reconstruction Department of the United States Army in 1918. The department consisted of physiotherapy, occupational therapy, and curative workshop divisions. Short intensive courses were arranged in recognized schools of physical education throughout the country to train women, called **Reconstruction Aides,** to perform physiotherapy, including massage, on wounded soldiers (McMillan, 1925, p. 10).

In his book, *A Practice of Physiotherapy* (1926), C. M. Sampson, MD describes the types of modalities used in the developing field of physiotherapy, including massage. Figure 2–4 is a photograph of a corner of the general massage section of an army hospital. It shows four operators, as practitioners were then called, working with soldiers who are seated in chairs, and lying or sitting on tables. Massage was applied to assist in rehabilitation.

Mary McMillan, who figured prominently in the development of the profession of physical therapy, received her special training in London at the National Hospital for Nervous Diseases, at St. Bartholomew's Hospital, and at St. George's Hospital with William Bennett. At the Southern Hospital in Liverpool, McMillan was in charge of massage and therapeutic exercises at Greenbank Cripples' Home. She came to the United States as Director of Massage and Medical Gymnastics at Children's Hospital in Portland, Maine. She later served as chief aide at Walter Reed Hospital and instructor of the special war emergency course at the Reed College Clinic for training reconstruction aides during World War I. McMillan was director of physiotherapy at Harvard Medical School while she was writing her book, *Massage and Therapeutic Exercise*, from 1921 to 1925.

Physical therapists trained for rehabilitation work during and after World Wars I and II continued to expand the field of physical therapy for treating a number of orthopedic conditions. They were called upon in the 1930–50s to treat victims of the polio epidemics of that time. But as Gertrude Beard

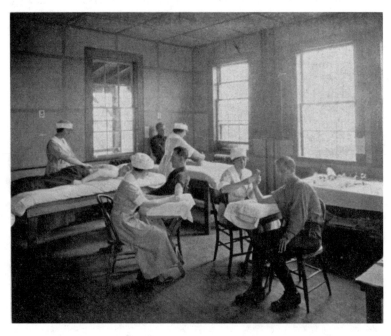

FIGURE 2–4. A corner of the general massage section of an army hospital from Sampson's book, *A Practice of Physiotherapy*, published in 1926.

noted, the amount of massage being prescribed by physicians in the United States declined in the decades following World War II. She speculates that this was due to the fact that massage is time consuming, sometimes strenuous, demands real skill, and the basis for prescribing it was largely empiric rather than scientific (Beard, 1964, p. 1). (For more information, read *Healing the Generations: A history of physical therapy and the American Physical Therapy Association*, edited by W. Murphy, 1995.)

Natural Healing

Massage and the Swedish movements were also practiced by proponents of natural healing, which was considered non-conventional therapy in the early 1900s. These practitioners used various natural remedies to treat different ailments and generally rejected the allopathic methods of drugs and surgery. The philosophy of natural healing includes the belief that humans are created with innate healing powers that can be facilitated by various natural methods such as rest, sunshine, heat and cold applied by water (hydrotherapy), exercise, massage, proper nutrition, laughter, and herbal remedies. Natural healing in the late 1800s and early 1900s also included magnetic healing, a form of energy work (Bilz, 1898).

The Battle Creek Sanitarium in Battle Creek, Michigan, run by **John Harvey Kellogg** (1852–1943), was a natural healing resort of the early twentieth century. Kellogg advocated a host of natural health practices he called "biologic living," including vegetarianism, physical exercise, sunshine, fresh air, colonic irrigation, various forms of bathing, and massage. There was no alcohol, no coffee, no tea, and no smoking. Kellogg and his brother invented the first cold cereal and started the breakfast cereal industry (Armstrong & Armstrong, 1991, pp. 107–111). Kellogg's book, *The Art of Massage*, was first published in 1895.

C. W. Post (1854–1914), of Post brand cereal fame, opened a competing sanitarium on the outskirts of Battle Creek called La Vita Inn. Post featured what he called "mental healing." In 1895 in a self-published book called *I Am Well*, Post offers this advice, which sounds much like relaxation techniques used today:

> Seek an easy position where you will not be disturbed. Relax every muscle, close your eyes and go into silence where mind is plastic to the breathings of Spirit, where God talks to son (Armstrong & Armstrong, 1991, p. 111).

Bernarr Macfadden (1868–1955) was a popular proponent of natural health practices, which he called *physical culture*. In the early 1900s, he opened a string of physical culture resorts in the East and Midwest. His *Physical Culture* magazine was launched in 1898 and was popular well into the 1930s. Macfadden's Physical Culture Training School in Chicago graduated "doctors" of hydropathy, kinesitherapy, and physcultopathy. His health regimen consisted of proper breathing, relaxation, diet, fasting, bathing, singing, exercise, and massage. He was considered a huckster by some, but was successful in bringing the tradition of natural health to the general public (Armstrong & Armstrong, 1991, pp. 203–213).

Swedish Massage

The heyday of Swedish massage was from about 1920 to 1950. During this time, the genre called **Swedish massage** came to include massage, Swedish movements, various forms of hydrotherapy, heat lamps, diathermy, and colonic irrigation. The focus was on health. "Reducing massage" was popular in the 1930–1940s, since massage was believed at that time to be a beauty aid that helped reduce fat on the thighs and waistline.

Practitioners were trained in private vocational schools called colleges, such as the College of Swedish Massage in Chicago. A typical women's class in "scientific massage technique" in the 1940s is shown in Figure 2–5. At this time, women and men were separated, and there was very little cross-gender legitimate massage outside of medical facilities (Benjamin, 1993).

Graduates of these colleges of Swedish massage often opened their own establishments, called **massage parlors** or health centers. In the 1920–1930s, the word *parlor* was simply a term for a functional room like a funeral parlor or beauty parlor. A *masseuse* was a female massage therapist, and a *masseur* was a male. Graduate masseuses worked in upscale beauty parlors such as Helena Rubenstein and Elizabeth Arden. Sometimes exercise classes were offered along with Swedish massage services. Graduates of colleges of Swedish massage could also find jobs at the YMCA, private health clubs, resorts, hospitals, and with professional sports teams. Many practitioners of Swedish massage were proponents of the tradition of natural healing and worked with alternative medical practitioners, especially chiropractors and naturopaths.

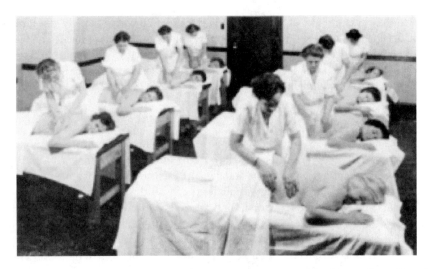

FIGURE 2–5. A women's class in "scientific massage techniques" from a catalog of the College of Swedish Massage in Chicago, circa 1940s.

SPORTS AND FITNESS

Sports Massage

Massage has been part of the sports and fitness scene since ancient Greek times. The **rubdown** was a well established practice by athletes in the United States and England in the late 1800s. A rubdown consisted of superficial skin friction with the hand, a brush, a coarse towel, or a horsehair glove. It was said that "Oxford athletes are never allowed to do cross country running without first rubbing their legs with horsehair gloves or with hands" (Pollard, 1902, p. 21).

H. Joseph Fay wrote about the use of massage in sports in 1916. In his book, *Scientific Massage for Athletes,* he describes massage as being used for ridding the muscles of wastes, which bring about fatigue and stiffness, and to produce additional growth of bone and muscle. He says that the practical trainer "works the meat, or muscle, between the hide and the bone so that it's in its highest state for exercise" (Fay, 1916, p. 20).

Harry Andrews, another trainer-masseur from that era, is shown in Figure 2–6 massaging an athlete's lower leg. Andrews believed that the "rubbing, stroking, pinching, and slapping . . . arouse the latent energy and reinvigorate the limbs, nerve centres, and muscular system generally" (Andrews, 1910, p. 22).

Massage performed by trainers was a familiar sight at college and amateur athletic events in the first part of the 20th century. Albert Baumgartner, a former trainer at the State University of Iowa, wrote *Massage in Athletics* in 1947. He describes massage as being used in preparation for a workout or competition, during rest periods between activities, for reconditioning or recuperation to revitalize the body, and in the treatment of minor injuries. Baumgartner also recognized the psychological benefits of massage to the athlete.

By the 1950s, massage had largely disappeared from the American sports scene. The profession of athletic training was growing, and trainers specialized in the prevention and treatment of athletic injuries using many of the methods of physical therapy. As physical therapists decreased their use of massage in the 1950s, so did athletic trainers.

In the 1970s, the tradition of massage for athletes was revived within the growing profession of massage therapy. Impressed by the success of European athletes who used massage in their training regimens, athletes in the United States began seeking massage to enhance performance and to complement other restorative methods. The American Massage Therapy Association launched a National Sports Massage Team in 1986 to promote massage for athletes. Sports massage was included as part of the official medical team at the centennial Olympics in Atlanta in 1996, and has been a presence at the Olympics ever since. Sports massage has become a specialty among massage therapists, and is popular for both amateur and professional athletes.

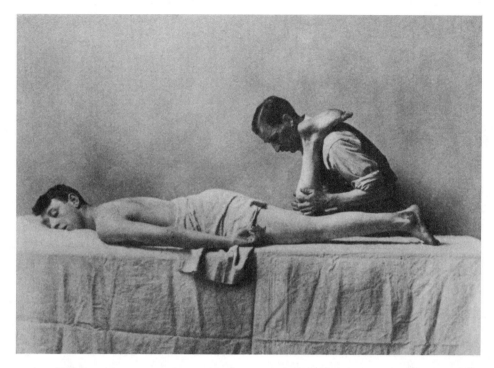

FIGURE 2–6. Harry Andrews, trainer and masseur, massaging the leg of an athlete circa 1910. From *Massage & Training* by Harry Andrews, published in 1910.

Fitness

Just as the ancient Greek gymnasia were not solely for elite athletes, YMCAs and health clubs offer various physical fitness activities for the general population. The YMCA tradition of exercise and massage was well established by 1915 when R. Tait McKenzie described the workouts at the "Y" as consisting of a mixture of Swedish gymnastics, German gymnastics, and games, ending with a bath and a rubdown (McKenzie, 1915, p. 70). By 1953, the health services at the YMCA offered massage and related services for general wellness. The scope of services offered was described by Frierwood:

> The technician uses massage, baths (shower, steam, electricity cabinet), ultraviolet irradiation (artificial and natural sunlight), infrared (heat), instruction in relaxation and in some cases directed exercise. The adult members secure a relief from tensions, gain a sense of well-being, give attention to the personal fitness and develop habits designed to build and maintain optimum health and physical efficiency throughout the lifespan. (1953, p. 21)

DECLINE AND REVIVAL IN THE 20TH CENTURY

In the 1950s, the practice of massage went into a period of decline. "Massage parlors" were used as cover for prostitution, ruining the image of legitimate practitioners. Other modalities were taking precedence in physical therapy, and the therapeutic value of massage was being questioned in professional publications. In the sports arena, trainers were specializing in injuries and the tradition of massage as a training aid was largely forgotten. It was a time of social conservatism, and the undressing and touching that happen in a massage session were uncomfortable for many in the general public. Most private massage schools closed down.

Esalen Massage in the 1970s

Two things happened in the 1960s to help revive the practice of massage: the **counterculture** and the **human potential movement.** Young people in the 1960s rejected the conservative, conformist, "untouchable" values of the 1950s, and began a search for a deeper meaning in life. Many became "hippies" and a culture counter to the mainstream was born. These were the post World War II baby boomers reaching young adulthood.

At the same time, a group of accomplished professionals started meeting at the Esalen Institute in Big Sur, California, in search of the limits of human potential. In the seminars at the Esalen Institute established in 1962, people explored their feelings in encounter groups, tried meditation, delved into various spiritual practices, learned physical exercises from Asia such as tai chi, and various forms of massage and bodywork. TV, movies, and popular magazines such as *Look* and *Life* brought knowledge of the Esalen experience to the American public. Americans were breaking out of the confines of the 1950s and exploring their potential in new ways (Leonard, 1988). (For more about the history of Esalen, go to *www.esalen.org.*)

A form of massage was developed at the Esalen Institute that was to affect the field of massage therapy dramatically. **Esalen massage** was not about technique, although it was loosely based on a simple form of Western massage that emphasized long flowing strokes, scented oils and incense. It was about making connection with the inner self, and with each other. It was not about professional massage at first, but about people connecting with each other on a deep level. As George Downing explained in his *Massage Book* (1972):

> The core of massage lies in its unique way of communicating without words . . . When receiving a good massage a person usually falls into a mental-physical state difficult to describe. It is like entering a special room until now locked and hidden away; a room the very existence of which is likely to be familiar only to those who practice some form of daily meditation . . . Trust, empathy and respect, to say nothing of a sheer sense of mutual physical existence, for this moment can be expressed with a fullness never matched by words (p. 1).

Many of those who embraced the ideals of the counterculture and the human potential movement tried Esalen massage as part of that experience. Others, searching for drugless spiritual or mystical experiences, studied Eastern philosophy and cultures. Many joined ashrams where they learned health practices of India, which include vegetarianism, meditation, yoga, and massage. Some studied Taoism, and tried health practices from China and Japan, including tai chi, chi kung, and shiatsu. China opened its doors to Western trade in 1972, and the ancient art of acupuncture was reintroduced to Western medicine.

Many of the values, as well as the practices, of the tradition of natural health and healing from earlier in the century were revived in the 1970s. Some of those who learned massage in ashrams, growth centers, or out of books wanted to try making a living doing massage professionally. Many still hold onto the values of the counterculture and resist efforts to "professionalize" the field of massage therapy. Others join professional associations and are active in legislative efforts, and in promoting research related to massage therapy.

The opening up to massage that happened in the 1960–1970s had a tremendous impact on the emerging profession of massage therapy. There was a significant growth in the number of practitioners and potential receivers of massage. The number of massage and bodywork training programs increased dramatically, and there was an infusion of youthful energy, spirit, and hope. The concepts of holistic health and healing were revived and expanded. There was openness to new ideas and diversity, and an expansion of thinking beyond Western science and medicine. The values of caring, heart, and connection became defining qualities of the work (Benjamin, 1996).

The cultural revolution of the 1960–1970s has affected health professions other than massage therapy. The **wellness movement,** undoubtedly influenced by the human potential movement, gained ground in the 1970s within the traditional fields of health, physical education, and recreation. The concept of wellness was promoted by people like John Travis, MD, who developed the illness/wellness continuum mentioned in Chapter 1.

Many hospitals today have picked up the concept, and offer "wellness programs" designed to teach good health habits and illness prevention. In the spirit of the wellness movement, they emphasize self-responsibility for health, and address holistic health, i.e., body, mind, emotions, and spirit.

In addition, methods that "touch" patients in a human way are being re-examined for their therapeutic value. For example, the American Nurses Association has recognized massage therapy as an official nursing subspecialty. The National Association of Nurse Massage Therapists (*www.nanmt.org*) is a member of the Nursing Organization Alliance (NOA). Many nurses have also adopted Therapeutic Touch, a form of energy work that has become a respected healing practice (*www.therapeutic-touch.org*).

MILESTONES AT THE TURN OF THE 21ST CENTURY

There were several noteworthy milestones for massage therapy in the 1990s and early 2000s. Most significant were an increase in research about massage therapy, a growing interest in CAM therapies by the U.S. government, the advent of a National Certification Examination for Therapeutic Massage and Bodywork, upgrading of curriculum standards for massage therapy programs, and a growing number of states in the United States licensing massage therapists.

The number of published research studies regarding massage therapy skyrocketed during the last decade of the 20th century. The **AMTA Foundation** was incorporated in 1992. A major part of their mission is to fund research about the efficacy of massage therapy. A database of massage therapy research was made available on their Web site in 2001 (*www.amtafoundation.org*).

The **Touch Research Institute** (TRI) was also created in 1992 at the University of Miami School of Medicine, with Tiffany Field as director. It was the first center in the world devoted to basic and applied research in the use of touch in human health and development. Information about the many studies sponsored by TRI can be accessed through their Web site (*www.miami.edu/touch-research*).

In addition, the first International Symposium on the Science of Touch was held in May 2002 in Montreal, Quebec, Canada. It was sponsored by the Canadian Touch Research Center. Presenters from all over the world participated in the event. Summaries of their presentations are available on line (*www.ccrt-ctrc.org*).

This increase in research and its availability to massage practitioners will help improve the quality of care given to clients and patients, and expand our understanding of the benefits of massage for different populations. It will also bolster the acceptance of massage therapy in an integrative health care system. Chapters 3 and 4 will review some of these study findings in more detail.

Public Policy

The Office of Alternative Medicine (OAM) was established within the U.S. National Institutes of Health (NIH) in 1992. Its charge was to explore "unconventional medical practices," and to recommend further research on the subject. *Alternative Medicine—Expanding Medical Horizons: A Report to the National Institutes of Health on Alternative Medical Systems and Practices in the United States* (1994) was published to summarize their findings.

The OAM was designated a Collaborating Center in Traditional Medicine by the United Nations World Health Organization in 1996. The status of the OAM was elevated to "center" in 1998, when it became the **National Center for Complementary and Alternative Medicine** (NCCAM). The NIH has subsequently awarded several grants for research projects on manual healing methods, including massage therapy (*www.nccam.nih.gov*).

The White House Commission on Complementary and Alternative Medicine issued its final report in March 2002. It made recommendations about coordination of CAM research, education of CAM practitioners, dissemination of information about CAM, and access to and delivery of CAM therapies. It urged the U.S. government to support research to determine which CAM therapies were effective for particular pathologies. The report also recognized the contribution of CAM approaches to wellness and health promotion (*www.whccamp.hhs.gov*).

Standards and Credentials

The **National Certification Examination for Therapeutic Massage and Bodywork** was first given in June 1992. Thus began the process of establishing valid credentials for massage therapists. Over 50,000 massage practitioners have become nationally certified since that time. The NCBTMB has developed massage therapy and specialty exams, and promoted the study of ethics via their recertification process, and Code of Ethics and Standards of Practice documents (*www.ncbtmb.org*).

In addition, in the United States an increasing number of states have passed occupational licensing laws for massage therapists. To date, 31 out of the 50 states have licensing laws. A list of states with massage licensing can be found in Appendix C. Check the American Massage Therapy Association Web site for the most up-to-date information about state licensing laws (*www.amtamassage.org*).

The **Commission on Massage Therapy Accreditation** (COMTA) received approval by the U.S. Department of Education in 2002, and the number of accredited massage therapy programs is growing. COMTA has initiated competency-based curriculum standards more clearly defining basic knowledge and skills for massage therapists (*www.comta.org*).

Consumers

Most importantly, consumers continue to receive massage for the whole range of goals outlined in the wellness massage pyramid. An article appeared in the *New England Journal of Medicine* in January 1993 titled "Unconventional Medicine in the United States." It was a report of a national survey that looked at the prevalence of the use of what was called "unconventional medicine," which included therapies such as chiropractic, acupuncture, relaxation techniques, herbal remedies, energy healing, hypnosis, spiritual healing, and massage therapy. Massage ranked third in alternative therapies used by the general public, with only relaxation techniques and chiropractic reported more frequently. The article concluded that the frequency of use of unconventional therapy in the United States is much higher than previously reported (Eisenberg et al., 1993, pp. 246–252). In a follow-up study of trends in alternative healthcare conducted in 1997, massage therapy was cited as one of the fastest growing CAM therapies in the United States (Eisenberg et al., 1998, pp. 1569–1575).

The American Massage Therapy Association reports increasing acceptance and use of massage therapy by consumers of all ages. In a 2002 Opinion Research study, 28% of adults reported having had a massage in the past 5 years, up from 17% in 1997. And a survey of medical practitioners ranked massage therapy highest (74%) among CAM approaches in terms of being perceived as always or usually effective. An increasing number of workplaces are offering massage as an employee benefit (AMTA 2002 "Demand for Massage Therapy"). The upcoming period in the history of massage therapy looks promising indeed.

SUMMARY

The history of massage is both ancient and global. It is used for health and healing in native and folk cultures all over the world. In the writings of the ancient civilizations of Sumer, China, India, Greece, and Rome we find descriptions of highly developed forms of massage. During the Middle Ages, classical Greco-Roman culture was preserved by Arabs in Turkey and the Near East, and monks in Ireland, and reintroduced into Europe during the Renaissance. The Turkish bath, which included a form of bodywork, was an evolution of the Greek gymnasium and Roman baths. Today's health clubs, with their workout facilities, swimming pools, steam rooms, whirlpools, and massage rooms, are part of this legacy.

Two men influential in the development of modern Western massage were Pehr H. Ling (1776–1839) of Sweden, and Johann G. Mezger of Amsterdam (1838–1909). Ling developed a system of active and passive movements to treat medical conditions and strengthen the body that in the late 1800s was called the Swedish Movement Cure in the United States. Mezger popularized the use of the familiar French terms for the Western massage technique categories of effleurage, petrissage, tapotement, and friction. In the 1900s the work of Ling and Mezger was further developed by their pupils, and found its way into conventional medicine, used both by nurses and physical therapists. Western massage was also an important part of the non-conventional healing methods of proponents of natural healing.

Swedish massage was very popular in the 1920–1940s. In its heyday Swedish massage was a set of therapies that included massage, Swedish movements, hydrotherapy, heat lamps, diathermy, and colonic irrigation. Swedish massage was offered at places like health clubs, the YMCA, resorts, reducing salons, and private establishments called massage parlors. Women massage therapists were called masseuses, and men were called masseurs.

Massage went through a period of decline in the 1950s. It was being used as a cover for prostitution, and its popularity in the United States as a health practice for the general public waned in the conservative climate of that decade. Massage was also losing credibility as a therapeutic modality within medical professions at that time.

Massage was revived as a valuable health and healing practice in the 1970s. The counterculture and human potential movement helped bring to light the benefits of massage as a holistic health practice. Esalen massage and sports massage raised public awareness, and helped invigorate the practice of massage. In addition, forms of massage from China and India came to the United States during this period.

In the 1990s and early 2000s, there were several noteworthy milestones in the history of massage therapy. There was an increase in scientific research about massage, and the creation of institutions to fund research and make results widely available via the Internet. The U.S. government began to develop public policy related to CAM therapies, and provide support for further study. Standards for massage therapists were raised with advent of national certification and USDE-recognized accreditation of training programs. The use and acceptance of massage continued to grow among consumers and other health professionals.

A look ahead . . .

Our understanding of the effects and benefits of massage continue to evolve. Chapter 3 presents some of the current theories about how massage enhances health, and reviews recent research on its efficacy.

REFERENCES

Alternative Medicine—Expanding Medical Horizons: A Report to the National Institutes of Health on Alternative Medicine Systems and Practices in the United States (1994). Available from the Office of Alternative Medicine, National Institutes of Health, 6120 Executive Blvd. #450, Rockville, MD 20892-9904.

AMTA (2002) *Demand for massage therapy use and acceptance increasing.* Retrieved: March 2003 (*http://amtamassage.org*).

Andrews, H. (1910). *Massage & training.* London: Health & Strength, Ltd.

Arano, L. C. (1976). *The medieval health handbook: Tacuinum sanitatis.* New York: George Braziller.

Armstrong, D., & Armstrong, E. M. (1991). *The great American medicine show: Being an illustrated history of hucksters, healers, health evangelists, and heroes from Plymouth Rock to the present.* New York: Prentice-Hall.

Baumgartner, A. J. (1947). *Massage in athletics.* Minneapolis, MN: Burgess.

Beals, K. R. (1978). Clubfoot in the Maori: A genetic study of 50 kindreds. *New Zealand Medical Journal, 88,* 144–146.

Beard, G., & Wood, E. C. (1964). *Massage principles and techniques.* Philadelphia: W. B. Saunders.

Benjamin, P. J. (1993). Massage therapy in the 1940's and the College of Swedish Massage in Chicago. *Massage Therapy Journal, 32*(4), 56–62.

Benjamin, P. J. (1996). The California revival: Massage therapy in the 1970–80's. Presentation at the AMTA National Education Conference in Los Angeles, CA, June 1996.

Benjamin, P. J. (2002). Shampooing—A journey to the East. *Massage Therapy Journal, 41*(2), 140–144.

Bilz, F. E. (1898). *The natural method of healing: A new and complete guide to health.* Translated from the latest German edition. Leipiz: F. E. Bilz.

Bohm, M. (1913). *Massage: Its principles and techniques.* Translated by Elizabeth Gould. Philadelphia: Lippincott.

Calvert, R. N. (2002). *The history of massage: An illustrated survey from around the world.* Rochester, VT: Healing Arts Press.

Chopra, D. (1991). *Perfect health: The complete mind/body guide.* New York: Harmony Books.

Cunliffe, B. (1978). *The Roman baths: A guide to the baths and Roman museum.* City of Bath: Bath Archeological Trust.

Downing, G. (1972). *The massage book.* New York: Random House.

Eisenberg, D. M., Kessler, R. C., Foster, C., Norlock, F. E., Calkins, D. R., & Delblanco, T. L. (1993). Unconventional medicine in the United States. *New England Journal of Medicine, 328*(4), 246–252.

Eisenberg, D. M., Davis, R. B., Ettner, S. L. et al. (1998). Trends in alternative medicine use in the United States, 1990–1997. *Journal of the American Medical Association, 280* (18), 1569–1575.

Fay, H. J. (1916). *Scientific massage for athletes.* London: Ewart, Seymour & Co.

Frierwood, H. T. (1953). The place of the health service in the total YMCA program. *Journal of Physical Education, 21.*

Georgii, A. (1880). *Kinetic jottings.* London: Henry Renshaw.

Grafstrom, A. (1904). *A text-book of mechano-therapy (massage and medical gymnastics), prepared for the use of medical students, trained nurses, and medical gymnasts.* Philadelphia: W. B. Saunders.

Graham, D. (1902). *A treatise on massage, its history, mode of application and effects.* Philadelphia: Lippincott.

Hoffa, A. (1978). *Technik der massage* (13th ed). Stuttgart, Germany: Ferdinand Enke. Translated for Fran Tappan by Ruth Friedlander.

Johnson, W. (1866). *The anatriptic art*. London: Simpkin, Marshall & Co.

Kellogg, J. H. (1923). *The art of massage*. Battle Creek, MI: Modern Medicine Publishing Co.

Kleen, E. A. (1921). *Massage and medical gymnastics*. New York: William Wood & Company.

Leboyer, F. (1982). *Loving hands: The traditional art of baby massage*. New York: Alfred A. Knopf.

Leonard, G. (1988). *Walking on the edge of the world: A memoir of the sixties and beyond*. Boston: Houghton Mifflin.

Ling, P. H. (1840a). The general principles of gymnastics. In *The collected works of P. H. Ling*. (1866). Stockholm, Sweden. Translated by Lars Agren and Patricia J. Benjamin. Unpublished.

Ling, P. H. (1840b). Notations to the general principles. In *The collected works of P. H. Ling*. (1866). Stockholm, Sweden. Translated by Lars Agren and Patricia J. Benjamin and published in *Massage Therapy Journal*, Winter 1987.

Ling, P. H. (1840c). The means or vehicle of gymnastics. Translated by R. J. Cyriax. In *American Physical Education Review*, 19(4), April 1914.

McKenzie, R. T. (1915). *Exercise in education and medicine*, 2nd ed. Philadelphia: W. B. Saunders.

McMillan, M. (1925). *Massage and therapeutic exercise*, 2nd ed. Philadelphia: W. B. Saunders.

Mennell, J. B. (1945). *Physical treatment*, 5th ed. Philadelphia: Blakiston.

M'Lean, T. (1814) *Picturesque representations of the dress and manners of the Chinese*. London: Howlett and Brimmer.

Monte, T., & the Editors of East West Natural Health (1993). *World medicine: The East West guide to healing your body*. New York: Putnam.

Murphy, W. (Ed.) (1995) *Healing the generations: A history of physical therapy and the American Physical Therapy Association*. Lyme, CT: Greenwich Publishing Group.

Murrell, W. (1890). *Massotherapeutics or massage as a mode of treatment*. Philadelphia: Blakiston.

Nissen, H. (1889). *A manual of instruction for giving Swedish movement and massage treatment*. Philadelphia: F. A. Davis.

Nissen, H. (1920). *Practical massage and corrective exercises with applied anatomy*. Philadelphia: F. A. Davis.

Ostrom, K. W. (1905). *Massage and the original Swedish movements*. Philadelphia: Blakiston.

Perrone, B., Stockel, H. H., & Krueger, V. (1989). *Medicine women, curanderas, and women doctors*. Norman, OK: University of Oklahoma Press.

Pollard, D. W. (1902). Massage in training. An unpublished thesis, International Young Men's Christian Association Training School, Springfield, MA.

Posse, N. (1895). *The special kinesiology of educational gymnastics*. Boston: Lothrop, Lee & Shepard.

Roth, M. (1851). *The prevention and cure of many chronic diseases by movements*. London: John Churchill.

Sampson, C. W. (1926). *A practice of physiotherapy*. St. Louis: C. V. Mosby.

Time-Life Books. (1987). *The age of god-kings: Timeframe 3000–1500 B.C.* Alexandria, VA: Time-Life Books.

Torres (no date). *The folk healer: The Mexican-American tradition of curanderismo*. Kingsville, TX: Nieves Press.

Wood, E. C., & Becker, P. D. (1981). *Beard's massage*, 3rd ed. Philadelphia: W. B. Saunders.

WEB SITES

www.amtafoundation.org American Massage Therapy Association Foundation

www.amtamassage.org American Massage Therapy Association

www.ccrt-ctrc.org Canadian Touch Research Center

www.comta.org Commission on Massage Therapy Accreditation

www.esalen.org Esalen Institute

www.nanmt.org National Association of Nurse Massage Therapists

www.ncbtmb.org National Certification Board for Therapeutic Massage and Bodywork

www.therapeutic-touch.org Nurse Healers-Professional Associates International

www.miami.edu/touch-research Touch Research Institute

www.nccam.nih.gov National Center of Complementary and Alternative Medicine

www.worldofmassagemuseum.org World of Massage Museum

www.whccamp.hhs.gov White House Commission on Complementary and Alternative Medicine

ADDITIONAL REFERENCES

Videos

"Esalen massage." (1999). Big Sur, CA: Esalen Institute. (*www.esalen.org*)

"Hawaiian lomi-lomi: Level 1" Venture, CA: Hawaiian Healing Arts. (*www.lomi-lomi.com*)

STUDY GUIDE

LEARNING OUTCOMES

Use the learning outcomes at the beginning of the chapter as a guide to your studies. Perform the task given in each outcome, either in writing or verbally into a tape recorder or to a study partner. This may start as an "open book" exercise, and then later from memory.

KEY HISTORICAL PEOPLE, KEY TERMS/CONCEPTS

To study key historical people, places, events, and forms of massage listed at the beginning of this chapter, choose one or more of the following exercises. Writing or talking about these stories will help you remember them better, and deepen your understanding of their significance.

1. Summarize the contributions of a key person in the development of massage at a particular period of time. Try to capture their contributions in one or two concise statements.

2. Make study cards by writing the name of a key historical person, place or event on one side of a 3 × 5 card, and details about them on the other. Shuffle the cards and read one side, trying to recite information from the other side.

3. Match key historical people to places and events or other people related to them in some way, and explain how they are related.

4. With a study partner(s), take turns telling the stories of key people, places or events in the history of massage. Telling the stories verbally to someone else can help you remember them, and help clarify details in your mind.

5. After each story in problem 4, ask each other questions to clarify the significance of the person, place, or event in the history of massage.

STUDY OUTLINE

The following questions test your memory of the main historical facts in this chapter. Locate the answers in the text using the page number given for each question.

Ancient and Global Heritage

1. The history of massage is both _____ and _____. (p. 20)

2. The exchange of ideas and practices among different cultures happens as the result of _____, _____, _____, _____, and _____. (p. 20)

3. Some of forms of massage and bodywork that continue to be performed in their traditional ways may be considered both _____ and _____ _____. (p. 20)

Native and Folk Traditions

1. An example of wellness massage practiced by people of the South Sea Islands for centuries is _____. (p. 21)

2. Hispanic healers called _____ use massage in their tradition of folk medicine developed in the 15th century when Catholic Spaniards came in contact with the _____ civilization in Mexico. (p. 21)

Ancient Civilizations

1. One of the oldest records describing rubbing for medicinal purposes was found on clay tablets written in _____ in 2100 BCE. (pp. 21–22)

2. Written over 2,500 years ago, _____ _____ is often cited as the first book written on Chinese medicine. (p. 22)

3. Traditional Japanese massage called _____ developed in Japan in the 6th century BCE when Chinese health and healing practices reached the islands. (p. 22)

4. Shiatsu is a modern form of Japanese bodywork developed in the _____ by _____ _____. (p. 22)

5. The traditional healing practices of India, called _____, can be traced back to the 5th century CE, and included forms of massage. (p. 23)

6. The ancient Greek medical writings of _____ mentioned massage used to treat sprains and dislocations. (p. 23)

7. Massage given to athletes in the Greek _____ used a lot of oil, and was given before and after exercises. (p. 23)

8. The _____ were communal gathering places where citizens of the Roman empire enjoyed cool and warm pools of water, steam rooms, and received a rigorous form of bodywork. (pp. 23–24)

9. The modern _____ is a legacy of the Greek gymnasium, Roman baths, and _____ baths. (p. 24)

Middle Ages and Renaissance Europe

1. During the Middle Ages, the practice of massage was kept alive in the _____ of Europe. (p. 24)

2. Classic Greek and Roman writings about the use of massage in medicine were preserved during the Dark Ages by the _____, and by the _____. (p. 24)

3. A book called the _____, translated from Arabic into Latin in the 11th century, is evidence of the early development of the philosophy of natural health and healing. (p. 24)

4. Classic Greek and Roman writings were brought back to Europe during the period called the _____. (pp. 24–25)

Western Massage

1. Western massage is a synthesis of techniques developed by _____ of Sweden and _____ of Amsterdam in the 1800s. (p. 25)

2. Pehr Ling developed a system of medical gymnastics to treat chronic ailments called the _____ _____ in the United States. (p. 25)

3. Ling's school in Stockholm, called the _____ _____, was founded in _____. (p. 26)

4. Johann Mezger categorized the many soft tissue techniques, calling them by the French terms _____, _____, _____, and _____. These, plus the technique of _____, make up the categories of Western massage. (p. 26)

5. Ling's medical gymnastics was brought to the United States by _____ of New York in _____. (p. 27)

Conventional and Natural Healing

1. Words used to describe massage technique in early conventional medical practice were _____, _____, and _____. (p. 27)

2. Massage and bodywork was called the _____ art by Walter Johnson in an 1866 book on the history of soft tissue manipulation. (p. 27)

3. Lucas-Championnière of France (c. 1880) advocated the use of soft tissue manipulation in the treatment of _____. (p. 27)

4. The Reconstruction Department of the United States Army was established in 1918 to help in the rehabilitation of soldiers wounded in (war) _____. Women trained to use massage, movements, and hydrotherapy in this effort were called _____. (p. 28)

5. _____ was a prominent figure in the history of physical therapy who trained Reconstruction Aides at the Walter Reed Clinic during World War I. She wrote *Massage and Therapeutic Exercise* while director of physiotherapy at _____ in the 1920s. (p. 28)

6. The director of the Battle Creek Sanitarium in Michigan in the late 1800s, and a famous advocate of natural healing, was _____. His book _____ was published in 1895. (p. 29)

7. A man named _____ popularized natural health practices in the late 19th and early 20th centuries through his resorts, *Physical Culture Magazine*, and radio shows. (p. 29)

8. The heyday of Swedish massage was from about _____ to _____. (p. 29)

9. Swedish massage practice consisted of Western massage, the Swedish movements, various forms of _____, _____, _____, reducing massage, and _____ irrigation. (p. 29)

10. Many Swedish massage practitioners in the early 20th century worked as natural healers, and with non-conventional doctors of _____ and _____. (p. 29)

Sports and Fitness

1. The _____ was a simple form of massage given to athletes in the late 1800s and early 1900s. (p. 30)

2. A book written in 1916 by H. J. Fay called _____ describes massage for recovery after athletic events. (p. 30)

3. Sports massage was revived by _____ in the (year) _____, and is now a popular specialty within the field. (p. 30)

4. Massage has been part of the health services at the _____, an American health and fitness institution, since the early 1900s. (p. 31)

Decline and Revival in the 20th Century

1. The _____ (decade) was a period of decline in the practice of massage in the United States. (p. 31)

2. Massage _____ were used as a cover for prostitution, ruining the image of legitimate massage practitioners. (p. 31)

3. A simplified version of Western massage developed in the 1970s that emphasized long flowing strokes and the sensual experience of scented oils, relaxing music, and incense was called _____ (p. 32)

4. Two important social movements in the development of the form of massage described in problem 3 were _____ and the _____. (p. 31)

5. A movement of the 1970s that had a major impact on health professions, including massage therapy, and that developed within the field of health, physical education, and recreation was the _____. (p. 32)

Milestones at the Turn of the 21st Century

1. A national organization whose mission is to advance massage therapy research is the _____ _____, incorporated in _____ (year). (p. 33)

2. The first center in the world devoted to research on the use of touch in human health was the _____ at the University of Miami. It was founded in _____ (year), and its first director was _____. (p. 33)

3. The U.S. National Institutes of Health (NIH) established the _____ in 1992 to explore unconventional medical practices. This was elevated to a center at NIH in 1998 called the _____. (p. 33)

4. The first National Certification Examination for Therapeutic Massage and Bodywork was given in _____ (year). (p. 33)

5. The Commission on Massage Therapy Accreditation received U.S. Department of Education recognition in _____ (year). (p. 34)

FOR GREATER UNDERSTANDING

The following exercises are designed to make history come alive by connecting it to the real world of human experience. The exercises will introduce you to primary sources for learning more about history, and help you gain a deeper understanding of the historical subjects covered in this chapter.

1. Choose one or two major figures introduced in this chapter, and research their lives and contributions to the development of massage therapy. Try to locate their original writings to read about their work in their own words.

2. Locate an old Turkish bath or spa in your community that is still in operation. Research its history, and visit the place, looking at its architecture and floor space. Receive a massage there if still available, or enjoy the baths. See if they have old photos or an archive. This is also a good vacation adventure.

3. Look through old newspapers, magazines, or playbills for advertisements related to the history of massage, e.g., Turkish baths, reducing salons, health clubs, massage parlors. From the 1890s to 1930s are good times to explore.

4. Visit an antique shop and look for things related to the history of massage, such as advertisements mentioned in problem 3, old books, electrical vibrators, or lotion and oil bottles that might have been used with massage.

5. Interview someone who remembers the 1950s and how massage was perceived at that time. Ask them

how their view of massage has changed over the years, and what has influenced that change. Share your interview with a study partner or group.

6. <u>Interview</u> someone who learned Esalen massage in the 1970s or early 1980s. Where did they learn it and what was their experience of it? How was it different from massage therapy today? Share your interview with a study partner or group.

7. <u>Interview</u> someone from a different culture who is familiar with massage as passed down within their family. How far back in time and where has it been practiced? Who did they learn it from? What was it like? How is it different or similar to Western massage?

8. <u>Interview</u> a nurse or physical therapist who was working in the 1950s, 1960s, or another period from the past. Ask them about how massage was used in health care at that time, and how it changed over the years. Report your findings.

9. Be alert to references about <u>massage in old movies</u>, especially from the 1930–1940s. Some movies set in historical periods also show massage as given at that time.

10. <u>Visit the website</u> of the World of Massage Museum (*www.worldofmassagemuseum.com*). Look at its mission and the content of its collection.

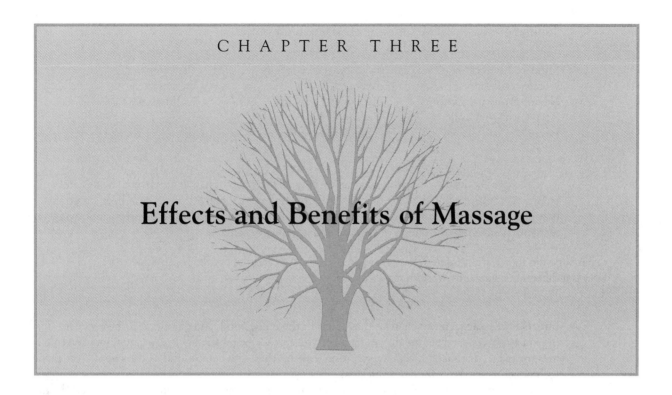

CHAPTER THREE

Effects and Benefits of Massage

LEARNING OUTCOMES

After studying this chapter, the student will have information to:

1. Explain the effects of massage at the tissue and organ system levels.
2. Explain the effects of massage at the organism level.
3. Describe the psychological effects of massage.
4. Explain various mechanisms for the effects of massage.
5. Describe how different massage techniques are applied for different effects.
6. Appreciate the holistic view of the effects of massage.
7. Discuss the beneficial effects of massage for everyone.
8. Discuss the beneficial effects of massage for special populations.

KEY TERMS/CONCEPTS

Adhesions	Character armor	Hyperemia
Analgesia	Effects of massage	Hypertonic
Anxiety reduction	Emotional release	Immunity
Benefits of massage	Endorphins	Ischemia
Body alignment	Energetic effects	Limbic system
Body awareness	Flexibility	Mechanical effects
Body-centered therapy	Holistic	Mental clarity

 MEDIALINK

A companion CD-ROM, included free with each new copy of this book, supplements the techniques presented in this chapter. Insert the CD-ROM to watch video clips of massage techniques being demonstrated. This multimedia feature is designed to help you add a new dimension to your learning.

Mind-body effects   Psychological effects   Tissue repair
Muscle relaxation   Reflex effects   Venostasis
Neural-gating mechanism   Relaxation response   Wellness massage
Pain-spasm-pain cycle   Sensory input
Posture   Thixotropy

Massage is valued for its ability to promote optimal body function, enhance overall health and well-being, and for its specific therapeutic effects. Through the years many theories have been proposed for how and why massage works. In this chapter we will explore some of those theories, and review research that examines the effects of massage and its many benefits.

EFFECTS OF MASSAGE

Effects of massage refer to changes that occur in the body, mind, and emotions of the recipient during a massage session. They are the outcomes of a session, for example, muscle relaxation, increased alertness, or reduced anxiety. Massage practitioners keep these effects in mind as they apply soft tissue techniques to accomplish therapeutic goals.

Different massage techniques are chosen for their specific effects, and are applied to elicit the desired response in the receiver. For example, tapotement has a stimulating effect if received for a short time and may have a sedating effect if received for a longer period of time. Effleurage applied slowly, rhythmically, and with light to moderate pressure usually has a relaxing effect, but applied briskly may feel invigorating.

Practitioners who know how to apply massage techniques to obtain specific effects will be more successful in achieving session or treatment goals. (Refer to *Outcomes-Based Massage* by Andrade & Clifford, 2001.) Information about Western massage techniques and how to apply them for specific effects is found in Part II, Western Massage.

The remainder of this chapter takes a systematic look at the effects of massage as understood in Western anatomy and physiology. The levels of organization found in standard anatomy and physiology textbooks provides a useful framework for studying the effects of massage, i.e., tissue level, organ system level, organism level. Psychological effects are discussed at the whole organism level. Effects that have practical implications from the wellness perspective will be highlighted. The potential effects of massage are summarized in Table 3–1.

TISSUE LEVEL EFFECTS

Massage improves the overall health of cells and tissues of the body, primarily by increasing blood and lymph circulation. The "milking" action of petrissage techniques and the sliding movements of effleurage are very effective in moving body fluids to facilitate natural processes. Increased fluid circulation improves delivery of oxygen and nutrients to tissue cells, and helps in removal of metabolic wastes and byproducts of the inflammatory process (Yates 1990).

Tissue Repair

Healing from tissue injuries such as burns, bruises, sprains, and wounds has three physiological phases. This **tissue repair** process consists of *inflammation* to stabilize the injured area, *regeneration* to restore the tissue structure, and *remodeling* for healthy scar formation. Massage can play an important role in the tissue repair process.

The initial reaction to injury, called inflammation, is designed to stabilize the situation and prepare damaged tissues for repair. Inflammation results in increased blood flow to the area causing redness, warmth, swelling, pain, and decreased function. The lymphatic system plays an important role in

Table 3–1 SUMMARY OF THE EFFECTS OF MASSAGE[a]

Physical Effects
Tissue Level

Enhance tissue repair and scar formation
Improve connective tissue health
  Improve pliability of fascia
  Break adhesions and separate tissues

Organ System Level

Integumentary system	Stimulate sensory receptors in skin
	Increase superficial circulation
	Remove dead skin
	Add moisture with oil or lotion
	Increase sebaceous gland secretions
	Facilitate healthy scar formation
Skeletal System	Promote good joint function
	Promote optimal joint flexibility and range of motion
	Promote proper skeletal alignment
Muscular System	"Milk" metabolic wastes into venous and lymph flow
	Promote specific and general muscle relaxation
	Promote optimal body flexibility
	Relieve myofascial trigger points
	Release myofascial adhesions
Nervous System	Stimulate parasympathetic nervous system (i.e. relaxation response)
	Reduce pain (e.g. neural-gating mechanism)
	Sharpen body awareness
Endocrine System	Release of endorphins (with nervous system)
Cardiovascular System	Increase general and local circulation
	Enhance venous return
	Reduce blood pressure and heart rate
	Increase red blood cells in circulation
Lymphatic System and Immunity	Increase lymph fluid movement
	Improve immune function via stress reduction
Respiratory System	Encourage diaphragmatic breathing
	Relax muscles of respiration
	Promotes good structural alignment and rib cage expansion
Digestive System	Digestion improved with relaxation
	Facilitate bowel movement
Urinary System	Enhances circulation to kidneys
	Increased urinary production and bladder tension
Reproductive System	Reproductive function improved with relaxation
	Promote general breast health

Organism Level

Growth and Development	Improve growth and development in infants
Pain Reduction	Relieve muscle pain from tension and poor circulation
	Deactivate myofascial trigger points
	Activate neural-gating mechanism
	Induce release of endorphins and enkephalins
Stress Reduction	Trigger relaxation response

Psychological Effects

Increase mental clarity
Reduce anxiety
Facilitate emotional release
Promote feelings of general well-being

[a]These effects do not occur during every massage session. The massage techniques used and the qualities of movement (e.g., rhythm, pacing, pressure, direction, duration) help determine which effects are likely to occur. The physical, mental, and emotional condition of recipients and their openness to massage might also have impact on which effects occur.

the resolution of inflammation by removing fluid that creates swelling and surveying that fluid for harmful microorganisms. The length of the inflammatory phase will vary depending on the severity of the initial trauma, and the strength of the individual's immune system. Massage is contraindicated in the immediate location of an injury during the inflammatory phase, especially in the presence of infection. Once the signs of inflammation subside, massage can be applied safely around the injury site.

In the regeneration phase, the tissue structure is rebuilt and restored. New tissue replaces damaged tissue of the same type. This involves removing damaged cells, excess fluids, and other byproducts of inflammation, as well as delivering the building blocks for new tissue formation. By improving general and local circulation, massage facilitates this transportation process.

Massage can also play a role in the remodeling phase of tissue repair by encouraging healthy scar formation. Deep transverse friction is used in rehabilitation to help form strong mobile scar tissue. Deep friction helps break interfiber adhesions by forcibly broadening the tissues. This in turn helps produce more parallel fiber arrangement and fewer transverse connections in the tissue that may inhibit movement (Cyriax & Cyriax, 1993). Subcutaneous scar tissue may be loosened by careful and persistent friction; however, further research is needed to establish whether deeper scarring in connective tissue can be realigned once it is formed.

A less understood role for massage in tissue repair is related to its promotion of stress reduction. A study reported in *Lancet,* a British medical journal, showed that wounds healed more slowing in people suffering from chronic stress. Researchers found that the stressed group had lower levels of interleukin-1 beta, an immune system substance known to play a role in wound repair (Greene, 1996, p.16). To the extent that massage reduces stress, it may help wounds heal faster.

Connective Tissue

Connective tissue is the most pervasive tissue in the body. It fills internal spaces, provides structural support, and is a vehicle for fluid transportation and energy storage. Three classifications of connective tissue are fluid (e.g., blood and lymph); supporting connective tissue (e.g., cartilage and bone); and connective tissue proper (e.g., ligaments, tendons, fascia). Some general connective tissue considerations and the nature of fascia will be discussed briefly in the following paragraphs.

Connective tissue has a property called **thixotropy,** which means that it becomes more fluid and pliable when it is mobile, and firmer when it is immobile. Pressing, friction, stretching, and other movements of massage raise the temperature and the energy level of the tissue slightly and create a "greater degree of sol (fluidity) in organic systems that are already there but are behaving sluggishly." (Juhan, 1987, pp. 69–70).

In addition to promoting healthy function, massage helps to *prevent* some connective tissue abnormalities and dysfunction. For example, massage techniques such as kneading and deep friction have been found to help prevent the formation of abnormal collagenous connective tissue called *fibrosis* (Yates, 1990).

Fascia is a connective tissue that surrounds all muscles, bones, and organs and helps to give them shape. Fascia literally holds the body together and can be thought of as continuous sheets of supportive tissue, which envelop the entire body and its parts. (For more detail about fascia read *The Endless Web: Fascial Anatomy and Physical Reality* by Schultz & Feitis, 1996.)

In healthy bodies, fascial tissues are pliable and move freely. With chronic stress, chronic immobility, trauma, or disease, this connective tissue may become thickened, rigid or may stick to other tissues forming adhesions. Adhesions result in restricted movement and impair the ability of the affected tissues to conduct exchanges of nutrients and cellular wastes. Massage can improve tissue function by helping to restore tissue pliability and break adhesions.

Certain massage techniques break **adhesions** formed when fascial tissues stick to each other or to other tissues. The simple mechanical action of some massage techniques separates tissues, for example, lifting, broadening, and applying a shearing force across the parallel organization of fibers. Kneading, skin rolling, deep transverse friction, broadening techniques, and myofascial techniques are examples of effective methods for separating and "unsticking" adhering tissues.

Chapter 12 provides more detailed information about massage for healthy fascia. The discussion of increased joint mobility and flexibility in the Muscular System section of this chapter has further information on connective tissue and massage.

ORGAN SYSTEM LEVEL EFFECTS

Massage has specific effects on the different organ systems of the body. In addition to keeping the organ tissues healthy and enhancing healing, massage can also improve the function of the system as a whole. And since organ systems interact in myriad ways, the effects of massage on any system impacts others as well. Overlapping function is especially obvious in certain system pairings such as muscular-skeletal, circulatory-lymphatic, nervous-endocrine, and respiratory-circulatory-muscular.

Integumentary System

The integumentary system includes the skin and its accessory structures such as hair, nails, and sebaceous and sweat glands. Sensory receptors in the skin detect touch, pressure, pain, and temperature and relay that information to the nervous system.

The skin is the primary point of contact between the giver and receiver of massage. One of the major effects of pressure to the skin is stimulation of the sensory receptors found here. This stimulation may have beneficial effects such as general relaxation, pain reduction, and body awareness. Good **body awareness** enhances a person's sense of integrity and wholeness, and is important for good mental and emotional health.

In order for the exocrine glands in the skin (i.e., sebaceous and sweat glands) to work properly, skin pores must be free from blockage. Pores may become blocked with substances like dirt, makeup, dried oils and sweat, or the accumulation of dead skin cells. Bathing with soap and water, and hydrotherapy such as whirlpool, steam room, and sauna, help open pores. Exfoliating, or removing dead skin cells by scraping or frictioning (i.e., with loofa, brush, or coarse towels) is an old health and beauty practice.

The friction of massage also increases the temperature of skin, which promotes perspiration and increases sebaceous oil secretions. Oil and lotion applied to the skin during massage add moisture needed to prevent further drying or cracking. This is especially beneficial in dry climates, on aging skin, and with certain dry skin conditions.

Massage can facilitate the formation of healthy scar tissue on the skin surface following lacerations, surgery incisions, or burns. Applying cross-fiber and with-fiber friction techniques to scars during the remodeling or scar maturation phase helps form strong mobile scars, break adhesions to underlying tissues, and reduce scar thickness.

Skeletal System

The skeletal system includes the bones of the skeleton, associated cartilage, ligaments, and other stabilizing connective tissue structures. In addition to general tissue health promoted by good circulation, massage and related joint movements help maintain good joint function and range of motion. Movement of the joints stimulates production of synovial fluid that keeps joints moving smoothly.

Optimal range of motion is achieved when the bones are in proper alignment and the tissues surrounding the joints are healthy, pliable, and relaxed. Joint flexibility (i.e., flex-ability) is enhanced with massage and stretching movements. Flexibility is discussed in greater depth in the Muscular System section of this chapter.

Proper body alignment is necessary for optimal functioning of the skeletal system. Maintaining alignment or body posture is discussed below as a function of the combined muscular and skeletal systems.

Muscular System

The muscular system includes skeletal muscles, associated connective tissue (i.e., fascia and tendons), and motor and sensory neurons related to movement. Proprioceptors, important sensory neurons that monitor the movement and position of the body in space, are located in the skeletal muscles and associated connective tissue.

The importance of muscular system health for overall wellbeing cannot be overestimated. It is through the musculature and the movement it produces that so many other health benefits derive: for example, good circulation, body heat, metabolism, kinesthetic awareness, and even emotional balance. Problems in the musculature cause untold pain, and reduced quality of life. It is not surprising that massage therapy is valued so highly for its role in maintaining good health and function of the muscular system.

Cellular Level Activity. Muscles maintain normal cellular level activity and balance through movement. Muscle contraction puts mechanical pressure on the veins and lymphatic vessels, thereby pushing fluids along and carrying away metabolic byproducts. As the muscles relax, fresh blood flows into them, bringing nutrients to the area. This balancing action is disturbed through under-activity or over-activity.

Under-activity disturbs balance, since the muscle contractions that provide the "milking" effect are less than needed for good fluid circulation. Waste products then accumulate in the muscle tissue, and the arrival of nutrients is slowed. When illness or injury results in muscular inactivity, massage can mimic the action of muscle contraction, thereby improving fluid circulation.

Over-activity, for example, from strenuous exercise or work, also disturbs balance at the cellular level. Insufficient time between contractions decreases the inflow of nutritive products and oxygen to muscle tissues. In addition, metabolic waste products are formed faster than they can be eliminated. Muscle tension increases and muscles shorten due to reduced cellular nutrition. Muscle tension worsens the situation by further limiting fluid circulation.

Massage given immediately after strenuous activity reduces muscle stiffness and soreness. A combination of effleurage (i.e., sliding) and petrissage (e.g., kneading, compression) flushes metabolic wastes, brings oxygen and nutrients to the area, and enhances tissue repair. These are important benefits of post-event, inter-event, and recovery sports massage (see Figure 3–1). (For further information on massage for athletes refer to *Understanding Sports Massage* by Benjamin & Lamp, 1996.) Also see the discussion on increased blood circulation in the Cardiovascular System section.

Muscle Relaxation. Massage is often used to relax **hypertonic** or tense muscles. There are several ways that **muscle relaxation** may be effected. Reduction of general muscle tension may be due in part to stimulation of the parasympathetic nervous system via relaxation massage. There may also be a conscious letting go of muscle tension by the higher brain centers as the recipient assumes a passive state during a massage session.

General muscle relaxation may also be traced to increased sensory stimulation that accompanies the application of massage techniques. Yates (1990) reasons that massage causes a massive increase in the **sensory input** to the spinal cord, which results in readjustments in reflex pathways, which leads to spontaneous normalization of imbalances of tonic activity between individual muscles and muscle groups. Residual muscle tension left over from past activity or emotional stress is released as the system balances itself (pp. 11–12). Thus, muscular relaxation results from the general application of a variety of basic massage techniques such as effleurage, petrissage, friction, tapotement, and vibration.

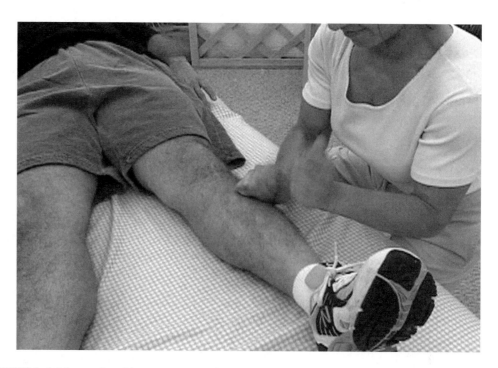

FIGURE 3–1. Massage for athletes improves performance.

Manual techniques may be applied to relax specific muscles. For example, in a technique called *muscle approximation*, the combined action of the muscular and nervous systems is utilized to reduce muscle tone. In this technique, the practitioner slowly and forcibly draws the attachments of the muscle closer together. This decreases stretch of the muscle spindles, which are composed of nerve filaments coiled around specialized muscle fibers. Muscle spindles cause contraction when muscles are suddenly elongated, i.e., stretch reflex. Approximation causes slack in the muscle, and is held until the muscle spindles stop firing and the muscle fibers relax. Approximation is useful for treating muscle spasms.

Another muscle relaxation method called the *origin and insertion technique* by Rattray is useful when direct work on the muscle belly is too painful. In the origin and insertion technique, cross-fiber and with-fiber friction is performed on the attachments of the targeted muscle in small segments until the muscle fibers relax. Eventually overall muscle tone is reduced. This works by stimulating sensory receptors called Golgi tendon organs located in tendons near muscle attachments. When Golgi tendon organs fire, they inhibit contraction of the associated muscle (Rattray 1994, pp. 43-44). Since muscular relaxation is one of the fundamental effects of massage, there are many other manual techniques for promoting muscle relaxation discussed throughout the text.

Increased Joint Mobility and Flexibility.   Flexibility refers to the degree of range of motion in a joint. It is a function of the combined muscular and skeletal systems with some nervous system involvement. Hypertonic muscles, scarring in muscle and connective tissues, myofascial adhesions, trigger points, and general connective tissue thickening and rigidity may all restrict movement at joints. Massage and passive joint movements can be used effectively to help maintain joint mobility and normal range of motion by addressing any abnormal conditions found in the soft tissues surrounding the joint.

In a study conducted by sport physical therapists and a massage therapist, massage was found to significantly increase range of motion in the hamstrings. The massage techniques used in the study were light and deep effleurage, stretching effleurage, petrissage (kneading), and friction (deep circular and deep transverse). Increased flexibility lasted for at least seven days after the massage (Crosman, Chateauvert, & Weisburg, 1985). Additional information on improving flexibility through joint movements may be found in Chapter 8.

Posture.   Proper body alignment or good posture is the combined function of the muscular, skeletal, and nervous systems. Poor posture usually results from a combination of factors such as ergonomically inadequate workstations or tools, injuries, or poor postural habits. Poor posture often leads to imbalances between muscle groups, hypertonic and shortened muscles, fascial adhesions, trigger points, and other problem conditions. Or vice versa: Muscle imbalances or pathologies may result in poor body alignment.

Some forms of massage and bodywork specifically focus on helping clients improve their body alignment. After analyzing the client's posture and identifying the probable cause of misalignment, massage and related joint movements are applied with the goal of proper alignment. This might involve strategies such as relaxing and elongating muscles with massage, lengthening muscle groups with stretching, or breaking fascial adhesions with myofascial techniques.

Nervous and Endocrine Systems

The nervous and endocrine systems work together, to coordinate organ system functions and respond to environmental stimuli. The nervous system controls relatively swift responses like those related to movement, while the endocrine system regulates slower responses such as metabolic rate. Nervous system anatomy consists of the central nervous system (i.e., brain and spinal cord), and peripheral nervous system (i.e., sensory receptors and motor neurons). A division of the nervous system that regulates the activity of smooth muscle, cardiac muscle, and glands is called the autonomic nervous system, which plays an important role in relaxation massage.

The endocrine system is composed of endocrine glands that secrete hormones that regulate important body processes such as cell growth and division, general metabolism, water loss and blood calcium levels.

Some of the effects of massage related to the nervous system have already been discussed. For example, stimulation of sensory receptors in the skin enhances body awareness, and plays an important role in muscle relaxation and pain reduction. The effects of massage on growth and development in infants are directly related to stimulation of the nervous system via the skin and through body movement.

Some massage and movement techniques use the nervous system to affect desired results. For example, some assisted stretching techniques deliberately activate proprioceptors in muscles to effect relaxation and elongation.

One of the most important effects of massage is its ability to elicit the relaxation response. This combined autonomic nervous system and endocrine system response is discussed below in more detail under the Organism Level, since it involves many organ systems as well as mental and emotional states.

Cardiovascular System

Cardiovascular system anatomy includes the heart, blood vessels (i.e., arteries and veins), and blood, which is considered a fluid connective tissue. The cardiovascular system is essentially a fluid transportation system for things like nutrients, waste products, dissolved gases, hormones, and cells and molecules for body defense.

The cardiovascular and lymphatic systems are transportation systems that rely specifically on the movement of fluids to carry out their functions. Good fluid circulation in these important body systems is a key to health at the cellular level.

The benefits of increased circulation include improved nutrient delivery and increased metabolic waste removal via the blood. It is also important for tissue repair, as building blocks for new tissues are brought to an area and damaged cells are removed. When pathogens enter the body, fluids deliver macrophages to attack the invaders and help prevent disease. The team action of these two body systems is succinctly described by Yates (1990):

> Increases in blood and lymph circulation are the most widely recognized and frequently described of the physiological effects of massage therapy. Changes in blood and lymph circulation are appropriately discussed together because they have effects in common on the clearance of metabolic wastes, and the by-products of tissue damage and inflammation, the absorption of excess of inflammatory exudate, and on the delivery of oxygen and nutrients to tissue cells (p. 20).

Blood Circulation.   Massage improves both general and local blood circulation. Several studies have shown that capillary vessel dilation and increased blood flow in an area occur with massage. Even light pressure was shown to have an effect (Wood & Becker, 1981, pp. 25–26).

Superficial friction produces **hyperemia** or increased local circulation in the skin and underlying connective tissue. As a result the skin appears red and feels warm. This effect is the result of the release of a chemical called *histamine* that causes dilation of capillaries in the area.

Deep effleurage and petrissage have specifically been shown to increase blood volume in an area. This increased flow is thought to last for some time after massage. For example, Bell (1964) reported that after a 10-minute massage of the calf, blood flow to the area doubled. This effect lasted 40 minutes. The benefits of increased circulation include improved nutrient delivery, and increased metabolic waste removal via the blood.

Venous Return.   The mechanical action of deep effleurage enhances venous flow in the limbs. This technique physically pushes blood through venous circulation.

The structure of veins dictates the direction of the application of deep stroking on the limbs. A dictum in classic Western massage states that deep stroking should always be "toward the heart," or moving distal to proximal.

Veins are low-pressure tubes. Movement of blood through them is aided by muscle contraction and by valves that prevent pooling due to the effects of gravity. Deep effleurage in the direction of the natural movement of blood enhances the flow. Applying massage in the opposite direction puts pressure on the valves and could possibly damage them.

Damage to valves results in a condition known as varicose veins. In varicose veins we find static, pooled blood. The constant pressure of pooled blood weakens the vein walls even further, causing a vicious cycle of pooling and weakening. Over time the veins become fragile. Under these conditions, massage could cause the vein to rupture, or release clots formed in the pools, into general circulation. Therefore, massage is locally contraindicated over superficial varicose veins, and generally contraindicated for someone with a history of blood clots.

The mechanical action of kneading and other forms of petrissage also assist in venous return, much the same way muscle contraction does during exercise. Compression of the tissues increases local circulation and blood in the capillaries is moved along toward the larger veins.

Venostasis is a condition in which the normal flow of blood through a vein is slowed or halted. Muscular inactivity can bring about venostasis, particularly in inactive or paralyzed limbs. Other causes for venostasis include varicose veins and pressure on the vessels from edema of the surrounding tissues. Massage given for this condition should first address the proximal aspects of an inactive limb before massage of the distal area. This ensures that the circulatory pathways are open enough to carry the venous flow from the distal area back toward the heart.

Blood Pressure.   Researchers Barr and Taslitz (1970) found that blood pressure is temporarily decreased for about 40 minutes after a massage session. The decrease in pressure is thought to result from a greater capacity for blood in the capillaries due to local vasodilation, and greater permeability of capillary walls. The more blood in the capillaries, the less in other vessels to cause pressure on vessel walls. Reduction in both systolic and diastolic pressure was duplicated in research by Cady and Jones (1997).

Also, as mentioned above, one of the long-term effects of eliciting the relaxation response regularly and learning to control stress is decreased blood pressure in individuals with hypertension. This saves wear and tear on the circulatory system and improves circulation overall.

Red Blood Cells.   Massage increases the number of circulating red blood cells, thereby increasing the oxygen carrying capacity of the blood. Red blood cells stored in the liver and spleen are thought to be discharged during massage, as well as RBC in stagnant capillary beds returned to circulation (Mitchell 1894; Pemberton 1939).

Lymphatic System and Immunity

The lymphatic system is made up of a network of lymphatic vessels, a fluid called lymph, and organs (i.e., lymph nodes) that contain a large number of lymphocytes. The lymphatic system functions to return fluids from body tissues to the blood; transport hormones, nutrients, and waste products from tissues into general circulation; and defend the body from infection and disease via white blood cells or lymphocytes.

Lymph Fluid Movement.   Lymph is a viscous fluid that moves slowly through the lymphatic vessels. These vessels are, for the most part, non-contractile. Lymphatic pressure is naturally lower, and lymph fluid movement slower than venous blood flow.

The movement of lymph through the capillaries, ducts, and nodes of the lymphatic system depends on outside sources such as the contraction of muscles, action of the diaphragm, and pressure generated by filtration of fluid from the capillaries. Lack of mobility due to a sedentary lifestyle, confinement to bed or a wheelchair, pain, or paralysis seriously interferes with flow of lymph fluid. It has been known for some time that massage techniques, especially effleurage and petrissage, mechanically assist general lymphatic flow (Drinker et al., 1941; Elkins et al., 1953; Mortimer et al., 1990). Special lymphatic massage techniques have been developed to maximize the effects of moving lymph through superficial capillaries. (For more detailed information on the lymph system related to massage, read *A Primer on Lymphedema* by Deborah G. Kelly, 2002; and *Compendium of Dr. Vodder's Manual Lymph Drainage* by Renato Kasseroller, 1998). Lymphatic massage is described in more detail in Chapter 14.

Immunity.   **Immunity** is defined as "the resistance to injuries and disease caused by specific foreign chemical compounds and pathogens" (Martini & Bartholomew 1999, p. 269). It is a complex phenomenon in which the lymphatic system plays an important part.

Massage affects immunity by enhancing the immune response, which is designed to destroy or inactivate pathogens, abnormal cells, and foreign molecules such as toxins. By improving lymphatic flow as described above, massage facilitates the transport of lymphocytes that participate in the immune response. This is a direct mechanical result of massage techniques like effleurage and petrissage that help move body fluids.

Massage also appears to improve immunity through a number of other mechanisms. Recent studies show massage to be associated with increased natural killer (NK) cells and increased CD4 cells, as well as decreased anxiety and cortisol levels. High cortisol levels inflict wear and tear on the body over time by inhibiting the production and release of white blood cells, blocking T and B cell function, and interfering with the production of interleukins, which are important for communication among white cells (Ironson, 1996; Zeitlin, 2000).

Respiratory System

The respiratory system includes the lungs and the passageways leading to the lungs (i.e., nose, nasal cavity and sinuses, trachea, bronchial tubes). It acts with the circulatory system to effect an exchange of gases between the body and the environment. The respiratory system relies on the diaphragm and other skeletal muscles to produce breathing.

Massage enhances respiratory function by improving general blood circulation, and encouraging relaxed diaphragmatic breathing. Massage can also address tension and shortening in skeletal muscles involved in respiration. To the extent that massage facilitates good posture, it helps achieve the structural alignment and rib cage expansion necessary for optimal vital capacity, i.e., the amount of air moved into or out of the lungs during a single respiratory cycle.

Digestive System

The digestive system consists of a muscular tube called the digestive tract (i.e., oral cavity, pharynx, esophagus, stomach, small intestine, large intestine, rectum and anus), and accessory organs including the salivary glands, gall bladder, liver and pancreas. Functions of the digestive system include ingestion, mechanical processing and chemical breakdown of food and drink, secretion, absorption of water and nutrients, and excretion of waste products.

Massage enhances digestion through eliciting the relaxation response, in which digestive activity is increased. One of the negative effects of stress accumulated over a long period of time is disruption of the normal digestive processes, which can cause indigestion. Relaxation massage as part of a stress reduction program helps prevent digestive maladies.

Abdominal massage has been used for decades to facilitate bowel movement in people suffering from constipation. The direct mechanical effects of massage move the contents of the large intestine, and initiate reflex effects that stimulate peristaltic movement (DeDomenico & Wood, 1997). Abdominal techniques of infant massage assist bowel and gas movement and help relieve distress. Abdominal massage for adults is described in Chapter 10, and for infants in Chapter 22.

Urinary System

The structures of the urinary system include the kidneys, ureters, urinary bladder, and the urethra. The primary function of the urinary system is removal of waste products from the blood, and their excretion out of the body. It also helps regulate blood volume and pressure, as well as blood composition.

Because massage enhances function of the cardiovascular system, it indirectly affects the urinary system, which filters the blood. Better circulation to the kidneys leads to improved blood filtration overall. In addition, one of the results of activation of the parasympathetic nervous system via relaxation massage is increased urinary production and bladder tension. It is not uncommon to have to go to the bathroom after receiving a relaxing massage.

Reproductive System

The male and female reproductive organs are not appropriate targets for therapeutic massage, although they do benefit from improved general cardiovascular function, as do all body systems. There is evidence that chronic stress can impair sexual function, so to the extent massage promotes relaxation it could be said to benefit the reproductive function.

There are specialized approaches to massage for pregnant women, and some massage therapists are trained to work with midwives and health care practitioners during delivery. They often combine Western massage techniques with others such as shiatsu or, in some cases, folk healing traditions. Chapter 22 describes preganancy massage. (Refer to *Mother-Massage: A Handbook for Relieving the Discomforts of Pregnancy* by E. Stillerman, 1992.)

Women's breasts contain mammary glands and lymphatic vessels surrounded by pectoral fat pads and other connective tissues. A layer of loose connective tissue separates the mammary complex from underlying muscle. Breast massage is a specialized skill that helps promote well-breast health, and is a complementary therapy for women undergoing treatment for breast cancer. (Refer to *Breast Massage* by Debra Curties, 1999.) Breast massage requires informed consent from the client, and may be beyond the legal scope of practice for some practitioners.

Occasionally in males, increased circulation to the groin area results in erection of the penis. This does not necessarily indicate sexual arousal. With no sexual arousal, the erection will subside naturally. This is the situation in the vast majority of cases.

However, if there is sexual arousal, it is advised to stop the session immediately, state your perception, and ask the client if your perception is correct. If you still believe that there is sexual arousal regardless of what the client says, or if you are uncomfortable, inform the client that the massage is over, and leave the massage room to allow the client to get dressed. The ethical issues with the client should be dealt with outside of the immediate massage environment.

ORGANISM LEVEL

The effects of massage at the organism level include phenomena that impact the person beyond the effects on any one or two organ systems. Important phenomena affected by massage include growth and development in infants, stress reduction, pain reduction, and certain psychological effects.

Growth and Development

Touch has been found to be essential for the proper growth and development of infants and children. Holding, cuddling, rocking, stroking, and other forms of touching are all necessary for infants to thrive. There is also evidence that adequate pleasurable tactile experience in early life can influence the development of personality traits such as calmness, gentleness, and non-aggressiveness (Brown, 1984, pp. 41–120; Juhan, 1987, pp. 43–55; Montagu, 1978, pp. 76–157).

The importance of stimulation to the skin for proper growth and development cannot be overestimated. The skin develops from the same primitive cells as the brain and is a prime sensory organ. Stimulation of the tactile nerve endings in the skin provides information about the outside world and helps the brain organize its circuitry for proper development. This is also true for movement and information received through the kinesthetic sense. Thus "the use of touch and sensation to modify our experience of peripheral conditions exerts an active influence upon the organization of reflexes and body image deep within the central nervous system" (Juhan, 1987, p. 40).

As infants learn about the world around them through touch and movement, they also learn about themselves and their own bodies. Juhan expresses this idea, "by rubbing up against the world, I define myself to myself" (Juhan, 1987, p. 34).

Massage is an excellent way to provide systematic and regular touching to growing infants (see Figure 3–2). The massage of infants has been practiced widely all over the world, and has been increasing in use in the United States as more caregivers become aware of its benefits. Chapter 22 describes infant massage in more detail.

Pain Reduction

Pain is defined in Taber's as "a sensation in which a person experiences discomfort, distress, or suffering due to irritation of or stimulation of sensory nerves, esp. pain sensors" (Thomas, 1985). **Analgesia,** or pain reduction, is one of the benefits of massage that follows from its ability to elicit the relaxation response, relieve muscle tension, and improve circulation.

Massage may be used effectively to reduce pain caused by certain conditions. For example, muscle relaxation and improved local circulation can help relieve pain associated with tense muscles and the accompanying **ischemia** or lack of blood supply. Massage may also be used to help interrupt a **pain–spasm–pain cycle** induced by hypertonic or tense muscles. By relaxing the muscle and relieving the pain of the spasm, the cycle is broken and healing can take place. The use of specific techniques such as approximation as described above can be very effective for this purpose (Kresge, 1983; Rattray, 1994; Yates, 1990).

It is also thought that massage reduces pain by activating the **neural-gating mechanism** in the spinal cord through increase in sensory stimulation. The theory is that by activating fast, large nerve

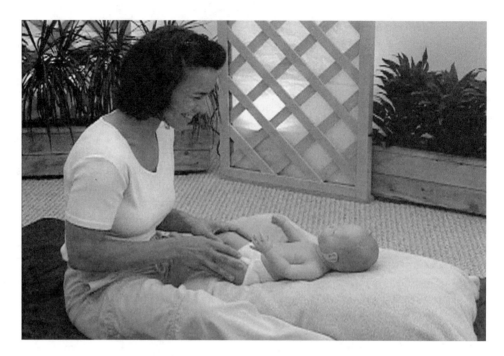

FIGURE 3–2. Massage for infants promotes growth and development.

fibers that carry tactile information, transmission from slower, smaller pain-transmitting nerve fibers is blocked. The perception of pain may be reduced for minutes or hours through the additional sensory input created by massage techniques. Activation of the neural-gating mechanism has been suggested as an explanation for the temporary analgesia associated with deep friction massage in the treatment of tendinous and ligamentous injuries (Yates, 1990).

Research by de Bruijn (1984) noted that the high degree of analgesia resulting from deep transverse friction is preceded by painful irritation of the affected tissues. De Bruijn concluded that friction massage was a promising treatment for soft tissue injuries since the eventual pain-reduction effect allowed the patient to use the affected tissue for better healing.

Myofascial trigger points (TP) are known to cause pain at the site of the TP, at satellite trigger points, and in muscles that lie within the reference zone of the TP. Massage (e.g., ischemic compression and muscle stripping) and stretching are therapies often used in deactivating trigger points (Travell & Simons, 1983, 1992). See Chapter 13 for further discussion of neuromuscular massage and the relief of trigger points.

There is also evidence that massage induces the release of neurochemicals called **endorphins** and enkephalins. These substances modulate pain-impulse transmission in the central nervous system and induce relaxation and feelings of general wellbeing. They are the body's natural painkillers. The mechanism involved in not clearly understood and may be a combination of psychological, as well as physical, reactions to massage (Yates, 1990).

Stress Reduction

Soothing massage is commonly recognized as an effective relaxation technique. It is one of several stress-management methods known to trigger the relaxation response. Other popular methods include meditation, guided imagery, progressive relaxation, abdominal breathing, hatha yoga, and biofeedback.

Back massage is especially effective for stress management, and its application for relaxation is described in more detail in Chapter 10. Several studies have confirmed the benefits of back massage for reducing stress in hospitalized patients (Bauer and Dracup 1987; Fakouri and Jones 1987; Fraser and Kerr 1993). The value of back massage for stress reduction is directly related to its ability to activate the parasympathetic nervous system, and elicit the physiological phenomenon called the **relaxation response.** Inducing the relaxation response counters the damaging effects of a chronic stress response by bringing balance to the body's systems.

Specific health benefits of the relaxation response cited by Robbins, Powers, and Burgess (1994, pp. 191–192) include:

- Decreased oxygen consumption and metabolic rate, less strain on energy resources
- Increased intensity and frequency of alpha brain waves associated with deep relaxation
- Reduced blood lactates, blood substances associated with anxiety
- Significantly decreased blood pressure in individuals with hypertension
- Reduced heart rate and slower respiration
- Decreased muscle tension
- Increased blood flow to internal organs
- Decreased anxiety, fear, and phobias, and increased positive mental health
- Improved quality of sleep

During the relaxation response, a person feels totally relaxed and is in a pleasant semi-awake state of consciousness.

Full-body massage consisting predominantly of effleurage and petrissage, with fewer specific techniques that cause discomfort, is very effective in eliciting the relaxation response. The qualities of such a session could be described as light, smooth, and flowing. The relaxing effects of this type of session may be enhanced with certain types of music, soft lighting, warm room temperatures, and minimum talking.

PSYCHOLOGICAL EFFECTS

The psychological effects of massage (i.e., on the mind and emotions) are less well understood than the physical effects, although they are related to the physical effects in many ways. The most well studied mental and emotional effects of massage include increased mental clarity, reduced anxiety, and feelings of general wellbeing. A phenomenon called *emotional release*, which is an interesting interface of body, mind, and emotions, may also occur during massage.

Mental Clarity

Two studies performed at the Touch Research Institute in Miami suggest that massage helps improve **mental clarity,** i.e., sharpening cognitive skills like solving problems, remembering information, or paying focused attention. In one study, 15-minute massage sessions were given to hospital personnel over a five-week period during their lunch hour. People reported feeling more relaxed, in better moods, and more alert after receiving massage. Similarly, students who received massage during finals week reported being more relaxed and less anxious and said that they remembered information better after an 8-minute massage session (Field 2000).

In a job stress study conducted in 1993, subjects received a 20-minute massage in a chair twice weekly for a month (see Figure 3–3). They reported less fatigue and demonstrated greater clarity of thought, improved cognitive skills, and lower anxiety levels. EEG, alpha, beta, and theta waves were also altered in ways consistent with enhanced alertness (Field, Fox, Pickens, Ironsong, & Scafidi, 1993).

Massage is used with athletes in pre-event situations to help spark the alertness necessary for competition. For pre-event readiness, sports massage sessions are 15–20 minutes in duration, have an upbeat tempo, and use techniques to increase circulation and joint mobility. Tapotement is frequently employed for stimulation (Benjamin & Lamp, 1996, pp. 67–68).

In each of the cases mentioned above, the massage sessions were relatively short—between 8 and 20 minutes. Increased mental alertness is most likely related to sensory stimulation and enhanced circulation to the brain. Improved mental clarity may also be the result of a calmer mind.

Reduced Anxiety

A consistent finding of research on massage is that it **reduces anxiety** significantly. This is true for the general public as well as for those with chronic diseases, and those hospitalized for different reasons. Anxiety is measured through subjective self-reporting instruments, as well as the more objective measure of cortisol levels in saliva and urine. Anxiety reduction would be an expected result of the relaxation response and action of the parasympathetic nervous system. It may also be related to the release of endorphins (Field 2000; Kaard & Tostinbo 1989; Rich 2002).

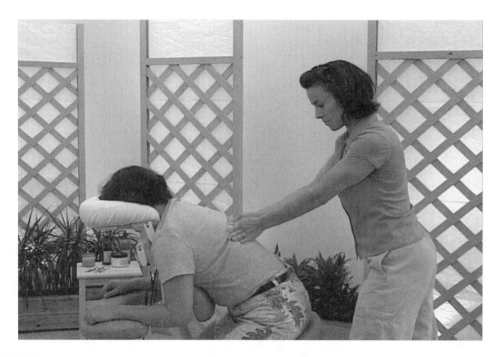

FIGURE 3–3. Seated massage increases mental clarity and alertness.

Emotional Release

A phenomenon called **emotional release** sometimes occurs during a massage session. Unexpressed emotions that are held in the receiver's body may come to the surface in various forms such as being tearful, feeling anger, fear, or grief. Although emotional release is a phenomenon familiar to many massage practitioners, relatively little is known about the mechanisms involved. It is possible that during deep relaxation, a person's natural psychological defenses are lowered, allowing them to feel or express emotions held inside.

Some forms of massage and bodywork specifically address the emotions, and practitioners are trained to deal with issues brought up during emotional release. Releasing unexpressed emotions can be an important step in a physical or psychological healing process. (Refer to *Where Healing Waters Meet: Touching Mind & Emotion Through the Body* (1989) and *Compassionate Touch: The Role of Human Touch in Healing and Recovery* (1993) by Clyde Ford, D.C.)

Massage practitioners should be considerate of their clients during an emotional release, and be good listeners, but be mindful of their own scope of practice. Clients should be referred to other health professionals as needed to resolve deep emotional problems.

Feelings of General Wellbeing

Stated in positive terms, massage is shown to increase feelings of general wellbeing. This likely involves the same mechanisms as anxiety reduction, that is, relaxation response and release of endorphins. Tactile pleasure associated with relaxation massage and simple caring touch may also contribute to feelings of wellbeing.

It is interesting to note that prolonged exposure to pain and other stressors has been shown to deplete the stores of endorphins, leading to an increased perception of pain and despair. To the extent that massage helps to manage pain and stress, and to release endorphins, it may contribute to a more positive outlook.

MECHANISMS OF MASSAGE

Several mechanisms have been identified to explain how the effects of massage are produced. Some of these theories are recognized within the Western biomedical model, while others are on the cutting edge of alternative and body–mind studies. The mechanisms presented here include mechanical, physiological, reflex, body–mind, and energetic. Table 3–2 outlines the mechanisms used to explain the effects of massage.

Table 3–2 MECHANISMS TO EXPLAIN THE EFFECTS OF MASSAGE

Mechanical Effects	The result of physical forces such as compression, stretching, shearing, broadening, and vibration of tissues. Occurs on the gross level of physical structure. *Examples:* venous return, lymph flow, breaking adhesions
Physiological Effects	Organic processes of the body on cellular, tissue, or organ system levels. *Examples:* activation of parasympathetic nervous system; release of endorphins
Reflex Effects	The result of pressure or movement in one part of the body having an effect in another part; or effects mediated through the nervous system. *Examples:* muscle relaxation, increased mental clarity, pain reduction, normalizing system function
Mind–Body Effects	The result of the interplay of body, mind, and emotions in health and disease processes. *Examples:* relaxation response, anxiety reduction
Energetic Effects	The result of balancing or improving the flow of energy within and around the body. *Examples:* Therapeutic Touch, Polarity Therapy, Asian Bodywork Therapy

Some effects are produced by more than one mechanism. For example, changes in local blood circulation during and after massage are thought to occur through direct physical and mechanical effects on vessels; circulatory changes mediated by the local release of vasodilator chemicals (e.g., histamine); or circulatory changes elicited by reflex responses of the autonomic nervous system to tissue stimulation. (Yates 1990).

Furthermore, a specific massage technique may produce a number of different effects. This is a further example of the holistic nature of human beings, and the complexity of effects produced by something seemingly simple like massage.

Mechanical Effects

Mechanical effects are the result of physical forces such as compression, stretching, shearing, broadening, and vibration of body tissues. These effects occur on the more gross level of physical structure. Examples of mechanical effects include enhanced venous return from deep effleurage; elongation of muscles by stretching; increased lymph flow from kneading and deep effleurage; and breaking tissue adhesions with deep transverse friction or myofascial massage.

Physiological Effects

Physiological effects refer to organic processes of the body. These effects involve biochemical processes at the cellular level, but may also occur at the tissue and organ system levels. Examples of physiologic effects include the various results of the relaxation response produced by activating the parasympathetic nervous system; decrease in anxiety by facilitating the release of endorphins; and proper development and growth in infants assisted by the tactile stimulation that occurs during massage.

Reflex Effects

Andrade and Clifford (2001) explain **reflex effects** as functional change mediated by the nervous system (p. 12). Sensory receptors in the skin and proprioceptors in muscles are stimulated by massage and joint movements, thereby eliciting reflex effects. Some examples of reflex effects are muscle relaxation, enhanced mental clarity, and pain reduction.

A different type of reflex effect forms the theoretical basis for a type of bodywork called *reflexology*. In this largely unexplained phenomenon, pressing or massaging one part of the body (e.g., ears, hands, or feet) is believed to have a normalizing effect on an entirely different part of the body. It is not clear if the apparent effects occur through the nervous system or some other mechanism. Chapter 15 explains more about reflexology.

Body–Mind Effects

Body–mind effects acknowledge the interplay of body, mind, and emotions in health and disease. This concept has a long tradition in natural healing, in most native cultures, and in healing traditions of China and India. Western medical science is beginning to confirm demonstrable links between our physical bodies and our mental and emotional states. The new science of psychoneuro-immunology has grown out of these studies.

The body–mind connection can be easily seen in the relaxation response, a physiological process involving the parasympathetic nervous system. The relaxation response is elicited by practices such as meditation, which quiets the mind, or by the tactile stimulation of massage. Other examples of body–mind effects of massage include reduction in anxiety and release of unexpressed emotions held in the body. The discussion of body–mind effects is continued below.

Energetic Effects

Massage and bodywork have been described as balancing, or improving the flow, of energy. What this energy is, and how it relates to the body, are yet to be determined in terms of Western science. However, there are ancient traditions of massage and bodywork, primarily from China and India, based on concepts of energy flow. Therapeutic Touch is a form of energy work adopted by many nurses that addresses the energy field of the recipient. Other popular forms of energy bodywork include polarity therapy and reiki (Claire, 1995).

There are many theories about how energy flows in and around the body, and many practitioners and receivers alike report "feeling" energy. Energy work is currently outside of the understanding and general acceptance of Western biomedicine, but it has persisted over time and is found to be useful by many people.

A HOLISTIC VIEW

Theoretically dividing the human organism into body, mind, and emotions is a useful exercise for discussing the effects of massage. Perhaps it is a product of Western thought and science to think of human beings as divided in this way. However, it should always be remembered that we live as whole or **holistic** persons, and that these effects interact with each other in complex ways to produce an overall effect that may be greater than the sum of its parts. Western medicine is just beginning to explore the holistic nature of human beings.

The Indivisible Body and Mind

The body and mind function as a single unit, i.e., in a holistic way. For example, emotions are felt in and expressed through the body. Love is felt deeply in the physical self, as is hate. Facial expressions are a window to our emotions. Mental and physical pain can be indistinguishable.

Physical manifestations of emotions include the blush of embarrassment, sweaty palms in nervousness, the clenched fist of anger, wide-eyed fear, and the quickened heartbeat of those in love. Some believe that body posture may be read for its emotional sources. For example, raised shoulders indicating fear; rounded shoulders carrying the weight of the world; or forward, hunched shoulders for self-protection and fear of being hurt (Dychtwald, 1977).

The connectedness of body and mind can be traced to our beginnings as an embryo. In the third week of life, there are three layers of cells. The outer layer, or ectoderm, eventually develops into the skin, brain, and nervous system. Thus the physical structures that allow us to feel physical sensations are from the same source as those through which we experience emotions. Juhan observes that "depending on how you look at it, the skin is the outer surface of the brain, or the brain is the deepest layer of the skin" (Juhan, 1987, p. 35).

This connection between the skin and the nervous system has profound implications when studying the effects of massage on the mind and emotions. In touching the outermost part of the physical body, we are able to touch the innermost parts of our patients and clients.

Research on touch has borne out this connection. For example, babies deprived of touch fail to develop properly and suffer retarded bone growth, failure to gain weight, poor muscular coordination, immunological weakness, and general apathy (Montagu, 1978). Massage, as a form of structured touch, has been used successfully to help premature infants gain weight and thrive (Field 2000).

Limbic System

The concept of the **limbic system** helps shed light on how the physical and emotional components of a person are related and how body memories are created. From a physiological perspective, the lymbic system is defined as follows:

> Limbic system—a group of structures within the rhinencephalon of the brain that are associated with various emotions and feelings such as anger, fear, sexual arousal, pleasure and sadness. The structures of the limbic system are the cingulate gyrus, the isthmus, the hippocampal gyrus, the uncus, and the hippocampus. The structures connect with various other parts of the brain (Anderson & Anderson, 1990).

Memory researchers have been able to trace the flow of information from touch receptors in the skin through the spinal cord and brain stem into different parts of the brain. This activates the limbic system to experience emotions related to the touch and to create memories or images of tactile experiences (Knaster, 1996, pp. 123–124).

There is the possibility, therefore, that memories are activated, as well as created, by touch. This has a variety of important implications for practitioners. For example, if the recipient of massage has experienced caring touch primarily in a sexual context, the touch of the practitioner might bring up feelings and memories that would be confusing and inappropriate during a session. Or a recipient who has been physically or sexually abused may have difficulty accepting healing touch without hardening against it. Touch may similarly be used to help in the healing and recovery process.

Character Armor

Wilhelm Reich (1897–1957) introduced the concept of **character armor,** or muscular tension caused by suppression of emotions. For example, unexpressed anger often causes tension in the muscles of the back and arms that would have been used to strike out. Or unexpressed grief may result in shallow breathing and stiffening of muscles used in crying. In the process of relaxing the affected muscles, the suppressed emotions may be felt by the recipient. Massage practitioners sometimes encounter such armoring and should be prepared to help the patient or client understand the release of emotions that sometimes happens.

The above discussion merely touches lightly on the complexity of the body, mind, and emotion relationship. Many of the concepts are in the theoretical stages of development. Research into the holistic nature of human beings is continuing to confirm and clarify ideas that have been little understood before in the context of Western medicine. In her book *Discovering the Body's Wisdom*, Mirka Knaster explores these ideas in more detail and offers a comprehensive introduction to the subject (1996).

Body-Centered Therapy

Massage has been called a **body-centered therapy,** since it works primarily through touch and movement of the body to enhance the overall wellbeing of the recipient. This concept includes the energetic aspect of the person as well, as, for example, in polarity therapy and Asian forms of bodywork.

Explained in Western scientific terms, massage produces effects on the parasympathetic nervous system, releases endorphins, stimulates sensory receptors, relaxes muscles, or gives pleasure. Any of these effects may, in turn, enhance the mental and emotional wellbeing of the recipient.

Practitioners experience the interconnectedness of human beings in many ways. For example, a practitioner may be focused on some physical aspect such as relaxing hypertonic muscles, and the recipient's experience might also have an emotional component such as painful memories of an accident that caused trauma to the area. A psychotherapist may witness the physical effects of stress, such as tension headaches, in their clients. Awareness of how the body, mind, and emotions interact will enable practitioners to better serve their clients.

BENEFITS OF MASSAGE FOR EVERYONE

When the effects of massage support general health and wellbeing or the ongoing healing process, there are **benefits** by definition. A general wellness or health massage aims to normalize body tissues and to optimize function. Everyone can benefit from the health-promoting effects of wellness massage.

The main intention in a general **wellness massage** is to elicit the relaxation response, promote muscular relaxation, and to enhance circulation of fluids, digestion, and elimination. The effects of general relaxation alone have an impact on many physiological and psychological aspects of health and wellbeing. Massage also provides healthy touch, which is a basic human need.

BENEFITS FOR SPECIAL POPULATIONS

The effects of massage may be especially beneficial for people with special needs. These benefits are the natural effects of a wellness massage tailored for a unique individual. For example, pregnant women who tend to have back and leg strain may find special benefit in the effects of massage related to muscle relaxation and improved circulation. Infants benefit from the extra tactile stimulation provided by regular massage for their normal growth and development. Chapter 22 discusses massage for mother and child. The elderly may find massage beneficial for mitigating the normal effects of the aging process and providing healthy caring touch (see Figure 3–4). Massage for healthy aging is discussed in Chapter 23.

Some practitioners are going to workplaces and providing wellness massage for people who sit at desks or similar workstations all day. Massage chairs are commonly used in this environment. The special chairs offer a convenient delivery model and give access to the upper body, which is stressed in office workers. Workplace wellness massage is described more fully in Chapter 25.

For centuries, athletes have benefited from massage as part of their training regimen. The intent of sports massage is to help athletes stay in top condition during strenuous training, prepare for competition, recover after competition, and recover from injury. See Chapter 21 for more information about sports massage.

People going through stressful life situations may benefit from the relaxing effects of massage. Massage may be used in psychotherapy treatment to help reduce anxiety as emotional issues are dealt with. Massage for mental and emotional wellness is also described in Chapter 4.

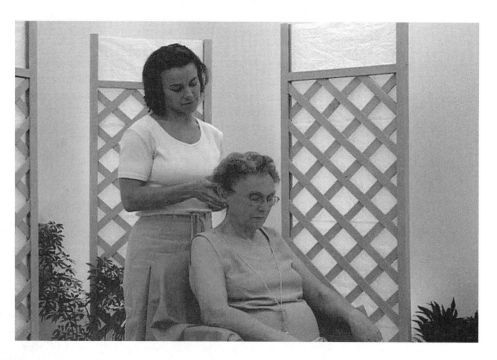

FIGURE 3–4. Massage promotes healthy aging.

People with life-threatening illnesses, those in hospices, and their caregivers may benefit from the psychological benefits of massage. Even those for whom treatment of a condition is not an option may improve the quality of their lives with massage, as explained in Chapter 24.

SUMMARY

Effects of massage refer to changes that occur in the body, mind, and emotions of the recipient during a massage session. Practitioners who know how to apply massage techniques to obtain specific results will be more successful in achieving session or treatment goals.

Massage improves the overall health of cells and tissues of the body. It assists the tissue repair process, especially in the regeneration and remodeling phases. Massage is contraindicated in the inflammation phase of tissue repair. To the extent that massage lowers stress it may help wounds heal faster.

Massage causes connective tissues to become more fluid and pliable, and prevents some connective tissue abnormalities and dysfunction. Certain massage techniques can "unstick" adhering fascial tissues.

Massage improves the overall functions of organ systems. Oil applied during massage moisturizes the skin, and massage stimulates sensory receptors, as well as exocrine glands. Cross-fiber massage techniques assist in healthy scar formation.

Massage promotes good joint mobility and flexibility, and proper alignment of the skeletal system. By improving local circulation, massage alleviates some of the negative effects of under-activity and over-activity of the muscular system. It can reduce muscle stiffness and soreness after strenuous activity, and relax hypertonic or tense muscles. Massage works through the nervous system to increase body awareness, relax muscles, and reduce pain.

Massage improves the function of the circulatory and lymphatic systems by helping to move fluids through the systems. It produces hyperemia locally, and increases blood volume in an area. Mechanical action of deep effleurage enhances venous flow in the limbs, and so deep stroking should always be towards the heart to prevent damage to valves in the veins. Massage can also play a part in decreasing blood pressure, and increasing the number of circulating red blood cells. Massage assists in movement of lymph fluid through the lymphatic system, and enhances immunity.

Massage improves respiratory system function by enhancing general circulation, relaxing muscles of respiration, and encouraging deep diaphragmatic breathing. Relaxation massage improves digestive system function, and abdominal massage is used to treat constipation.

Massage can address the needs of pregnant women, and breast massage is a specialty used for well-breast health and as complementary treatment for breast cancer. Men can experience non-sexual erection of the penis during massage due to increased circulation in the groin area.

On the organism level, massage enhances growth and development of infants. It has pain reduction effects, and can elicit the relaxation response. Psychological effects of massage include increased mental clarity, reduced anxiety, emotional release, and increased feelings of general wellbeing. Mechanisms through which the effects of massage are produced include mechanical, physiological, reflex, body-mind, and energetic.

The connection of body, mind, and emotions has profound implications when studying the effects of massage. In touching the outermost part of the physical body we are able to touch the innermost parts of our patients and clients. Massage is called a body-centered therapy, since it works primarily through touch and movement to create its effects.

Everyone can benefit from the general health promoting effects of massage. Special populations also benefit from massage planned to address their special needs.

A look ahead . . .

Practitioners in several health professions use massage and related bodywork approaches to treat specific medical conditions. Chapter 4 looks at the clinical applications of massage, and some of the research that supports its use in treatment.

REFERENCES

Anderson, K. N. & Anderson, L. E. (1990). *Mosby's pocket dictionary of medicine, nursing & allied health*. St. Louis: C.V. Mosby Company.

Andrade, C., & P. Clifford. (2001) *Outcomes-based massage*. Philadelphia: Lippincott Williams & Wilkins.

Barr, J. S., & N. Taslitz. (1970) Influence of back massage on autonomic functions. *Physical Therapy*, 50.

Bauer, W. C., & Dracup, K. A. (1987). Physiological effects of back massage in patients with acute myocardial infarction. *Focus on Critical Care, 14*(6), 42–46.

Bell, A. J. (1964). Massage and the physiotherapist. *Physiotherapy, 50*, 406–408.

Benjamin, P. J., & Lamp, S. P. (1996). *Understanding sports massage*. Champaign, IL: Human Kinetics.

Brown, C. C., ed. (1984). *The many facets of touch*. Johnson & Johnson Baby Products Company.

de Bruijn, R. (1984). Deep transverse friction: Its analgesic effect. *International Journal of Sports Medicine, 5*(suppl.), 35–36.

Cady, S. H., and G. E. Jones. (1997) Massage therapy as a workplace intervention for reduction of stress. *Perceptual and Motor Skills, 84*(1), 157–158.

Claire, T. (1995). *Bodywork: What type of massage to get, and how to make the most of it*. New York: William Morrow.

Crosman, L. J., Chateauvert, S. R., & Weisburg, J. (1985). The effects of massage to the hamstring muscle group on range of motion. *Massage Journal*, 59–62.

Curties, D. (1999). Breast massage. Toronto: Curties-Overzet Publications.

Cyriax, J. H., & Cyriax, P. J. (1993). *Illustrated manual of orthopedic medicine*, 2nd ed. Boston: Butterworth & Heinemann.

DeDomenico, G., & Wood, E.C. (1997) *Beard's Massage*, 4th ed. Philadelphia: W.B. Saunders.

Drinker, C. K., & Yoffey, J. M. (1941). *Lymphatics, lymph and lymphoid tissue: Their physiological and clinical significance*. Cambridge: Harvard University Press.

Dychtwald, K. (1977). *Body-mind*. New York: Jove Publications.

Elkins, E. C., Herrick, J. F., Grindlay, J. H., et al. (1953). Effects of various procedures on the flow of lymph. *Archives of Physical Medicine, 34*, 31.

Fakouri, C., & Jones, P. (1987). Relaxation ℞: Slow stroke back rub. *Journal of Gerontological Nursing, 13*(2), 32–35.

Field, T. (2000). *Touch therapy*. London: Churchill Livingstone.

Field, T. M., Fox, N., Pickens, J., Ironsong, G., & Scafidi, F. (1993). Job stress survey. Unpublished manuscript. Touch Research Institute, University of Miami School of Medicine. Reported in *Touchpoints: Touch Research Abstracts, 1*(1).

Ford, C. W. (1989). *Where healing waters meet: Touching mind & emotion through the body*. Barrytown, NY: Station Hill Press.

Ford, C. W. (1993). *Compassionate touch: The role of human touch in healing and recovery*. New York: A Fireside/Parkside book.

Fraser, J., & Kerr, J. R. (1993). Psychophysiological effects of back massage on elderly institutionalized patients. *Journal of Advanced Nursing, 18*, 238–245.

Greene, E. (1996). Study links stress reduction with faster healing. *Massage Therapy Journal, 35*(1), 16.

Ironson, G., Field, T. et al. (1996). Massage therapy is associated with enhancement of the immune system's cytotoxic capacity. *International Journal of Neuroscience, 84*: 205–217.

Juhan, D. (1987). *Job's body: A handbook for bodywork*. Barrytown, NY: Station Hill Press.

Kaard, B., & Tostinbo, O. (1989). Increase of plasma beta endorphins in a connective tissue massage. *General Pharmacology, 20*(4), 487–489.

Kasseroller, R. (1998). *Compendium of Dr. Vodder's Manual Lymph Drainage*. Heidelberg: Karl F. Haug Verlag.

Kelly, D. G. (2002) *A primer on lymphedema*. Upper Saddle River, NJ: Prentice Hall.

Knaster, M. (1996). *Discovering the body's wisdom*. New York: Bantam.

Kresge, C. A. (1983). Massage and sports. In O. Appenzeller & R. Atkinson (eds.), *Sports medicine: Fitness, training, injuries* (pp. 367–380). Baltimore: Urban & Schwarzenberg.

MacKenzie, J. (1923) *Angina pectoris*. London: Henry Frowde and Hodder and Stoughton.

Martini, F. H. & Bartholomew, M. S. (1999). *Structure & Function of the Human Body*. Upper Saddle River, N.J.: Prentice-Hall.

Mitchell, J. K. (1894). The effect of massage on the number and haemoglobin value of the red blood cells. *American Journal of Medical Science, 107*, pp. 502–515.

Montageu, A. (1978). *Touching: The human significance of the skin*, 2nd ed. New York: Harper & Row.

Mortimer, P. S., Simmonds, R., Rezvani, M., et al. (1990). The measurement of skin lymph flow by isotope clearance: Reliability, reproducibility, injection dynamics, and the effects of massage. *Journal of Investigative Dermatology, 95*, 666–682.

Pemberton, R. (1939). Physiology of Massage. In *American Medical Association Handbook of Physical Therapy*, 3rd ed. Chicago: Council of Physical Therapy.

Rattray, F. S. (1994). *Massage therapy: An approach to treatments*. Toronto, Ontario: Massage Therapy Texts and MA Verick Consultants.

Rttray, F., & L. Ludwig (2000). *Clinical massage therapy: Understanding, assessing and treating over 700 conditions.* Toronto, Canada: Talus Incorporated.

Rich, G. J. (2002) *Massage therapy: The evidence for practice.* New York: Mosby.

Robbins, G., Powers, D., & Burgess, S. (1994). *A wellness way of life,* 2nd ed. Madison, WI: Brown & Benchmark.

Schultz, R. L., & R. Feitis (1996). *The endless web: Fascial anatomy and physical reality.* Berkeley, CA: North Atlantic Books.

Stillerman. E. (1992). *Mother-Massage.* New York: Delta/Delcorte.

Thomas, C. L. (ed.) (1985). *Taber's cyclopedic medical dictionary.* Philadelphia: F. A. Davis.

Travell, J. G., & Simons, D. G. (1983). *Myofascial pain and dysfunction: The trigger point manual.* Baltimore: Williams & Wilkins.

Travell, J. G., & Simons, D. G. (1992). *Myofascial pain and dysfunction: The lower extremities.* Vol. 2. Baltimore: Williams & Wilkins.

Wood, E. C., & Becker, P. D. (1981). *Beard's massage,* 3rd ed. Philadelphia: W. B. Saunders.

Yates, J. (1990). *A physician's guide to therapeutic massage: Its physiologic effects and their application to treatment.* Massage Therapists Association of British Columbia, Vancouver, BC, Canada.

Zeitlin, D., et al. (2000). Immunological effects of massage therapy during academic stress. *Psychosomatic Medicine, 62,* 83–87.

ADDITIONAL REFERENCES

Videos

"Anatomy and Pathology for Bodyworkers." Santa Barbara, CA: Real Bodywork. (*www.deeptissue.com*)

STUDY GUIDE

LEARNING OUTCOMES

Use the learning outcomes at the beginning of the chapter as a guide to your studies. Perform the task given in each outcome, either in writing or verbally into a tape recorder or to a study partner. This may start as an "open book" exercise, and then later from memory.

KEY TERMS/CONCEPTS

To study key words and concepts listed at the beginning of this chapter, choose one or more of the following exercises. Writing or talking about ideas helps you remember them better, and explaining helps deepen your understanding.

1. Write a one- or two-sentence explanation of each key word and concept.
2. Make study cards by writing the explanation from problem 1 on one side of a 3 × 5 card, and the key word or concept on the other. Shuffle the cards and read one side, trying to recite either the explanation or word on the other side.
3. Pick out two or three key words or concepts and explain how they are related.
4. With a study partner, take turns explaining key words and concepts verbally.
5. Make up sentences using one or more key words or concepts.
6. Read your sentences from problem 5 to a study partner, who will ask you to clarify your meaning.

STUDY OUTLINE

The following questions test your memory of the main concepts in this chapter. Locate the answers in the text using the page number given for each question.

Effects of Massage

1. Changes in the body, mind, and emotions of the recipient as a result of soft tissue manipulation and related techniques are called _____. (p. 42)

2. Practitioners who know how to apply massage techniques to obtain specific effects will be more successful in achieving _____. (p. 42)

Tissue Level Effects

1. Massage promotes the overall health of tissues, primarily through increased blood and lymph _____. (p. 42)

2. Massage is _____ during the inflammation phase of tissue repair. (p. 44)

3. During the regeneration phase of tissue repair, massage removes _____, and transports _____ to the affected area. (p. 44)

4. During the remodeling phase of tissue repair, massage helps in healthy _____ formation. (p. 44)

5. A study showed that wounds heal more slowly in people suffering from _____. (p. 44)

6. The property of connective tissue whereby it become more pliable when it is mobile is called _____. (p. 44)

7. The type of connective tissue that surrounds all muscles, bones, and organs, and gives them their shape is called _____. (p. 44)

8. When fascial tissues stick together, _____ _____ are formed. (p. 44)

Organ System Level Effects

Integumentary System

1. Benefits of stimulating the sensory receptors in the skin with massage include _____ _____. (p. 45)

2. Friction that occurs with massage helps keep _____ free from blockage. (p. 45)

3. Oil and lotion applied with massage _____ _____ the skin. (p. 45)

Skeletal System

1. Movement of the joints stimulates production of _____. (p. 45)

2. Optimal range of motion is achieved when the bones are in _____. and the tissues surrounding the joints are _____. (p. 45)

Muscular System

1. Muscular *under-activity* caused by illness or injury results in _____ _____. (p. 46)

2. Massage techniques that simulate _____ _____ can alleviate negative effects of muscular *under-activity*. (p. 46)

3. Muscular *over-activity* such as from strenuous exercise can cause _____ _____. (p. 46)

4. Massage techniques that increase blood flow, for example _____ and _____, can alleviate negative effects of *over-activity*. (p. 46)

5. General muscle relaxation may be elicited by massage through activation of the _____ nervous system, by conscious release of _____, or by increased sensory _____. (p. 46)

6. Muscles that are tense and in a state of partial contraction are said to be _____. (p. 46)

7. The muscle relaxation technique in which the practitioner slowly and forcibly draws the muscle attachments together is called _____. (p. 47)

8. The muscle relaxation technique in which cross-fiber and with-fiber friction is performed on the attachments of the targeted muscle is called _____. (p. 47)

9. Movement at joints is restricted by _____ _____ _____. (p. 47)

10. Proper body alignment is commonly called _____. (p. 47)

11. Massage and joint movements can improve posture by _____ and _____ shortened muscles, lengthening muscle groups with _____, and unsticking fascial _____ that are contributing to posture distortion. (p. 47)

Nervous and Endocrine Systems

1. An example of a massage and joint movement technique that utilizes the nervous system to effect desired results is _____. (p. 48)

2. The _____ occurs with activation of the parasympathetic nervous system, which has ef-

fects on skeletal muscles as well as several other organ systems. (p. 48)

Cardiovascular System

1. Superficial friction massage can cause release of a chemical called _____. that leads to capillary vessel dilation and _____ _____ in skin and underlying connective tissue. (p. 48)

2. Increase in the amount of blood in an area is referred to as _____. (p. 48)

3. A condition in which normal blood flow in the veins is slowed or halted is called _____. (p. 49)

4. Venous return is facilitated by the mechanical action of these massage techniques: _____ _____. (pp. 48–49)

5. The dictum in classic Western massage that deep effleurage should always be _____ reflects the thought that valves in the larger veins would be damaged if blood flow were forced backwards against them. (p. 49)

6. Blood pressure may be temporarily decreased during massage. This is thought to be the result of _____. (p. 49)

7. The number of circulating red blood cells may be (choose one: increased or decreased) with massage. (p. 49)

Lymphatic System and Immunity

1. Movement of lymph through the lymph vessel system depends on outside sources such as _____ _____. (p. 49)

2. Resistance to injuries and disease caused by foreign substances is called _____. (p. 49)

3. Massage improves immunity through these effects: _____ _____. (pp. 49–50)

Respiratory System

1. Respiratory system function is enhanced by massage through improved _____ to the lungs, encouraging deep _____ breathing, and relieving tension and shortening in _____ involved in respiration. (p. 50)

2. By facilitating good posture, massage and bodywork helps clients achieve the _____ and _____ needed for optimal vital capacity. (p. 50)

Digestive System

1. Activation of the parasympathetic nervous system in relaxation massage (choose one: increases or decreases) digestive activity. (p. 50)

2. The stimulation of bowel movement through abdominal massage is useful for normal digestion function as well as treatment for _____. (p. 50)

3. Bowel movements stimulated through massage are the result of direct _____ effects, as well as reflex stimulation of _____ movement of the large intestine. (p. 50)

Urinary System

1. The kidney function enhanced by increased circulation is _____ of the blood. (p. 50)

2. Parasympathetic nervous system activation (choose one: increases or decreases) urinary output and bladder tension. (p. 50)

Reproductive System

1. Male and female genitals are not _____ _____ for therapeutic massage. (p. 50)

2. There is evidence that chronic stress (choose one: improves or impairs) sexual function. (p. 50)

3. Breast massage is a specialized skill that promotes well-breast health. Breast massage requires _____ _____ from the client, and may be beyond the _____ of some practitioners. (pp. 50–51)

Organism Level Effects

1. Stimulation of the _____ in the skin and muscle tissue is essential for proper growth and development of infants. (p. 51)

2. Lack of blood supply to an area is called _____. (p. 51)

3. Massage can provide increased sensory input that blocks slower pain-transmitting nerve impulses. This is called the _____ mechanism. (p. 51)

4. Myofascial trigger points can be deactivated by massage techniques such as _____ _____ and _____. (p. 52)

5. Pain may also be modulated by the release of neuro-chemicals called _____ and _____

_____ that induce relaxation and feelings of wellbeing. (p. 52)

6. Relaxation massage is known to elicit the _____ Response by activating the parasympathetic nervous system. (p. 52)

7. Psychological effects of massage include improved mental _____, _____ anxiety, emotional _____, and increased feeling of wellbeing. (p. 53)

Mechanisms of Massage

1. Effects of massage that are the result of physical forces such as compression, stretching, and vibration of body tissues are called _____ effects. (p. 55)

2. Functional changes mediated by the _____ system are called reflex effects. (p. 55)

3. Effects of massage involving organic processes at the cellular, tissue and organ system level are called _____ effects. (p. 55)

4. Body-mind effects acknowledge the interplay of _____, _____, and _____ in health and disease. (p. 56)

5. Theories of energy effects of bodywork are currently outside of purview of _____; however, they have persisted over time and have been found useful by many people. (p. 56)

A Holistic View

1. A _____ view of massage appreciates that we live as whole beings, and the separate effects of massage interact in complex ways to produce an overall effect that may be greater than the sum of its parts. (p. 56)

2. The connection of mind and body can be traced to our beginnings as embryos, when the outer layer of cells or ectoderm eventually develops into the _____, _____ and _____ system. (p. 56)

3. Research on infant massage demonstrates the need for touch for proper _____ and _____. (p. 57)

4. The limbic system is group of structures in the brain related to the experience of _____, and in the formation of _____ memories. (p. 57)

5. Character _____ is a concept used to explain muscular tension caused by suppressed emotions. (p. 57)

6. Massage is considered a _____ therapy since it works primarily through touch and movement of the body to produce holistic effects in the recipient. (p. 57)

Benefits for Everyone

1. Effects of massage that support general health and well-being are _____ by definition. (p. 58)

2. Massage provides health touch, which is a basic _____. (p. 58)

Benefits for Special Populations

1. People with special needs that can benefit from massage include _____ _____. (p. 58)

2. Even if massage is not an appropriate _____ _____ for a certain medical condition, it may provide other health _____ that improve the lives of those living with the condition. This is the essence of the wellness perspective. (p. 59)

FOR GREATER UNDERSTANDING

The following exercises are designed to take you from the realm of theory into the real world. They will help give you a deeper understanding of the subjects covered in this chapter. Action words are underlined to emphasize the variety of activities presented to address different learning styles, and to encourage deeper thinking.

1. Write a brief personal health history for the past 1 or 2 years. Using the information in this chapter, identify any areas that might have benefited (or did benefit) from receiving massage. Discuss your conclusions with a study partner or group.

2. Interview a family member or friend, and complete problem 1 for their case.

3. Choose a special population to study. List their special needs that result from their unique situation. If possible, interview someone from that population. Using the information in this chapter, identify any areas that might have benefited (or did benefit) from receiving massage.

4. For the special population studied in problem 3, identify a nonprofit organization that offers support. Read

their brochures or check out their Web sites for information on their mission and services. Do they recommend massage as being beneficial for the population? Write a letter to the organization providing evidence of the benefits of massage for the population and encouraging their recommendation. The letter may actually be sent or just written as a learning exercise.

5. Choose one particular effect of massage to study in more depth. Search several sources for further information including anatomy and physiology textbooks, and the AMTA Foundation research database. Discuss your findings with a study partner or group.

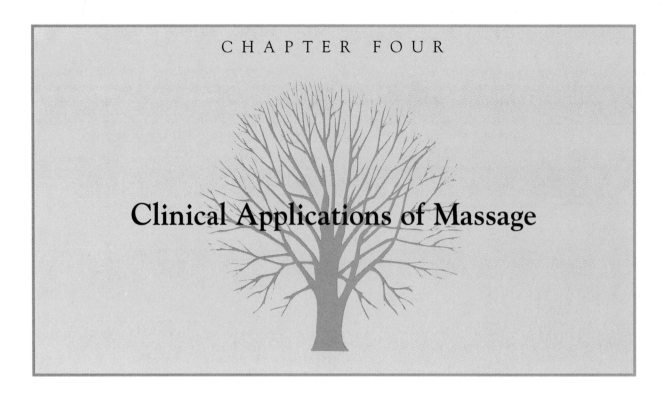

CHAPTER FOUR

Clinical Applications of Massage

LEARNING OUTCOMES

After studying this chapter, the student will have information to:

1. Define clinical massage therapy.
2. Locate research about clinical massage therapy.
3. Explain Yates' principle-based theory of massage treatment.
4. Discuss three major clinical approaches to massage.
5. Describe the benefits of massage in treating specific pathologies.
6. Discuss the benefits of massage for hospitalized patients.
7. Discuss the benefits of massage for cancer patients.
8. Explain how massage improves development of preterm infants.
9. List applications of massage in pediatric care.
10. Explain how massage benefits people with conditions worsened by stress.
11. Discuss the benefits of massage for people with psychiatric disorders.
12. Describe therapeutic touch and its potential as a clinical approach.
13. Explain how massage is used to complement chiropractic care.

KEY TERMS/CONCEPTS

Clinical massage therapy	Evidence-based	Palliative care
Complementary	Indicated	Principle-based therapy
Contraindicated	Integrated health care	Research literacy
Direct therapeutic effects		

 MEDIALINK

A companion CD-ROM, included free with each new copy of this book, supplements the techniques presented in this chapter. Insert the CD-ROM to watch video clips of massage techniques being demonstrated. This multimedia feature is designed to help you add a new dimension to your learning.

CLINICAL MASSAGE THERAPY

Massage has been used to treat human ailments since ancient times, and is currently being integrated into a number of medical settings as a complementary therapy. The term **clinical massage therapy** describes applications of massage for the treatment of pathologies. The growing interest in massage for treatment has led to an increase in research studies about its efficacy.

Two centers for the study of touch therapies have been established: the Touch Research Institute (TRI) at the University of Miami School of Medicine in Florida, and the Canadian Touch Research Center in Montreal. In addition, the AMTA Foundation research database lists thousands of studies about the benefits of massage and its clinical uses. The National Library of Medicine search service called PubMed offers access to studies about massage reported in over 4,000 health-related journals. Table 4–1 lists some major sources of information about clinical applications of massage.

VALUE OF RESEARCH

In the emerging **integrated health care** scene, those therapies for which there is more scientific research will more likely be used. These are called **evidence-based,** since research provides some verifiable objective evidence for their effectiveness. As stated in the Forward to Touch Therapy (Field 2000):

> One of the principal requirements of modern health care provision can be summed up by the term, "evidence-based." It is no longer sufficient for any therapeutic approach to simply rely on a long history of use, or popularity, or widespread availability, to justify its continued acceptance (especially if insurance reimbursement is anticipated) (pp. vii).

Evidence from scientific studies can more clearly substantiate the benefits of massage in treating certain diseases, as well as identify contraindications. Applications of clinical massage therapy will become safer and more effective as the result of research.

Table 4–1   SOURCES OF INFORMATION ABOUT CLINICAL APPLICATIONS OF MASSAGE

Institution Web sites	Touch Research Institutes (TRI) at the University of Miami School of Medicine www.miami.edu/touch-research
	Canadian Touch Research Centre (CTRC) www.ccrt-ctrc.org
	National Center for Complementary and Alternative Medicine (NCCAM) at the National Institutes of Health, Washington, DC www.nccam.nih.gov
Massage research database Web sites	Massage Therapy Research Database AMTA Foundation www.amtamassage.org/foundation/dbase.htm
	National Library of Medicine www.ncbi.nlm.nih.gov/PubMed
Books	*Clinical Massage Therapy* by Fiona Rattray and Linda Ludwig (Toronto, Canada: Talus Incorporated, 2000)
	A Massage Therapist's Guide to Pathology, 2nd ed., by Ruth Werner (Philadelphia: Lippincott, Williams & Wilkins, 2002)
	A Physician's Guide to Therapeutic Massage by John Yates (Toronto, Canada: Curties-Overzet, 2004)
	Making Sense of Research: A Guide to Research Literacy for Complementary Practitioners by Martha Brown Menard (Toronto, Canada: Curties-Overzet Publications, 2003)
	Massage Therapy: The Evidence for Practice by Grant Jewell Rich (Philadelphia: Mosby, 2002)
	Pathology A to Z—A Handbook for Massage Therapists, 2nd ed., by Premkumar (Calgary, Canada: VanPub Books, 2000)
	Touch Therapy by Tiffany Field (Philadelphia: Churchhill Livingston, 2000)

It has been argued that the nature of massage as a holistic therapy makes it unsuited for scientific inquiry. For example, many practitioners distrust the formula approach to massage used in research to minimize variables in treatment. They understand the importance of varying the approach for the unique individual receiving the massage. Nevertheless, there are certain aspects of massage and its effects that can be measured objectively and provide valuable information to practitioners.

Knowledge gained from research is essential to an approach to treatment that Yates calls **principle-based therapy.** Principle-based massage is in contrast to recipe-based or formula massage, in which each client receives exactly the same treatment (i.e., same techniques applied in same way) for a particular condition. Yates describes the foundation of principle-based therapy as the creation of an overall treatment plan directed toward the achievement of specific treatment goals. Such a plan takes into consideration the condition being treated, tissue involvement, and most importantly in terms of research, the therapeutic potential of different treatment methods. Principle-based therapy also allows for variation:

> Appropriate treatment techniques and modalities are selected, integrated and adapted as necessary to achieve specific effects and are modified according to the changing physiological and psychological state of the patient as treatment proceeds. Treatment is therefore patient-centered rather than technique-centered (Yates 1999, pp. 3–4).

Research takes on practical importance for the selection of techniques based on their healing potential. It can help sort out which massage techniques or approaches are most effective for particular pathologies. Research is most useful for adding to our understanding of the applications of massage, not as a means for developing recipes for treatment. A deeper level of knowledge complements those aspects of massage therapy practice that are intuitive and artful.

Research literacy is important for all massage therapists, especially those in clinical settings. Research literacy includes understanding the scientific method, locating research articles, and reading, analyzing, and evaluating specific studies. (The book to study is *Making Sense of Research: A Guide to Research Literacy for Complementary Practitioners* by Martha Brown Menard, 2003.)

CLINICAL APPROACH

Massage is **indicated** for treating a particular injury or illness if it contributes to the alleviation of the diagnosed condition, or helps ease its symptoms. Massage may be **contraindicated,** or not advisable, if its use as a form of treatment would be detrimental to the client. The word *patient* is most often used to describe a person being treated. However, the word *client* is gaining ground in clinical settings to infer a degree of empowerment on the part of the person receiving treatment. Rattray and Ludwig define client "as a person who is able to make choices about health care" (2000, p. ix).

There are three useful ways of thinking about the clinical benefits of massage therapy, i.e., for its complementary, palliative, or direct therapeutic effects. For example, massage is sometimes indicated as **complementary** to a primary treatment method to enhance its effectiveness and create a more favorable environment for healing. This is especially true for massage designed to help clients relax and reduce anxiety, thereby improving the body's own healing process.

Massage may also be used as **palliative care** to reduce symptoms and discomfort associated with certain diseases or with their treatment. For example, massage has been successful in reducing some of the negative side effects of cancer treatment. By helping to make patients more comfortable, massage is indirectly involved in the healing process. Massage may also be indicated for its more **direct therapeutic effects** such as for relieving constipation, relaxing hypertonic muscles, or for healthy scar formation.

Clinical massage therapy includes Western massage as well as specialized soft tissue manipulation techniques developed to address specific body structures or organ systems. These specialized approaches include neuromuscular massage (i.e., trigger point therapy), deep transverse friction, myofascial massage, lymphatic massage, breast massage, and an energy approach called Therapeutic Touch.

The remainder of this chapter will discuss some of uses of massage in medical settings and some of the promising research that has been done on its clinical applications. It is just a sampling of the growing amount of information available, and points to areas where the study of the clinical applications of massage has been strong.

MUSCULO-SKELETAL PATHOLOGIES

Massage is routinely incorporated into the rehabilitation of musculo-skeletal injuries by physical therapists, athletic trainers, and massage therapists. It is also frequently used as a complement to chiropractic.

Massage is particularly effective in relieving muscle tension, increasing flexibility and range of motion, promoting healthy scar tissue, and reducing muscular pain. These direct therapeutic effects on the muscular system were discussed in Chapter 3.

Deep transverse friction has been especially effective in the treatment of repetitive strain injuries (RSI) such as tendinitis/tenosynovitis, (i.e., inflammation of tendons and tendon sheaths), and bursitis (i.e., inflammation of the fluid sacs around joints). Deep friction techniques increase local circulation, help separate adhesions, and have an analgesic or pain reducing effect (de Bruijin, 1984; Hammer, 1993).

Pain caused by hypertonic muscles can be relieved with massage. For example, tension headaches resulting from tense and shortened cervical muscles have been successfully treated with massage (Puustjarvi, K. et al., 1990). Massage has also been effective in treating subacute chronic low back pain (Cherkin et al, 2001; Preyde, 2000). These findings are particularly encouraging since tension headaches and low back pain afflict so many people in the modern world.

Neuromuscular and myofascial massage are specialized techniques that relieve myofascial pain and dysfunction. Chapters 12 and 13 discuss these techniques in more detail.

Fibromyalgia

Fibromyalgia syndrome (FMS) is a chronic condition characterized by widespread muscle pain and stiffness, and tenderness at specific body sites. The pain and fatigue associated with FMS can be debilitating. Other common symptoms of this syndrome are disturbed sleep, severe headaches, and osteoarthritis. Mental and emotional problems such as anxiety and depression often accompany FMS. Although there is no known cure for FMS, massage can address many of its symptoms. The general effects of massage that offer relief are reduction of stress and anxiety, more restful sleep, more positive outlook, improved circulation, and relief for sore and stiff muscles (Sunshine et al, 1996; Field, 2000).

CARDIOVASCULAR AND LYMPHATIC PATHOLOGIES

Relaxation massage may be beneficial in treating some cardiovascular pathologies such as hypertension (high blood pressure), and cardiac arrhythmia (Curtis, 1994; Longworth 1982). It not only reduces heart rate and blood pressure, but also reduces anxiety which helps give the patient a more positive outlook and improved feelings of wellbeing.

A study by nurses Bauer and Dracup (1987) found that back massage consisting of effleurage had a positive effect on the perception of relaxation and comfort reported by patients with acute myocardial infarction. Although they could not confirm improvement in the pathology, the massage had no apparent detrimental effects.

In another study, patients hospitalized in a cardiovascular unit of a large medical center in New York City who received Therapeutic Touch had a significantly greater reduction in anxiety scores than those who received casual touch or no touch (Heidt, 1981). A fuller discussion of Therapeutic Touch can be found later in this chapter.

Edema and Lymphedema

Edema, or excess interstitial fluid in the tissues, is not a disease, but rather a condition of fluid buildup or swelling. The edema itself can cause pain from increased fluid pressure, and from the buildup of toxins due to decreased circulation (Premkumar 1999).

Edema may occur with minor muscular injuries such as strains and sprains, or with conditions that cause venostasis such as varicose veins or prolonged standing (e.g., swollen feet or ankles). Petrissage and effleurage applied with light to moderate pressure distal to proximal can help reduce these types of edema in the limbs.

Lymphedema is a specific type of edema caused by poor lymph circulation, for example, after removal of lymph nodes during cancer surgery. Massage in general, and lymphatic massage in particular, are useful methods of reducing edema in the extremities. The beneficial effects of manual lymph drainage for patients with chronic and postmastectomy lymphedema continues to be confirmed. It has been noted that permanent and regular treatment is necessary for these conditions (Badger, 1986; Bunce et al., 1994; Kurz et al., 1978; Zanolla et al., 1984). Lymphatic massage is discussed further in Chapter 14.

A note of caution: Massage is contraindicated in cases of edema due to chronic cardiac, kidney, or liver problems.

IMMUNE FUNCTION

One of the basic positive effects of massage is improvement in immune function, as noted in Chapter 3. One of the first major studies to link massage and improved immunity was conducted by the Touch Research Institute in 1996. In a group of HIV-positive men who received daily massage for a month, the majority had significant increase in the number and activity of NK cells. The men showed reduced anxiety and stress, lower cortisol levels, as well as increased serotonin levels during the month of massage.

> Given that elevated stress hormones (catecholamines and cortisol) negatively affect immune function, the increase in NK activity probably derived from the decrease in these stress hormones following massage therapy (Field 2000, pp. 201–205).

To the extent that massage helps reduce stress and thus improves immune function, it can be considered an important disease prevention measure. Health problems caused by compromised immunity include frequent infections, autoimmune disorders, and possibly, cancer (Corwin, 1996; Field, 2000).

RESPIRATORY PATHOLOGIES

Massage is used as a complementary therapy for people with respiratory conditions such as chronic bronchitis, emphysema, and asthma. The benefits of massage for these patients include anxiety reduction and relaxation that deepens breathing patterns, relaxation and lengthening of muscles tense from labored breathing, and reduced fatigue overall. Passive movement of the rib cage, as well as percussion on the back and chest, can help loosen mucus for more productive coughs.

Children with asthma have been the subjects of several recent research projects. In one study, children with asthma were found to have lower anxiety, improved attitude towards the asthma condition, and increased peak airflow after regular massage by their parents. Over a one-month period, these children had fewer asthma attacks. The study suggested that daily massage may lead to improved airway tone, decreased airway irritability, and better control of asthma in children (Field, 2000, pp.179–186).

In another study, asthma, bronchitis, and emphysema patients received a form of bodywork called Trager Psychophysical Integration®, which consists of gentle painless, passive movements. Focus was on the neck, abdomen and chest wall. After treatment, improvement was found in forced vital capacity, respiratory rate, and chest expansion. Patients reported general relaxation and decrease in anxiety and tension (Witt & MacKinnon, 1986).

An increase in thoracic gas volume, peak flow and forced vital capacity was found in 4 out of 5 COPD patients receiving a combination of massage and myofascial trigger point therapy, i.e., neuromuscular massage. The neuromuscular techniques were specifically directed to improve the function of chronically hypertonic muscles involved in breathing (Beeken et al., 1998).

Note that the studies cited above used different massage therapy approaches to achieve their positive results. The overall objectives were to reduce stress, improve diaphragmatic breathing, relax and lengthen the muscles of respiration. Studies help identify specific techniques that are effective for these goals.

ANXIETY REDUCTION IN HOSPITALIZED PATIENTS

The ability of massage to elicit the relaxation response and reduce anxiety accounts for much of its value as a complement to standard medical treatment. Nurses in particular have found massage useful in caring for patients hospitalized for a variety of conditions.

For example, back massage was found to be an effective, noninvasive technique for promoting relaxation and improving communication with elderly, institutionalized patients. The nurses who conducted the study noted the potential of massage for reducing the common dehumanizing effects of institutional care (Frazer and Kerr, 1993). Those results were confirmed by another study of slow stroke back rub for the elderly by two other nurses, Fakouri and Jones (1987).

Another study by nurses examined the effects of therapeutic massage on hospitalized cancer patients. Primary techniques used were effleurage, petrissage, and trigger point therapy. They found that massage therapy significantly reduced the patients' perceived level of pain and anxiety, while enhancing their feelings of relaxation. Objective physiologic measures, i.e., heart rate, respiratory rate, and blood pressure, tended to decrease, providing further indication of relaxation (Ferrell-Torry and Glick, 1993).

MASSAGE FOR CANCER PATIENTS

Massage was once listed as a general contraindication for cancer patients. It is now recognized as a valuable complementary therapy, and cancer patients who receive massage are reporting relief from a number of physical, mental and emotional discomforts related to the disease and its treatment.

General benefits of massage especially important to cancer patients include reduced stress and anxiety, improved sleep, improved immune system function, pain relief, and the comfort of caring touch (Rhiner et al 1993; Sims 1986; Weinrich & Weinrich 1990).

Cancer patients who undergo surgery may benefit from the effects of massage related to faster recovery from anesthesia, faster wound healing, separation of adhesions around incisions, healthy scar formation, and reduction of edema and lymphedema. Massage has also been linked to reduced pain and less need for pain medication. Hospitalized patients find relief from muscle soreness caused by prolonged bed rest. Improved circulation from massage helps prevent pressure and bed sores.

Massage has also been found to reduce some of the negative side effects of radiation and chemotherapy such as fatigue, nausea, diarrhea, loss of appetite, and insomnia (MacDonald, 1995). However, the timing of massage in relation to treatment can be important; for example, the patient may be overtaxed and negative side effects worsened if massage is received too soon after a bout of chemotherapy.

The benefits of massage on the emotional level can be significant. Massage can help a cancer patient deal with depression, and offer pleasant social interaction providing relief from isolation. It can help reestablish a positive body image, and reclaim the body as an ally. It empowers patients to participate in their healing process, and helps rebuild hope (Chamness, 1996; Rattray 2000).

Breast massage is increasing in use as a clinical application for women who have experienced breast cancer. It is especially useful for post-mastectomy patients, including for general wound healing, healthy scar formation, and treating lymphedema. (Refer to *Breast Massage* by Debra Curties, 1999).

The concern about metastasis, or that massage may spread cancer, is still real in some cases. For example, massage should be avoided completely around the site of a tumor, or where a tumor has recently been removed. Massage practitioners should consult the patient's physician to assess the potential for harm from massage, and to get advice on how to proceed safely. (Refer to *Massage Therapy & Cancer* by Debra Curties (1999); and *Medicine Hands: Massage Therapy for People with Cancer* by Gayle Macdonald (1999)).

PEDIATRIC CARE

Massage is being used increasingly in the care of hospitalized children, from infants to adolescents. Many of the uses of massage in pediatric care are similar to uses for adults, e.g., rehabilitation and anxiety reduction. A unique benefit for infants is the tactile stimulation provided by massage, which is essential for proper growth and development.

Much of the recent interest in massage for children has been generated by the work of Tiffany Field, PhD, who in 1991 founded the Touch Research Institute (TRI) at the University of Miami School of Medicine, Department of Pediatrics. The research being performed at TRI on a variety of pediatric conditions can be reviewed on their Web site.

Preterm Infants

Building on research done in the 1970s, Field found that preterm infants who received tactile stimulation during their stay in the transitional care nursery setting experienced greater weight gain, increased motor activity, more alertness, and improved performance on the Brazelton Neonatal Behavioral Assessment Scale. Tactile stimulation was applied by gentle stroking of the head and neck, across the shoulders, from upper back to the waist, from the thighs to the feet, and from the shoulders to the hands. Additional stimulation was provided by passive flexion/extension movements of the arms and legs (Field et al., 1986).

Subsequent research has shown that massage also benefits cocaine-exposed preterm infants. In addition to better weight gain, massaged infants showed significantly fewer postnatal complications and stress behaviors than the control infants did (Wheeden et al., 1993).

Pediatric Applications

A review of some of the research being done at TRI demonstrates the broad range of situations in which massage is found to be a useful treatment for children. Descriptions of the research for the results below, and for many other studies, can be found in the book *Touch Therapy* by Tiffany Field (2000) and on the TRI Web site (www.miami.edu/touch-research.)

- **Asthmatic children:** 20-minute massages given to asthmatic children by their mothers for one month resulted in decreased anxiety levels and improved mood for both children and parents; the children's cortisol levels decreased; and they had fewer asthma attacks and were able to breathe better.
- **Autistic children:** After one month of massage therapy, the autistic children were less touch sensitive, less distracted by sounds, more attentive in class, related more to their teachers, and received better scores on the Autism Behavior Checklist and on the Early Social Communications Scales.
- **Diabetic children:** A pilot study showed that as a result of massage given to diabetic children by their parents, both children and parents showed lower anxiety and less depressed mood levels; the children's insulin and food regulation scores improved, and blood glucose levels decreased to the normal range.
- **Depressed adolescent mothers:** After 10 massage sessions over a five-week period, depressed adolescent mothers reported lower anxiety; showed behavioral and stress hormone changes, including decreases in anxious behavior and in pulse and salivary cortisol levels; and a decrease in urine cortisol levels, suggesting lower stress levels.
- **Infants of depressed adolescent mothers:** Full-term infants born to depressed adolescent mothers were given 15 minutes of massage two times a week for six weeks. These infants gained more weight, showed greater improvement on emotionality, sociability, and soothability temperament dimensions and on face-to-face interaction ratings, and had greater decreases in urinary stress catecholamines/hormones (norepinephrine, epinephrine, cortisol) than the controls who were simply rocked.
- **Children with posttraumatic stress disorder:** Children traumatized by Hurricane Andrew were massaged at their schools two times a week for one month. The massaged children had less depression, lower anxiety levels, and lower cortisol (stress hormone) levels than children in the control group.

Although further research is needed to substantiate much of what has been found to date, massage appears to be a promising adjunct to treatment of children with a variety of disorders.

PSYCHOLOGICAL ASPECTS OF TREATMENT

Massage is used to address the psychological and emotional problems of patients receiving medical treatment. For example, several of the studies mentioned in this chapter found massage to be beneficial in the reduction of the anxiety of patients hospitalized for serious medical conditions.

Massage may also help in the treatment of patients with medical conditions significantly worsened by stress. For example, in a study by Joachim (1983), patients with chronic inflammatory bowel disease, ulcerative colitis, or Crohn's disease (ileitis) who received massage for relaxation had fewer episodes of pain and disability from the disease.

Massage may also help patients hospitalized for psychiatric reasons. In a study by Field et al. (1992), hospitalized depressed and adjustment-disorder children and adolescents who received massage were less

depressed and anxious and had lower saliva cortisol levels (an indication
tients who watched relaxation videotapes.

Psychotherapy patients not hospitalized may also benefit from the
stress and anxiety reduction, improved body awareness, and the abili
sexual touch. For example, some massage therapists work with psych
survivors of sexual and physical abuse. Massage has been found to be b
reconnect with their bodies, develop a more compassionate relation'
experience their bodies as a "source of groundedness and eventual.,
good things instead of a bad thing" (Benjamin, 1995, p. 28).

THERAPEUTIC TOUCH

Therapeutic Touch is a form of manual therapy in which the energy field of the recipient is rebalanced, thus promoting health and healing. Although it does not fall directly into the category of soft tissue massage, it is performed by many massage practitioners and integrated into their work. It has found special acceptance by nurses, who find it effective in caring for patients.

Therapeutic Touch was developed by Dolores Krieger, PhD, RN, in the 1970s. She explains the technique as one of centering; then placing the hands in the recipient's energy field to detect a break in energy flow, pressure, or dysrhythmias; then rebalancing or repatterning the energy field by sweeping hand movements a few inches above the skin. She explains what happens as a profound relaxation response that has a positive effect on the immune system, which allows self-healing to reassert itself (Karpen, 1995).

Kreiger explains that Therapeutic Touch has been found to have more effect on some conditions than others. For example, it seems to have a positive effect in working with fluid and electrolyte imbalances, dysfunctions of the autonomic nervous system, lymphatic and circulatory dysfunctions, and musculoskeletal problems. She further explains that:

> Some collagen dysfunctions respond, such as rheumatoid arthritis, but lupus is resistant. Within the endocrine system, the thyroid, adrenals, and ovaries respond, but there is little success with the pituitary and variable success with the pancreas in treating diabetes. In psychiatric disorders, manic depressives and catatonics respond, but there has been little success with schizophrenics. (Karpen, 1995)

Therapeutic Touch was found to have potential in the treatment of tension headache pain (Keller & Bzdek, 1986). Therapeutic Touch has also been used successfully to help reduce the stress of hospitalized children (Kramer, 1990). Research and articles about Therapeutic Touch can be found in nursing journals such as the *American Journal of Nursing* and *Nursing Research*. Further information about Therapeutic Touch research is available from Nurse Healers–Professional Associates, which was established in 1977 under the leadership of Dolores Kreiger (see Appendix A). The NH-PA is a voluntary, nonprofit cooperative whose international exchange network facilitates the exchange of research findings, teaching strategies, and developments in the clinical practice of Therapeutic Touch (www.therapeutic-touch.org).

COMPLEMENT TO CHIROPRACTIC

Chiropractic care is gaining increasing recognition as an effective treatment for certain conditions. Massage is often given as a complement to chiropractic care to help prepare the body for chiropractic adjustments, to relieve tension and pain in muscles and related soft tissues, and to prevent future musculoskeletal misalignment.

The term *chiropractic adjustment* is used here to mean a technique in which bones and joints are manipulated to return the body to proper alignment. This often involves a forceful thrusting movement or manipulation. Such adjustments are performed on *subluxations*, a condition of misalignment in a joint, which often results in structural, nervous system, and chemical dysfunctions.

Local massage is sometimes used in preparation for an adjustment. Massage relieves muscle tension and warms up the soft tissues in the area, making joints more pliable and more easily adjusted. Massage may be given along with heat and ultrasound in this preparatory routine.

A general massage (1 half to 1 hour long) may also be good preparation for an adjustment. In addition to preparing the immediate area of concern, it helps induce general relaxation and accustoms the recipient to touch. The recipient may be more receptive to other hands-on treatment in such a relaxed state. Massage after an adjustment may help the muscles remain relaxed and prevent a tightening reaction to the treatment. Regular massage may help adjustments last longer by keeping muscles relaxed and lengthened.

Therapeutic massage may also be used to address some of the muscular problems that bring patients for adjustments. These include nerve constriction due to tight muscles, poor circulation, trigger points, damaged tissues, and the pain–spasm–pain cycle. Massage used with ice can help relieve muscles in spasm. Recent research shows massage to be an effective treatment for low back pain (Cherkin et al., 2001; Preyde, 2000).

SUMMARY

The term *clinical massage therapy* refers to applications of massage for the treatment of pathologies. In an integrated health care system, therapies that are evidenced-based, i.e., supported by scientific research, are more likely to be used. Research on clinical applications of massage is available through centers for the study of touch, and on the Internet in research databases. Research literacy is important for massage practitioners in clinical settings.

Knowledge gained from research is essential to a principle-based approach to massage therapy. In the principle-based approach, massage techniques are chosen, applied, and adapted to reach treatment goals. This is in contrast to a recipe-based approach, where the same techniques are applied in every case.

Massage is indicated for injuries and illness if it contributes to their alleviation, or helps ease symptoms. Three useful ways of thinking about the clinical benefits of massage are for its complementary, palliative, or direct therapeutic effects.

Massage has been found effective in relieving musculo-skeletal conditions such as repetitive strain injuries, tension headaches, and low back pain. It relieves symptoms of fibromyalgia. Massage is used in treatment of cardiovascular and lymphatic disorders such as hypertension, edema, and lymphedema. It improves immune function, which is important in the treatment of many diseases.

Massage is a useful complementary therapy for people with respiratory conditions such as chronic bronchitis, emphysema, and asthma. Several different massage therapy approaches have been studied for their effects on people suffering from COPD.

Massage has been used effectively as a palliative measure to reduce anxiety in hospitalized patients, as well as reduce pain and improve communication. Benefits of massage for cancer patients include reduced stress and anxiety, faster recovery from surgery, and reduction of the side effects from cancer treatment. Emotional benefits for cancer patients include help in dealing with depression, reestablishing a positive body image, and rebuilding hope.

Massage has been used successfully in pediatric care for children with asthma, autism, diabetes, depression, and posttraumatic stress disorder. It helps preterm infants gain weight and develop more normally.

Massage is an effective complement to treatment of conditions worsened by stress. It relieves the anxiety and stress of psychiatric patients.

Therapeutic Touch is a form of manual therapy that rebalances the energy field of the patient. It has been found effective in treatment of fluid and electrolyte imbalances, dysfunction in the autonomic nervous system, and lymphatic and circulatory disorders. Nurses have been particularly involved in the development of Therapeutic Touch and its use with patients.

Massage is an effective complement to chiropractic care. It helps prepare the body for adjustment, and addresses some of the muscular problems of chiropractic patients.

A look ahead . . .

While massage has many beneficial effects, there are certain circumstances in which it should be modified or avoided altogether for the health and safety of the recipient. Chapter 5 presents guidelines for endangerment sites, contraindications, and cautions for giving massage.

REFERENCES

Badger, C. (1986). The swollen limb. *Nursing Times* (England), *82*(31), 40–41.

Bauer, W. C., & Dracup, K. A. (1987). Physiological effects of back massage in patients with acute myocardial infarction. *Focus on Critical Care, 14*(6), 42–46.

Beeken, J., et al. (1998). Effectiveness of neuromuscular release massage therapy on chronic obstructive lung disease. *Clinical Nursing Research, 7*(3), 309–325.

Benjamin, B. E. (1995). Massage and body work with survivors of abuse: Part I. *Massage Therapy Journal, 34*(3), 23–32.

Bunce, I. H., Mirolo, B. R., Hennessy, J. M., et al. (1994). Post-mastectomy lymphedema treatment and measurement. *Medical Journal* Australia, *161*, 125–128.

Chamness, A. (1996). Breast cancer and massage therapy. *Massage Therapy Journal, 35*(1, Winter).

Cherkin, D. C., Eisenberg, D. et al. (2001). Randomized trial comparing traditonal Chinese medical acupuncture, therapeutic massage, and self-care education for chronic low back pain. *Archives of Internal Medicine 161*(8), 1081–1088.

Corwin, E. J. (1996). *Handbook of pathophysiology.* Philadelphia: Lippincot.

Curties, D. (1999). *Breast Massage.* Toronto, Canada: Curties-Overzet Publications.

Curties, D. (1999). *Massage Therapy and Cancer.* Toronto, Canada: Curties-Overzet Publications.

Curtis, M. (1994). The use of massage in restoring cardiac rhythm. *Nursing Times* (England), *90*(38), 36–37.

de Bruijn, R. (1984). Deep transverse friction; its analgesic effect. *International Journal of Sports Medicine, 5*, 35–36.

Fakouri, C., & Jones, P. (1987). Relaxation ℞: Slow stroke back rub. *Journal of Gerontological Nursing, 13*(2), 32–35.

Ferrell-Torry, A. T., & Glick, O. J. (1993). The use of therapeutic massage as a nursing intervention to modify anxiety and the perception of cancer pain. *Cancer Nursing, 16*(2), 93–101.

Field, T. (2000). *Touch Therapy.* London: Churchill Livingston.

Field, T. M., Morrow, C., Valdeon, C., et al. (1992). Massage reduces anxiety in child and adolescent psychiatric patients. *Journal of the American Academy of Child and Adolescent Psychiatry, 31*(1), 125–131.

Field, T. M., Schanberg, S. M., Scafidi, F., et al. (1986). Tactile/kinesthetic stimulation effects on preterm neonates. *Pediatrics, 77*(5), 654–658.

Frazer, J., & Kerr, J. R. (1993). Psychophysiological effects of back massage on elderly institutionalized patients. *Journal of Advanced Nursing, 18*, 238–245.

Hammer, W. I. (1993) The use of transverse friction massage in the management of chronic bursitis of the hip and shoulder. *Journal of Manipulation and Physical Therapy, 16*(2), 107–111.

Heidt, P. (1981). Effect of therapeutic touch on anxiety level of hospitalized patients. *Nursing Research, 30*(1), 32–37.

Joachim, G. (1983). The effects of two stress management techniques on feelings of well-being in patients with inflammatory bowel disease. *Nursing Papers, 15*(5), 18.

Karpen, M. (1995). Dolores Kreiger, PhD, RN: Tireless teacher of Therapeutic Touch. *Alternative & Complementary Therapies,* April/May, 142–146.

Keller, E., & Bzdek, V. M. (1986). Effects of therapeutic touch on tension headache pain. *Nursing Research, 35*(2), 101–106.

Kramer, N. A. (1990). Comparison of therapeutic touch and casual touch in stress reduction of hospitalized children. *Pediatric Nursing, 16*(5), 483–485.

Kurz, W., Wittlinger, G., Litmanovitch, Y. I., et al. (1978). Effect of manual lymph drainage massage on urinary excretion of neurohormones and minerals in chronic lyphedema. *Angiology, 29*, 64–72.

Longworth, J. D. (1982). Psychophysiological effects of slow stroke back massage in normotensive females. *Advances in Nursing Science 4*, 44–61.

Macdonald, G.(1999). *Medicine Hands: Massage Therapy for People with Cancer.* Tallahassee, FL: Findhorn Press.

MacDonald, G. (1995). Massage for cancer patients: A review of nursing research. *Massage Therapy Journal,* Summer, 53–56.

Menard, M. B. (2003). *Making sense of research: A guide to research literacy for complementary practitioners.* Toronto: Curties-Overzet Publications.

Premkumar, K. (1999). Pathology A to Z: A handbook for massage therapists. 2nd Ed. Calgary, Canada: Van Pub Books.

Preyde, M. (2000). Effectiveness of massage therapy for subacute low-back pain: A randomized controlled trail. *CMAJ, 162*(13), 1815–1820.

Puustjarvi, K., Airaksinen, O., & P.J. Pontinen (1990). The effects of massage in patients with chronic tension headache. *Acupuncture Electrotherapy Research, 15*(2), 159–162.

Rattray, F. and L. Ludwig (2000). *Clinical massage therapy: Understanding, assessing and treating over 700 conditions.* Toronto, Canada: Talus Incorporated.

Rhiner, M., Ferrell, B. R., Ferrell, B. A., & Grant, M. M. (1993). A structured non-drug intervention program for cancer pain. *Cancer Practice, 1*, 137–143.

Sims, S. (1986). Slow stroke back massage for cancer patients. *Nursing Times, 82*, 47–50.

Sunshine, W., Field, T., et al. (1996) Fibromyalgia benefits from massage therapy and transcutaneous electrical stimulation. *Journal of Clinical Rheum.* 2(1), 18–22.

Weinrich, S. P., & Weinrich, M. C. (1990). The effect of massage on pain in cancer patients. *Applied Nursing Research, 3,* 140–145.

Wheeden, A., Scafidi, F., Field, T., et al. (1993). Massage effects on cocaine-exposed preterm neonates. *Developmental and Behavioral Pediatrics, 14*(5), 318–322.

Witt, P. L., MacKinnon, J. (1986). Trager psychosocial integration: A method to improve chest mobility of patients with chronic lung disease. *Physical Therapy,* 66(2), 214–217.

Yates, J. (1999). *A physician's guide to therapeutic massage: Its physiological effects and treatment applications,* 2nd edition. Vancouver, BC: Massage Therapists' Association of British Columbia.

Zanolla, R., Monzeglio, C., Balzarini, A., & Martino, G. (1984). Evaluation of the results of three different methods of postmastectomy lymphedema treatment. *Journal of Surgical Oncology, 26,* 210–213.

WEB SITES

AMTA Foundation *(www.amtafoundation.org)*

Canadian Touch Research Center *(ccrt-ctrc.org)*

National Library of Medicine *(ncbi.nlm.nih.gov/PubMed)*

Nurse-Healers–Professional Associates International *(www.therapeutic-touch.org)*

Touch Research Institute *(www.miami.edu/touch-research)*

ADDITIONAL REFERENCES

Videos

"Cancer massage video." Canada Institute of Palliative Massage. Nelson, British Columbia, Canada: Sutherland Massage Productions. *(www.sutherlandmassageproductions.com)*

"AIDS massage video." Canada Institute of Palliative Massage. Nelson, British Columbia, Canada: Sutherland Massage Productions. *(www.sutherlandmassageproductions.com)*

"Massage for children with Down Syndrome." Canada Institute of Palliative Massage. Nelson, British Columbia, Canada: Sutherland Massage Productions. *(www.sutherlandmassageproductions.com)*

S T U D Y   G U I D E

LEARNING OUTCOMES

Use the learning outcomes at the beginning of the chapter as a guide to your studies. Perform the task given in each outcome, either in writing or verbally into a tape recorder or to a study partner. This may start as an "open book" exercise, and then later from memory.

KEY TERMS/CONCEPTS

To study key words and concepts listed at the beginning of this chapter, choose one or more of the following exercises. Writing or talking about ideas helps you remember them better, and explaining helps deepen your understanding.

1. Write a one- or two-sentence explanation of each key word and concept.

2. Make study cards by writing the explanation from problem 1 on one side of a 3 × 5 card, and the key word or concept on the other. Shuffle the cards and read one side, trying to recite either the explanation or word on the other side.

3. Pick out two or three key words or concepts and explain how they are related.

4. With a study partner, take turns explaining key words and concepts verbally.

STUDY OUTLINE

The following questions test your memory of the main concepts in this chapter. Locate the answers in the text using the page number given for each question.

Value of Research

1. Applications of massage for the treatment of pathologies are called _____ massage therapy. (p. 67)

2. Therapies for which there is supportive scientific research are called _____ - based. (p. 67).

3. In recipe-based therapy, every patient receives the _____. (p. 68)

4. In principle-based therapy, appropriate treatment techniques are _____, _____ _____, and _____ as necessary to achieve specific effects. (p. 68)

5. Research is most useful when it adds to our understanding of the effectiveness of certain massage applications, and not as a means of developing _____ for treatment. (p. 68)

6. Research literacy includes understanding the _____ method, locating _____ _____, and reading, analyzing and evaluating _____. (p. 68)

Clinical Approach

1. Massage is considered _____ to a primary treatment to enhance its effectiveness and create a more favorable environment for healing. (p. 68)

2. Massage is considered _____ care when it reduces discomforts related to a disease or its treatment. (p. 68)

3. Massage has _____ effects for treating a number of pathologies. (p. 68)

Musculo-Skeletal Pathologies

1. Direct therapeutic effects related to musculo-skeletal pathologies include _____, _____, _____, and _____. (p. 69)

2. Deep transverse friction is used effectively in treatment of _____ strain injuries. (p. 69)

3. Massage is an effective treatment for hypertonic muscles, e.g., in _____ and _____. (p. 69)

4. Symptoms of fibromyalgia relieved with massage include _____ _____. (p. 69)

Cardiovascular and Lymphatic Pathologies

1. Cardiovascular pathologies for which massage is beneficial include _____ and _____. (p. 69)

2. Hospitalized heart patients experienced reduced _____ with massage. (p. 69)

3. Edema, the condition of excess _____ _____ in the tissues, can be relieved with massage. (p. 69)

4. Massage may be contraindicated in cases of edema due to chronic _____, _____ _____, or _____ problems. (p. 70)

Immune Function

1. Massage is thought to be of benefit to clients who are HIV positive because of its _____ effects. (p. 70)

2. Massage can be an important _____ measure for health problems that result from compromised immune function. (p. 70)

Respiratory Pathologies

1. Respiratory conditions for which massage is a good complementary therapy include _____, _____, and _____. (p. 70)

2. Massage and bodywork techniques studied for their effectiveness in treating respiratory conditions include _____, _____, and _____. (p. 70)

3. _____ techniques on the back and chest, and rib cage _____ techniques are effective in helping to produce productive coughs. (p. 70)

Anxiety Reduction in Hospitalized Patients

1. Nursing studies have found massage to be an effective complement to treatment for hospitalized patients, particularly its _____ and _____ effects. (pp. 70–71)

2. Massage holds potential for reducing the _____ effects of institutional care. (p. 71)

Massage for Cancer Patients

1. General effects of massage especially beneficial for cancer patients include _____, _____, _____, _____, and _____. (p. 71)

2. Massage can reduce some of the negative side effects of cancer treatments, such as _____ and _____. (p. 71)

3. The benefits of massage after cancer surgery include _____. (p. 71)

4. Emotional benefits of massage for cancer patients may include _____, _____, _____, _____, and _____. (p. 71)

5. _____ massage benefits women who have had breast cancer by enhancing post-mastectomy wound healing, and healthy scar formation. (p. 71)

6. Lymphatic massage helps reduce _____ that often accompanies mastectomy. (p. 71)

Pediatric Care

1. Tactile stimulation of preterm infants through massage enhances _____, _____, _____, and _____ (pp. 71–72)

2. Massage has been found to be an effective complementary treatment for children with a variety of medical conditions including _____,

_____, _____, and _____. (p. 72)

Psychological Aspects of Treatment

1. Massage can be a valuable complement to treatment for people with diseases induced by or aggravated by _____. (p. 72)

2. The effects of massage that can benefit psychiatric patients include _____, _____, _____, and receiving pleasurable non-sexual _____. (p. 73)

Therapeutic Touch

1. Therapeutic Touch is an _____ approach to manual therapy developed by a nurse, Dolores Krieger, in the 1970s. (p. 73)

2. Theories about the mechanisms of Therapeutic Touch range from the physiological (e.g., _____), to those beyond the realm of science (e.g., _____ the patient's energy field). (p. 73)

Complement to Chiropractic

1. Massage can help _____ a person for a chiropractic adjustment, relieve tension and pain in soft tissues as a _____ to chiropractic treatment, and help _____ future musculo-skeletal misalignment. (pp. 73–74)

FOR GREATER UNDERSTANDING

The following exercises are designed to take you from the realm of theory into the real world. They will help give you a deeper understanding of the subjects covered in this chapter. Action words are underlined to emphasize the variety of activities presented to address different learning styles, and to encourage deeper thinking.

1. Choose a specific pathology to study. Locate research studies about the effectiveness of massage in treating that pathology. Write a review of the research that you find.

2. Choose one research study to read, analyze and evaluate. Present your findings and conclusions to a study partner or group.

3. Choose a specific pathology to study. Locate information about contraindications and cautions related to the pathology. Identify implications for giving massage to a person with the pathology studied. Discuss with a study partner or group.

4. Interview someone who is receiving massage as treatment for a particular pathology. Ask them to identify the benefits they feel from receiving massage. Compare this with conventional wisdom and available research.

5. Interview a massage practitioner who specializes in clinical applications, or the director of a clinical massage setting. Ask them about the types of pathologies they see in their practices and the benefits patients receive from massage. Report to a study partner or group.

6. Develop plans for a research study related to a specific pathology.

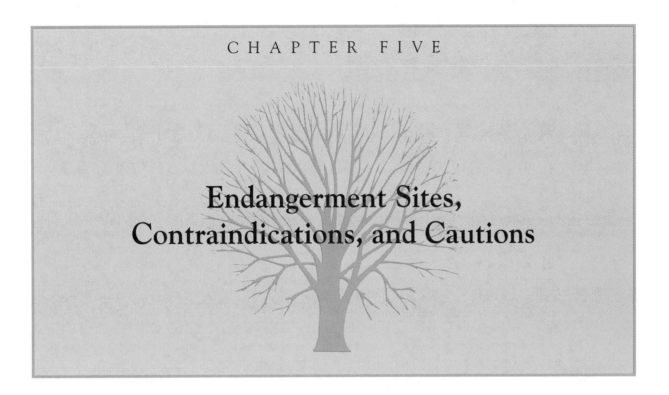

CHAPTER FIVE

Endangerment Sites, Contraindications, and Cautions

LEARNING OUTCOMES

After studying this chapter, the student will have information to:

1. Locate major endangerment sites.
2. Discuss the general principles of safety around endangerment sites.
3. Distinguish between general and regional contraindications for massage.
4. List and explain the general principles for contraindications and cautions for massage.
5. Discuss considerations related to medications.
6. Explain the concept of person-centered massage.
7. Identify sources of information about endangerment sites and contraindications for massage.

KEY TERMS/CONCEPTS

Caution
Contraindications
Do no harm
Endangerment site

General contraindications
Health history
Local contraindications
Medications

Person-centered massage
Professional library
Regional contraindication

 MEDIALINK

A companion CD-ROM, included free with each new copy of this book, supplements the techniques presented in this chapter. Insert the CD-ROM to watch video clips of massage techniques being demonstrated. This multimedia feature is designed to help you add a new dimension to your learning.

DO NO HARM

One of most basic rules of giving therapeutic massage is to **do no harm.** Guidelines for helping you make decisions about what to do and what to avoid, to protect the health and safety of your clients will be presented in this chapter. Topics addressed will include endangerment sites, contraindications, cautions, and resources for further information.

The variety of massage approaches used today complicates the issue somewhat. These forms vary from deep tissue structural massage of the physical body to light work affecting the energy within and around the physical body. An endangerment site or a contraindication in one form of bodywork may be considered perfectly safe for a different form.

This chapter will focus on endangerment sites, contraindications, and cautions that are important when giving Western massage and forms that use similar techniques. This includes all techniques applied to the physical body that involve pressing, stroking, friction, kneading, tapping, and vibrating. Chapters devoted to other types of massage and bodywork will address contraindications and cautions for that particular type of work.

Knowledge of Western anatomy and physiology is essential to ensure the safety of the person receiving massage and bodywork. It is particularly important to know the location of major nerves and blood vessels, glands, and visceral organs. Endangerment sites, contraindications, and cautions will be discussed in this chapter in terms of Western science and pathologies.

ENDANGERMENT SITES

Endangerment sites are areas of the body where delicate structures are less protected and, therefore, may be more easily damaged when receiving massage. Caution is required when performing massage on or around endangerment sites. The following paragraphs identify the location of endangerment sites, and describe cautions when working in those areas. Figure 5–1 shows the general location of endangerment sites on the anterior and posterior body.

Anterior Neck.   The anterior neck is the triangular area on the front of the neck defined by the sternocleidomastoid (SCM) and includes the sternal notch, which is the depression found on the superior aspect of the sternum. Delicate structures located in the anterior neck region are the carotid artery, jugular vein, vagus nerve, larynx, and thyroid gland. Deep pressure on any of these structures is dangerous.

Pressure within the anterior triangle of the neck, including the depression formed by the sternal notch, should be avoided entirely in most forms of massage. Some advanced techniques address cervical muscles from the anterior neck, but they should be performed only by experienced therapists with special training. The gentle superficial stroking during lymphatic massage and non-contact forms of energy work are possible exceptions to the no-touch rule.

Great care should be taken when performing neck massage on the elderly due to the likelihood of atherosclerosis and the potential for dislodging a thrombus that could lead to stroke. Too much pressure from massage could also cause further damage to blood vessels in the area. Only light pressure should be used on the neck, if massage is applied to the neck at all.

Vertebral Column.   The vertebral column protects spinal cord of the central nervous system. The spinous processes of the cervical, thoracic and lumbar vertebrae can be felt along the middle of the neck and back. Massage techniques that apply heavy pressure or that involve thrusting or percussion movements should not be performed directly over the spinous processes.

Thoracic Cage.   The thoracic cage consists of the ribs and sternum. The thoracic cage is relatively flexible to allow for breathing, and ribs 1–10 attach to the sternum with cartilage. The lower tip of the sternum called the xiphoid process is a slender piece of bone that can break under pressure and be driven into the liver, causing severe damage. Avoid strong pressure or impact over the sternum overall, and especially the xiphoid process. Heavy pressure over the anterior and lateral surfaces of the rib cage should also be avoided, especially in the elderly.

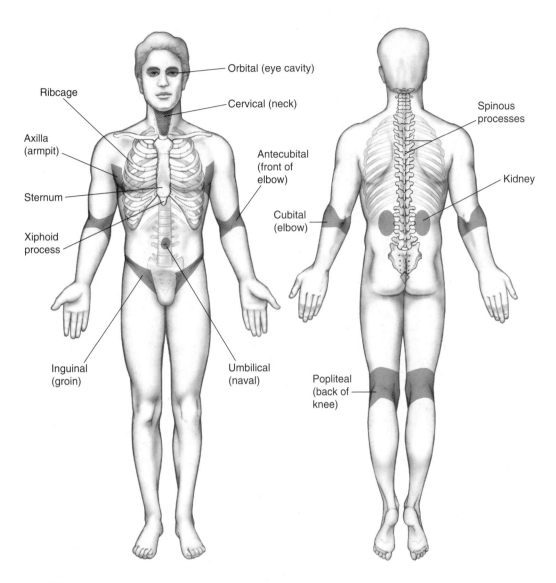

FIGURE 5–1. Endangerment sites—anterior and posterior views.

Axilla.   Delicate circulatory and nervous structures are relatively exposed in the axilla or armpit area. These include the brachial artery, axillary artery and vein, cephalic vein, and the nerve complex of the brachial plexus. Deep pressure in this area should be approached with caution.

Elbow.   Two places around the elbow area require caution. One is the space just medial to the olecranon process where the ulnar nerve is relatively exposed. This is the "funny bone" area that causes sharp pain when hit. The second area is the anterior surface, or fold, of the elbow. This area is similar to the popliteal fossa found posterior to the knee as described later on. Vulnerable structures found in this area include the brachial vein and artery, median cubital vein, and median nerve. These structures are all close to the surface and unprotected by muscle. Moderate broad pressure may be applied to the area, but deep specific pressure should be restricted to the surrounding muscles and their attachments.

Umbilicus.   The umbilicus or "belly button" is a sensitive area superficial to the descending aorta and abdominal aorta. Avoid direct heavy pressure to the umbilicus.

Kidney Area.   The kidneys are located on either side of the spine generally at the level between the 3rd lumbar and 12th thoracic vertebrae. They are positioned behind the parietal peritoneum and against the deep muscles of the back. Superficial or deep stroking and pressing techniques may be applied carefully to the muscles of the back located in the kidney area. However, only very light pressure should be used when performing percussion techniques over this area.

Inguinal Area.   The inguinal or groin area is located roughly where the thigh and the trunk meet on the anterior side of the body. The femoral nerve and major blood vessels to the lower extremities cross there, i.e., femoral artery, great saphenous and femoral veins. When the thigh is flexed, a depression is created in the area exposing the more delicate structures. Great care should be taken when applying deep pressure into this area, for example, when reaching for the iliopsoas. This should be attempted only by students under supervision and by practitioners with advanced training.

Popliteal Fossa.   The muscles of the posterior lower extremity cross the knee laterally and medially, leaving the center space relatively unprotected. This is the popliteal fossa. The popliteal artery and vein and the tibial nerve are located there. Avoid heavy specific pressure over this area. Follow the muscles around the popliteal fossa when massaging them.

Eyes.   Take great care when working around the eyes. Be careful not to slip and hit the eyeball by accident. Only the very lightest pressure is used when stroking the eyelid.

Major Veins in Extremities.   Major veins in the extremities are being included under endangerment sites because structural damage can occur to the valves within the veins if deep effleurage is applied improperly. Always apply deep flushing effleurage to the arms and legs from distal to proximal, that is, toward the heart, and with the flow that opens the valves.

GENERAL PRINCIPLES FOR SAFETY AROUND ENDANGERMENT SITES

Here are some general principles to keep in mind to protect the receiver's body from structural damage during massage. Remember, your first responsibility is to do no harm.

1. Always adjust the pressure you use to match the part of the body, the condition of the tissues, and the person you are working on. Any part of the body can be damaged if too much pressure is used.
2. Avoid heavy pressure anyplace where nerves, blood vessels, or lymph vessels are close to the surface or are unprotected by muscle or bone.
3. Be careful around joints where delicate structures are less protected by skeletal muscle.
4. If you feel a pulse, it means that you are on a major artery. Move to a different place immediately.
5. If the receiver feels searing, burning, shooting, electrical sensations, "pins and needles," or numbness, you may be pressing on a nerve. Move to a different place immediately.
6. Any abnormal structure is a potential endangerment site. Get information about structural abnormalities, and proceed with caution when you are sure it is safe to do so.
7. Always work with awareness, and when in doubt, do not take a chance that might lead to injury.

CONTRAINDICATIONS

Contraindications are conditions or situations that make the receiving of massage inadvisable because of the harm it might do. In the treatment model, a contraindication is "any symptom or circumstance indicating the inappropriateness of a form of treatment otherwise advisable" (Thomas, 1985). For **general contraindications,** avoid massage altogether. For **regional** or **local contraindications,** avoid only the specific area of the body affected.

Cautions are areas of potential danger that require thoughtful consideration and possible modifications of technique application. Cautions may or may not involve a pathology.

Practitioners should be alert to possible contraindications and cautions for every client. A **health history** taken during the initial visit will provide information about previous conditions or situations to be aware of and current health status. Appendix E contains health history forms for general wellness massage, as well as treatment-oriented sessions. Practitioners should check with regular clients at every session to see if their health status has changed in significant ways, especially if they are known to have a condition that is a contraindication or for which special cautions apply.

Knowledge of normal anatomy and physiology, as well as the nature of common pathologies, is important for the massage practitioner. Such knowledge may help prevent a well-meaning practitioner from causing harm. Those performing clinical applications need to be especially well versed in the pathologies that they are treating.

Be sure you fully understand the origin of any symptom of disease reported by a client. This will help in the selection of appropriate techniques and of positioning to best support the health of the massage recipient. If a client reports having a condition or disease that you are not familiar with, use your professional resources (see below) to get more information before proceeding with the massage.

Some general principles can be used to help determine whether receiving massage might be harmful. Some of the more common conditions and situations encountered in a massage practice are listed below.

PRINCIPLES FOR CONTRAINDICATIONS AND CAUTIONS

1. **Severe Distress.** *Do not perform massage when the recipient is experiencing severe distress.* For example:
   - Feels physically ill or nauseated
   - Is in severe pain
   - Has a fever
   - Has been seriously injured recently

2. **Acute Inflammation.** *Do not perform massage in the presence of acute inflammation.* Signs of inflammation are redness, heat, swelling, and pain. Any diagnosed condition that ends in "itis" is either a general or local contraindication.
   For example:
   - **Appendicitis.** Massage will spread inflammation throughout abdomen; avoid massage entirely.
   - **Rheumatoid arthritis.** Avoid massage over acutely inflamed joints (local contraindication); use caution even when not acute. Avoid traction of joints and spine.
   - **Phlebitis.** Inflammation of a vein; completely avoid site of disease, usually the legs.
   - **Locally inflamed tissues.** Signs are redness, heat, swelling, and pain. Avoid the surrounding area. On limbs, work proximal to the affected area.

3. **Loss of Structural Integrity.** *Understand the physician's recommendations and the relevant anatomy and physiology in cases where there is a loss of integrity in an area.*
   For example:
   - **Over recent surgery.** Only those specifically trained to work with scar tissue should attempt this work.
   - **Around burns.**
   - **Recent fractures.** Wait for physician's approval before performing massage in the area of recent fracture.
   - **Artificial joint replacements.** Check recommended restrictions in range of motion in replaced joints.

4. **Skin Conditions.** *Do not touch areas of the skin where there is a pathologic condition that is contagious or that may be worsened or spread by applying pressure or rubbing.*
   For example:
   - **Rashes**
   - **Boils**
   - **Athlete's foot**
   - **Herpes simplex (e.g., cold sores)**
   - **Impetigo.** A skin infection usually caused by staph or strep.
   - **Allergies.** Clients with skin allergies, may react negatively to certain oils or lotions used during massage. Check with recipient for substances to avoid, and be alert to skin reactions during the session.

5. **Decreased Sensation.** *Use extreme care in amount of pressure used when the client has decreased sensation.* Recipients cannot give accurate feedback regarding pressure and may also have

abnormal vasomotor response to the massage. May be due to stroke, diabetes, spinal cord injury, or medication.

6. **Increased Sensitivity to Touch.** *Massage only to recipient's tolerance or comfort when there is increased sensitivity to touch.* Clients who are ticklish or who have ticklish areas (e.g., feet) generally find light superficial stroking unpleasant and annoying. They may respond well to deeper, slower pressure, or to percussion techniques on the ticklish area.

7. **Cardiovascular Disorders.** *For clients with cardiovascular system disorders, research the condition carefully, including getting a physician's recommendation if serious.* Be aware of medications the client is taking and their potential as contraindications for massage.
   For example:
   - **High blood pressure.** If high, even with treatment, avoid circulatory massage.
   - **Low blood pressure.** Someone with low blood pressure may be more susceptible to fainting after receiving massage either on a table or on a massage chair. Be sure that such a client gets up slowly from a horizontal position.
   - **Cardiac arrhythmias or carotid bruit.** Avoid lateral and anterior neck.
   - **Severe atherosclerosis.** Massage only with the physician's permission, and then only very superficially.
   - **Severe varicose veins.** Tissues easily damaged and tendency to clotting; avoid massage of the area.
   - **Stroke.** Avoid circulatory massage, especially massage of neck. Blood thinners are usually prescribed after stroke, so use light pressure with all soft tissue manipulation.

8. **Spreading Disease by Circulation.** *Do not perform circulatory massage when there is a pathologic condition that might be spread through the lymph or cardiovascular systems.*
   For example:
   - Blood poisoning (lymphangitis). Inflammation of the lymphatic vessels; appears as steaks of red on the skin.
   - Malignant melanoma. A cancerous mole or tumor that metastasizes or spreads easily through the bloodstream or lymph system.
   - Swollen glands (i.e., lymph nodes). The immune system may be attempting to filter out bacteria or other pathogens, and draining them may cause an infection to spread.

9. **Bleeding and Bruising.** *Do not perform massage near an area where there is bleeding or bruising.*
   For example:
   - A bruise; avoid pressure to immediate area.
   - Whiplash or other acute trauma. Any situation in which there is tearing of tissue and where there may be bleeding into the tissue during the first 24 to 48 hours after the trauma; avoid massage in area, and if severe trauma avoid massage totally (see principle 1 above).

10. **Edema.** *Be sure of cause of edema before proceeding with massage.* Acute edema resulting from trauma, edema from inflammation due to bacterial or viral infection, pitted edema indicating tissue fragility, lymphatic obstruction due to parasites, and edema due to deep vein thrombosis are all contraindications for massage (Rattray, 2000). In cases of general edema caused by cardiac, liver, or kidney disease, avoid massage altogether.

11. **Compromised Immunity.** Be especially careful with personal and environmental hygiene when a client's immune function is depressed, e.g., after organ transplant when immune system is depressed with medication, with AIDS/HIV, or chronic fatigue syndrome.

12. **Osteoporosis.** Osteoporosis is a disease in which bones become fragile, brittle, and fracture easily. Avoid deep pressure and vigorous joint movements with a client with diagnosed osteoporosis, someone whom you suspect to have the disease, or those in a high-risk category (e.g., small, sedentary postmenopausal women; frail elderly; or someone with hyperkyphosis or "dowager's hump."

13. **Personal Appliances**
   - **Contact Lenses.** If a client is wearing contact lenses, take special care when working around the eyes to avoid pressure on the lenses and to avoid dislodging or moving the lenses. If using a face cradle when the recipient is prone, make sure that no pressure is put on the recipient's eyes. Taking the contact lenses out during massage is preferable.
   - **Hearing Aid.** If a client wears a hearing aid, be careful not to dislodge it while massaging around the ears. If it is turned on, massage on the head or around the ears may make a lot

of noise and be annoying. Remember that a client with severe hearing loss will not be able to hear you ask for feedback, or give directions. Be sure they can see you if you talk to them.

MEDICATIONS

Medications are used by an increasing number of people for a variety of ailments. This includes prescription, as well as over-the-counter, drugs. This also includes medications for short-term use, for example, common cold medications and pain-killers (analgesics) like aspirin; and longer term use, for example, heart medications or antidepressants. Massage practitioners need to be more aware of what their clients are taking, and understand the implications for massage therapy. Table 5–1 lists some of the most common considerations for massage and medications.

A client's medication may affect the scheduling of massage sessions, the length of sessions, techniques used and their application, or client behavior. Types of medications that require caution include, but are not limited to, those that alter sensation (e.g., numbing); affect the blood and circulation (e.g., prevent clotting, regulate blood sugar level); compromise tissue integrity (e.g., corticosteroids), or alter mood (e.g., depressants, antidepressants). Check with the health care provider who prescribed the medication if in doubt. (For more detailed guidelines on massage and medications, refer to *Massage Therapy & Medications: General Treatment Principles* by Randal S. Persad, 2001.)

Persons under the influence of alcohol or recreational drugs should not receive massage. These drugs alter sensation, affect mood, and in many cases, reduce good judgment.

Table 5–1   GUIDELINES FOR MASSAGE AND MEDICATIONS

The following chart summarizes some important points to consider when working with clients taking medication. If in doubt, check with clients and their health care providers about potential for harm and how to avoid it.

Scheduling of Sessions
- Massage **after** the client's scheduled dosage if the medication is needed for condition stability, i.e., to ensure maximum bioavailability of the medication. For example, with insulin-dependent diabetics, chronic pain clients, epileptic patients.
- Massage **before** or **shortly after** the client's scheduled dosage if medication decreases the client's perception of pain and their ability to give accurate feedback. For example, clients taking drugs like non-steroidal anti-inflammatories, narcotic analgesics, and central nervous system depressants.

Session Length
- <u>Shorten</u> the session if the medication significantly depletes the energy level of the client, causing abnormal fatigue. For example, clients taking hypertension medications, anti-anxiety drugs, and many antidepressants.
- <u>Shorten</u> the session if the medication significantly decreases the emotional stability of the client, causing them to feel emotionally volatile or easily overwhelmed. For example, clients taking corticosteroids (long term), or medications that have side effects that cause mood fluctuations, anxiety, or depression.

Selection of Massage Techniques
- **For drugs that alter clotting mechanisms,** e.g., anticoagulants, platelet inhibitors, and aspirin and other non-steroidal anti-inflammatories—Avoid high-pressure techniques like muscle stripping, deep kneading, ischemic compression, and cross-fiber friction.
- **For drugs that alter protective responses,** e.g., centrally acting muscle relaxants, narcotic analgesics, anti-anxiety drugs—Avoid deep massage, tense-relax stretching, and any technique that requires accurate client feedback for safe application.
- **For drugs that compromise tissue integrity,** e.g., corticosteroids, long-term use or injected directly into joints or tissues—Avoid deep pressure techniques, heavy tapotement, forced stretching, skin rolling and wringing.
- **For drugs that mask pain responses,** e.g., anti-inflammatories, analgesics—Rely less on client feedback and more on observation and palpation to determine appropriate pressure and technique applications.
- **For drugs that alter a client's cooperativeness,** or **make them less communicative,** e.g., narcotic analgesics and anti-anxiety medications—Take time to ask questions as needed for accurate health histories and ongoing feedback during massage.

Information from **Massage Therapy & Medications: General Treatment Principles** by Randall S. Persad (Toronto, Canada: Curties-Overzet Publications, 2001.)

PERSON-CENTERED MASSAGE

It is easy to lose sight of the person when there is pathology involved. From the wellness perspective, massage can be thought of as person-centered rather than pathology-centered. In other words, practitioners may give massage to people with pathologies, but the people are more than their pathologies. In fact, practitioners often find themselves working around pathologies.

This may be the case when a person has a condition for which deep or vigorous massage is contraindicated. A light massage may be appropriate to add an element of care, comfort, and stress reduction as a complement to standard medical care. For example, there would be few pathologies for which stroking the hand or head of an elderly person is contraindicated.

Most of the contraindications and cautions mentioned above are based on common sense, given some knowledge of anatomy, physiology, and pathology. If the giver of massage is motivated by sincere concern, is gentle in giving, and is receptive and responsive to feedback from the recipient, the experience will most likely be a healthy one for both people. Even in the hands of a child, massage given with love and sensitivity can be supportive and helpful.

RESOURCES

Personal professional libraries should include some basic resources for information about conditions and pathologies commonly encountered in massage practices. This information can provide insights into possible contraindications and cautions, and implications for performing massage. Pathologies may also be researched at a local library, a library at a school of medicine, and on the Internet. See Table 4–1, Sources of Information about Clinical Applications of Massage.

A basic **professional library** for massage practitioners should include a good anatomy and physiology text, an atlas of human anatomy, a general pathology text, and a medical dictionary. Pathology books written especially for massage therapists have been published recently, and are valuable references that include special considerations for massage including contraindications and cautions. (Refer to *Clincal Massage Therapy*, by Fiona Rattray and Linda Ludwig (2000); *Massage Therapist's Guide to Pathology*, by Ruth Werner (2000); *Pathology A to Z—A Handbook for Massage Therapists*, by Kalyani Premkumar (1999).)

Practitioners working with special populations should have applicable references for basic information. There are books available on massage with specific populations (e.g., pregnant women, children, elderly, cancer patients). An up-to-date general reference book for common medications and their effects and side effects would also be useful.

One of the best resources for information may be the recipient himself or herself. Recipients are often very knowledgeable about their own pathologies, especially if they have lived with a chronic condition for some time. The recipient's health care providers may also serve as valuable resources when there is any doubt as to the safety of someone receiving massage.

SUMMARY

One of the most basic rules of giving therapeutic massage is to do no harm. Massage practitioners should be aware of endangerment sites, contraindications and cautions to ensure the health and safety of clients.

Endangerment sites are areas of the body where delicate structures are less protected and therefore more easily damaged when receiving massage. Endangerment sites include the anterior neck, vertebral column, thoracic cage, axilla, elbow, umbilicus, kidney area, inguinal area, popliteal fossa, eyes, and the major veins in the extremities. General principles for performing massage related to endangerment sites include adjusting pressure to avoid damage, care around joints, avoiding pressure directly on major arteries and nerves, care around abnormal structures, and always working with awareness.

Contraindications are conditions that make receiving massage inadvisable because of the harm it might do. For general contraindications, massage should be avoided altogether. For local or regional contraindications, only the specific area of the body affected should be avoided. Cautions are areas of potential danger that require thoughtful consideration and possible modifications of technique application.

Acute distress and acute inflammation are general contraindications for massage. Other contraindications and cautions include loss of structural integrity, skin problems, decreased sensation, increased sensation, cardiovascular disorders, diseases spread by circulation, bleeding and bruising, edema, compromised immunity, osteoporosis. Take caution with clients wearing contact lenses and hearing aids.

Clients may be taking medications including prescription and over-the-counter drugs. A client's medication may affect the scheduling of massage sessions, the length of sessions, techniques used and their application, or their behavior. Types of medications that require caution include those that alter sensation, affect the blood and circulation, compromise tissue integrity, or alter mood. Persons under the influence of alcohol or recreational drugs should not receive massage since they alter sensation, affect mood, and reduce good judgment.

From the wellness perspective, massage can be thought of as person centered. Practitioners may give massage to people with pathologies, but the people are more than their pathologies.

Personal professional libraries should include an anatomy/physiology text, atlas of human anatomy, a pathology book, medical dictionary, and books specific to special populations encountered in practice. Access to the Internet is useful for finding information about specific pathologies. The recipient him- or herself and caregivers are also good sources of information about safety for receiving massage.

A look ahead . . .

Establishing and maintaining a successful massage practice involves many factors, including developing good client relationships and creating a therapeutic environment. Longevity is secured by self-care measures that preserve your own health and wellbeing. Effective application of massage requires an understanding of various performance elements. Chapter 6 describes general principles for giving massage that provide the context for performing healing massage techniques.

REFERENCES

Persad, R. (2001). *Massage Therapy & Medications*. Ontario, Canada: Curties-Overzet Publications.

Premkumar, K. (1999) *Pathology A to Z–A handbook for massage therapists*. Calgary, Canada: VanPub Books.

Rattray, F., and Ludwig, L. (2000). *Clinical massage therapy: Understanding, assessing and treating over 70 conditions*. Toronto, Canada: Talus Incorporated.

Thomas, C. L., ed. (1985). *Taber's cyclopedic medical dictionary*. Philadelphia: F. A. Davis.

Werner, R. (2000). *Massage therapist's guide to pathology*, 2nd ed. Philadelphia: Lippincott Williams & Wilkins.

STUDY GUIDE

LEARNING OUTCOMES

Use the learning outcomes at the beginning of the chapter as a guide to your studies. Perform the task given in each outcome, either in writing or verbally into a tape recorder or to a study partner. This may start as an "open book" exercise, and then later from memory.

KEY TERMS/CONCEPTS

To study key words and concepts listed at the beginning of this chapter, choose one or more of the following exercises. Writing or talking about ideas helps you remember them better, and explaining them helps deepen your understanding.

1. Write a one- or two-sentence explanation of each key word and concept.

2. With a study partner, take turns explaining key words and concepts verbally.

3. Make up sentences using one or more key words or concepts.

4. Read your sentences to a study partner, who will ask you to clarify your meaning.

STUDY OUTLINE

The following questions test your memory of the main concepts in this chapter. Locate the answers in the text using the page number given for each question.

1. One of most basic rules of giving therapeutic massage is to _____ harm. (p. 80)

2. An endangerment site or contraindication in one form of massage and bodywork may be considered _____ for a different form. (p. 80)

Endangerment Sites

1. Endangerment sites are areas of the body where delicate structures are _____ and, therefore, may be more easily _____ when receiving massage. (p. 80)

2. Endangerment sites for Western massage on the anterior part of the body include _____ _____. (pp. 80–82)

3. Endangerment sites for Western massage on the posterior part of the body include _____ _____. (pp. 80–82)

4. Deep effleurage or stroking should always move from _____ to _____ to avoid damage to the valves in the large veins. (p. 82)

General Principles of Safety around Endangerment Sites

1. Always adjust the pressure you use to match the _____, the _____, and the _____ you are working on. (p. 82)

2. Avoid _____ pressure over nerves, blood vessels, and lymph vessels close to the body surface. (p. 82)

3. Move off of the spot if you feel a _____, or if the client reports _____ sensations indicating pressure on a nerve. (p. 82)

4. Proceed with _____ around abnormal structures. (p. 82)

5. Always work with _____, and do not take a chance that may lead to _____. (p. 82)

Contraindications

1. Contraindications are conditions or situations that make receiving massage inadvisable because of the _____. (p. 82)

2. Avoid massage altogether for _____ contraindications. (p. 82)

3. Avoid the area affected for _____ or _____ contraindications. (p. 82)

4. Cautions are areas of potential danger that require _____ and possible modifications of _____. (p. 82)

5. A client _____ should be taken to identify possible contraindications and cautions. (p. 82)

Principles for Contraindications

1. Severe distress is a general contraindication for massage, for example, _____, _____, _____, and _____. (p. 83)

2. Acute inflammation is a general or local contraindication for massage, e.g., any condition that ends in "_____." (p. 83)

3. Loss of structural integrity occurs with surgery, _____, _____, and _____. (p. 83)

4. Avoid massage near a _____ skin condition, or when massage would make a skin condition worse. (p. 83)

5. _____ may prevent a client from giving accurate feedback regarding pressure, so use care in amount of pressure used during massage. (p. 83)

6. _____ to touch calls for massage only to recipient's tolerance level. (p. 84)

7. Avoid massage when there is pathology that might spread through blood or lymph _____ _____. (p. 84)

8. Bruising is a _____ contraindication. (p. 84)

9. In cases of edema from infection, deep vein thrombosis, and general edema from cardiac, liver, or kidney disease _____. (p. 84)

10. A client's compromised immunity calls for extra care in personal and environmental _____. (p. 84)

11. Avoid _____ on clients with diagnosed osteoporosis, or frail clients in high-risk categories. (p. 84)

Medications

1. A client's medications may affect the _____ and _____ of massage sessions, techniques used, their method of application, and client _____. (p. 85)

2. Types of medications that require caution include those that _____, _____, _____, and _____. (p. 85 ; Table 5–1)

3. Clients under the influence of recreational drug or alcohol should not receive massage since these drugs _____, _____ _____. (p. 85)

Person-Centered Massage

1. From a wellness perspective, massage can be thought of as _____- centered rather than *pathology-centered*. (p. 86)

2. Light massage that adds care, comfort and stress reduction may be appropriate even for someone for whom more vigorous massage is _____ _____. (p. 86)

Resources

1. Resources for information on pathologies and conditions can be found _____, _____, _____. (p. 86; Table 4–1)

2. Every massage practitioner should have a personal _____ for looking up information related to contraindications and cautions. (p. 86)

3. The client himself or herself may be one of the best sources of information about their condition and relevant _____ when they are receiving massage. (p. 86)

FOR GREATER UNDERSTANDING

The following exercises are designed to take you from the realm of theory into the real world. They will help give you a deeper understanding of the subjects covered in this chapter. Action words are underlined to emphasize the variety of activities presented to address different learning styles, and to encourage deeper thinking.

1. On yourself, or working with a study partner, explore the surface anatomy of the major endangerment sites. Carefully and safely feel the structure of the area and visualize the tissues, and anatomical structures underneath the skin. Imagine how deep specific structures are to the surface and how exposed to pressure. Use an anatomy book or atlas as an aid to visualization.

2. Choose a specific pathology to study. Locate information about contraindications and cautions related to the pathology. Identify implications for giving massage to a person with the pathology studied. Discuss with a study partner or group.

3. Interview someone who receives massage regularly and who has the pathology studied in problem 2. Ask them to identify any restrictions related to massage

that they are aware of related to their pathology. Compare this with information you have located. Explain to them what you found out related to contraindications and cautions.

4. Interview a massage practitioner who specializes in clinical applications, or the director of a clinical massage setting. Ask them about the types of pathologies they see in their practices and the cautions they take in working with those clients. Report to a study partner or group.

5. Interview a person taking one or more medications. List the medications they take and the related pathology that they are being treated for. Identify modifications you would make in a massage session with this person. Discuss your session plan with a study partner or group.

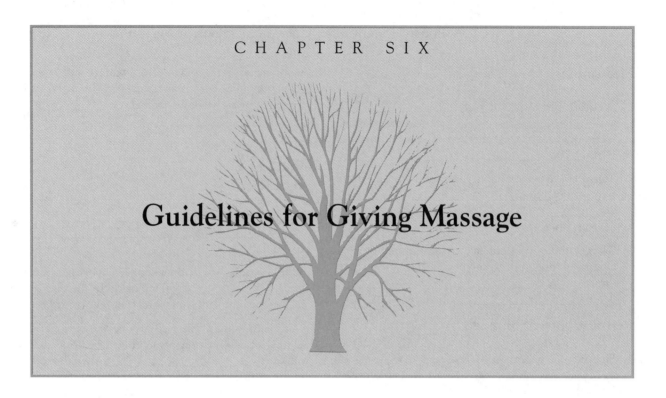

CHAPTER SIX

Guidelines for Giving Massage

LEARNING OUTCOMES

After studying this chapter, the student will have information to:

1. Establish good therapeutic relationships.
2. Maintain professional boundaries.
3. Project a professional demeanor.
4. Appreciate the significance of touch in massage.
5. Be aware of gender considerations in a massage practice.
6. Demonstrate the use of informed consent.
7. Apply the seven-step intervention model.
8. Engage in appropriate level of talk during massage.
9. Maintain confidentiality of client information.
10. Comply with HIPAA standards regarding client records.
11. Create an ideal physical environment for massage.
12. Choose topical substances used in massage.
13. Provide for client safety and comfort.
14. Take physical and emotional self-care measures.
15. Analyze the elements of massage performance.

 MEDIALINK

A companion CD-ROM, included free with each new copy of this book, supplements the techniques presented in this chapter. Insert the CD-ROM to watch video clips of massage techniques being demonstrated. This multimedia feature is designed to help you add a new dimension to your learning.

KEY TERMS/CONCEPTS

Air quality	Lighting	Self-care
Boundaries	Liniment	Side-lying position
Cleanliness/neatness	Lotion	Sound
Confidentiality	Oil	Specificity
Counter-transference	Pacing	Standards of practice
Cross-gender massage	Positioning	Supine position
Direction	Pressure	Tenting
Draping	Professional demeanor	Therapeutic relationship
Dressing arrangements	Prone position	Topical substances
Dual relationships	Reclining position	Touch
Emotional release	Rhythm	Transference
Feedback	Room temperature	Verbal interaction
Informed consent	Routine	
Intervention Model	Same-gender massage	

Guidelines for providing safe, effective massage and bodywork are presented in this chapter. They take into consideration the nature of the therapeutic relationship, the physical environment, the comfort and safety of the recipient, self-care for the practitioner, and the performance of the massage itself. These guidelines are relevant no matter what specific form, approach, or style of massage and bodywork you practice.

THE THERAPEUTIC RELATIONSHIP

The **therapeutic relationship** involves an implicit agreement regarding the roles of the massage practitioner and the client. The role of the practitioner is to provide massage within the scope of practice of their training and credentials. The role of the client is to receive massage, participate in the therapy, and fulfill financial and appointment obligations within the agreement.

Maintaining clarity about the roles in the therapeutic relationship is achieved by keeping professional **boundaries.** A boundary is defined as "a limit that separates one person from another," and its function is "to protect the integrity of each person." Keeping good boundaries includes practicing within personal limitations, not exploiting the relationship for personal gain, limiting the impact of transference and counter-transference, avoiding dual relationships, not engaging in any sexual activity, and respecting the client's freedom of choice and self-determination (NCBTMB Standards of Practice).

McIntosh (1999) identifies some common mistakes related to boundaries. The first involves going outside of your area of expertise, for example, claiming to provide treatment beyond your training, or advertising expertise in some skill after a weekend workshop, giving advice outside of the scope of practice, or delving into emotional problems without training in psychotherapy. Another mistake is losing the distinction between personal and professional lives; for example, going out socially with clients, or mutual sharing of personal lives.

Boundaries within most health care settings are usually well established. However, boundaries in the context of a private massage practice, or in a spa, health club, or similar non-medical setting need to be carefully maintained by the practitioner.

Dual Relationships

A **dual relationship** is any relationship other than the primary one of practitioner and client. For example, if your client is also your friend, a tenant, an employer, or your stockbroker, there is potential for conflict in the practitioner–client relationship. Dual relationships can end in confusion of roles and weakening professional boundaries. Dual relationships should be avoided if possible, and entered into only with caution.

Transference and Counter-Transference

Transference happens when clients respond to practitioners as they might have responded to an important person from their childhood, e.g., parent, teacher, or other authority figure. They *transfer* those positive or negative feelings onto the practitioner. It is an unconscious, irrational phenomenon.

Counter-transference is similar, except that practitioners transfer feelings from their past onto the client. In both cases, the feelings have little to do with the actual relationship with the massage practitioner and client. The boundaries between the present and the past become blurred.

In a typical case of transference, a client might "fall into the illusion that we are wiser and somehow better than they are," or try too hard to please us as they would a parent. Transference can also manifest as sexual feelings or "crushes." Maintaining good professional boundaries, and awareness of the potential confusion, can help keep clarity in these situations. (For a comprehensive discussion of the practitioner–client relationship refer to *The Educated Heart* by Nina McIntosh, 1999; and *The Ethics of Touch* by Ben Benjamin and Cherie Sohnen-Moe, 2003.)

PROFESSIONAL DEMEANOR

The **professional demeanor,** i.e., appearance and behavior of the practitioner, are important in putting the receiver of massage at ease. Your demeanor should inspire confidence and a sense of safety, and help establish the professional nature of the relationship. This is especially important in a relationship based primarily on touch.

Clothing should be neat, clean, modest, and comfortable, allowing freedom of movement. Avoid clothing that may be sexually suggestive such as tight pants, short shorts, and shirts that expose the chest or midriff. Jewelry should be minimal. Avoid rings that might scratch the client, and dangling bracelets and necklaces.

The practitioner should be free from offensive odors. This includes odors from the body and clothes, and strong perfumes and colognes. Some practitioners bathe or change shirts during the day to stay fresh. After a spicy meal, or just a long day, you may want to consider a breath freshener. Smokers should be particularly aware to eliminate odors on their clothes, hands, and breath.

Language used by the practitioner also sets the tone of the professional relationship. Practitioners should speak in a way that can be clearly understood, avoiding unduly technical and scientific language and jargon. Practitioners should speak to the understanding and educational level of the receiver. However, care should be taken in referring to the body, and sexually suggestive words and expressions avoided.

The physical contact inherent in massage establishes a close relationship between practitioner and receiver. This relationship should be understanding and sympathetic, but never personal.

TOUCHING ANOTHER PERSON

It has been observed that "touch is our most social sense," because it implies interaction with another person. Human beings have an innate touch hunger. Touch is essential for proper growth and development in infants, and for well being at all stages of life. Touch deprivation has been linked to increased stress, physical violence, sleep disturbance, and suppressed immune response. (For further information about the importance of touch read *Touching: The Significance of the Human Skin* by Ashley Montagu, 1978; and *Touch* by Tiffany Field, 2001).

Touch is the primary mode of personal interaction during massage. It is essential that the practitioner be knowledgeable about the psychosocial implications of touch, as well as its physical nature. Practitioners giving massage need to be skilled in touch.

More Basic than Technique

Touch is more basic than technique. To touch means "to come into contact with." In massage, that contact happens on a physical and an energetic level, and is achieved primarily through the hands of the practitioner. From the holistic perspective, you touch the whole person, and what may seem to be only physical touch often has profound effects on the mind, emotions, and spirit of the receiver.

Touch can communicate care and compassion, confidence, calmness, focus, and skillfulness. It can also convey anxiety, apprehension, anger, distractedness, disinterestedness, and lack of confidence. Practitioners should always be aware of their state of being, because whatever it is, it will be communicated through touch to a sensitive receiver. Prepare yourself to give massage by being aware of your intention to be caring and compassionate, and by becoming calm and focused.

A unique feature of touch is that when you touch another person, you are touched yourself. When you are giving touch, you are also receiving touch. This is one reason why giving massage can be such a rewarding experience. However, this can also necessitate some self-care. For example, a practitioner who comes in contact with someone who is experiencing grief, anger, anxiety, or extreme stress can pick up some of the negative effects of these emotions. Self-care techniques like meditation, talking to a colleague, or consciously "washing away" negative energy after a session can limit the degree to which you are affected by the negative "vibes" of your clients. It is important to take care of yourself, while you remain a source of care and compassion for your clients.

Touch and the Therapeutic Relationship

Comfort levels with touch vary for a number of reasons. People from different cultural backgrounds will have different experiences with and attitudes toward touch. For example, studies have shown that people from Great Britain and northern Europe experience touch less in social interaction than those from Mediterranean countries such as Spain, Italy, and Greece (Montagu, 1978).

Appropriate touch in one situation or with one client may be inappropriate in other circumstances. The practitioner must cultivate an awareness of their own, and each client's, comfort with touch. The practitioner's challenge is to create an openness to the touch of massage.

The practitioner should be clear about the difference between friendly, caring, and even affectionate touch and sexual touch. Sexual touch is never appropriate in a professional setting.

Many men and women have been the victims of physical and sexual abuse. Many more have endured the traumatic stress of natural disaster, war, or other disturbing events. These people need special care regarding touch. The practitioner should be aware of each receiver's reaction to touch, and ensure that he or she feels safe and comfortable.

It is possible that the receiver of massage may interpret your touch in a way that was not intended. He or she may project his or her own issues regarding touch onto you. Your touch may be perceived as abusive or sexual when you had no such intention. When that transference happens, clear verbal communication is essential to clear up any misperceptions. Clear professional boundaries are especially important in a therapeutic relationship based on touch.

PERMISSION TO TOUCH

When a person agrees to receive massage from a practitioner, there is an implicit permission to touch. However, when the touch occurs in certain areas, especially those that feel vulnerable, there should be an *explicit* permission to touch that specific area for therapeutic purposes. This is true for areas like the upper or inner thigh, the lower abdomen, and around breast tissue in women.

Informed Consent

In an **informed consent** statement, the practitioner explains what they are going to do (e.g., massage the abdomen), why they are doing it (i.e., therapeutic intention), what the client should expect, and asks permission to touch the area. The client should clearly understand that they have the option of saying "no" either before or at any time during the proposed action. The elements of informed consent are summarized in Table 6–1.

In cases where the recipient has suffered physical or sexual abuse, there may be additional vulnerable areas. For example, if someone has been physically abused with beatings on the back of the legs and buttocks, these may be emotionally sensitive areas to be considerate of and receive permission to work on. You may not know beforehand about these situations, so it is wise to be aware of the client's reactions to touch throughout the session.

Informed consent is a good idea at any time the recipient might be unpleasantly surprised. For example, communicate with the recipient before going deep into the tissues, or pressing into painful

Table 6–1   ELEMENTS OF INFORMED CONSENT

Used when the massage practitioner plans to touch a vulnerable body area (e.g., upper or inner thigh, lower abdomen, or breast tissue in women), or plans to apply a technique that may feel strange or cause unusual or increased pain.

1. Explain what you propose to do.
2. Explain your intent.
3. Describe what the client should expect.
4. Give the client the option to say no either before beginning or at any time during the application. Be alert to nonverbal as well as verbal signals.
5. Ask permission to touch the area.

Examples
Intended action: To massage into the muscle attachments on the inner thigh.

1. "I would like to massage your upper thigh thoroughly, including the inner thigh."
2. "This will help relax those tense muscles in your legs. The muscle attachments are at the knee and the pelvis."
3. "I'll secure the drape around the groin so that you will be covered appropriately, and will just massage up to the drape. The inner thigh can be sensitive, so it may feel strange to you."
4. "At any time, if you don't like how it feels, let me know and I'll stop."
5. "Is it OK to go ahead?"

Intended action: To apply pressure to sensitive points on the cervical muscles.

1. "I'd like to press some of the sensitive spots on your neck."
2. "I suspect that they are trigger points causing your tension headaches. Pressing the points helps de-activate and relieve them."
3. "You will feel pain if I press directly on a trigger point, and it may also refer pain into your head. I will ask for feedback on the location of the points, and the amount of pressure I'm using."
4. "If the pressure seems to be too much, let me know and I'll reduce it. And we can stop at any time."
5. "Is it OK to begin?"

trigger points. If you sense that the recipient is uncomfortable physically or emotionally with your touch, it is best to ask permission to continue.

GENDER CONSIDERATIONS

Because of its basis in touch and the interpersonal nature of massage, there are certain considerations related to gender to be aware of. These may be peculiar to a person's cultural background, or to the professional setting. Professional demeanor, good boundaries, and good verbal communication skills will help make the following situations less troublesome. This is true regardless of the gender of the practitioner and the receiver.

Cross-gender massage has become more common. When women give massage to men, or men to women, they need to be especially clear about the non-sexual nature of their work and establish clear professional boundaries. Sexualizing the professional relationship by either party is unacceptable, and if allowed by the practitioner, is unethical.

Same-gender massage may also be an issue for some clients. In some cases, a client or patient may unconsciously transfer their personal aversion to homosexual orientation to the practitioner–client relationship. This presents problems in a same-gender situation, whether the practitioner is homosexual or not. In Western culture, touch is often equated with sexual touch, so that any touch by another person may have sexual overtones. Practitioners need to be mindful of this cultural dilemma. This poses special problems when nurturing and compassion are called for. Practitioners need to meet the needs of their clients in a way that is comfortable and acceptable.

Male practitioners working with women clients should be mindful that most cases of sexual harassment and abuse are committed towards women. Chances are high that some of the women recipients of massage have such histories. It is also possible that the women may not identify this past experience as a problem in the present. Men must approach all women as possible survivors of abuse and must be aware of and especially sensitive to their need for clear boundaries.

Needless to say, any of the considerations mentioned above could apply to either gender. Clear boundaries and professional demeanor are keys to addressing these gender considerations.

INTERVENTION MODEL

During the massage itself, if a client touches you inappropriately, appears to be sexually aroused, makes comments of a sexual nature, or otherwise appears to sexualize the situation, apply an intervention model. Steps in the seven-step **intervention model** include:

1. Stop the session using assertive behavior.
2. Describe the behavior you are concerned about.
3. Ask the client to clarify their behavior.
4. Re-state your intent and professional boundaries.
5. Evaluate the client's response.
6. Continue or discontinue the session as appropriate.
7. Document the situation.

(For further discussion refer to *The Ethics of Touch* by Ben Benjamin and Cherie Sohnen-Moe, 2003.)

It is important not to ignore client misbehavior. A practitioner should never continue the session if they feel that the client is sexualizing the massage. The seven-step intervention model is summarized in Table 6–2.

TALKING AND FEEDBACK

Whether, and how much, **verbal interaction** should go on during a massage session depends on the purpose of the session and the needs of the receiver. The practitioner should be aware of the amount and nature of talking taking place, and structure the session in the best interests of the receiver.

When relaxation is a primary goal, talking should be kept to a minimum. Silence allows receivers to sink further into a relaxed state and be quietly with themselves. They are more likely to be receptive to the relaxing effects of music playing and to the "letting go" that happens during relaxation. A soft voice should be used for necessary communications.

People who are nervous about receiving massage, especially for the first time, may need more verbal interaction. The practitioner may want to give more direction, describe what he or she is doing and ask for frequent feedback to help put the person at ease.

Certain types of techniques require frequent **feedback** on pain level for the safety of the recipient, and for information on the effectiveness of techniques. For example, the receiver may give feedback to

Table 6–2   SEVEN-STEP INTERVENTION MODEL

Used when the client's behavior is inappropriate; for example, if they sexualize the session in any way.

1. Stop the session using assertive behavior.
2. Describe the behavior you are concerned about.
3. Ask the client to clarify their behavior.
4. Re-state your intent and professional boundaries.
5. Evaluate the client's response.
6. Continue or discontinue the session as appropriate.
7. Document the situation.

help pinpoint the precise location of trigger points, or to determine how much to stretch a muscle safely. Feedback can take different forms. A receiver whose face winces in pain, or whose muscles tighten up, or who gives a deep sigh is offering feedback on his or her state of being. The practitioner should be aware of this nonverbal feedback and use it during the flow of the session.

Sometimes a recipient will experience what is called an **emotional release.** Suppressed emotions may be stored in our bodies, and these feelings may be released in a massage session as a person is touched, or as the recipient relaxes and lets down emotional defenses. This may be as simple as a sigh or crying. Practitioners should not attempt to delve into the meaning of such a release of emotions, but should simply be present and supportive.

Practitioners can also give useful feedback to recipients. For example, they may call the receiver's attention to a muscular holding pattern or mention when a formerly tense muscle relaxes. In this way, a person can become more aware of his or her own body.

Talking may also be of a more social nature. This should be kept to a minimum in most cases during a session. An exception may be an elderly person who has little other social contact and wants to talk, or a person who has recently experienced something upsetting and needs to talk about it. Careful judgment is needed in instances like these to prevent crossing professional boundaries.

Practitioners should avoid talking to receivers about their own lives and troubles. A good rule of thumb is to follow the lead of the receiver by listening and responding only to the receiver's questions or comments. This helps you determine whether the interaction is coming from your own or the receiver's needs. You should not get your needs met at the expense of the therapeutic relationship. Practitioners should be especially mindful of their scope of practice and not delve into psychotherapy unless properly trained. It may be useful to keep a referral list for receivers who ask for help finding a psychotherapist.

Practitioners should develop skill in recognizing and establishing the amount and nature of verbal interaction that is best in a given situation. Since the primary mode of communication in massage is touch, usually less talk is better.

CONFIDENTIALITY

In a professional relationship, there is an implicit trust that the practitioner will keep information about the receiver confidential. The ethical principle of **confidentiality** is based on the client's right to privacy. This includes information found on a health history form; information told to the practitioner during a session, or before or after a session; and observations about a client related to physical, mental, or emotional condition. It is a matter of respecting the privacy of the receiver, and in medical settings, confidentiality is a legal matter.

There are exceptions to the general rule of confidentiality, for example, talking to another health professional about a receiver's condition in order to serve him or her better. A practitioner receiving professional supervision may discuss a case with a supervisor. Confidential information may also be divulged if required by law, or in cases of emergency.

In non-medical settings such as health clubs, salons or spas, confidentiality is a matter of professional standards, and respect for the receiver. It is considered unethical to gossip about a client or to give information about him or her without permission.

The National Certification Board for Therapeutic Massage and Bodywork has published a **Standards of Practice** that addresses issues related to professionalism, confidentiality, roles and boundaries, and prevention of sexual misconduct. The standards give more detail about acceptable professional behavior. The standards of practice can be found on the Internet (www.ncbtmb.org).

HIPAA PRIVACY RULE

In 1996, the U.S. Congress passed the Health Insurance Portability and Accountability Act. The HIPAA Privacy Rule is a federal standard designed to protect the medical records of individuals. In general, HIPAA requires a health care provider to inform patients/clients about their privacy rights and how their information can be used. Providers must adopt and implement privacy procedures, and train employees to comply. In an office or clinic, a person must be designated as responsible for seeing that privacy policies are followed.

Patients/clients should be able to see their records, and obtain copies upon request. They may ask for corrections to records if they find mistakes.

Patient/client records must be secured, and kept away from anyone who does not need to see them. For example, records should be kept in locked file cabinets preferably in isolated records rooms, and passwords needed to access client files on the computer. Patients/clients must give written consent for use and disclosure of information for treatment, payment, and health care operations.

HIPAA is administered by the U.S. Department of Health & Human Services (HHS), and enforcement and complaints are handled by the HHS Office of Civil Rights (OCR). Information about HIPAA can be found on the HHS website at (www.hhs.gov/ocr/hipaa).

THE PHYSICAL ENVIRONMENT

Massage Tables and Chairs

Massage tables are specially designed for the needs of the massage practitioner. A massage table should be adjustable in height and have a removable, adjustable face cradle. Tables vary in length, width, and type of padding and covering (e.g., soft or hard vinyl). A typical portable massage table and a face cradle are shown in Figure 6–1a,b.

The type of table you choose depends on the type of work you do, and the setting. For example, if you work in a setting in which tables are rarely moved, you may want a stationary table for its stability. If you carry your table from place to place, you will want a lightweight portable table. If you do sports massage, you may want a narrow table. Some shiatsu practitioners get up on the table for better leverage, and so a wider table is more practical. There are special tables for pregnant clients, and tables with hinges that permit a reclining or partial sitting position.

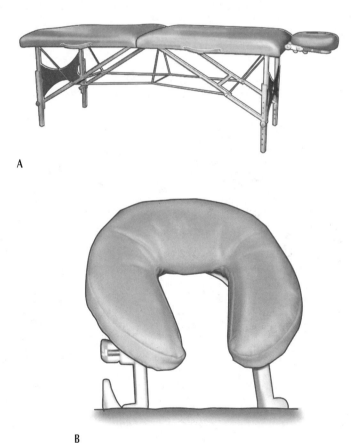

A

B

FIGURE 6–1. Massage table and face cradle. **A.** Adjustable massage table. **B.** Adjustable face cradle.

Your table is an important investment. To see a variety of tables, you may want to visit a massage supplies showroom, or a trade show or convention, or check table manufacturers on the Internet. A good quality table is a wise investment.

The massage chair is specially designed to provide maximum comfort while receiving massage in a seated position while fully clothed. Chairs usually have a seat, knee rests, armrest, chest cushion, and face cradle. There should be adjustments for the chest cushion and the face cradle. A typical massage chair is shown in Figure 6–2a,b. This type of massage chair was introduced in the 1980s, and chairs are continually undergoing improvement in design.

Whenever possible, practitioners should use equipment specially designed for massage. However, sometimes practitioners have to improvise in less than ideal situations. For example, massage may be given to people in wheelchairs, to the bedridden elderly or ill, to workers at their desks, or even at poolside at a swim meet. In these circumstances, care should be taken to ensure the safety and comfort of the receiver while providing for good body mechanics for the practitioner.

The Massage Space

Massage is given in a variety of settings, including private offices, chiropractic clinics, health clubs, spas or salons, training rooms, medical clinics and hospitals, nursing homes, and hospices. On-site massage in special massage chairs is given in commercial businesses and other public places. Whatever the location, there are certain factors in the environment that will help maximize the benefits of the session. Important factors to consider include the room temperature, air quality, lighting, sound, dressing arrangements, and overall cleanliness and neatness.

The **room temperature** should be warm enough so that the receiver is comfortable. When the receiver is partially or fully unclothed under a drape, a comfortable room temperature is usually around 75°F. Receivers often get cold during massage as they relax. Ways to help keep them warm include an electric mattress pad underneath the bottom sheet, a heat lamp overhead, or a blanket on top. Turning up the heat in the room is a less desirable solution, because the practitioner may then get overheated while working.

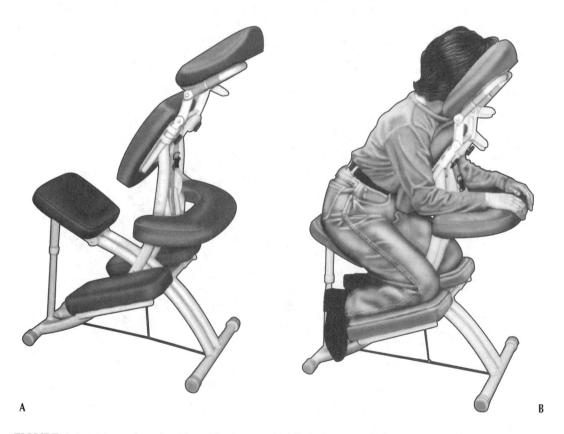

A   B

FIGURE 6–2. Massage chair. **A.** Adjustable massage chair. **B.** Recipient positioned in massage chair.

Air quality should be fresh and pleasant, and rooms well ventilated. This may be a challenge in some places like hospitals or beauty salons where strong odors are present, or in buildings where smoking is allowed. Also consider allergens such as pollen and animal hair. Electric air cleaners may be used, and in the summer, air conditioners can help keep air fresh. However, when using an air conditioner, be mindful of the warmth of the room.

Lighting is an important consideration. Soft and indirect lighting are more restful than harsh and direct lighting. Overhead lighting may shine in the receiver's eyes when he or she is supine on a table, as will the sun if doing massage in an outdoor setting such as at a spa or at an athletic event. In places where overhead lighting cannot be controlled, you may provide the receiver with a light shield for the eyes when he or she is supine.

Sound can help create a peaceful and healing environment, or a stimulating one. Music elicits certain emotions and is often used to create a particular effect. In general, popular and vocal music should be avoided if the intent is to relax. Use of popular music may also confuse the professional relationship, since it is normally heard in social situations. Numerous CDs and tapes are available with music specifically designed for relaxation, and some specifically for massage.

Sometimes it is desirable to have a background of more stimulating music, for example, when the receiver must go back to work immediately, or for an athlete receiving massage just before an event. Music that is stimulating, while not stressful or frenetic, is appropriate in these situations. The receiver's taste in music should be taken into consideration and a variety of choices made available.

For some people, silence, or a fish tank bubbling in the background, is most restful. Fish tanks are known to have a relaxing effect on most people. There are also machines that produce "white noise" to mask annoying outside noises.

Dressing arrangements should be convenient and provide a private space for receivers to disrobe and get onto the table. If there is only one table in a room, then the practitioner may simply leave the room while the recipient is disrobing. In a situation where there is more than one table in the room, such as in a training room or clinic, gowns may be provided for the receivers to use when walking from the dressing area to the massage table. Robes are often provided for this purpose at spas.

It is generally considered a breach of professional boundaries for recipients to be seen naked as they are preparing for massage. Exceptions are in cases where the person receiving massage needs assistance dressing, such as with the elderly or disabled. Even in these cases, care should be taken to preserve the modesty of the recipient as much as possible.

Overall **cleanliness** and **neatness** of the space where massage is given should be maintained. Not only does this provide a sanitary environment for the recipient, it helps create a calm, peaceful, and cheerful atmosphere. Oil bottles should be neatly arranged and wiped clean, and clean linens neatly stacked or stored away. Used sheets and towels should be placed in a closed container and kept out of sight. Floors should be cleaned, carpets vacuumed frequently, and furniture dusted.

There may be local health department regulations concerning sanitation in places where massage is provided. These may include the materials used on the floor, how sheets and towels are stored, and how floors should be cleaned.

TOPICAL SUBSTANCES

Many forms of massage and bodywork use some kind of topical substance to enhance their effects or to minimize skin friction during the application of techniques. These are classified as liniments, oils, lotions, or combinations of these.

Liniments have been used for centuries for sore and stiff muscles and for sprains and bruises. They are particularly popular with athletes. A **liniment** is a liquid or semi-liquid preparation for rubbing on or applying to the skin for therapeutic purposes. Liniments are typically counter-irritating and contain ingredients like camphor, menthol, and turpentine. Herbal preparations might contain rosemary, wild marjoram, or cayenne pepper. Since they contain irritants, rubbing with them too vigorously may cause blistering. If liniments are used, they are usually rubbed onto the skin after massage of an area.

Oils serve as a lubricant to minimize uncomfortable skin friction during sliding and kneading techniques. Certain vegetable oils may also add moisture and nutrients to the skin. Commonly used vegetable oils include almond, olive, and grape seed. Mineral oils are sometimes used, and are generally washed out of sheets more easily than vegetable oils. Vegetable oils trapped in sheets can spoil and turn rancid, causing sheets to have an unpleasant odor. However, some consider vegetable oils healthier for both the giver and the receiver of massage.

Jojoba (pronounced *ho-ho-ba*) is an oil-like substance made from seeds of the jojoba plant found in the North American desert. Native Americans used jojoba for skin and hair care. Many massage practitioners use jojoba either by itself or in combination with lotions, because it is hypoallergenic and healthy for skin, and washes out of sheets easily.

Practitioners choose their oils based on a number of factors. These include properties such as the "feel" of the oil (e.g., thick or thin), inherent nutrients, and scent. Unscented oils are available. Massage oils should be of a high quality and cold pressed. Oils developed specially for massage can be purchased from suppliers.

Lotions are semi-liquid substances containing agents for moisturizing the skin or for therapeutic purposes such as reducing itching or local pain. Lotions are absorbed into the skin, unlike oils, which tend to stay on top of the skin. Lotions are good for situations in which lubrication is desired for a warm-up phase, but more friction is desired later in the session. Those who don't like the feel of oil on their skin may prefer lotions. Lotions also tend to be more water soluble than oils and are, therefore, more easily washed out of sheets.

Practitioners experiment with different topical substances and concoct combinations of substances to get the properties that best enhance their work. They frequently mix different oils, or lotions and oils.

Some substances are more likely to cause allergic reactions. Also, some skin types are more easily irritated. Scent can be an important consideration. People going back to work after massage may desire an unscented substance. Men usually prefer different scents than women. Care should be taken in choosing a topical substance for each unique client or patient.

POSITIONING AND DRAPING

Positioning

Placing the receiver in a comfortable and safe position on the table, called **positioning,** is essential for effective application of massage. The recipient's position can also allow easier access to particular muscles or regions of the body.

The receiver should not have to exert muscular effort to stay in position or to hold draping in place. Various size bolsters, pillows, or rolled towels are used to support body areas and position receivers properly.

In the **supine position** (i.e., face up), a bolster under the knees takes pressure off of the lower back, and a neck roll provides support in the cervical area. In the **prone position** (i.e., face down), support is put under the ankles to ease pressure on them, and small cushions may be placed under the shoulders for women and men with large chests. The face cradle is adjusted for comfort and better access to the cervical area. See Figures 6–3, 6–4, and 6–5.

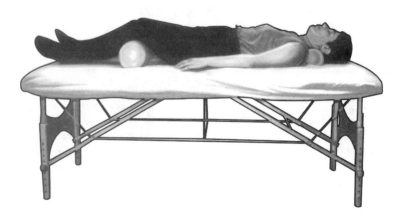

FIGURE 6–3. Supine position. Placement of bolsters under the knees and neck.

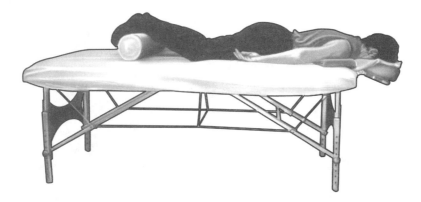

FIGURE 6–4. Prone position. Placement of bolsters under ankles and shoulders, head supported by face cradle.

In the **side-lying position,** support is provided for the superior leg and arm, and under the head. In the **reclining** or semi-supine position, a backrest is created either by adjusting a special hinged table, or by propping the recipient up with bolsters. A bolster is placed under the knees to prevent them from over-extension. See Figures 6–6 and 6–7.

Draping

Covering the body during massage, or **draping,** serves to protect the receiver's modesty, provide clear professional boundaries, and keep the receiver warm. Skill in draping helps the receiver feel safe and allows for maximum relaxation. Draping should be substantial enough to provide a sense of safety and modesty. The use of thin sheets or narrow small towels may leave the recipient feeling exposed and uncomfortable.

When clients remove their clothing and are draped for massage, some general guidelines apply. The genitals and women's breasts should be draped at all times. Mutual consent or familiarity between practitioner and receiver are not good reasons to ignore this guideline. An exception might be during breast massage, but only after special training and with informed consent from the client. Draping can be adjusted to allow access to areas close to the genitals or breasts (e.g., attachments to the adductors or

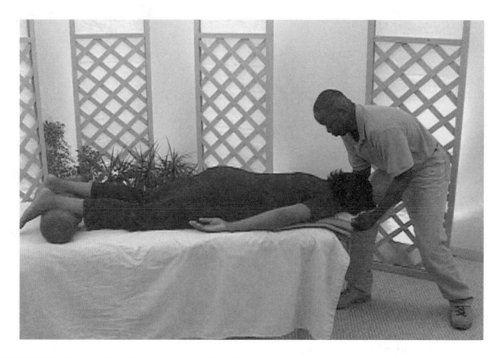

FIGURE 6–5. Face cradle adjustment for comfort of receiver.

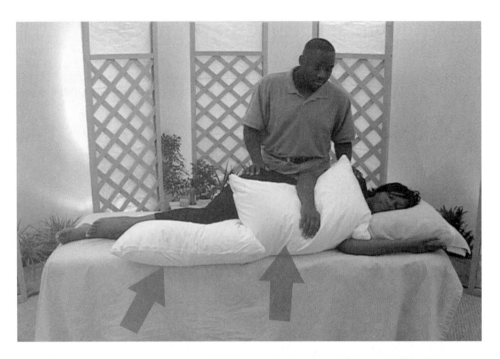

FIGURE 6–6. Side-lying position. Placement of bolsters under the superior leg, arm, and head.

pectoralis major muscle), while maintaining clear professional boundaries. This should be done only with informed consent.

Draping with a sheet provides maximum coverage. The part to be massaged is uncovered and then recovered during the session. Skillful tucking will enhance the security of the drape and prevent inadvertently exposing the receiver. Figure 6–8a–c demonstrates undraping the arm prior to massage.

Preserve the client's modesty when undraping the leg. The leg is lifted at the thigh. The drape is pulled underneath and securely tucked around the hip. Figures 6–9a,b and 6–10a–c demonstrate undraping and securing the drape for the leg.

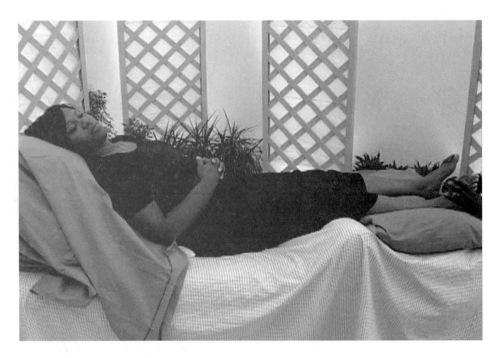

FIGURE 6–7. Reclining position. Back supported and placement of bolster under the knees.

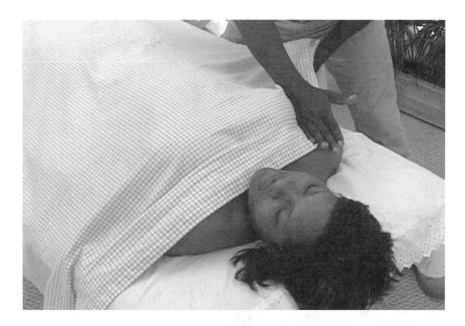

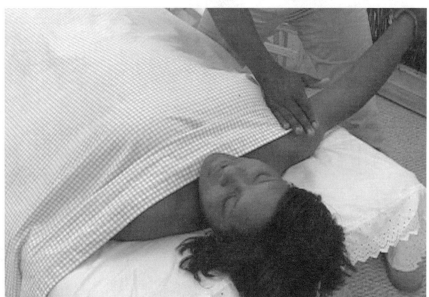

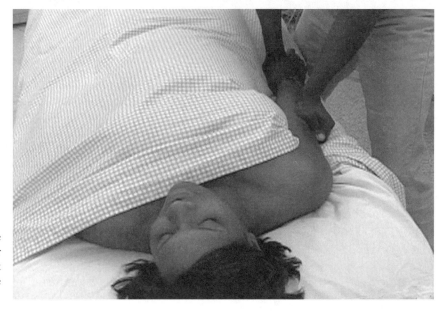

FIGURE 6–8. Draping for massage of arm. **A.** Undraping the arm prior to massage. **B.** Lift arm and tuck sheet underneath. **C.** Arm on table ready for massage.

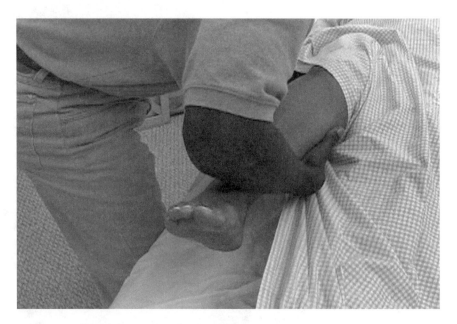

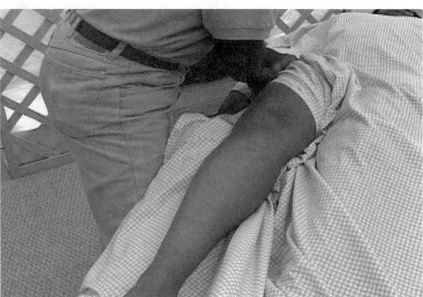

FIGURE 6–9. Draping for massage of leg in supine position. **A.** Lift leg and pull drape underneath. **B.** Secure drape around hip.

Prior to massage of a woman's abdomen or chest area, the breasts are draped with a towel. This is done with informed consent. To begin, a towel is placed over the breasts on top of the sheet. Either you or the client can hold the towel in place as you pull the sheet down to the waist, exposing the upper chest and abdomen. The towel remains covering the breasts. Tuck the sheet around the recipient's hips. Figure 6–11a,b demonstrates proper draping for woman's breasts.

When the receiver is changing from the supine to the prone position, or vice versa, the sheet should be held in place while the person turns over under it. This **tenting** technique allows the receiver to turn over and avoid getting wrapped up in the sheet. Care should be taken not to expose the receiver to the practitioner or to others who might be in the room. See Figure 6–12.

Large towels may also be used for draping. The same general guidelines for modesty apply whatever type of drape is used.

In some situations, receivers do not remove their clothes and draping is unnecessary. For example, receivers usually remain clothed during pre-event and post-event sports massage, chair massage, and some shiatsu and other energy-balancing sessions.

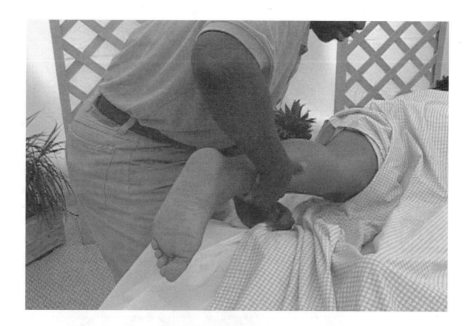

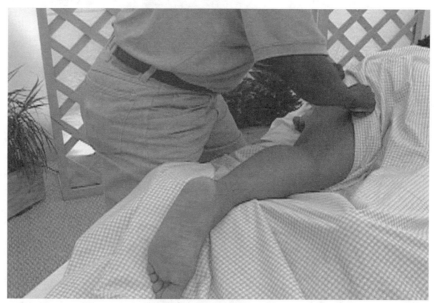

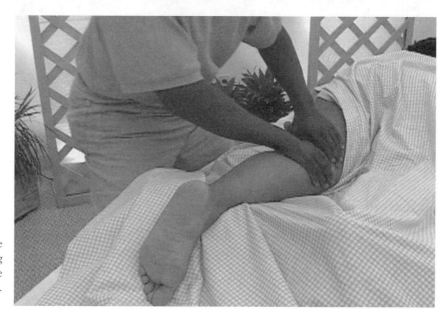

FIGURE 6–10. Draping for massage of leg in prone position. **A.** Lift leg and pull drape underneath. **B.** Secure drape around upper leg and hip. **C.** Massage undraped leg.

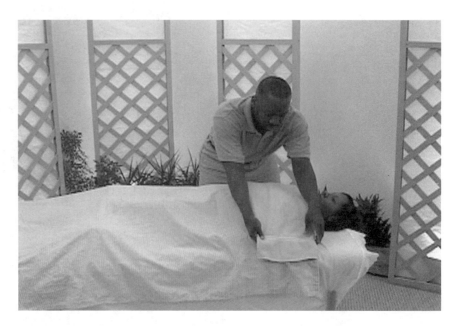

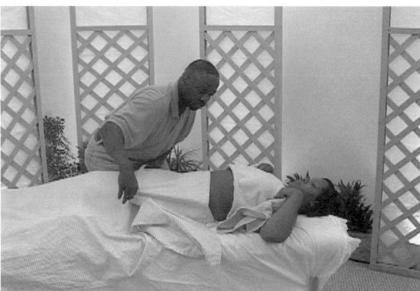

FIGURE 6–11. Draping for a woman's chest. **A.** Place towel over the breasts, and hold the towel in place. **B.** Pull the sheet down to expose the chest and abdomen. Towel remains in place. Tuck the sheet under the hips.

PHYSICAL SELF-CARE FOR THE PRACTITIONER

Physical self-care is essential for the wellbeing and longevity of the massage practitioner. In addition to general health practices, practitioners need to pay special attention to their hands and wrists, posture, and body mechanics. Scheduling of sessions should also be taken into consideration.

Hand and Wrist Care

The hands are the primary means for giving massage. Nails should be clipped so short that they cannot be seen if the hands are held up with the palm toward the face. Rings and bracelets should be avoided, since they might scratch or distract the receiver. Hands should be washed thoroughly before and after every session. This will help protect both the giver and receiver of massage from communicable diseases. Practitioners who smoke should be especially careful to remove odors from their hands. The hands should always be warm and dry before touching the receiver. If necessary, they can be warmed beneath a heat lamp, by hot water, or by rubbing them briskly together. Hands may be dried with a towel or by applying powder to them.

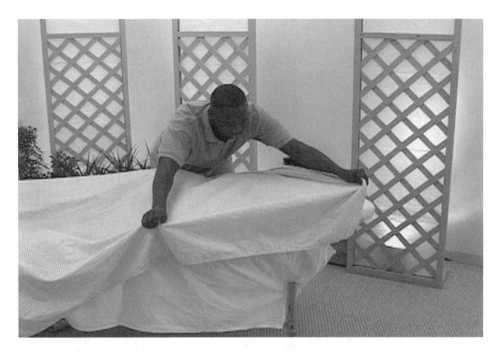

FIGURE 6–12. Creating a tent for turning from prone to supine or vice versa. Pin one side of the sheet against the table with the leg or hip, and lift the sheet so that the recipient can turn over underneath the sheet.

Practitioners can protect themselves from injuries to the hands, arms, and back with conditioning exercises, proper hand position and body mechanics during massage, the use of a variety of techniques, and adequate time for rest between sessions. Common injuries sustained by massage practitioners include tendinitis and tenosynovitis, damage caused by overuse and repetitive strain, and nerve impingement injury (e.g., carpal tunnel and thoracic outlet syndromes). A conditioning program should include exercises to strengthen the upper body, especially the hands, wrists, and arms. Flexibility may be maintained through regular stretching. (The books to read for injury prevention are *Body Mechanics for Manual Therapists* by Barbara Frye, 2000, and *Body Mechanics and Self-Care Manual* by Marian W. Dixon, 2001.)

In applying techniques, strain on finger, thumb, and wrist joints should be minimized. The thumb is especially vulnerable to misuse during high-pressure techniques like trigger point work. Stacking the joints is a protective technique in which pressure is applied along the line of the bones, and through joints, as opposed to being applied at a right angle or across the joint. Figure 6–13a shows correct thumb alignment for applying direct pressure. Avoid applying pressure with the thumb abducted since this puts strain on the joint, as shown in Figure 6–13b.

Wrists should be kept in a neutral position (i.e., neither flexion nor extension) as much as possible when applying techniques (see Figure 6–14). When applying compression techniques, avoid hyperextension at the wrist. If reinforcing one hand with the other during compression techniques, place the top hand directly over the metacarpals, and *not* over the bent wrist. Correct and incorrect positions for compression are demonstrated in Figure 6–15a–c.

Consider the use of the elbow or a special massage tool to apply direct sustained pressure when working in heavily muscled areas. Chapter 13 offers useful suggestions for applying direct pressure safely. The forearm can be used to apply broad effleurage to the thighs or to the back, as demonstrated in Figure 6–16.

Good Body Mechanics

Good body mechanics will minimize shoulder and back problems. First, be sure your table is at the proper height for you. A table too high or too low can cause poor body mechanics and put undue strain on your body. To determine a good table height, stand facing the table with your hands at your sides, as shown in Figure 6–17. Adjust the legs so that your knuckles touch the tabletop. Notice your

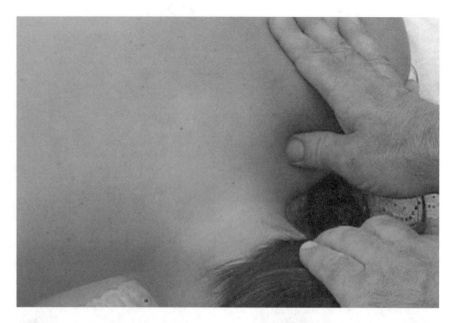

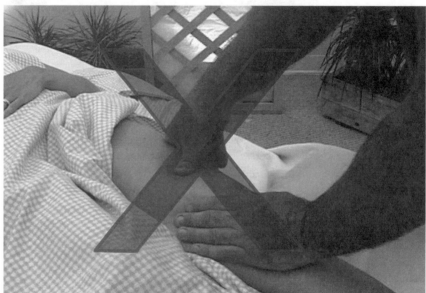

FIGURE 6–13. Correct thumb position when applying pressure. **A.** Correct thumb-wrist alignment for applying direct pressure. **B.** Incorrect position with thumb abducted will cause injury to the joints.

alignment when performing massage at that height. Further adjust the table up or down as needed to keep good alignment of back and neck.

Keep your back and neck in alignment during the session, and bend your knees to lower your body. Avoid bending your back excessively (see Figure 6–18), which puts strain on your back and neck.

Martial arts stances, for example from tai chi, are very effective for keeping good alignment when giving massage. They help take the strain off of your back by using the legs to generate power. These stances not only help keep the back in alignment, but also position you to use body leverage to apply deep pressure.

When facing the head or foot of the table, use a forward leaning stance. Good body alignment and leg position for the forward leaning stance are demonstrated in Figure 6–19a,b. Notice that the front leg is bent more than the rear leg, and pressure is applied as you lean slightly into the technique by shifting the weight from one leg to the other.

When facing the table directly, a side-to-side, or horse, stance is effective. Figure 6–20a,b demonstrates body and foot alignment for the horse stance.

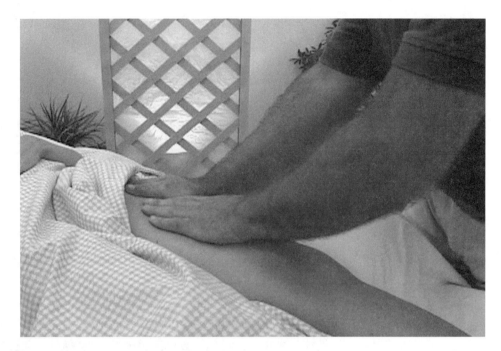

FIGURE 6–14. Wrist in neutral position while performing effleurage.

Sitting on a chair or stool while massaging the receiver's head, hands, and feet also helps minimize strain on the body. Sit near the edge of the seat with your feet flat on the floor and upper body in good alignment. The height of the chair should be adjusted to allow you to keep your wrists in a neutral position. See Figure 6–21a,b.

Avoiding Strain

The warming-up phase of a massage session not only prepares the client for massage, but may also help warm up the practitioner's hands and body. Including a variety of techniques in a session also helps minimize repeated strain on a particular joint or body area of the practitioner.

There are techniques for relaxing tense muscles that cause less strain to the practitioner's body, for example, positional release techniques and some forms of energy work. Techniques that strain the practitioner's body should be alternated with less stressful techniques to provide a resting phase to a session. At the end of a session, the hands are often hot or feel "charged" with energy. Running cold water on the hands after washing them is helpful.

The number of massage sessions any practitioner can perform safely in one day depends on the type of massage performed, his or her strength and fitness, and the quality of his or her body mechanics. Someone just starting out doing massage must build the strength and stamina to perform the work safely. A sudden drastic increase in the number of sessions performed per week may lead to strain, pain, and possible injury.

The following are guidelines for scheduling sessions for a week. They take into account how much work you can expect to perform and maintain your own health and wellbeing. Generally, you should schedule *no more than:*

- Five 1-hour sessions in one day, if you work four days per week
- Four 1-hour sessions in one day, if you work five days per week
- Twenty hours per week total

Furthermore, you should:

- Have 15- to 20-minute breaks between sessions
- Have at least a 30-minute break after three consecutive one-hour sessions
- Do no more than four one-hour sessions in one day, if the type of massage is strenuous

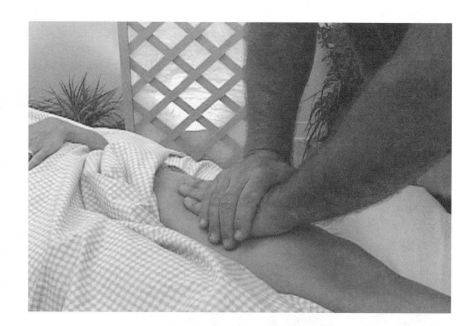

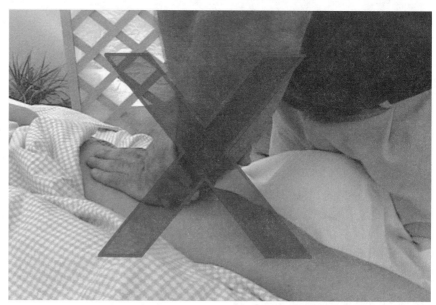

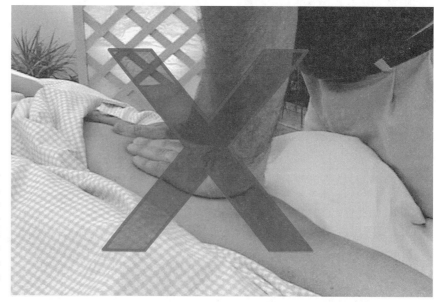

FIGURE 6–15. Correct wrist position while performing compression. **A.** Correct wrist position for compression techniques. **B.** Incorrect position with wrist hyperextended will cause wrist injury. **C.** Incorrect position with pressure directly on the wrist with the other hand will cause wrist injury.

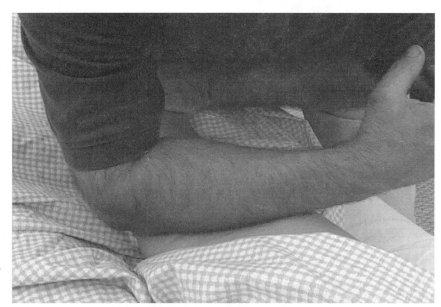

FIGURE 6–16. Use of forearm for performing effleurage on the hamstring muscles.

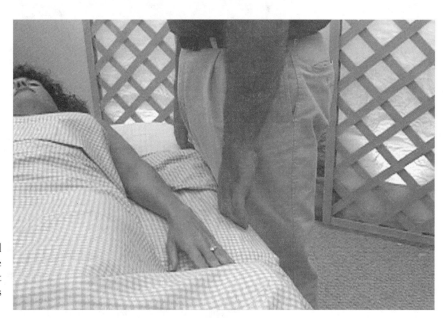

FIGURE 6–17. Determining a good table height. Stand facing the table with your hands at your sides. Adjust the table lags so that your knuckles touch the table top.

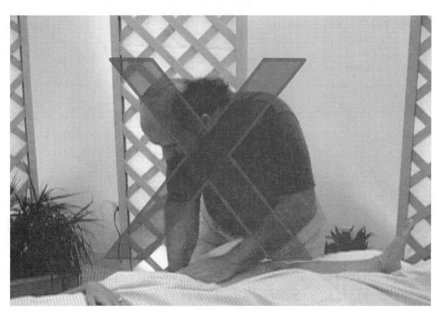

FIGURE 6–18. Incorrect body alignment with back bent and head forward.

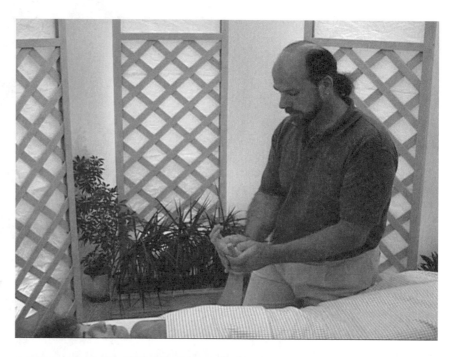

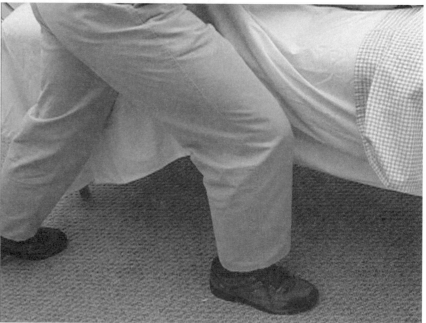

FIGURE 6–19. Good body mechanics when facing the head or foot of the table. **A.** Head and back in alignment. **B.** Legs and feet in forward leaning stance.

If you have a private massage practice, you will also need time to clean linens, keep client or patient records, do financial bookkeeping, and perform other chores related to having your own business.

EMOTIONAL SELF-CARE

Emotional self-care is often overlooked, but it is equally important to prevent stress and burnout. Establish and maintain clear professional boundaries. The practitioner's job is to help patients or clients, not to rescue them from their life's problems. It is useful to have a fellow practitioner with whom to discuss upsetting situations. Peer and professional supervision can help you keep clear boundaries and sort out confusing situations that come up in the practitioner–recipient relationship.

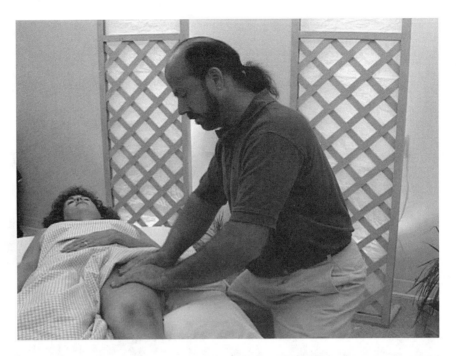

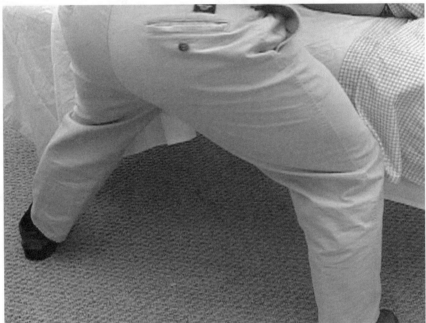

FIGURE 6–20. Good body mechanics when facing table directly. **A.** Head and back in alignment. **B.** Legs and feet in horse stance.

PERFORMANCE ELEMENTS

Length of the Session

Session lengths vary depending on the goals and the setting in which it is given. For example, massage sessions for general health purposes last from 30 to 90 minutes, with 60 minutes the most common. This is typical at a health club, spa, or private massage therapy practice. Chair massage given to employees of a business may last 15–20 minutes. Athletes may receive pre-event massage for 15 minutes and general maintenance massage for 30 minutes to 1 hour. Massage that is part of a larger therapy session (e.g., physical therapy) may last as little as 10 minutes. Guidelines for session length will be given for each type of massage described later in this book.

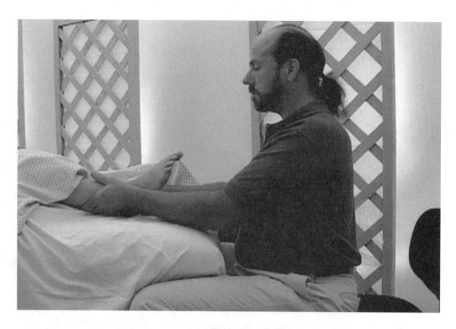

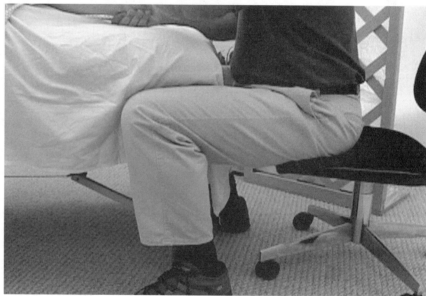

FIGURE 6–21. Good body mechanics for sitting on chair while performing massage. **A.** Sit with back and head in alignment. **B.** Sit near edge of chair with feet flat on floor.

Amount of Lubricant

Generally speaking, you should use the least amount of lubricant needed to get the job done. Too much lubricant prevents firm contact, and the hands will only slip and slide over the surface of the skin. This is especially true when doing more specific work on small areas and when friction is used. Too little lubricant can cause skin irritation, especially in people with thick hair on the arms, legs, or chest, and in people with fair skin. More oil may be used when warming up an area with sliding movements and then wiped off for techniques that are best performed with less lubricant. Recipients of massage may benefit from extra lubricant to relieve dry skin. Additional lotion or oil may be applied after massaging a particular body area as a moisturizer.

The face is an area where little, if any, lubricant should be used. Care should be taken not to get oil or lotion in the hair when working on the neck. Recipients may want to wear surgical or shower caps to keep lubricants out of the hair.

Lubricant should be absorbed into the skin, or wiped off of the skin, before clothes are put back on. Some substances can stain clothes, or certain scents may be difficult to wash out. Rubbing with a dry towel will remove most lotions and oils, and alcohol may be used when more thorough removal is desired.

Sequence of Techniques and Routines

Individual techniques are rarely performed in isolation, but are blended into sequences for the desired effects. Deep specific techniques should be preceded and followed by superficial warming ones. Smooth transitions between techniques give a skillful feel to a session.

Routines are regular sequences of techniques performed in almost the same way each time. A routine may also include a regular sequence of body sections addressed during a session. Experienced practitioners usually establish a routine way of working, which they vary depending on the needs of the receiver.

Routines are useful to establish a smooth pattern of working and are an effective way to learn new massage techniques. Routines will be presented for some of the different approaches discussed later in this book.

Specificity and Direction

Much of massage is performed in a general way and over larger areas of the body. For example, long sliding strokes are often performed over the whole back, and muscle *groups* are kneaded and stretched as opposed to individual muscles. This more general way of applying techniques is appropriate for effects such as warming an area, eliciting the relaxation response (a total body reaction), or relaxing a muscle group.

The **direction** of technique application may be expressed in terms of general anatomical terminology (e.g., proximal, distal, medial, lateral), or in relation to a specific body structure (e.g., toward the muscle attachment).

For example, when performing deep sliding strokes to a limb, always move in the direction of venous flow, that is, distal to proximal. Moving fluids away from the heart, or against venous flow, can cause backflow of blood, which can damage the valves in the veins.

Lighter sliding movements using superficial pressure may be performed proximal to distal. These are used as return strokes between deep sliding movements to the limbs distal to proximal. They may also be used when finishing an area before going to the next area of the body.

Massage practitioners are said to be working with **specificity** if they focus their use of techniques on a specific condition and in a small area (e.g., relieving a trigger point with thumb pressure, or deep transverse friction on a tendon). This requires thorough knowledge of anatomic structures and good palpation skills.

Pressure, Rhythm, and Pacing

Pressure, rhythm, and pacing describe different qualities of applying massage techniques. These qualities will vary with the desired effect of the session, of a sequence of techniques, or of a single technique.

Pressure is related to the force used in applying techniques and to the degree of compaction of tissues as the technique is applied. The amount of pressure used in any one situation will depend on the intended effect and the tolerance or desires of the recipient. Generally speaking, when working an area, pressure should be applied lightly at first then more deeply if desired, then finishing lightly. This allows tissues to be warmed and prepared gradually, and the body to adjust better to the cessation of deep pressure. If too much pressure is used too quickly on a specific area, tissue damage and bruising may result. Too light pressure may cause tickling, and too deep pressure may elicit a tensing response. Both effects are undesirable.

Rhythm refers to a recurring pattern of movement with a specific cadence, beat, or accent. Rhythm may be described as smooth, flowing, or uneven. Rhythm is important when applying techniques generally and in sequence, as with sliding movements and kneading. Working specifically slows or stops the rhythm, as when you slow down to press a trigger point or acupoint. Each massage practitioner has his or her own rhythm for working, which is developed over time. A smooth, flowing, and regular rhythm helps to elicit relaxation in the receiver. An uneven rhythm may be stimulating, or in some cases distracting, to a receiver. Avoid breaking contact with the skin once a session has begun. Abruptly taking the hands off of the body can be unpleasant to the recipient.

Pacing refers to the speed of performing techniques. Generally, a slower pace is more relaxing, while a faster pace more stimulating. Choice of pace depends on the desired effect.

It is the skillful blending of all of these performance elements that comprise the art of massage.

SUMMARY

The therapeutic relationship involves an implicit agreement regarding the roles of the practitioner and the receiver of massage. Professional boundaries help keep those roles clear. Maintaining boundaries involves avoiding dual relationships, being aware of the potential effects of transference and counter-transference, and staying within your scope of practice.

Professional demeanor also helps establish the professional nature of the relationship, and inspires confidence. The practitioner's clothing is neat, clean, and modest, and jewelry minimal. The practitioner and the surrounding space are free of offensive odors. Professional tone is set through appropriate language.

Touch is the primary mode of interaction during massage. From a holistic perspective, what may seem to be only physical touch can have profound effects on the mind, emotions, and spirit. Knowledge of the human need for touch and its cultural implications gives the practitioner insight for better understanding clients and patients. Practitioners prepare to give massage by being aware of intention to be caring and compassionate, and by becoming calm and focused. Self-care techniques can help limit the degree to which practitioners absorb negative "vibes" from receivers.

It is the practitioner's challenge to create openness in the receiver to the touch of massage. Factors like cultural background and history of abuse need to be considered when putting receivers at ease. Practitioners must remain aware of the potential for transference and counter-transference related to touch. Sexual touch is never ethical in a professional setting.

Permission to touch should be sought before massaging vulnerable areas. Informed consent involves describing the proposed action, explaining its intent and what to expect, and asking permission to proceed. The recipient always has the option of saying no, either before or during the application.

Cross-gender situations necessitate special clarity about the non-sexual nature of massage. Clear boundaries and professional demeanor are keys to addressing gender considerations that arise during a massage session. The seven-step intervention model is a procedure for responding to misbehavior by a client.

The appropriate level of verbal interaction during massage depends on the purpose of the session and the needs of the receiver. Getting feedback from the receiver to ensure their health and safety is desirable. Practitioners should remain present and supportive if a receiver experiences an emotional release, and remain clear about the limits of their scope of practice. Since the primary mode of communication in massage is touch, usually less talk is better.

Information about the client or patient is kept confidential. Exceptions include consultation with another health professional, in emergencies or as required by law. The HIPAA Privacy Rule is a federal standard to protect confidentiality of medical records.

A good massage table is adjustable for height and has an adjustable face cradle. Massage chairs are specially made for massage of clothed clients and also have many adjustments. Good massage equipment is a wise investment.

Important factors to consider in setting up the massage space are comfortable room temperature, fresh air quality, indirect lighting, peaceful sounds, private dressing arrangements, and overall cleanliness and neatness. Topical substances used in massage include liniments, oils, and lotions. Practitioners may mix ingredients to get properties that enhance their work. A wide selection of topical substances is available from manufacturers.

Receivers are positioned on the table for comfort, safety, and access to areas to be massaged. Table positions include supine, prone, side-lying, and reclining. The body is draped with a sheet for modesty and warmth. The genitals and women's breasts are draped at all times. Body regions are uncovered before being massaged and recovered afterward. In some situations such as sports events and for chair massage, receivers remain clothed and draping is not used.

The practitioner's hands are clean, nails trimmed, and jewelry that might scratch the receiver removed. Injury to hands is avoided by conditioning exercises, proper technique and adequate rest. Injury to thumbs is minimized by applying pressure through the joints and not while the thumb is abducted. Wrists are held in neutral position, and hyperextension and pressure on wrists avoided.

Good body mechanics involves keeping the back and neck in good alignment, and using the legs to generate power. Martial arts stances, such as the forward-leaning and horse stances, are effective for keeping good body alignment. Table height is adjusted to facilitate healthy body mechanics.

A healthy schedule for massage includes no more than 20 one-hour sessions per week and no more than five in one day. Adequate breaks between sessions helps avoid strain on the body. Emotional self-care helps prevent stress and burnout.

Session lengths vary depending on the goals of the session and the setting, and range from 15 to 90 minutes. One hour is a typical time for full-body table massage. Chair massage given on site generally lasts 15–20 minutes.

The amount of lubricant used for massage depends on the substance used and the techniques performed. Generally speaking, use the least amount needed to get the job done.

Massage techniques are performed in sequences for specific effects. Practitioners develop routine ways of working that are varied to address each client's needs. Elements of technique application include direction, specificity, pressure, rhythm, and pacing. It is the skillful blending of these performance elements that comprise the art of massage.

A look ahead . . .

The guidelines outlined in this chapter support the actual application of techniques. Chapter 7 describes in detail the Western massage technique categories of effleurage, petrissage, tapotement, friction, and vibration.

REFERENCES

Benjamin, B. E., and Sohnen-Moe, C. (2003) *The ethics of touch*. Tucson, AZ: SMA Inc.

Dixon, Marian W. (2001). *Body mechanics and self-care manual*. Upper Saddle River, NJ: Prentice Hall.

Field, T. (2001). *Touch*. Cambridge, MA: The MIT Press.

Frye, B. (2000). *Body mechanics for manual therapists: A functional approach to self-care and injury prevention*. Stanwood, WA: Freytag Publishing.

McIntosh, N. (1999). *The educated heart: Professional guidelines for massage therapists, bodyworkers and movement teachers*. Memphis, TN: Decatur Bainbridge Press.

Montagu, A. (1978). *Touching: The human significance of the skin*, 2nd ed. New York: Harper & Row.

National Certification Board for Therapeutic Massage and Bodywork (2000) *Standards of Practice*. Retrieved March 2003 (*www.ncbtmb.org*).

WEB SITES

HIPAA Privacy Guidelines (www.hhs.gov/ocr/hipaa)

National Certification Board for Therapeutic Massage and Bodywork (www.ncbtmb.org)

S T U D Y   G U I D E

LEARNING OUTCOMES

The learning outcomes for this chapter list skills developed by successful massage practitioners. For each outcome, discuss the guidelines and key points to remember when developing the skill listed. This can be in writing, or discussed with a study partner or group.

KEY TERMS/CONCEPTS

To study key words and concepts listed at the beginning of this chapter, choose one or more of the following exercises. Writing or talking about ideas helps you remember them better, and explaining them helps deepen your understanding.

1. Write a one- or two-sentence explanation of each key word and concept.

2. Find key words or concepts that are related in some way. Explain the relationship. For example: "*Liniments, lotions,* and *oils* are all topical substances used in massage." Or "Guidelines for the *therapeutic relationship* are outlined in *standards of practice.*"

3. Repeat problem 2 for groups of 3–5 words or concepts.

4. Pair each key word with one of the learning outcomes. For example: "Air quality is a part of 10: Create an ideal physical environment for massage." Go on to explain the guidelines related to the word; for example, "The air in the massage space should be fresh . . ."

STUDY OUTLINE

The following questions test your memory of the main concepts in this chapter. Locate the answers in the text using the page number given for each question.

The Therapeutic Relationship

1. The _____ involves an implicit agreement regarding the roles of the massage practitioner and the client. (p. 91)

2. Clarity about roles is maintained by keeping _____. (p. 91)

3. A _____ relationship is any relationship other than the primary one of practitioner and client. (p. 91)

4. When clients unconsciously bring unresolved feelings from their past into the practitioner–client relationship, it is called _____. (p. 92)

5. When practitioners unconsciously bring unresolved feelings from their past into the practitioner–client relationship, it is called _____. (p. 92)

Professional Demeanor

1. The practitioner's appearance and behavior help establish a good therapeutic relationship by _____ _____. (p. 92)

2. Professional clothing is _____, _____, and _____. (p. 92)

3. Offensive odors such as _____, _____, and _____ should be eliminated. (p. 92)

4. The practitioner's language should avoid _____, as well as unduly _____

language and jargon; and speak to the _____ level of the client. (p. 92)

5. The relationship between giver and receiver should be understanding and sympathetic, but never _____ _____. (p. 92)

Touching Another Person

1. Human beings have an innate touch _____ _____. (p. 92)

2. To touch means _____ _____. (p. 92)

3. From the holistic perspective, what seems to be simple physical touch often has profound effects on the _____, _____, and _____ of the receiver. (p. 92)

4. Touch can communicate _____, _____, _____, and _____. (p. 93)

5. Examples of self-care for preventing absorption of a client's negative "vibes" are _____, _____, and _____. (p. 93)

6. Comfort levels with touch vary among clients because _____ _____. (p. 93)

7. _____ touch is never appropriate in a professional setting. (p. 93)

Permission to Touch

1. Informed consent is a process initiated when _____. (p. 93)

2. Informed consent includes _____, _____, _____, and _____. (Table 6–1)

3. For informed consent the client should clearly have the option of _____ to the proposed action. (pp. 93–94)

Gender Considerations

1. In cross-gender and same-gender massage, be clear about the _____ nature of massage therapy, and establish clear _____. (p. 94)

2. Many people, especially women, have been victims of _____ and _____, and have special needs for clear _____. (p. 94)

Intervention Model

1. The intervention model is used when _____ _____. (p. 95)

2. The steps in the seven-step intervention model are
   (a) _____, (b) _____,
   (c) _____, (d) _____,
   (e) _____, (f) _____,
   (g) _____. (Table 6–2)

Talking and Feedback

1. The degree of verbal interaction that goes on during a massage session depends on _____ and _____. (p. 95)

2. When relaxation is the goal, talking should be _____. (p. 95)

3. Verbal and non-verbal communication that gives the practitioner information from the receiver about the massage performance is called _____. (p. 95)

4. Emotional release is the result of _____ _____. (p. 96)

5. During emotional release, the practitioner's reaction is to _____, and *not* to _____. (p. 96)

6. An exception to the "minimal talk during massage" guideline might be _____ _____. (p. 96)

7. A good way to avoid letting your own life come into the talk during massage is to _____ _____. (p. 96)

Confidentiality

1. Confidentiality is an ethical principle in the professional relationship based on the client's right to _____. (p. 96)

2. Confidential information about the client or patient includes _____, _____, and _____. (p. 96)

3. Exceptions to the general rule of confidentiality are _____ and _____. (p. 96)

4. It is considered unethical to give out information about a client without _____ _____. (p. 96)

5. The National Certification Board for Therapeutic Massage and Bodywork has adopted a document called _____ that gives detailed guidelines about professional ethical behavior. (p. 96)

HIPAA Privacy Rule

1. HIPAA stands for the _____ _____ act. (p. 96)

2. HIPAA was designed to protect the _____ of individuals. (p. 96)

3. Clients should be able to see their _____, and ask for _____ if they find mistakes. (p. 97)

4. According to HIPAA, client records must be kept in _____ file cabinets, preferably in _____ records rooms. (p. 97)

5. Clients must give _____ consent for use and disclosure of information for _____, _____, and _____. (p. 97)

The Physical Environment

1. Essential features of a massage table are adjustable _____ and _____. (p. 97)

2. The type of massage table you choose depends on _____ and the _____. (p. 97)

3. A typical massage chair consists of a _____, _____, _____, _____, and _____.
(p. 98)

4. A comfortable temperature for a massage room is approximately _____ degrees. (p. 98)

5. A _____ can help remove dust, mold, and other allergens from a room. (p. 99)

6. Lighting for massage should be _____ and _____. (p. 99)

7. Sound, including music, can help create a _____ and _____ environment, or a _____ one. (p. 99)

8. When clients are _____ or _____, it is appropriate to help them disrobe and get onto the table. (p. 99)

9. Used sheets and towels should be kept _____ _____. (p. 99)

Topical Substances

1. Ingredients commonly found in liniments include _____, _____, _____, _____, _____, and _____. (p. 99)

2. Liniments are usually applied (choose one: before, during, after) a massage. (p. 99)

3. Vegetable oils commonly used for massage include _____, _____, _____, and _____. (p. 99)

4. Practitioners choose the oils the use for their _____, _____, and _____. (p. 100)

5. Lotions are absorbed into _____, unlike oils, which tend to stay on _____. (p. 100)

Safety and Comfort of the Receiver

1. The purpose of positioning the receiver is _____, and _____. (p. 100)

2. In the supine (i.e., face-_____) position, bolsters are placed under the _____, and _____. (Figure 6–3)

3. In the prone (i.e., face-_____) position, a bolster is placed under _____ to take pressure off of the _____. (Figure 6–4)

4. In the side-lying position support is provided for _____, _____, and _____. (Figure 6–6)

5. Draping during massage serves to _____, _____, and _____. (p. 101)

6. Body areas to be draped at all times include _____ and _____. (p. 101)

7. A technique to use when the receiver is turning from prone to supine is called _____. (p. 104)

Physical Self-Care for the Practitioner

1. Practitioners can protect themselves from hand, arm, and back injuries by _____, _____, _____, and _____. (p. 107)

2. A protective technique in which pressure is applied through a straight line of joints is called _____ the _____. (p. 107)

3. Avoid pressure with the thumb (choose one: abducted or adducted). (p. 107)

4. When applying compression with the palms, avoid _____ of the wrist. (p. 107)

5. When reinforcing one hand with the other during compression, the top hand should be placed over the _____. (p. 107)

6. Bend your _____ to lower your body when performing massage. (p. 108)

7. When facing the head or the foot of the table, use a _____ stance. (p. 108)

8. Pressure is applied by _____, not by using the arms. (p. 108)

9. The maximum number of one-hour massage sessions that can be done safely in a week is _____. (p. 109)

Emotional Self-Care

1. Emotional self-care is important to prevent _____ and _____. (p. 112)

2. Strategies for emotional self-care include _____ _____. (p. 112)

Performance Elements

1. The length of a massage session is determined by _____. (p. 113)

2. Use the least amount of lubricant needed to _____. (p. 114)

3. Too much lubricant can _____. (p. 114)

4. Deep specific techniques should be preceded and followed by _____ ones. (p. 115)

5. Sequences of techniques performed in almost the same way each time are called _____. (p. 115)

6. The direction of technique application is expressed in general anatomical terms, for example, proximal, _____, _____, and _____. (p. 115)

7. Massage practitioners are working with _____ _____ if they focus their techniques on a particular anatomical structure. (p. 115)

8. A _____, _____, _____ rhythm helps evoke relaxation. (p. 115)

9. It is the skillful blending of performance techniques that comprise the _____ of massage. (p. 115)

FOR GREATER UNDERSTANDING

The following exercises are practical applications of the guidelines presented in this chapter. Action words are underlined to emphasize the variety of activities presented, and to encourage advanced skill development. These exercises can be done with a study partner or group, or in class.

1. Analyze a professional relationship you have with a doctor, lawyer, psychotherapist, religious leader, or teacher. Is it similar to the therapeutic relationship described in this chapter? Do they have a professional demeanor? How is it similar or different from a massage practitioner? Discuss your observations.

2. Receive a massage from a professional practitioner. Notice how they establish a therapeutic relationship and maintain professional boundaries. Was there anything that seemed unprofessional to you? Discuss your observations.

3. Receive a massage from a professional practitioner. Afterwards, analyze the amount and content of talking that occurred in the session. Did their communication enhance or detract from the experience for you? Write down your observations giving specific examples. Discuss with a study partner or group.

4. Look through a magazine written for massage practitioners (e.g., Massage Therapy Journal (AMTA), Massage & Bodywork (ABMP), Massage magazine). Critique photographs of massage practitioners, pointing out examples of professional and unprofessional images. Present and discuss your findings.

5. Interview two people with cultural backgrounds different from yourself. Ask them about touch in their cultures. For example: How do people greet each other? How much do they touch when they talk? Walk together? Other occasions? Are there restrictions related to touch between men and women, two adults of the same gender, or between people of different ages? Compare and contrast the cultures. How might a client's touch background affect his/her openness to massage, and how would this affect your behavior as the massage practitioner? Present and discuss your findings.

6. Role play a situation that calls for informed consent. Have observers critique your performance. Repeat the situation using their suggestions.

7. Role play a situation that calls for the intervention model. Have observers critique your performance. Repeat the situation using their suggestions.

8. Visit the Web sites of two different table manufacturers. Create a comparison chart of the features of their most basic massage table, and of options available.

9. Repeat problem 8 for a massage chair.

10. Envision your massage practice over the next five years. Describe your ideal massage table in detail. Visit Web sites, showrooms, or consult brochures. Determine which table is best for you and its approximate cost.

11. Visit a facility that offers massage (e.g., private office, spa, health club, beauty salon, rehabilitation clinic, hospital, nursing home). Describe in detail the elements of the space such as temperature, air quality, lighting, sound, dressing arrangements, and cleanliness. How is it conducive to massage? How could it be made better? Discuss your findings in a group or class, and compare experiences.

12. Each person in a group or class brings a different liniment, oil or lotion used for massage. Compare ingredients of these products. Perform massage techniques with the substances, noting how they feel and how they enhance the massage technique. Choose your favorite and discuss your choice with the group.

13. Practice placing a study partner in different positions, (e.g., supine, prone, side-lying, and reclining) using bolsters and other props as needed. Adjust the face-cradle when they are prone. Using their feedback, rearrange the position or use of bolsters for maximum comfort. Practice on different size people and different body types. Identify factors to consider with different people.

14. <u>Practice</u> sheet draping with a recipient in different positions (e.g., supine, prone, side-lying, and reclining). Uncover and recover different body parts. Practice draping women's breasts. <u>Get feedback</u> from the recipient on how they feel. Do you seem confident? Do they feel safe and their modesty preserved?

15. <u>Videotape</u> yourself performing massage for about 10 minutes. <u>Analyze</u> your performance for good hand and wrist care, and general body mechanics. Get feedback from observers. Re-tape your performance, making corrections.

16. <u>Practice</u> performing massage with the table at different heights. <u>Identify</u> the height at which you can best maintain good body mechanics. <u>Get feedback</u> from observers.

17. <u>Practice</u> different massage techniques with different amounts of lubricant. <u>Determine</u> the right amount for each technique performed. Identify factors that had an impact on your judgment, e.g., your intent, the type of lubricant, or skin condition of the recipient. <u>Discuss</u> your findings with a group.

18. <u>Perform</u> a sequence of massage techniques varying the pressure, rhythm, and pacing. <u>Get feedback</u> from the recipient regarding how the variations felt and their effect.

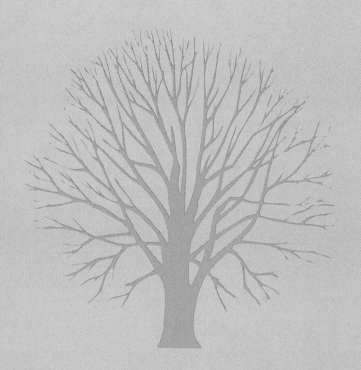

II

Western Massage

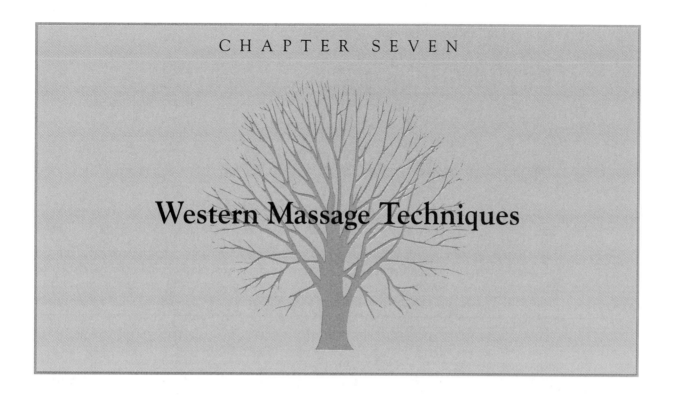

CHAPTER SEVEN

Western Massage Techniques

LEARNING OUTCOMES

After studying this chapter, the student will have information to:

1. Describe the Western massage technique categories.
2. Choose different techniques for their effects.
3. Perform variations of basic techniques.
4. Vary rhythm, pacing, and pressure for different effects.

KEY TERMS/CONCEPTS

Swedish massage
Western massage
Western massage techniques
Effleurage
  basic sliding effluerage
  stripping
  shingles effleurage
  bilateral tree stroking
  three-count stroking of
    trapezius
  horizontal stroking

Mennell's superficial
  stroking
nerve strokes
knuckling
Petrissage
  basic two-handed kneading
  one-handed kneading
  alternating one-handed
    kneading
  circular two-handed
    petrissage

alternating fingers-to-
  thumb petrissage
skin rollling
compression
rolling
Friction
  superficial warming friction
  sawing
  deep friction
  deep transverse friction
  Cyriax friction

MEDIALINK

A companion CD-ROM, included free with each new copy of this book, supplements the techniques presented in this chapter. Insert the CD-ROM to watch video clips of massage techniques being demonstrated. This multimedia feature is designed to help you add a new dimension to your learning.

Tapotement	pincement	shaking
hacking	quacking	jostling
rapping	squishes	Touch without movement
cupping	Vibration	passive touch
clapping	electric vibrator	direct pressure
slapping	fine vibration	ischemic compression
tapping	light effleurage with vibration	

WESTERN MASSAGE

Western massage is the basis of massage therapy performed in North America and Europe today. It is the most common form of massage found in spas, health clubs and private practice, and is the foundation for therapeutic applications within the professions of massage therapy, physical therapy, and nursing.

Today's Western massage traces its origin to the 19th century and the work of Pehr Ling of Sweden and Johann Mezger of Amsterdam. It is the legacy of people like Ling (Swedish movements), Mezger (classic massage), Kellogg (massage in natural healing), McMillan (massage in physical therapy), and many others. **Swedish massage** is a form of Western massage popular for over 100 years. See Chapter 2 for a more detailed view of the history of Western massage in conventional medicine and natural healing.

The effects, benefits, and indications for Western massage are understood in terms of Western concepts of anatomy and physiology and Western notions of health and disease. This is in contrast to Chinese medicine and Ayurveda (India). The techniques of Western massage are recognized as valuable for improving circulation of blood and lymph, relaxing muscles, improving joint mobility, inducing general relaxation, and promoting healthy skin. See Chapters 3 and 4 for a more thorough discussion of massage and Western science.

WESTERN MASSAGE TECHNIQUES

Western massage techniques fall into seven categories: effleurage, petrissage, friction, tapotement, vibration, touch without movement, and joint movements. The first five techniques are the classic massage categories, and the last two complete the picture of massage therapy as practiced today. These are the same categories used by J. Harvey Kellogg in the early 20th century to describe the "procedures of massage" (Kellogg 1929). The categories of Western massage are useful for thinking about how techniques are performed, their physiological effects, and common uses.

This chapter will describe the techniques of soft tissue manipulation, while joint movements will be described in Chapter 8. Keep in mind that there is an endless number of variations of massage techniques, and that the ones presented in this text are merely representative of many possibilities. Always perform techniques taking into consideration endangerment sites, contraindications and cautions, as described in Chapter 5, and using good hand and body mechanics, as presented in Chapter 6.

EFFLEURAGE

Effleurage techniques slide or glide over the skin with a smooth, continuous motion. Pressure may be light to moderate, as when applying oil or warming an area, or may be deep, as when facilitating venous return in heavily muscled areas. Experienced practitioners can perform effleurage in many different ways to suit the body area and to evoke specific effects.

Effleurage is perhaps the most versatile of the Western techniques and is used most frequently. For example, effleurage is usually used to begin a session, especially when oil or lotion is applied. It accustoms the receiver to the touch of the practitioner. It is used as a connecting or transition technique. It is often performed as a break from more specific techniques, to move gracefully from one area to another, to conclude work on an area, or to end the session.

While performing effleurage, a practitioner skilled in palpation can assess the general condition of the soft tissues and the firmness and shape of the musculature. Sensitive fingers may find areas of tension or holding. In some cases where there is pain, effleurage may be the only technique employed.

Effleurage can affect the recipient's body and mind in a variety of ways. The qualities of pressure, pacing, and rhythm may be varied for different effects. For example, when effleurage is performed with moderate pressure, slowly and smoothly on the back, it may stimulate the parasympathetic nervous system and evoke the relaxation response. It enhances venous return in the limbs when performed with moderate to deep pressure moving distal to proximal. Deep effleurage may also provide a passive stretch to a muscle group.

VARIATIONS OF EFFLEURAGE

Basic sliding effleurage is performed with the palms and fingers of the hands, the thumbs, fists, or forearms. When using the palms and fingers, mold the hands to the surface of the body. This provides full contact, as shown in basic effleurage of the leg in Figure 7–1. The thumbs may be used in small places like between the metatarsals of the foot, as in Figure 7–2. More pressure may be applied using the forearms or fists in broad places like the back and hamstrings, as seen in Figure 7–3.

Stripping is a type of basic sliding effleurage performed with deep pressure along the length of the muscle fibers, typically done with the thumb. See Figure 7–4. It is commonly performed on the long muscles in the arms and legs, and on the cervical muscles. Stripping is specific to a particular muscle and usually follows the muscle to its site of attachment. If the muscle is wider than the thumb, stripping is performed in parallel lines to cover the entire muscle. Stripping separates and helps lengthen muscle fibers. It is a useful technique to follow direct pressure to trigger points.

Shingles effleurage refers to alternate stroking, first one hand then the other in continuous motion, with the strokes overlaying each other like shingles on a roof. One hand always remains in contact with the receiver as the other hand is lifted. This gives the feeling of unbroken contact. Shingles effleurage is commonly applied to the back with hands parallel to the spine and to the direction of movement as shown in Figure 7–5. It may also be performed with hands perpendicular to the spine and to the direction of movement.

Bilateral tree stroking traces a pattern reminiscent of branches growing out from both sides of the trunk of a tree. It is usually performed on the back starting with the hands on either side of the spine, and moving laterally across the shoulders or around the sides as far as you can reach. This movement is repeated as you progress to cover the entire back. It may be performed standing at the head and progressing from the shoulders toward the hips as shown in Figure 7–6. It may also be done standing at the side moving from hips to shoulders.

Three-count stroking of the trapezius is performed in three strokes, alternating hands with each movement. Count one begins at the origin of the lower trapezius and moves toward its insertion in the shoulder. Count two begins just as the first stroke concludes, moving from the origin of the middle trapezius toward the insertion. As soon as the first hand has completed its slide over the lower trapezius, it lifts and crosses over to the origin of the upper trapezius to begin count three. Count three moves

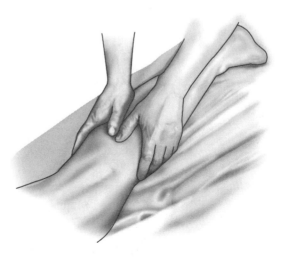

FIGURE 7–1. Basic sliding effleurage using the palms of the hands provides full contact with the leg.

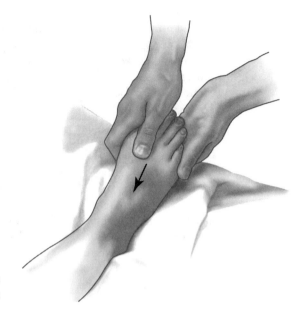

FIGURE 7–2. Basic sliding effleurage using the thumb gets into the small spaces between the metatarsals of the foot.

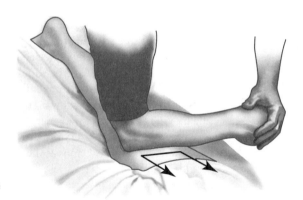

FIGURE 7–3. Basic sliding effleurage using the forearm applies broad, deep pressure to an area.

FIGURE 7–4. Stripping is performed with deep pressure along the length of a muscle to its attachment. Parallel strips are applied to cover the entire muscle width.

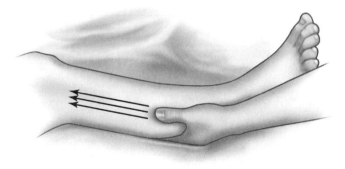

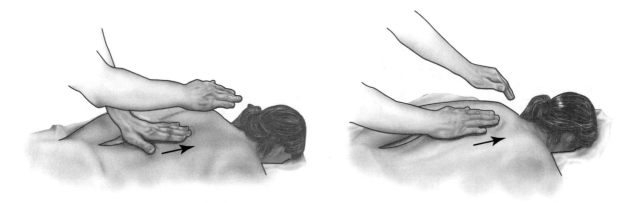

FIGURE 7–5. Shingles effleurage with hands parallel to the spine and to the direction of movement.

laterally to the insertion to complete the sequence. Figure 7–7 shows how the stroke is performed from the opposite side. The entire three-count sequence is repeated several times. This particular method of stroking the whole trapezius is rhythmic and relaxing when well done. It must be timed so that in spite of the lost contact as each hand is raised, the receiver feels unbroken contact.

Horizontal stroking is usually applied to broad, rounded areas like the thigh, abdomen, or lower back. The movement is across the width of the body part, rather than over the length. Horizontal stroking may be considered a hybrid form of effleurage and petrissage because in addition to sliding, there may be a lifting and pressing motion.

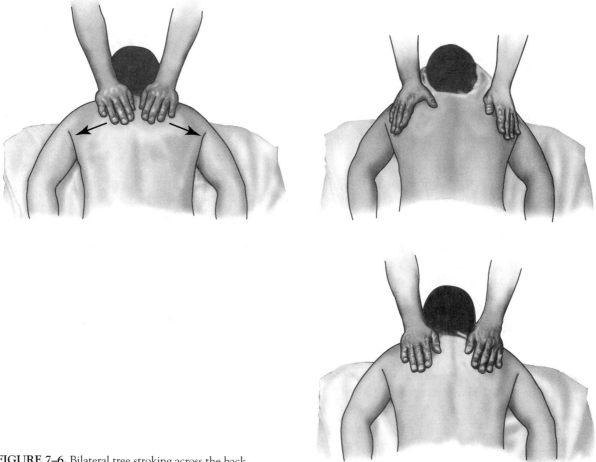

FIGURE 7–6. Bilateral tree stroking across the back.

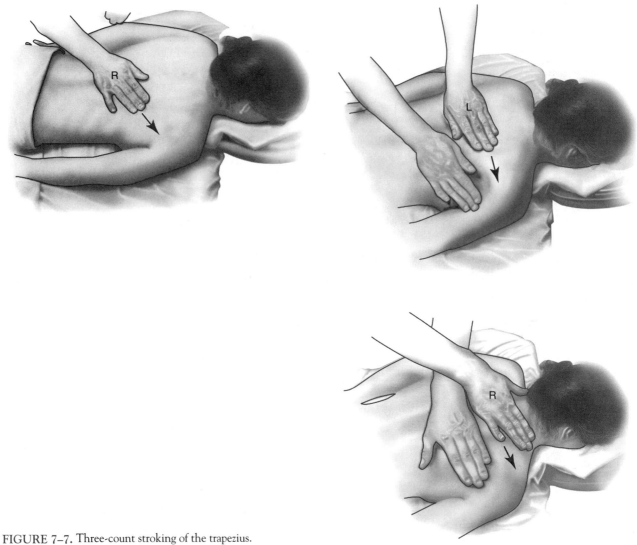

FIGURE 7–7. Three-count stroking of the trapezius.

To perform horizontal stroking on the lower back, stand facing the table at the side of the receiver near the waist. Place your hands lightly on the receiver's back, one hand on each side with the fingers of both hands pointing away from you, as shown in Figure 7–8. Slide both hands toward the spine using firm pressure, and then continue the movement all the way to the other side. One hand will move forward and one hand backward, crossing at the spine. The motion is then reversed without changing the position of the hands. As the hands slide from side to side, they execute a lifting and pushing together of the soft tissues. No pressure should be placed over the spinous processes as the hands pass over them. Greatest pressure comes with the lift and push together of the tissues as the hands move upward and inward to meet and cross over.

Mennell's superficial stroking is very light effleurage usually performed on a limb, moving in one direction either centripetally (distal to proximal) or centrifugally (proximal to distal), but never in both directions. To perform it on the arm with the recipient prone, slide your hand from the recipient's wrist to the shoulder while maintaining full contact and using the lightest pressure possible. See Figure 7–9. Return to the starting position through the air just over the skin surface in a controlled even rhythm. Take the same time to perform the return movement as the stroke that contacts the receiver. This is a gentle relaxing technique.

Nerve strokes are another very light effleurage movement. They are performed with the fingertips gently brushing the skin. They may also be done on top of the drape. Nerve strokes can go in any direction and are often used when finishing a section of the body or when ending the session. A few seconds of nerve strokes are usually enough to create a relaxing effect.

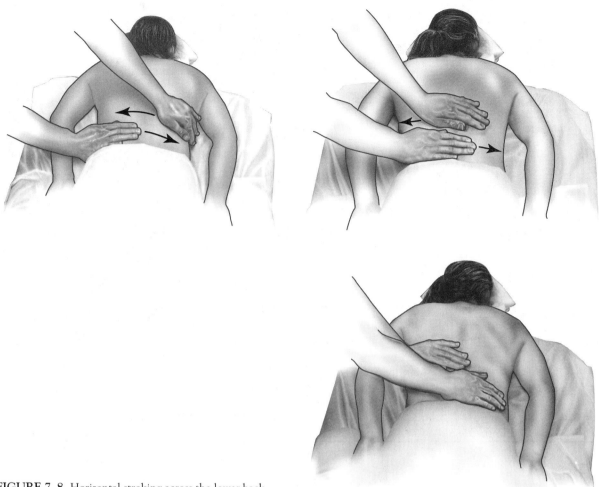

FIGURE 7–8. Horizontal stroking across the lower back.

Knuckling is an effleurage variation taught by Hoffa in which the pressure is first applied with the back of the fingers in a loose fist, gradually turning the fist over as it slides over the skin, and finishing with the palm of the hand. See Figure 7–10. Hoffa describes knuckling further.

> Gradually bring the hand from plantar (flexion) to dorsal (hypertension) flexion. Pressure is not contin-uous, but swells up and down, starting lightly and becoming stronger, then decreasing again in pressure. The hand must not adhere to the part but should glide over it lightly. Knuckling should only be used where there is enough room for the hand to be applied (Hoffa 1900).

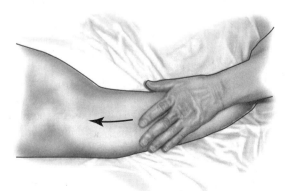

FIGURE 7–9. Mennell's superficial stroking over the arm with the recipient prone.

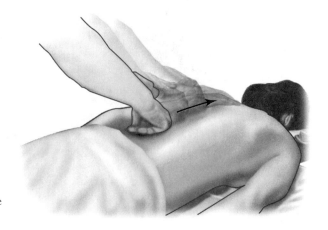

FIGURE 7–10. Knuckling effleurage (knuckle to palm) performed on the back.

PETRISSAGE

Petrissage techniques lift, wring, or squeeze soft tissues in a kneading motion or press or roll the tissues under or between the hands. Petrissage may be performed with one or two hands, depending on the size of the muscle or muscle group. There is minimal sliding over the skin except perhaps in moving from one area to another when using lubricant. The motions of petrissage serve to "milk" a muscle of accumulated metabolites (waste products), increase local circulation, and assist venous return. Petrissage may also help separate muscle fibers and evoke muscular relaxation.

Before performing petrissage, prepare and warm an area, usually with effleurage. Use only a small amount of oil or lotion when warming up the area, since too much lubricant will make it difficult to grasp the tissues during petrissage. If you are working without lubricant, light compressions may be used to warm an area.

Care should be taken to avoid pinching or bruising the tissues and to not work too long in one area. Adjust the amount of pressure used to match the condition of the recipient. Muscular and physically strong receivers will enjoy harder pressure, while less pressure should be used for smaller or frail individuals.

Variations of Petrissage

Basic two-handed kneading is performed by lifting, squeezing, and then releasing soft tissues with hands alternating in a rhythmical motion. Graham (1884) described the fingers and hands as slipping on the skin during kneading, while Kellogg (1929) discouraged letting the hands slide. In basic kneading, tissues are lifted with the whole hand in firm contact as shown in Figure 7–11, rather than with just the fingertips. The movement is a lifting away from the underlying bone. Two-handed kneading works well on the larger muscles of the arms, shoulders, and legs.

One-handed kneading may be used on smaller limbs, for example, arms and children's legs. Place your hand around the part, picking up the muscle mass using the whole hand. The kneading movement may be described as circular—grasping the tissues on the up motion, and relaxing the hand on the down motion without losing contact. As with two-handed kneading, the rhythm should be slow and regular. Progression to a new position should follow three or four repetitions in the same place. In general, the movements should be performed distal to proximal, and effleurage may be interspersed with petrissage or may follow it, to enhance venous return.

The biceps is a good place to practice one-hand kneading. Grasp the biceps with one hand as shown in Figure 7–12. Let the muscle belly fit firmly into the palm of the hand while the thumb and fingers apply pressure and lift as they begin the kneading motion.

Alternating one-handed kneading may be used to work flexors and extensors at the same time. For example, on the upper arm, grasp the biceps with one hand and the triceps with the other hand. Alternate lifting and squeezing first the biceps and then the triceps in an even rhythm. See Figure 7–13. Perform this technique rapidly when stimulation is desired.

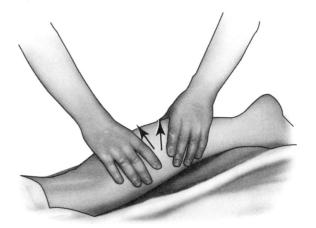

FIGURE 7–11. Basic two-handed kneading. Tissues are lifted with the whole hand in firm contact.

Circular two-handed petrissage is best performed on broad, flat areas like the back. This technique may be applied to one side of the spine after warming the area using deep effleurage. Stand facing the receiver from the side and near the hips and be ready to move along toward the head while performing the technique. Place both hands firmly on one side of the receiver's back, with the hand nearest the hips ready to start the movement over the upper portion of the gluteals. Each hand will describe a counterclockwise circle, timed so that when the hands pass each other, the soft tissues are picked up and pressed between the hands. The hands are almost *flat* as they shape themselves to the contours of the back. Pick up tissues between the hands (not with the hands) as they pass each other as shown in Figure 7–14. After about three repetitions of this technique in one place, slide the lower hand up to where the upper hand has just been working, while the upper hand slides to a new position closer to the head. Eventually, the technique progresses from lower back to upper back, ending over the shoulders. This technique may also be performed on the forehead using the thumbs.

Alternating fingers-to-thumb petrissage is very useful for following the direction of the fibers of the more superficial muscles such as the trapezius. In this technique, the soft tissues are pressed between the thumb of one hand and the first two fingers of the other hand. The hands alternate back and forth with an even rhythm.

To perform the technique, the fingers of one hand pick up the tissues and press them against the opposite thumb. At the same time, the thumb is moving toward, and pressing the tissues against, the fingers of the opposite hand. See Figure 7–15. This same motion is repeated alternating hands and working from the distal to the proximal (or lateral to medial) aspects of each muscle.

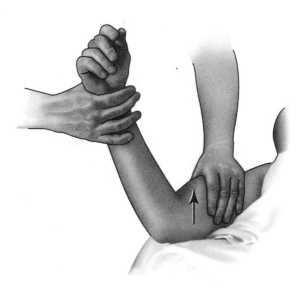

FIGURE 7–12. One-handed kneading. Tissues are lifted with the whole hand in firm contact.

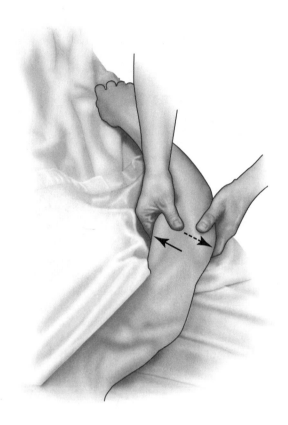

FIGURE 7–13. Alternating one-handed kneading. Alternate lifting and squeezing biceps and triceps in an even rhythm.

Skin rolling is a technique in which the skin and subcutaneous tissue are picked up between the thumb and the first two fingers and gently pulled away from the deeper tissues. Once the skin is pulled away, the thumbs may push forward, lifting the tissues in a smooth, continuous motion and causing a rolling effect. Skin rolling stretches the underlying fascia and increases superficial circulation. It is considered a basic myofascial massage technique. It is often performed on the back, but may be applied to almost any part of the body. Figure 7–16 shows skin rolling on the back.

In **compression** techniques, tissues are pressed or rolled against underlying tissues and bone in a rhythmic motion. The effects are similar to other petrissage techniques as the tissues are compressed under the hands. Figure 7–17 shows compression using the palm of one hand, while the other hand pro-

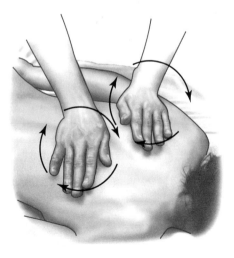

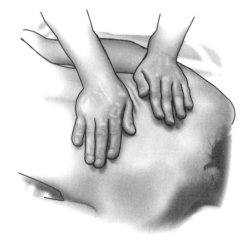

FIGURE 7–14. Circular two-handed petrissage. Tissues are picked up between the hands as they pass each other.

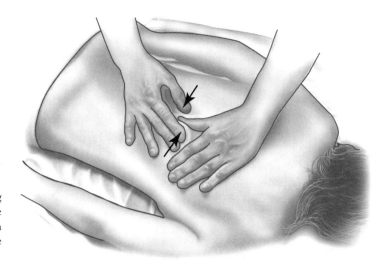

FIGURE 7-15. Alternating fingers-to-thumb petrissage. The soft tissues are pressed between the thumb of one hand and the fingers of the other hand.

vides additional force from above. Note that the heel of the top hand is placed so that it does not put pressure on the wrist of the bottom hand. The compressing force is applied through the palms, as you lean into the movement with your body weight. Avoid using just your arms and shoulders to perform compression techniques. Review the principles of good hand and body mechanics for compression in Chapter 6. A variation useful in working the buttocks is compression with a fist.

Rolling is a form of petrissage performed on the limbs. Grasp the limb lightly on opposite sides between the palms of the hands. The muscles of the limb are compressed against each other as the hands press in and perform an alternating back-and-forth motion. Rolling progresses from proximal to distal. In addition to compressing tissues, rolling causes movement in the shoulder or hip joint. The larger your hands are in proportion to the limb, the easier rolling is to perform.

FRICTION

Friction is performed by rubbing one surface over another repeatedly. For example, the hand is used to rub the skin for superficial warming, as in a traditional rubdown. The resistance to the motion provided by the surfaces creates heat and stimulates the skin.

Friction may also be created between the skin and deeper tissues. In *deep friction*, the practitioner's fingers do not move over the skin, but instead move the skin over the tissues underneath. Deep friction addresses one small area at a time and adds specificity to the massage by affecting specific structures, such as a particular section of a muscle or tendon. Cross-fiber, parallel, and circular friction are common forms of deep friction.

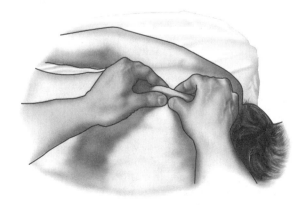

FIGURE 7-16. Skin rolling. Superficial tissues are picked up and gently pulled away from deeper tissues.

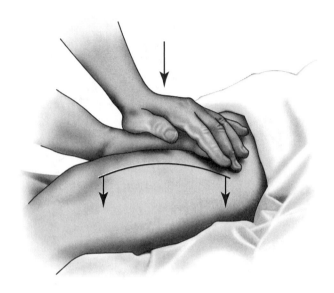

FIGURE 7–17. Compression using reinforced palm. The heel of the top hand is placed to avoid putting pressure on the wrist of the bottom hand.

Variations of Friction

In **superficial warming friction,** the palm or some other part of the practitioner's hand is rubbed briskly over the skin. This generates heat and stimulates superficial circulation. Variations of warming friction use different parts of the hands to create the friction. Greater pressure may be applied to affect deeper tissues such as when using the knuckles (Figure 7–18) and in **sawing,** also called ulnar friction (Figure 7–19). Warming friction is best done "dry" or with little lubricant, since oil or lotion reduces the amount of resistance between the two surfaces and thus reduces the amount of friction.

Deep friction is used to create movement between the deeper tissues and helps keep them from adhering to one another. For example, tissues of the musculoskeletal system are designed for smooth and efficient movement and should slide over each other without sticking. With lack of movement, stress, or trauma to an area, muscle fibers may stick together or tendons stick to tissues they come in contact with. Deep friction can help keep tissues separated and functioning smoothly.

Deep friction may also be used to create movement in tissues around joints such as the ankle and knee, reach into small spaces like the suboccipital region, or be used in areas that lack muscle bulk such as on the head. Areas that don't lend themselves well to petrissage (e.g., at tendonous attachments) may be massaged with deep friction. See Figure 7–20.

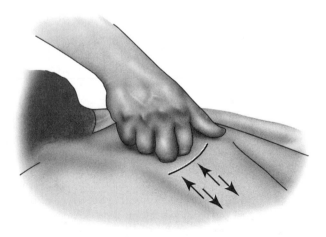

FIGURE 7–18. Warming friction using the knuckles. The first two knuckles move back and forth on the skin to create friction in the area to be warmed.

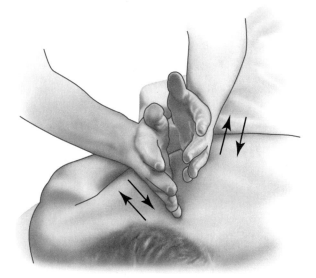

FIGURE 7–19. Warming friction created with a sawing motion, i.e., ulnar friction. The ulnar sides of the hands move back and forth on the skin to create friction in the area to be warmed.

   Deep friction may be performed in a cross-fiber, parallel, or circular motion. Cross-fiber refers to deep friction applied across the direction of the fibers, while parallel friction is applied in the same direction as the fibers. Circular friction is performed using circular movements, which move the underlying tissues in many directions. Figure 7–21 shows cross-fiber friction being applied to the paraspinal muscles.

   Deep friction is performed with the tips of the fingers, the thumb, or the heel of the hand, depending on the size of the surface to be covered. For example, small tendons in places such as the wrist or around the ankle may be frictioned with the fingertips. In Figure 7–22, circular friction is applied with the heel of the hand to free up the broad iliotibial band on the side of the leg.

   Before deep friction is applied, the area must be warmed up thoroughly, usually with effleurage and petrissage. The lubricant used in the warming-up phase may have to be wiped off before performing friction, to allow the practitioner's hands to move the skin without sliding over it. Deep friction is a three-dimensional technique. Practitioners must be keenly aware of the depth at which they are

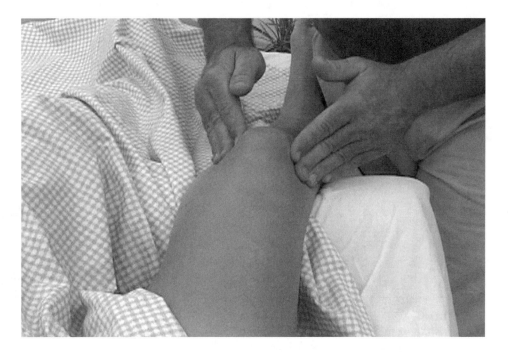

FIGURE 7–20. Circular friction around the knee with the fingertips.

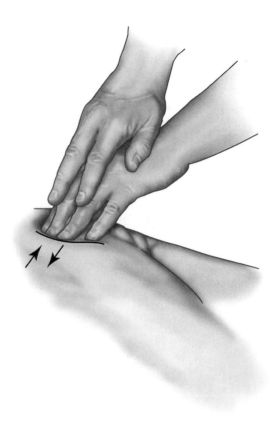

FIGURE 7–21. Cross-fiber friction to the paraspinal muscles. Friction is created by moving the skin and superficial tissues over the deeper tissues underneath.

working, and the depth of the tissues they wish to affect. If the tissues are just beneath the skin, then lighter pressure may be effective. If the tissues are deep or under other tissues, then you must "work through" the more superficial tissues. It is helpful to visualize the tissues in cross-section and to develop palpation skills that will allow you to feel the layers of tissue. Care must be taken in applying deep pressure. Do not try to "muscle through" more superficial tissues, but instead soften them layer by layer. This process takes patience and sensitivity.

Friction Used in Rehabilitation

Deep transverse friction or **Cyriax friction** is a specific type of cross-fiber friction that is applied directly to the site of a lesion. It is used to facilitate healthy scar formation at an injury site. The mechanical action across tissues causes broadening and separation of fibers. Deep transverse friction encourages a

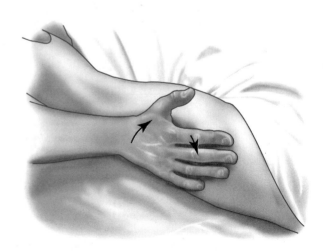

FIGURE 7–22. Circular friction to the broad iliotibial band. The heel of hand is used to create friction between the skin and the underlying tendon, and between the tendon and underlying muscles.

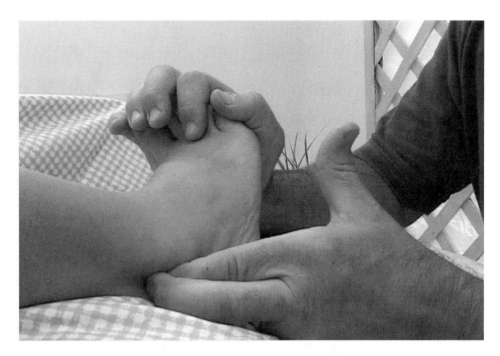

FIGURE 7–23. Deep transverse friction (i.e., Cyriax friction) on an ankle ligament.

more parallel fiber arrangement of scar tissue and fewer cross-connections that limit movement. See Figure 7–23.

James Cyriax popularized the use of deep transverse friction in injury rehabilitation. In the *Illustrated Manual of Orthopedic Medicine* (1993), the following principles were given for treating muscle and tendon lesions:

- The fingers and skin move together to affect deep tissues.
- The effect of friction is most important, not the amount of pressure used.
- The movement must be over the precise site of the lesion.
- The tissue must be in the appropriate tension.
- Do 6 to 12 sessions of 20 minutes each on alternate days for best results.

In addition to promoting healthy scar formation, circular and cross-fiber friction around an injury site can help keep normal tissues from adhering to the scarred area. Such adhering of tissues may cause chronic pain or inflammation. This is especially important where there is a large wound, such as in a cesarean section or other surgery.

TAPOTEMENT

Tapotement consists of a series of brisk percussive movements following each other in rapid, alternating fashion. Tapotement has a stimulating effect and is pleasant to receive if performed skillfully. The most common forms of tapotement are hacking, rapping, cupping, clapping, slapping, tapping, and pincement.

The movement of tapotement is light, rapid, and rhythmic. The hands should "bounce off" of the surface as they make contact, lightening the impact. The recipients should not feel like they are taking a beating, but should feel pleasantly stimulated. The percussive sound itself can be pleasing and can add to the therapeutic effect. Different hand positions create different sounds, and different parts of the body sound different when struck. Quacking and squishes described below are nontraditional forms of tapotement that make distinctive, interesting sounds.

Tapotement takes a certain rhythmic ability and much practice to master. The effort to learn it, though, is well worth while for the diversity it can bring to your work. Experiment with varying rhythms and hand positions for different effects.

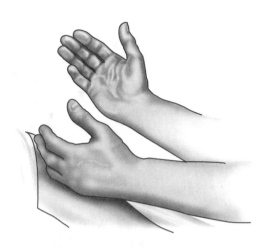

FIGURE 7–24. Hacking. Tapotement performed with the ulnar side of relaxed hands.

Tapotement is often used in finishing either a section of the body, a side of the body, or the session itself. Because it can be stimulating if received for a short period of time, tapotement is useful in situations in which the receiver must be alert when leaving the session. For example, it may be used if the receiver must drive directly after a session or go back to work. Athletes benefit from tapotement before a competition. Some people simply like the tingling and alive feeling that tapotement can leave with them.

While performing tapotement, the amount of force to use and the degree of stiffness of the hands depends on the area receiving the technique. Heavily muscular areas like the back and thighs can withstand more force, while more delicate areas like the head need a light touch. When performing tapotement over a broad area, as in ending a session with tapotement over a whole side of the body, the amount of force used will vary as you move from one section to another.

Variations of Tapotement

Hacking is performed with the hands facing each other, thumbs up. The striking surface is the ulnar surface of the hand and sometimes the sides of the third, fourth, and fifth fingertips. See Figure 7–24. The wrists, hands, and fingers should be held loosely during the rapid percussion movement. Alternate hitting with the left and right hands. Performed correctly, the effect of hacking is one of pleasant stinging and stimulation.

To practice hacking, shake your hands letting the wrists, hands, and fingers relax and "flip up and down." No attempt should be made to hold the fingers together or the hands and wrists in any particular position. If relaxation is complete, you will notice that the hands fall into a neutral plane of mo-

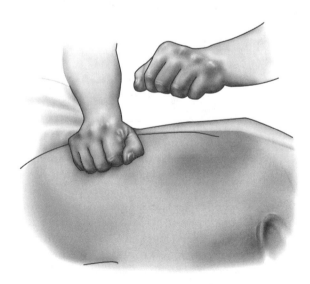

FIGURE 7–25. Rapping. Tapotement performed with the knuckles of a loosely closed fist, as if rapping lightly on a door.

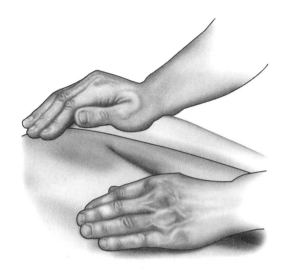

FIGURE 7–26. Cupping. Tapotement performed with the outside rim of a cupped hand.

tion that neither supinates nor pronates the forearms. Move the hands rapidly alternating one up and one down keeping the hands relaxed and shaking them. Practice on the back moving from the hips to the shoulder, and then back to the hips again. Never hit hard over the kidneys.

A similar movement, called **rapping,** may be performed using lightly closed and loosely held fists. The fists may be held palms down as in rapping on a door as shown in Figure 7–25. In side-rapping (sometimes called *beating*), the striking surface is the ulnar side of the fist. Keep the force of the blows light and "rebounding" in effect rather than jarring.

Cupping and **clapping** are applied with the same rhythmic, rapidly alternating force. For both techniques, cup the hand so that the thumb and fingers are slightly flexed, and the palmar surface contracted. The thumb is held tightly against the first finger. For *cupping*, strike the body surface with the outside rim of the cupped hand, keeping the palm contracted, as shown in Figure 7–26. There will be a hollow sound. A sight vacuum is created with each blow, which some believe may loosen broad flat areas of scar tissue or fascial adhesions. Cupping is also used for loosening congestion in the respiratory system.

Let the palm contact the body surface for **clapping.** This produces a less hollow sound and provides a broader contact surface. **Slapping** is performed with an open hand, the fingers held lightly together. Strike gently and briskly with the palmar surface of the fingers, rather than with the whole hand.

Tapping is done with the ends of the fingers. Sharp, light taps are done either with the edge of the fingernails or padding of the fingers. See Figure 7–27.

Pincement is a rapid, gentle movement in which superficial tissues are picked up between the thumb and first two fingers. It might be described as "plucking." A rhythm is established alternating left and right hands. See Figure 7–28.

Quacking is done with the palms together and fingers loosely apart. The striking surface is the lateral edges of the tips of the fourth and fifth (little) fingers as shown in Figure 7–29. As the fingers hit the bony surface, they come together, making a quacking sound.

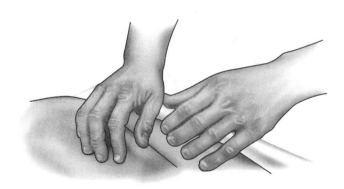

FIGURE 7–27. Tapping. Tapotement performed with the fingertips of a relaxed hand.

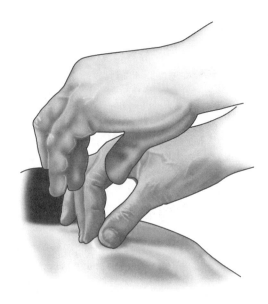

FIGURE 7–28. Pincement. Tapotement performed by gently picking up superficial tissues between the thumb and first two fingers with a light rapid movement.

Squishes are done with the hands loosely folded, making an air pocket with the palms. The striking surface is the back of one of the hands. As the back of the hand hits, the palms push out the air between them, creating a "squishing" sound.

VIBRATION

Vibration may be described as an oscillating, quivering, or trembling motion, or movement back and forth or up and down performed quickly and repeatedly. The vibration may be fine, and applied to a small area with the fingertips. Or it may be coarse, and involve shaking a muscle belly back and forth.

Vibration over the abdomen is sometimes used to stimulate the organs of digestion and elimination. Coarse vibration, in the form of jostling, may be used to help a recipient become aware of holding tension, to bring greater circulation to a muscle, and to help it relax. Fine vibration techniques impart an oscillating motion to the soft tissues and have a stimulating effect. They may also numb or relax specific muscles.

Electric vibrators may be used to impart fine vibration to tense muscles. The motion of vibration can be sustained for a longer period of time with a machine than if performed by hand. There are many types of hand-held electric vibrators. Some impart a coarser vibration, others a finer oscillation. One type of vibrator straps to the back of the hand and causes vibration in the fingers. This allows the

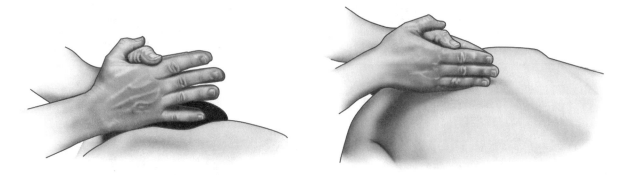

FIGURE 7–29. Quacking. Tapotement performed with the hands together and fingers loosely apart. Fingers come together as the little finger strikes, making a "quacking" sound.

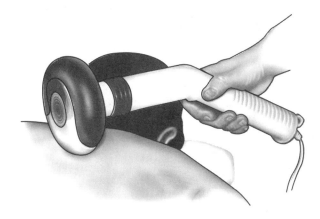

FIGURE 7–30. Fine vibration applied with a hand-held electric vibrator.

practitioner to stay in direct contact with the receiver and perform another technique such as light effleurage or friction. A standard hand-held vibrator is shown in Figure 7–30. A still finer vibration may be created by sound waves. There are devices that impart a lower frequency wave than ultrasound and are within the scope of practice of most practitioners.

Variations of Vibration

A **fine vibration** or trembling motion is imparted through the fingertips, but generated by the forearm. To practice fine vibration, place one hand on a muscle with the fingertips slightly apart. The trembling movement comes from the whole forearm, through the elbow, and the wrist and finger joints are kept in a fixed position. The elbow should be slightly flexed. This vibrating motion should be more in and out than side to side. The fingers remain in contact with the same spot during the vibration and are then lifted off of the skin and replaced to a new spot. Heavy pressure should be avoided. Fine vibration on the abdomen is shown in Figure 7–31.

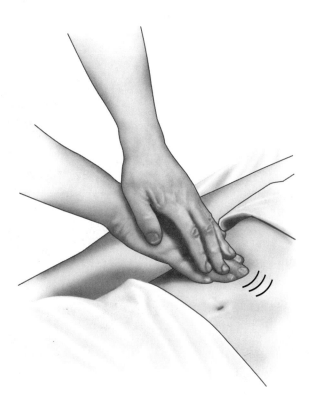

FIGURE 7–31. Vibration applied with fingertips to the abdomen.

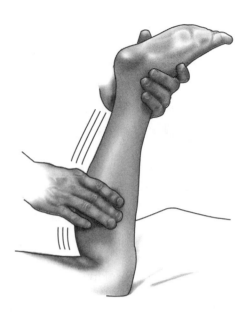

FIGURE 7–32. Shaking. A form of coarse vibration to a muscle or muscle group.

Light effleurage with vibration may be used for a soothing effect. While performing a light effleurage movement, add a sight vibration back and forth with the fingertips. Pressure can be so light that there is slight contact between the hand and the skin. It is a light brushing movement. In cases of hypersensitive nerves, this technique has been credited with having a soothing effect.

Shaking is a coarse form of vibration that can assist muscular relaxation. For example, a muscle such as the biceps or gastrocnemius may be grasped with one hand and shaken gently back and forth. Figure 7–32 shows shaking of the muscles of the leg.

In **jostling** the upper leg, two hands are used, one on each side of the leg. In this case, the muscle movement is back and forth from hand to hand as shown in Figure 7–33. It is helpful at times to jostle the entire limb gently to mobilize the surrounding joints and encourage relaxation and "letting go" of the whole area.

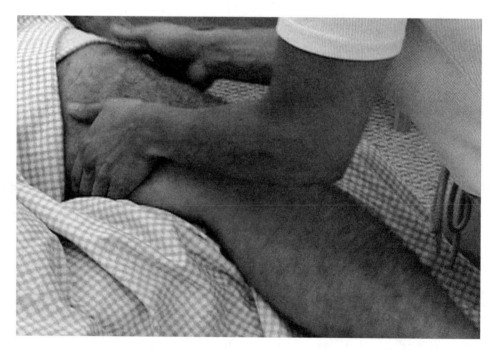

FIGURE 7–33. Jostling. A form of coarse vibration that includes mobilizing joints.

TOUCH WITHOUT MOVEMENT

Touch without movement is a unique massage technique category. It is defined by touch with the hands, but without any visible movement. Touch without movement is not casual or social touch, but is skilled touch with intention. Kellogg cautions that this is not ordinary touch, but "touch applied with intelligence, with control, with a purpose; and simple as it is, is capable of producing decided physiological effects" (p. 52).

Passive Touch

Passive touch is simply laying the fingers, one hand, or both hands lightly on the body. Passive touch may impart heat to an area, having a calming influence on the nervous system, or as some believe, help balance energy. Historically, the effects of passive touch have been attributed to "hypnotic" or "electrical" effects, "magnetism," and "subtle qualities of manner, a peculiar softness of the hand, or other personal quality not easy to describe" (Kellogg, 1929, p. 53). The use of passive touch to balance energy is more fully developed in systems of massage outside of classic Western systems.

Passive touch is often used to begin or end a session, or before turning over. It is used effectively for its calming effects when applied to the feet or to the head, as shown in Figure 7–34 and 7–35.

Direct Pressure

Direct pressure, also called direct static pressure, may be applied with a thumb, finger, knuckle, or elbow. Tissues are compressed using light to heavy pressure. Once tissues are compressed, the technique is held for 5–30 seconds, depending on the intent. There is no movement after the initial compression.

Although this text categorizes direct pressure as touch without movement, it might also be considered "static friction," or a form of compression. **Ischemic compression,** a form of direct pressure applied with enough force to cause blanching, causes vasodilation upon release of pressure, thus increasing local circulation. Ischematic compression is used to treat trigger points as described in Chapter 13.

Pressure should be applied slowly and carefully to avoid bruising or damaging tissues. Direct pressure is often preceded by warming the area with effleurage or rhythmic compressions, and followed with effleurage to "smooth out" the area or transition to another place. Figures 7–36 and 7–37 show two different uses for direct pressure.

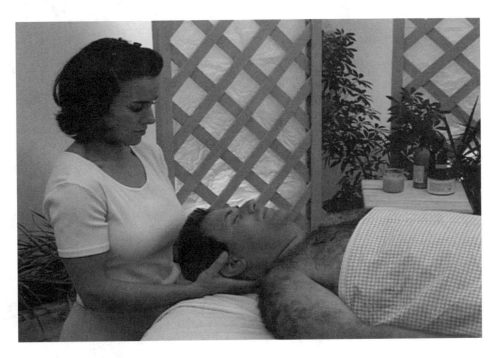

FIGURE 7–34. Passive touch by holding the head lightly.

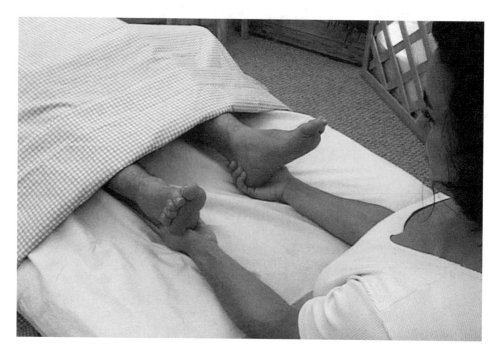

FIGURE 7–35. Passive touch by holding the feet lightly.

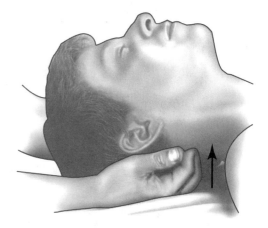

FIGURE 7–36. Direct pressure to suboccipital muscles. Fingers press up into the cervical muscle attachments along the occipital ridge.

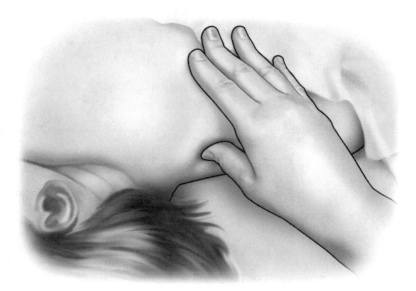

FIGURE 7–37. Ischemic compression (i.e., direct pressure) to a trigger point in the trapezius muscle.

Direct static pressure to various points is known to relieve pain, diminish congestion, and help muscles relax. Theories about how it works have evolved over the years and include the concepts of zone therapy, motor points, stress points, reflex points, trigger points, and acupressure points. The intentions of practitioners using direct static pressure may differ, and the amount of pressure used, location of areas pressed, and duration of pressure may also vary.

SUMMARY

Western massage is the most common form of massage found in spas, health clubs, and private practice, and is the foundation for therapeutic applications within the professions of massage therapy, physical therapy, and nursing. It is the legacy of historical figures such as Pehr Ling of Sweden, Johann Mezger of Amsterdam, J. Harvey Kellogg of the United States, and Mary McMillan of Britain and the United States. Swedish massage is a popular form of Western massage.

Western massage is understood in terms of Western science, and Western beliefs about health and disease. It is recognized as valuable for improving circulation, relaxing muscles, improving joint mobility, inducing general relaxation, and promoting healthy skin.

Western massage techniques fall into seven broad categories: effleurage, petrissage, friction, tapotement, vibration, touch without movement and joint movements. There are an endless number of variations of massage techniques, and the ones presented in this text are merely representative of many possibilities. Soft tissue techniques will be described in this chapter, while joint movements will be described in Chapter 8.

Effleurage techniques slide or glide over the skin with a smooth continuous motion. Effleurage is used to begin a session, apply lubricant, accustom the receiver to touch, connect or transition from one body region to another, assess the condition of tissues, and conclude work on an area. The application of effleurage, e.g., pressure, rhythm, pace, is varied for different effects. Variations of effleurage include basic sliding effleurage, stripping, shingles effleurage, bilateral tree stroking, three-count stroking of the trapezius, horizontal stroking, Mennell's superficial stroking, nerve strokes, and knuckling.

Petrissage techniques lift, wring, or squeeze soft tissues in a kneading motion, or press or roll the tissues under or between the hands. Petrissage is used to increase local circulation, "milk" tissues of accumulated waste products, assist venous return, separate muscle fibers, and evoke muscular relaxation. When applying petrissage, avoid pinching or bruising tissues, and working too long in one area. Variations of petrissage include basic two-handed kneading, one-handed kneading, alternating one-handed kneading, circular two-handed petrissage, alternating fingers-to-thumb petrissage, skin rolling, compression, and rolling.

Friction is performed by rubbing one surface over another repeatedly. Superficial friction is used for warming tissues, and is performed by rubbing the palms briskly over the skin. Deep friction is used to separate tissues, break adhesions, form healthy scar tissue, or to create movement in less-muscled areas such as around joints and over the head. Deep friction is performed in cross-fiber, parallel, or circular motion. Cyriax friction is a form of deep cross-fiber friction used in injury rehabilitation.

Tapotement consists of a series of brisk percussive movements following each other in rapid, alternating fashion. Tapotement is used for stimulation, and as a finishing technique. Variations of tapotement include hacking, rapping, cupping, clapping, slapping, tapping, pincement, quacking, and squishes.

Vibration is an oscillating, quivering, or trembling motion, or movement back and forth or up and down performed quickly and repeatedly. Fine vibration is applied with the fingertips, or with an electric vibrator. Coarse vibration is applied with the whole hand over a larger area and includes light effleurage with vibration, shaking, and jostling.

Touch without movement is defined by touch with the hands, but without any visible movement. Touch without movement is used to impart heat, have a calming effect, or balance energy. Variations of touch without movement include passive touch and holding. Direct pressure, e.g., ischemic compression, is applied to points for a number of effects including to relieve pain, diminish congestion, relax muscles, and stimulate points according to zone therapy, motor points, stress points, reflex points, trigger points, or acu-point theories.

A look ahead . . .

While soft tissue manipulation techniques are the most recognizable aspect of massage, joint movements are equally important for their therapeutic effects and have always been an important part of Western massage. Chapter 8 describes mobilizing and stretching techniques within the scope of massage therapy for each region of the body.

REFERENCES

Cyriax, J. H., & Cyriax, P. J. (1993). *Illustrated manual of orthopedic medicine*, 2nd ed. Boston: Butterworth & Heinemann.

Graham, D. (1884). *Practical treatise on massage*. New York: Wm. Wood and Co.

Hoffa, A. J. (1900). *Technik der massage*, 3rd ed. Verlagsbuchhandlung, Stuttgart: Ferdinand Enke. As translated by F. M. Tappan and Ruth Friedlander.

Kellogg, J. H. (1929). *The art of massage: A practical manual for the nurse, the student and the practitioner*. Battle Creek, MI: Modern Medicine Publishing Co.

STUDY GUIDE

LEARNING OUTCOMES

Use the learning outcomes at the beginning of the chapter as a guide to your studies. Perform the task given in each outcome using the information in the chapter. This may start as an "open book" exercise, and then later from memory.

KEY TERMS/CONCEPTS

To study key techniques listed at the beginning of this chapter, choose one or more of the following exercises. Writing or talking about ideas helps you remember them better, and explaining helps deepen your understanding. Some exercises are designed to sharpen your focus on the details of performing the techniques.

1. Write a description of the six technique categories presented in this chapter. Describe how they differ from each other.

2. Demonstrate technique variations while explaining them verbally to a study partner.

3. Describe how each technique might be used in a massage session, e.g., for warming tissues, as a transition technique, or for ending a session.

4. Explain the physiological/psychological effects of each soft tissue technique variation.

STUDY OUTLINE

The following questions test your memory of the main concepts in this chapter. Locate the answers in the text using the page number given for each question.

Western Massage

1. Western massage is the basis of most massage therapy performed in _____ and _____ today. (p. 126)

2. Today's Western massage traces its origin to the work of _____ of Sweden and _____ of Amsterdam in the 19th century. (p. 126)

3. The effects, benefits and indications of Western massage are explained in terms of Western _____ and _____, and Western notions of _____ and _____. (p. 126)

4. The seven technique categories of Western massage include the five classic massage categories of _____, _____, _____, _____,

and _____, plus _____
and _____. (p. 126)

5. The number of technique variations within each category are _____. (p. 126)

Effleurage

1. Effleurage techniques _____
or _____ over the skin with a
smooth continuous motion. (p. 126)

2. Effleurage has many uses in a massage session, including to _____, _____,
_____, or _____. (p. 126)

3. The effects of effleurage depend on the manner of application, but may include _____,
_____, or _____ (p. 127)

Petrissage

1. Petrissage techniques _____, _____,
or _____ soft tissues in a kneading
motion, or _____ or _____
the tissues under or between the hands. (p. 132)

2. Petrissage is used to "milk" muscles of _____,
increase local _____, relax
_____, and broaden or separate
_____. (p. 132)

3. Pressure used during petrissage should vary according
to the condition of _____, and should
avoid _____ or _____. (p. 132)

4. Kneading or lifting types of petrissage include basic
_____, _____,
_____, _____,
and _____. (pp. 132–134)

5. Pressing petrissage techniques include
_____, and _____. (pp. 134–135)

Friction

1. Friction is performed by rubbing one surface over
_____ repeatedly. (p. 135)

2. _____ friction generates heat on
the skin by brisk rubbing over the skin surface, and is
done best with little or no lubricant. (p. 135)

3. Superficial friction variations are created by
varying the part of the hand used, for example
_____, or by using a back and forth
_____ motion with the ulnar side of
the hand. (p. 136)

4. Deep friction creates movement between
_____ tissues and helps to keep
them from _____ to each other. (p. 136)

5. Deep friction is performed either in
_____ fiber, _____
fiber, or _____ motion. (p. 137)

6. Deep friction is used for specific attention to small
areas, and areas around _____ and
on _____. (p. 137)

7. Tissues should be warmed thoroughly before performing deep friction, and pressure should be monitored
carefully to avoid _____. (p. 137)

8. _____ friction is a specific type of
cross-fiber friction applied directly to the site of a lesion, and is used to aid healthy _____ formation, and in healing of _____. (p. 138)

9. _____ is a specific application of
deep transverse friction used in rehabilitation. (p. 138)

Tapotement

1. Tapotement consists of a series of brisk _____
movements following each other in light, rapid, rhythmic, alternating fashion. (p. 139)

2. Hands should _____ the surface
of the body providing pleasant stimulation, and avoid
_____ that feels uncomfortable. (p. 139)

3. Tapotement is used when finishing _____
or _____ of the body, or to
_____ the session, or when
_____ rather than sedation is
desired. (p. 140)

4. Variations of tapotement are achieved by altering
_____ and include hacking, rapping, cupping, clapping, slapping, tapping, pincement,
quacking, and squishes. (p. 140)

Vibration

1. Vibration may be described as an _____,
_____, or _____
motion, or movement back and forth or up and
down performed _____ and
_____. (p. 142)

2. Vibration can be _____, _____,
or _____ depending on how it is
performed. (p. 142)

3. Fine vibration or trembling motion is imparted by the
fingertips, but generated by _____.
(p. 143)

4. Various types of _____ vibrators may be used for fine vibration. (p. 142)

5. _____ is coarse vibration of an individual muscle or muscle group, and used for relaxation. (p. 144)

6. _____ is a variation of shaking with movement back and forth from hand to hand, usually of a limb. It causes movement in related joints. (p. 144)

Touch Without Movement

1. Touch without movement is a unique massage technique category. It is not casual or social touch, but _____ with _____. (p. 145)

2. _____ is simply laying the fingers, one hand, or both hands lightly on the body. It may

impart _____, have a _____ effect, or help balance _____. (p. 145)

3. When applying direct pressure, there is no _____ after the initial compression of tissues. (p. 145)

4. Ischematic compression is a form of direct pressure applied with enough pressure to cause _____ of tissues. After pressure is released, local _____ is increased. (p. 145)

5. Direct pressure has a variety of uses including relieving _____, diminishing _____, and helping muscles _____. (p. 145)

6. Different types of "point" therapy that involve direct pressure include _____, _____, _____, _____, and _____. (p. 147)

FOR GREATER UNDERSTANDING

The following exercises are designed to take you from the realm of theory into practical applications. They will help give you a deeper understanding of the techniques covered in this chapter. Action words are underlined to emphasize the variety of activities presented to address different learning styles, and to encourage deeper thinking.

1. One person performs a key massage technique variation, while another observes. The observer verbally describes the hand and body position of the person performing the technique.

2. Evaluate how closely their performance matches the written descriptions and illustrations in the book and CD video. Instruct the giver on how to alter their performance to more closely resemble the technique as illustrated.

3. After completing problems 1 and 2, experiment with variations on the technique.

4. Videotape your performance of each of the technique variations. Watching the video, analyze your hand and body mechanics. Perform the techniques again, correcting mechanics. (You may substitute an observer for the videotape).

5. Watching a video of a full-body Western massage (or portion of a session), identify the techniques as you

observe them. Identify broad technique categories, and any specific variations you see. (You may substitute a live performance for the video.)

6. Watching a video of a full-body Western massage (or portion of a session), identify how the techniques are being used in the session, e.g., warming, transition, ending, and for their different effects, e.g., circulatory, muscle relaxation, general relaxation. (You may substitute a live performance for the video.)

7. Watching a video of a full-body Western massage (or portion of a session), become aware of the richness of techniques used, i.e., how many variations and combinations of techniques the practitioner applies. Watch two or more sessions and compare them.

8. Receive a massage and pay attention to the feel of the different techniques, naming them in your mind as they are applied. Notice how they are used by the practitioner.

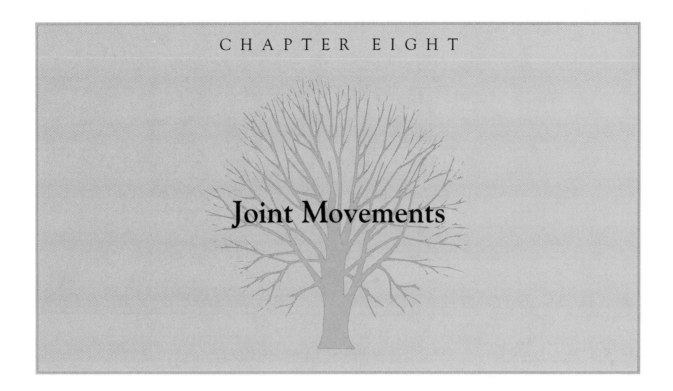

CHAPTER EIGHT

Joint Movements

LEARNING OUTCOMES

After studying this chapter, the student will have information to:

1. Describe the different categories of joint movements.
2. Compare mobilizing techniques and stretching.
3. Perform three methods of stretching: static, contract-relax-stretch, using reciprocal inhibition.
4. Explain the therapeutic benefits of joint movements.
5. Apply the general principles for joint movements.
6. Perform joint movement techniques for different areas of the body.

KEY TERMS/CONCEPTS

Assisted movements
Contract-relax-stretch (CRS)
Free active movements
Joint manipulations/
    adjustments

Normal range of motion
Mobilizing techniques
Passive movements
Reciprocal inhibition
Resisted movements

Static stretch
Stretching
Swedish movements

MEDIALINK

A companion CD-ROM, included free with each new copy of this book, supplements the techniques presented in this chapter. Insert the CD-ROM to watch video clips of massage techniques being demonstrated. This multimedia feature is designed to help you add a new dimension to your learning.

JOINT MOVEMENT TECHNIQUES

Neck

Mobilizing Techniques
simple mobilizing movements
finger push-ups
melt-down
wavelike movement

Stretches
lateral flexion
rotation
forward flexion
cross-arm stretch

Shoulder Girdle

Mobilizing Techniques
wagging
shaking
passive shoulder roll
scapula mobilizing (prone)

Stretches
horizontal flexion
overhead stretch

Elbow

Mobilizing Techniques
pronation and supination
circling the forearm

Stretching
overhead stretch

Wrist

Mobilizing Techniques
passive movement through full
   range of motion
waving

Stretches
hyperextension
flexion

Hand

Mobilizing Techniques
passive movements of all joints
figure-eights
scissoring

Stretches
hyperextension of fingers and
   wrist
flexion

Chest

Mobilizing Techniques
rocking rib cage

Stretches
overhead stretch

Hip

Mobilizing Techniques
rhythmic rocking of straight
   leg
passive movement through full
   range of motion

Stretches
knee to chest flexion
straight leg flexion
diagonal adduction with flexed
   knee
straight leg hyperextension in
   side-lying

Knee

Mobilizing Techniques
wag
leg toss
circling the lower leg

Stretches
heel to buttocks

Ankle

Mobilizing Techniques
dorsiflexing foot with thumb
   pressure to bottom
passive movement through full
   range of motion
side to side mobilizing

Stretches
dorsiflexion
plantar flexion

Foot

Mobilizing Techniques
figure eights of toes
scissoring metatarsals
straightening toes with
   effleurage

Stretches
hyperextension of toes
foot widening at metatarsals
interlocking finger and toes

OVERVIEW OF JOINT MOVEMENTS

Western massage traditionally includes joint movements, as well as soft tissue manipulation. Pehr Ling's original system of medical gymnastics included passive movements of both the soft tissues and joints (Roth 1851). The term **"Swedish movements"** was commonly used in the United States to refer to joint movements up through the 1950s.

Categories of Joint Movements

Joint movements are categorized as active (i.e., free, assisted, and resisted) and passive (McMillan, 1925). **Free active movements** are performed entirely by a person without assistance from a practitioner. In **assisted movements,** recipients initiate the movement, while practitioners help them perform the movement. In **resisted movements,** practitioners offer resistance to the movement, thereby challenging the muscles used. **Passive movements** refer to movements initiated and controlled by the practitioner, while the recipient remains totally relaxed and passive.

Mobilizing techniques or joint mobilizations, within the context of massage therapy, are passive movements performed within the normal range of joint movement. Mobilizing techniques are nonspecific movements of the joints and surrounding soft tissues that free up motion at the joints involved. They can be easily integrated into a massage routine.

Stretching is a type of passive joint movement that is performed to the limit of the range of motion, with a slight stretch beyond. It is used to increase flexibility at the joint, as it elongates the muscles and connective tissues that cross the joint. Stretching may also be used for muscle relaxation.

Joint manipulations or adjustments (sometimes called *chiropractic adjustments*) are <u>not</u> within the scope of massage therapy. By joint manipulations and adjustments, we mean techniques that take a joint beyond its normal range of motion and that are specific attempts to realign a misaligned joint, or free a frozen joint, usually using a thrusting movement. They should be performed only by those trained to do so within their legal scope of practice. "Cracking" necks and backs and "popping" toes are potentially dangerous and should not be performed as part of standard Western massage.

In this chapter, we will describe simple passive joint movements that fall under the categories of nonspecific joint mobilizing techniques and stretching. These movements may be incorporated into a general massage session or might be used for specific therapeutic goals.

Uses of Joint Movements

Practitioners use joint movements for a variety of reasons including to stretch surrounding soft tissues, increase range of motion, stimulate production of synovial fluid, increase kinesthetic awareness, stimulate muscle relaxation, and build muscle strength. Both active and passive joint movements are applied to increase flexibility, and improve posture and body alignment. Athletes find joint movements particularly beneficial for improving performance, preventing injuries, and for rehabilitation.

Some contemporary systems of bodywork, such as Trager Psychophysical Integration®, use joint movements to affect the nervous system, re-educate muscles, and integrate function. Receivers can also learn to let go of tension they are unconsciously holding onto during passive joint movement. Joint movement adds a kinetic dimension to a massage session and provides diversity of technique.

GENERAL PRINCIPLES OF JOINT MOVEMENTS

Massage practitioners should be familiar with the bony structure and muscles that move each joint. Together these determine the movements possible at the joint. **Normal range of motion** refers to the degree of movement commonly found at a joint, and is useful knowledge to generally assess the degree of flexibility at a joint. Knowing the normal limitations to movement at each joint will decrease the likelihood of inadvertently damaging a joint or the surrounding tissues, and increase safety for the recipient.

Caution is advised in cases of abnormality of the bony structure, hypermobility, recent injury, and diseases of the joints such as bursitis and arthritis. A past trauma may have caused some unusual conditions around a joint, including shortening or loss of muscle tissue, scarring in connective tissues, and abnormal joint structure. Sometimes "hardware," such as metal pins and plates, is present from past injuries. Joint replacements are becoming more common, and movement around artificial joints may be restricted. Hip and knee replacements are important to know about, especially in the elderly. Take the time to learn about the condition from up-to-date medical references, the recipient, from available medical records, or from the recipient's physician to ensure a safe application of joint movements. Remember that massage and joint movements are contraindicated when acute inflammation is present.

Palpation skills are very important for learning how joints move. Practitioners can learn much about the condition of the joint and surrounding tissues from the kinesthetic feel of the movement. Sensations like "drag" and "end feel" offer clues to restrictions to normal range of motion, areas of tightness, patterns of holding, and the limits of stretches. Drag refers to resistance felt as the soft tissues around a joint are stretched, and end feel refers to resistance as the limit of the stretch is approached.

The stretches described in this chapter are passive movements applied as **static stretches.** Avoid sudden, forceful, or bouncing movements while performing the stretches. Move the part being stretched into position and hold at the limit of movement, which is determined by feeling for the point of resistance. Use feedback from the recipient for safety. The recipient should feel the stretch, but not feel pain. Hold for 10–15 seconds, and then try to increase the stretch. The muscles will often relax after a short time, allowing further stretch (30–45 seconds overall).

Stretches can be facilitated with techniques called **contract-relax-stretch (CRS),** and contract-relax-stretch using **reciprocal inhibition.** In CRS, the practitioner gets into position to perform the stretch, but first asks the client to contract the muscle to be stretched against a resistance (resisted movement). Immediately following the muscle's relaxation, the stretch is applied.

When reciprocal inhibition is used, the practitioner gets into position to perform the stretch, but first asks the client to contract the target muscle's antagonist against a resistance. The target or agonist muscle relaxes as its antagonist contracts. Immediately following the antagonist's relaxation, the stretch is applied.

Breathing may be used to help the recipient relax during a stretch. The body is more relaxed during exhalation than during inhalation, and holding the breath causes tension in the musculature and restricts movement. So it is better to stretch a muscle on the exhalation. Once you and the recipient are in position to apply a stretch, ask her to "take a deep breath and then let it out slowly." During the exhalation, apply the stretch.

The following is a summary of the general guidelines for performing passive joint movements:

- Stay within the normal range of motion of the joint.
- Qualities of mobilizing techniques are smooth, free, and loose.
- Warm surrounding soft tissues before stretching.
- Use breathing to enhance a stretch.
- Stay within the comfort range of the recipient.
- Be aware of abnormality of joint structure and adapt movements accordingly.

JOINT MOVEMENT TECHNIQUES

Neck

Structure and Movement.   The "neck" is a general term for the region between the head and the trunk. It includes the seven cervical vertebrae and the surrounding soft tissues. The cervicals are the smallest, most delicate vertebrae and are designed to allow for a lot of movement but not bear a lot of weight. They are arranged vertically with an anterior convex curve.

The musculature in the neck region is complex with deeper, smaller muscles entirely within the neck, and larger and more superficial muscles attaching superior and inferior. The bony and muscular structures allow a variety of movements including flexion, extension, hyperextension, lateral flexion, and rotation.

Mobilizing Techniques.   Mobilizing techniques for the neck are performed when the recipient is lying supine. The mobilizing movement occurs between the cervical vertebrae and in the suboccipital region. All of the following examples may be performed with the practitioner seated at the head of the recipient. It is useful to have an adjustable stool or chair on wheels so that you can get in good position, for both leverage and self-care.

Simple mobilizing movements of the neck may be performed by lifting the head slightly off the table, and moving the neck into lateral flexion, rotation, forward flexion, or hyperextension. Be sure to have a firm grip on the head. You may have to remind the recipient to relax, since it takes great trust to let someone hold and move your head. You may also assure them that you will not "crack" their neck, and that such manipulations are not part of this type of mobilization. Keep the movements small at first and gradually increase the range of motion as the recipient allows.

Finger push-ups may be used to produce gentle movement between the cervical vertebrae. First warm up the neck muscles with effleurage and circular friction along each side. Straighten the neck, so that the recipient is directly face up. Simply place the fingers at the base of the neck on either side, palms up, and push up with the fingers, applying direct pressure. Move your hands about an inch at a time along the neck, pressing up at each spot as you move along. You will feel movement between the vertebrae and notice movement at the head. Variations of finger push-ups include alternating pressing from side to side. The rhythm would be to press right, press left, move along; press right, press left, move along; repeating the sequence along the neck, moving toward the head.

The melt-down is a variation of the finger push-up applied in the suboccipital region. Place your hands, palms up, under the recipient's head, with fingers along the suboccipitals. Lift the head with the hands, and then lower the wrists to the table, while leaving the head balanced on the fingertips. Usually within 5–10 seconds, the neck muscles relax, the suboccipital tissues "melt," and the head hyperextends. You will notice the recipient's head falling back, and your fingers will be deep into the suboccipital space. This pressure usually feels good to the recipient. Finish by gently pulling on the occiput to straighten any hyperextension remaining from the movement.

A wavelike movement may be created in the neck by simply applying deep effleurage on both sides at the same time, moving from the base to the suboccipital region. You exaggerate the natural curve of the neck by pressing up as you slide along. The neck will return to its normal curve as you finish the movement. (See Figure 9–21.) At the end of the movement, give a gentle pull on the occiput to straighten any hyperextension remaining from the movement. The *wave* is a good technique to use to detect tension in the neck. The wavelike motion will not occur if the recipient is unconsciously holding tension in the neck or if the neck muscles are shortened and tight.

Stretches.   Massage and simple mobilizing techniques are used to warm up the neck thoroughly before applying stretches. The following stretches may be performed when the recipient is lying supine on a table.

A stretch in lateral flexion helps lengthen the muscles on the sides of the neck. Place the head in position to one side at a point where you feel the tissues just starting to stretch. The head placement, either face up or turned to the side, will determine which muscles are stretched most. Place one hand on the shoulder and the other on the side of the head. You can create a gentle stretch of tissues by pushing the head and shoulders in opposite directions as shown in Figure 8–1. Guide the recipient to exhale as you apply the stretch. The head will move to a position of greater lateral flexion as the upper trapezius relaxes and lengthens. Repeat on the other side.

Range of rotation may be enhanced with a simple stretch. Position the head face up so that the neck is straight. Then rotate the head to one side, keeping the neck vertically aligned. Gently push the head into greater rotation, stretching the neck muscles. Repeat on the other side.

Position the head face up to stretch the neck in forward flexion. Lift the head with one hand, and with the other hand, reach under the head and across to the tip of the shoulder. The head rests on the

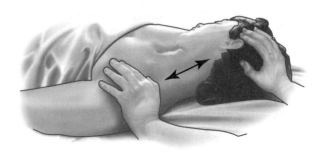

FIGURE 8–1. Stretch of trapezius and cervical muscles with neck in lateral flexion.

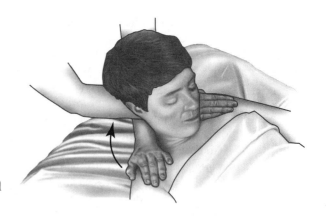

FIGURE 8–2. Cross-arm stretch of cervical muscles with neck in forward flexion.

forearm. Reach under that arm with the free hand and place it on the other shoulder. The head should be cradled safely at the place where the forearms cross, as shown in Figure 8–2. Slowly stretch the neck into forward flexion. Stand during this movement for best leverage.

The **cross-armed stretch** may also be performed with the head rotated. This will stretch neck muscles at a different angle. After forward flexion, return to the starting position and turn the head to one side. Repeat the forward flexion to each side with the head in rotation. For safety, be sure that the stretch is pain free.

Shoulder Girdle

Structure and Movement.   The shoulder girdle is a complex region that can be defined in different ways. For our purposes, the shoulder girdle will be defined as including the glenohumeral, acromio-clavicular, and scapulocostal joints. The glenohumeral joint is classified as a ball-and-socket joint, and the acromioclavicular joint as diarthrodial nonaxial. The scapulocostal juncture may be described as a gliding joint of the scapula with the rib cage separated by muscles and a bursa (Cailliet, 1981, p. 2).

The shoulder girdle is the most mobile area of the body. Movements possible in the shoulder girdle include the upper arm movements of flexion, extension, hyperextension, abduction, adduction, rotation, and horizontal flexion. Movements of the scapulae themselves include elevation, depression, upward and downward rotation and tilt, and retraction and protraction. The entire shoulder girdle is structured to accomplish circumduction.

Mobilizing Techniques.   Mobilizing movements of the shoulder girdle may be performed with the recipient in supine, prone, side-lying, or seated position. Mobilizing the joints of the shoulder may be accomplished indirectly by movement of the arm or by movement of the scapula.

To mobilize the shoulder girdle with the recipient in the supine position, take hold of the hand and lift and wag the arm as shown in Figure 8–3. While **wagging** the arm, there will also be movement at the wrist and elbow. **Shaking** is performed by creating a slight traction of the arm toward the feet, holding onto the hand and leaning back as shown in Figure 8–4. Loosely shake the arm up and down. Movement will be felt at the wrist, elbow, and shoulder.

The **passive shoulder roll** may be used for mobilizing the shoulder. Hold onto the upper arm with one hand close to the glenohumeral joint, and the other hand at the tip of the shoulder. Simply move the shoulder through the full range of motion possible in the supine position. The quality of movement should be smooth, free, and loose. This same technique is effective in the prone, side-lying, and seated positions. Figure 8–5 shows the passive shoulder roll with the recipient supine.

With the recipient prone, **scapula mobilizing** may be accomplished using pressure applied at the top of the shoulder. Position the recipient's arm on the table with elbow bent and hand near the waist. Then place your hand on top of the shoulder near the tip and pressing lightly toward the feet. The scapula will move and lift if the attached muscles are relaxed as shown in Figure 8–6. Don't force the movement, but encourage relaxation by gentle motions and reminding the recipient to let go of tension in the area. Once the medial border lifts, you may apply effleurage to massage the muscles that attach there.

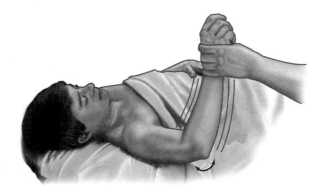

FIGURE 8–3. Wagging: an arm and shoulder mobilizing technique.

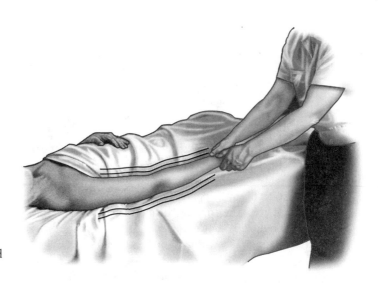

FIGURE 8–4. Shaking: an arm and shoulder mobilizing technique.

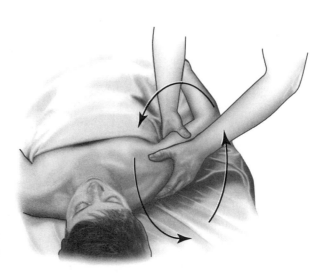

FIGURE 8–5. Passive shoulder roll. Mobilizing technique for the shoulder with recipient in supine position.

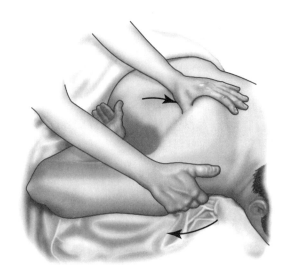

FIGURE 8–6. Scapula mobilizing technique. Move and lift the scapula by pulling back at the shoulder.

Stretches.   Use massage and mobilizing technique to warm up the shoulder girdle before stretching. Shoulder girdle stretches are effective in the supine, prone, and side-lying positions. The muscles of the shoulder girdle are stretched primarily with movements of the upper arm.

In the supine position, a stretch in **horizontal flexion** may be performed by moving the arm over the chest. This elongates the muscles that attach to the medial border of the scapula, including the rhomboids, as well as the posterior shoulder muscles. Hold onto the recipient's lower arm near the wrist with one hand, while the other hand reaches under to the medial border of the scapula. Stretch the arm over the chest and enhance the stretch by gently pulling back on the scapula at the same time. See Figure 8–7.

A very pleasant stretch may be applied with the recipient's arms extended overhead. This **overhead stretch** may be performed one arm at a time or both arms at the same time. For a two-arm stretch, simply place the arms overhead, grasping the forearm near the wrist. Lean back to create the stretch at the shoulder, as shown in Figure 8–8. This technique stretches all of the muscles of the shoulder girdle, including the latissimus dorsi and pectoral muscles.

A similar stretch may be applied with the recipient seated in a massage chair. Grasp the forearm with both hands and move the arm overhead to a position in line with the angle of the body. You should be facing in the same direction as the recipient. Lift the arm upward and give it a gentle shake as shown in Figure 8–9.

Elbow

Structure and Movement.   The elbow is formed by the junction of the distal end of the humerus and the proximal ends of the radius and the ulna. Movements of the humeroulnar joint are limited to flexion and extension. The bony structure of the joint further limits the range of motion in extension.

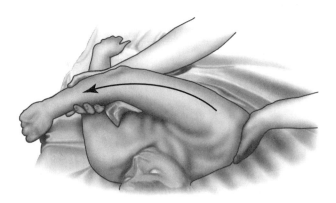

FIGURE 8–7. Stretching the shoulder muscles with arm in horizontal flexion.

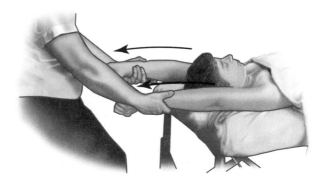

FIGURE 8–8. Overhead stretch for the shoulder muscles. Lean back to create the stretch using your body weight.

What we think of as the point of the elbow is the olecranon process of the ulna. The movements of pronation and supination of the forearm (palm-down and palm-up) occur as the head of the radius rotates over the surfaces of the capitulum of the humerus and the radial notch of the ulna. At the same time, the distal ends of the radius and ulna glide over one another.

Mobilizing Techniques.   Movements at the elbow are limited by the structure of the joint. **Wagging** of the arm as described above offers some mobilization at the elbow. You may also **pronate and supinate the forearm** by holding the hand and turning it alternately palm up and palm down.

To perform a simple mobilizing technique at the elbow, bend the arm at the elbow so that it is perpendicular to the table. Hold the arm just below the wrist. Trace a circle with the hand (i.e., **circling the forearm**) creating movement at the elbow as shown in Figure 8–10.

Stretches.   Stretches of muscles that cross the elbow are accomplished largely by stretching the whole arm as in the **overhead stretch** of the shoulder described above. If the biceps muscles are shortened, the stretch is created by simply straightening out the arm at the elbow.

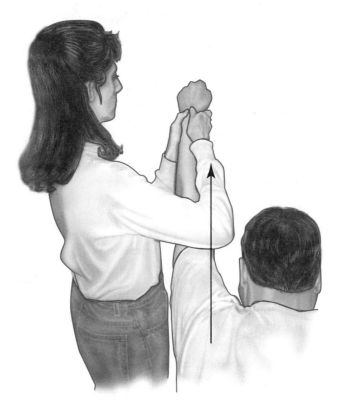

FIGURE 8–9. Overhead stretch of the shoulder muscles. Recipient in a massage chair.

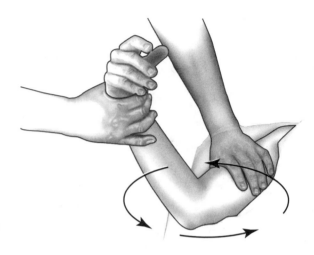

FIGURE 8–10. Circling the forearm to create movement at the elbow.

Wrist

Structure and Movement.   The wrist joint is formed by the union of the slightly concave surface of the proximal row of carpal bones with the distal end of the radius and the midcarpal joint. What people commonly call the "wrist bone" is actually the distal end of the ulna. Movements possible at this juncture include flexion, extension, hyperextension, radial and ulnar deviation (side-to-side movement), and circumduction.

Mobilizing Techniques.   Mobilizing of the wrist are best performed with the recipient supine. The soft tissues in the wrist area may be warmed up with small effleurage movements with the thumbs prior to mobilizing and stretching. A useful starting position for basic mobilizing techniques and stretching is achieved by clasping the recipient's hands, palms facing and fingers interwoven. The recipient's elbow is bent and may be resting on the table. In the hand-clasp position, you may move the hand through its entire range of motion at the wrist including flexion, extension, hyperextension, side-to-side in radial and ulnar deviation, and circumduction. Keep the passive movement well within the possible range of motion.

A light, quick mobilizing technique may be performed at the wrist with a **waving** movement. Face the head of the table and hold the forearm just proximal to the recipient's wrist (palm down) with both of your hands, the thumbs on top and index fingers below. Use the remaining fingers to cause the hand to *wave*, by pressing up against the heel of the hand quickly and repeatedly, letting gravity help it fall between times. Movement at the wrist also occurs during less specific mobilizations, including wagging the arm as shown in Figure 8–3, and supination and pronation of the forearm.

Stretches.   Flexion and hyperextension are the major stretches performed at the wrist. Figure 8–11 shows stretching the flexors of the forearm by **hyperextending at the wrist.** Press down gently on the palm side of the fingers to create the stretch. Now **flex the hand at the wrist** and press down on the back side of the hand to create a stretch of the extensors of the forearm as shown in Figure 8–12. During these stretches, be careful to approach the limit of motion slowly.

Hand

Structure and Movement.   Joints within the hand and distal to the wrist include the metacarpophalangeal juncture (i.e., knuckles) and the small joints between phalanges. The second through fifth fingers each have three phalanges with two joints, while the thumb has just two phalanges with one joint. The joint between the carpal and metacarpal of the thumb is designed to allow freer movement than similar junctures of the carpals and metacarpals. Movement may also occur between metacarpals. Movements of the fingers include flexion, extension, abduction, and adduction. The hand as a whole is capable of holding and grasping objects.

Mobilizing Techniques.   Perform mobilizing techniques of the hand joints very carefully, matching the force used to the size and strength of the hand you are working with. Warm the muscles in the recipient's hands with effleurage and light frictions before performing mobilizing techniques and stretches.

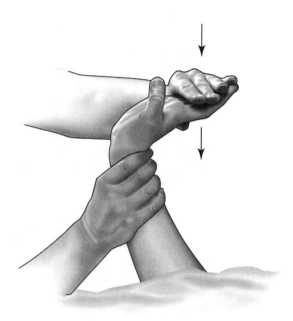

FIGURE 8–11. Stretching the flexor muscles
of the forearm by hyperextending the wrist.

Mobilizing the knuckles, one at a time may be achieved making **figure eights.** Hold the recipient's hand with one of your hands, his fingers pointing toward you, palm down. With your other hand, grasp the fifth (little) finger firmly near the knuckle and move in a small figure eight pattern two or three times, mobilizing the joint. See Figure 8–13. Repeat for each knuckle joint. A similar, but lighter, mobilizing of the knuckles may be achieved by grasping the fingers more distally. Perform the figure eights as described above.

You can mobilize the tissues between the metacarpals with a **scissoring** motion. With the recipient's palm down, take hold of knuckles of the fifth and fourth fingers as shown in Figure 8–14. Simply move one knuckle up and the other down at the same time, alternating in a scissoring motion. Repeat along all of the knuckles.

Stretches.   There are a few simple stretches for the joints of the hand. Perform them slowly and with care. The fingers can be **hyperextended** at the knuckles. Interlace your fingers with the recipient's, palm to palm, placing the tips of your fingers just below the recipient's knuckles. Gently press between the metacarpals, bending the fingers into hyperextension. This movement may also cause the metacarpals to spread out, stretching the tissues between them.

Taking the whole hand into **hyperextension** can stretch all of the flexor muscles within the hand and the wrist flexors in the forearm. Hold the forearm with one hand and, with the other hand, press back on the phalanges, causing hyperextension at the knuckles and at the wrist. Gently stretch the tissues of the hand and the forearm. See Figure 8–11.

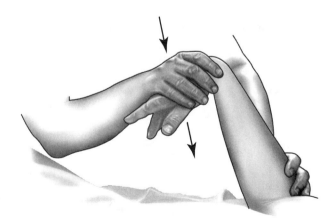

FIGURE 8–12. Stretching the extensor
muscles of the forearm by flexing the wrist.

Chest

Structure and Movement.   The "chest" is a common term for the area on the front and sides of the upper body generally defined by the ribs, sternum, and clavicle. It is the part of the thorax accessible when lying supine. The entire thorax, including the chest, expands and contracts with the inhalation and exhalation of breathing. The pectoral muscles are located on the chest.

Mobilizing Techniques.   The rib cage may be mobilized by **gentle rocking** from the side. Stand facing the side of the table in line with the rib cage. Put one hand on top of the other and place them on the rib cage as shown in Figure 8–15. Gently rock the rib cage by repeatedly pushing and then letting up the pressure in a rhythmic manner. Move around on the rib cage to mobilize different areas. You will feel the elastic quality of the rib cage as it springs back after you push.

If you can reach far enough with your arms, you can cause movement in the chest from both sides. Facing the head of the table, reach over with one hand to the far side of the chest, fingers pointing down toward the table. Place the other hand on the near side, fingers pointing up. See Figure 8–16. Gently rock the rib cage by alternating pulling with the far hand and pushing with the near hand. Establish a smooth rhythm to encourage relaxation of the surrounding musculature.

Stretches.   There are no highly movable joints on the chest itself. However, the pectoral muscles of the shoulder girdle attach there. Use the overhead stretch of the arms as shown in Figure 8–8 to lengthen the pectorals.

Hip

Structure and Movement.   The hip joint is a typical ball-and-socket joint formed by the articulation of the head of the femur with the deep cup-shaped acetabulum of the pelvis. The large muscles that move the hip joint are located primarily on the thigh and the buttocks. The iliopsoas is a strong hip flexor that attaches to the lumbar vertebrae and inner surface of the ilium and the lesser trochanter of the femur. Movements possible at the hip joint include flexion, extension, hyperextension, abduction, adduction, diagonal abduction and adduction, outward and inward rotation, and circumduction.

Mobilizing Techniques.   Most hip movements are performed with the recipient in the supine position. Mobilizing techinques are an excellent way to affect the deeper muscles that move the hip.

With the recipient supine, remove the bolster from under the knees. The legs should be straight and slightly apart. Stand facing the thigh at the side of the table. **Gently rock the leg** into rotation by placing the hands palms down on the top of the thigh and pressing down and away. See Figure 8–17.

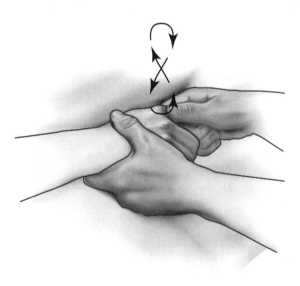

FIGURE 8–13. Figure 8s at the knuckles of the hand.

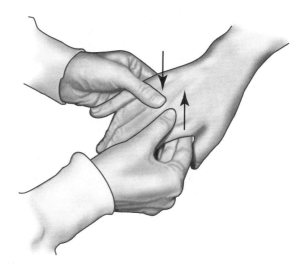

FIGURE 8–14. Scissoring motion to create movement between the metacarpals of the hand.

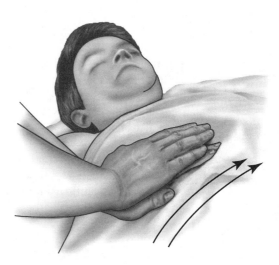

FIGURE 8–15. Placement of hands for mobilizing the rib cage from one side.

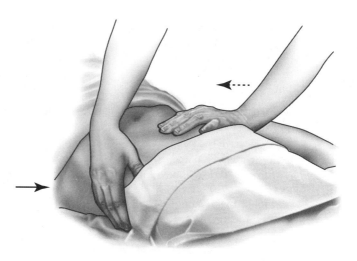

FIGURE 8–16. Placement of hands for mobilizing the rib cage from both sides.

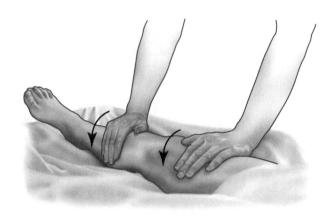

FIGURE 8–17. Rocking the leg to create rotation in the hip joint.

The leg will usually rotate back, especially if the gluteals are tight. The foot will wag from side to side if performed properly. Repeat with a rhythmic rocking motion.

To **move the hip through its full range of motion,** bend the leg, placing the foot in one hand, and using the other hand for support at the knee. See Figure 8–18. Let the knee trace a circle as the hip flexes, adducts diagonally, extends, abducts diagonally, and goes round again in circumduction. The movement should be smooth and loose.

Stretches.   The muscles that move the hip can be stretched in many directions. The following are a few simple yet useful stretches for the hip joint.

A stretch for the gluteals may be applied with the hip in flexion by pressing the **knee toward the chest** (supine position). See Figure 8–19. The hamstrings may be stretched with the leg straight and in flexion as shown in Figure 8–20. To enhance the stretch and involve all of the gluteal and leg muscles, dorsiflex the foot while you bring the leg perpendicular to the table, and then as far toward the chest as possible.

Diagonal adduction of the thigh while lying supine will also stretch the gluteals. Bring the knee toward the chest, and then let it cross the body diagonally as shown in Figure 8–21. The shoulders remain flat on the table, while the supine twists and the hip muscles stretch. This is also a good stretch for the lower back.

The flexors may be stretched from the prone or side-lying position. With the recipient prone, stand at the side of the table facing the head. Bend the leg at the knee and grasp the thigh from underneath; the lower leg can rest against your shoulder. Lift the knee off the ground, putting the hip into hyperextension. You may anchor the hip with the other hand. This stretch takes some strength and is most easily performed if the recipient is smaller than you are.

The **stretch into hyperextension** can be more easily performed with the recipient in side-lying position. Stand behind the recipient facing the table at the hip. Cradle the upper leg with one arm while you stabilize the trunk with the other. Pull the upper leg back into hyperextension as shown in Figure 8–22. Because you are pulling the leg back, instead of lifting it up, this technique is more efficient and takes less strength. It primarily stretches the quadriceps and iliopsoas muscles.

Knee

Structure and Movement.   The knee is classified as a hinge joint and is formed by the articulation of the distal end of the femur with the proximal end of the tibia. A large sesamoid bone embedded in the connective tissues that cross the joint forms the knee cap or patella. The major movements of the knee joint are flexion and extension. Some minor inward and outward rotation of the tibia is possible when the knee is flexed in a non–weight-bearing situation.

Mobilizing Techniques.   The knee joint is best mobilized with the recipient in the prone position. For a simple mobilizing technique, stand facing the side of the table at the knee. Pick up the leg near the ankle with both hands, so that the lower leg is perpendicular to the table. Lift the leg slightly off the table and **wag** it back and forth. This also mobilizes the hip joint.

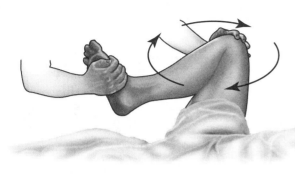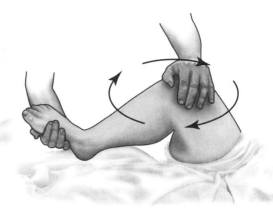

FIGURE 8–18. Moving the hip through its full range of motion.

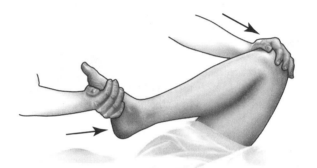

FIGURE 8–19. Stretching the gluteals by bringing knee to chest.

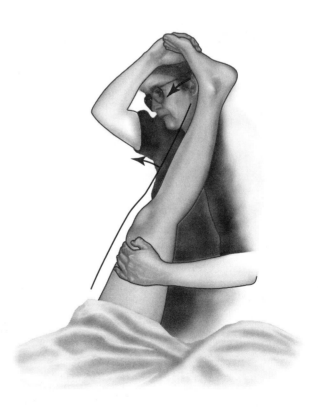

FIGURE 8–20. Stretching the hamstrings with straight leg flexion.

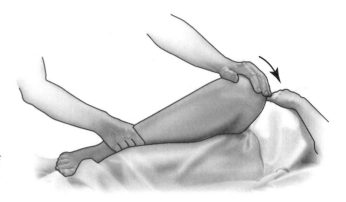

FIGURE 8–21. Stretching the muscles of the hip and lower back with diagonal adduction of the bent leg.

Another simple mobilization at the knee involves tossing the lower leg back and forth from hand to hand. This **leg toss** technique helps the recipient learn to relax and let go of tension in the legs. After the leg toss, you may perform a different knee mobilization by **circling the lower leg.** Place one hand on the thigh to steady it and grasp the lower leg near the ankle with the other hand. Make small circles with the lower leg. Stay well within the small range of this circular motion.

Stretches.   A few of the stretches for the hip joint, performed with a straight leg, also stretch muscles that cross the knee. See Figure 8–20. An additional stretch for the knee extensors can be created with the recipient in the prone position by bringing the **heel of the foot toward the buttocks.** See Figure 8–23.

Ankle

Structure and Movement.   The ankle is a hinge joint formed by the junction of the talus with the malleoli of the tibia and fibula. The structure is bound together with many ligaments for stability. The tendons of muscles of the lower leg that attach to the foot all pass over the ankle. They are bound neatly at the ankle by a band of connective tissue called the retinaculum. Movements possible at the ankle include dorsiflexion (flexion), plantar flexion (extension), pronation (eversion and abduction), and supination (inversion and adduction).

Mobilizing Techniques.   When the recipient is prone, the ankle may be accessed by lifting the lower leg so that the foot comes off the table. For **mobilizing with dorsiflexion,** stand at the feet facing the end of the table. Lift one leg and place both hands on the foot, thumbs on the bottom of the foot. Lean into the foot with the thumbs in the arch, moving the foot into dorsiflexion as shown in Figure 8–24. Repeat the mobilization several times in a rhythmic manner, changing the location of the thumbs to affect different spots on the feet.

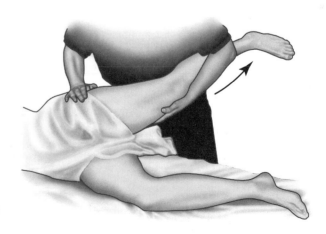

FIGURE 8–22. Stretching the hip flexors with the recipient side-lying.

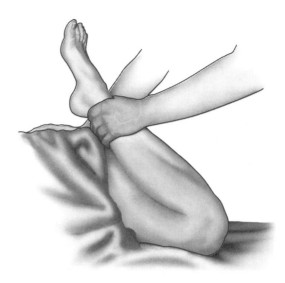

FIGURE 8–23. Stretching the quadriceps by bring-ing the heel of the foot toward the buttocks.

With the lower leg lifted so that it is perpendicular to the table, the ankle can be put through a full range of motion. Grasp the bottom of the foot from above and move the ankle through dorsiflex-ion, pronation, plantar flexion, and supination in a circular movement. This is also an excellent posi-tion from which to apply **simple dorsiflexion** and **plantar flexion.**

With the recipient supine, the ankle can be mobilized by placing the heels of the hands on the foot just under the malleoli of the tibia and fibula (ankle bones) and pressing in alternation one side and then the other. The movement is rapid, and causes the heel of the foot to move from side to side at the articulation of the talus and malleoli of the tibia and fibula. (See Figure 9–12.)

Stretches.   Stretches at the ankle are primarily performed in dorsiflexion and plantar flexion and may easily be done with the recipient prone or supine. Stretches may be applied from any of the positions mentioned for mobilizations. Simply move the foot into dorsiflexion or plantar flexion and take it to the limit of range of motion. Figure 8–25 shows the ankle and foot stretching in **plantar flexion.** This movement helps elongate the foot flexors located on the front of the lower leg and may be felt across the top of the foot.

Foot

Structure and Movement.   The foot may be described as an elastic arched structure made up of 26 bones and designed for support and propulsion. A foot has 7 tarsal bones (i.e., calcaneus, talus, navicular, cuboid, and 3 cuneiforms), 5 metatarsals, and 14 phalanges. There is a longitudinal arch, which ex-tends from the heel to the heads of the 5 metatarsals, and a transverse arch, which extends side to side formed by the anterior tarsal bones and the metatarsals. The intertarsal joints are irregular joints and

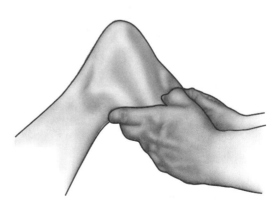

FIGURE 8–24. Dorsiflexion of the foot with direct pressure to bottom of foot with the thumbs.

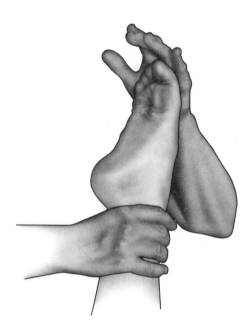

FIGURE 8–25. Stretching the flexors of the foot in plantarflexion. Lower leg perpendicular to the table.

allow slight gliding movements, and the interphalangeal joints of the toes are hinge joints that allow for flexion and extension.

Mobilizing Techniques.   Mobilizing techniques for the feet are similar to those for the hands. They are best performed with the recipient supine. The soft tissues in the feet may be warmed up with small sliding effleurage movements with the thumbs or fingers, and compressions with the fist on the bottom of the foot.

Hold the foot steady with one hand and with your other hand, grasp the fifth (little) toe firmly near the knuckle and move in a small **figure eight** pattern two or three times, mobilizing the joint. Repeat for each knuckle joint. You can mobilize the tissues between the metatarsals with a **scissoring** motion. Take hold of knuckles of the fifth and fourth toes. Simply move one knuckle up and the other down at the same time, alternating in a scissoring motion. Repeat for all of the metatarsals.

Sometimes the toes curl under due to shortening of the toe flexors that are located on the bottom of the feet. The toes can be **mobilized into extension using effleurage** along the underside of the toes. This is usually performed with the thumbs. Do not "pop" or pull on the toes forcefully straightening them out, which is uncomfortable to most recipients and dangerous.

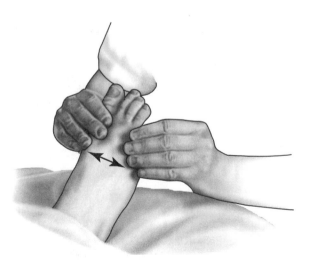

FIGURE 8–26. Creating space between metatarsals by pulling sides of foot away from each other.

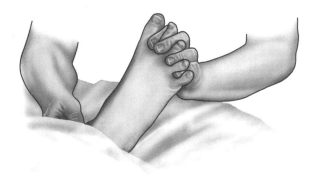

FIGURE 8–27. Creating space between metatarsals by interlocking fingers with recipient's toes.

Stretches.   There are a few stretches for the intrinsic tissues of the foot itself. As described above, you can plantar flex the foot from either the prone or supine positions, stretching the tissues on the top of the foot, including the extensor muscles. The toes alone may easily be stretched back at the ball of the foot or pressed forward for a stretch. The foot may be spread stretching the spaces between the metatarsals, and the muscles that run across them. Simply grasp both sides of the foot and pull in opposite directions, **widening the foot and stretching** related tissues as shown in Figure 8–26.

You may also **interlock your fingers between the toes** of the foot. This in itself is usually enough to spread the toes and metatarsals into a stretch. See Figure 8–27. It will be ineffective if your hands are too small in relation to the recipient's foot, and may be painful if your hands are relatively big.

Since the foot is a small part of the body with many joints, it can be massaged thoroughly rather quickly combining soft tissue techniques with mobilizations and stretches. Joint movements help recipients regain a sense of their feet as having moving parts and help sharpen their kinesthetic sense. This is important especially for those who live in cultures where shoes are worn all day.

SUMMARY

Western massage traditionally includes joint movements as well as soft tissue techniques. Joint movements may be categorized as active (free, assisted, resisted) and passive. During passive joint movements the practitioner initiates and controls the movement, while the recipient remains totally relaxed and passive.

Mobilizing techniques are passive movements performed within the normal range of joint movement. Stretching is a type of passive joint movement that is performed to the limit of the range of motion, and then slightly beyond, to increase flexibility at the joint. Stretching approaches include static stretch, contract-relax-stretch, and using reciprocal inhibition. Mobilizing techniques and stretches can be easily integrated into a massage routine.

Joint manipulations or adjustments that involve thrusting movements are not within the scope of massage therapy. They should be performed only by those trained to do so within their legal scope of practice. Joint movements within the scope of massage therapy include simple passive and active joint movements, which fall into the categories of non-specific mobilizing and stretching techniques.

General guidelines for performing joint movements safely are as follows: Stay within the normal range of motion of the joint; qualities of movement for mobilizing techniques are smooth, free, and loose; warm the surrounding soft tissues before stretching; use breathing to enhance the stretch; stay within the comfort range of the recipient; be aware of any abnormality of joint structure and adapt movements accordingly.

The areas of the body for which passive joint movements are effective include the neck, shoulder girdle, wrists, hands, chest, hips, knees, ankles, and feet. Practitioners should have practical knowledge of the structure and the movement possible at each joint to ensure the safety of the recipient during joint movements.

Joint movements are used for a variety of reasons including to stretch surrounding soft tissues; increase joint range of motion; stimulate production of synovial fluid; increase kinesthetic awareness; induce muscle relaxation; and build muscle strength. Some contemporary systems of bodywork use joint movements to affect the nervous system, reeducate muscles, and integrate function. Receivers can learn to let go of tension during passive joint movements. Joint movements add a kinetic dimension to a massage session and provide diversity of technique.

A look ahead . . .

Massage techniques and joint movements are combined and applied to achieve the therapeutic goals of a massage session. In many settings (e.g., health club, spa, private practice) massage is offered in one-hour full-body sessions that focus on general health and wellbeing. Chapter 9 describes a typical full-body massage.

REFERENCES

Cailliet, R. (1981). *Shoulder pain*, 2nd ed. Philadelphia: F. A. Davis.
McMillan, M. (1925). *Massage and therapeutic exercise*. Philadelphia: W. B. Saunders.
Roth, M. (1851). *The prevention and cure of many chronic diseases by movements*. London: John Churchill.

S T U D Y   G U I D E

LEARNING OUTCOMES

Use the learning outcomes at the beginning of the chapter as a guide to your studies. Perform the task given in each outcome using the information in the chapter. This may start as an "open book" exercise, and then later from memory.

KEY TERMS/CONCEPTS

To study the key concept and terminology listed at the beginning of this chapter, choose one or more of the following exercises. Writing or talking about ideas helps you remember them better, and explaining them helps deepen your understanding. Some exercises are designed to sharpen your focus on the details of performing the techniques.

1. Write a one-sentence explanation of the different categories of joint movements: active, passive, assisted, resisted. Demonstrate and explain them to a study partner or group.

2. Explain the difference between mobilizing techniques and stretches. Demonstrate the difference on one or two joints.

3. Perform a specific stretch using static, contract-relax-stretch, and reciprocal inhibition. Explain the de-

tails of the three stretching approaches to a study partner or group.

4. Demonstrate mobilizing techniques for major joints in the body. With a study partner lying clothed on a massage table, start at the head and move clockwise around the body. Name and describe the movements as you perform them.

5. Repeat problem 4 for stretches of major joints.

STUDY OUTLINE

The following questions test your memory of the main concepts in this chapter. Locate the answers in the text using the page number given for each question.

Joint Movements

1. Joint movements are categorized into _____ (i.e., without practitioner assistance), and _____ (i.e., initiated and controller by practitioner) movements. (p. 153)

2. In _____ movements, the client initiates the movement, while the practitioner helps in completion of the movement. (p. 153)

3. In _____ movements, the practitioner provides resistance to the active movement of the client. (p. 153)

4. Mobilizing techniques or joint mobilizations, in the context of massage therapy, are passive movements performed within _____ of joint movement. (p. 153)

5. _____ is a type of passive joint movement that is performed to the limit of range of motion, and used to elongate muscles and tendons. (p. 153)

6. Three different approaches to stretching a joint include _____ stretch, contract- _____- stretch, and _____. (p. 154)

7. Joint movements are used to stretch _____, increase range of _____, enhance _____ awareness, stimulate _____ relaxation, build muscle _____, and improve _____. (p. 153)

8. Some contemporary forms of bodywork use joint movement to affect the _____ system, i.e., re-educate muscles and integrate function (e.g., Trager Psychophyscial Integration). (p. 153)

9. Joint _____ or _____ intended to realign a misaligned joint by sudden thrusting movements, and characterized by "popping" or "cracking" at the joints, are <u>not</u> within the _____ of massage therapy. (p. 153)

General Principles of Joint Movements

1. Stay within the _____ range of motion of the joint when performing joint movement techniques. (p. 153)

2. Mobilizing techniques can be characterized as smooth, _____, and _____. (p. 154)

3. Warm surrounding _____ before stretching. (p. 154)

4. Use breathing to enhance a stretch, _____ holding the breath, and time the stretch to the client's (choose one: inhalation or exhalation). (p. 154)

5. Stay with the _____ range of the recipient during joint movements. (p. 154)

6. Be aware of _____ of joint structure and adapt movements accordingly. (p. 154)

JOINT MOVEMENTS

Neck

1. The neck is a general term for the region between the head and the trunk, which includes the seven _____ vertebrae and surrounding _____. (p. 154)

2. Mobilizing techniques of the neck are performed best with the recipient (choose one: prone or supine, or side-lying). (p. 154)

3. Simple mobilizing techniques of the neck may be performed by lifting the head slightly off the table, and moving the neck through its full _____. (p. 155)

4. Finger push-ups may be used to produce a gentle movement between the _____. (p.155)

5. The melt-down is a variation of the finger push-up used primarily in the _____ region. (p. 155)

6. A _____ movement can be created in the neck by applying deep effleurage on both sides at the same time, traveling from the base of the neck to the suboccipital space. (p. 155)

7. Neck stretches include lateral _____, _____, forward _____, and cross- _____ stretch. (pp. 155–156)

Shoulder Girdle

1. The shoulder girdle is a complex structure and the most mobile area of the body. It includes the gleno-_____, acromio-_____, and scapulo-_____ joints. (p. 156)

2. Mobilizing techniques for the shoulder girdle may be performed with the recipient in the _____, _____, _____, or _____ position. (p. 156)

3. Mobilizing the joints of the shoulder may be accomplished indirectly by movement of the _____ or by movement of the _____. (p. 156)

4. Mobilizing techniques for the shoulder when the recipient is prone include _____, _____, direct mobilizing, and _____ mobilizing. (p. 156)

5. Stretches to the shoulder in supine include horizontal _____, and the over _____ stretch. (p. 158)

Elbow

1. Movements of the elbow are limited to _____, _____, _____, and _____. (p. 158)

2. Mobilizing the elbow may be performed by _____ and _____ of the hand, or _____ the forearm with upper arm immobilized. (p. 159)

3. Stretches of muscles that cross the elbow are accomplished largely by stretching the whole arm, as in the _____ stretch for the shoulder. (p. 159)

Wrist

1. Movements of the wrist include flexion, extension, _____ extension, radial and ulnar _____, and _____. (p. 160)

2. Mobilizing movements of the wrist include (choose one: passive or resisted) movement of the wrist through its *full range of motion*, and waving. (p. 160)

3. Flexion and _____ are the most common stretches of the wrist. (p. 160)

Hand

1. Movements of the hand distal to the wrist involve movements of the fingers, i.e., flexion, extension, _____, _____; movements between the meta _____; and the more complex movements of the _____. (p. 160)

2. Mobilizing techniques for the hand include passive movements of all joints; _____ at the knuckles; _____ between metacarpals. (pp. 160–161)

3. Stretches of the hand involve _____ at the knuckles _____ and _____ at the wrist. (p. 161)

Chest

1. The chest is a general term for the front and sides of the _____, *generally* defined by the _____, _____, and _____. (p. 162)

2. Mobilizing the rib cage is performed in supine by gentle _____ from side to side. (p. 162)

3. Stretch of the arm muscles that attach to the chest may be accomplished by the _____ stretch. (p. 162)

Hip

1. The large muscles of the hip are located on the upper _____ and _____. (p. 162)

2. Movements possible at the hip joint itself include flexion, _____, hyper _____, ab _____, ad _____, diagonal _____ and _____, outward and inward _____; and _____. (p. 162)

3. Rhythmic _____ of the straight leg with recipient in supine position is a mobilizing technique of the hip joint. (p. 162)

4. The hip joint can be taken through its full range of motion using _____ movement. (p. 164)

5. Some useful stretches of the hip joint with recipient in supine include knee to _____ flexion, straight _____ flexion, diagonal _____ with knee flexed. (p. 164)

Knee

1. The knee is a hinge joint, and its movements are largely limited to _____ and _____. (p. 164)

2. The knee is best mobilized with the recipient in the _____ position. Simple mobilizing techniques include the _____ toss, _____ the lower leg at the knee. (p. 164)

3. Some stretches of the _____ leg also stretch the muscles that cross the knee. (p. 166)

4. Bringing the heel of the foot towards the buttocks (flexion) will stretch the _____ muscles of the thigh. (p. 166)

Ankle

1. The ankle is a hinge joint, and its movements include _____ flexion (flexion), _____ flexion (extension), _____ (eversion/abduction), and _____ (inversion/adduction). (p. 166)

2. Mobilizing techniques at the ankle include thumb pressure to bottom of foot while _____ flexing the ankle (prone); _____ movement of the ankle through full range of motion (prone); side to side mobilizing of the ankle using _____ (supine). (pp. 166–167)

3. Stretches at the ankle primarily involve _____ and _____ flexion. (p. 167)

Foot

1. The foot itself is a complex structure with two types of joints (i.e., _____ and _____) and two arches (i.e., _____ and _____). Movement can occur at the articulation of any of the (number) _____ bones. (p. 167)

2. Mobilizing techniques for the foot are similar to those for the hands, and are applied easiest with the recipient in _____ position. These include figure _____ with the toes; _____ between metatarsals; and straightening toes with _____ along the underside of phalanges. (p. 168)

3. Stretches for the foot include _____ flexion; _____ of the toes; foot widening at the _____; and interlocking _____ (giver) and _____ (receiver). (p. 169)

FOR GREATER UNDERSTANDING

The following exercises are designed to take you from the realm of theory into practical applications. They will help give you a deeper understanding of the techniques covered in this chapter. Action words are underlined to emphasize the variety of activities presented to address different learning styles, and to encourage deeper thinking.

1. For each of the stretches covered in the chapter, name muscles involved, and locate their attachments on a skeleton. If possible, perform the joint movements on the skeleton and observe how the bones move in relation to each other.

2. One person performs mobilizing techniques on a joint, while another observes. The observer verbally describes the hand and body position of the person performing the technique.

3. For problem 2, the observer evaluates the giver's body mechanics, and offers suggestions on how they might be improved.

4. In a group of three, one person talks another through performing a particular stretch to a receiver lying on the massage table. He or she describes step by step how the technique is performed. Include static, contract-relax-stretch, and reciprocal inhibition.

5. Videotape your performance of mobilizing techniques. Watching the video, analyze your body mechanics. Perform the technique again, correcting body mechanics.

6. Perform active versions of the passive movements (mobilizing techniques and stretches) covered in this chapter. Include static, contract-relax-stretch, and reciprocal inhibition techniques.

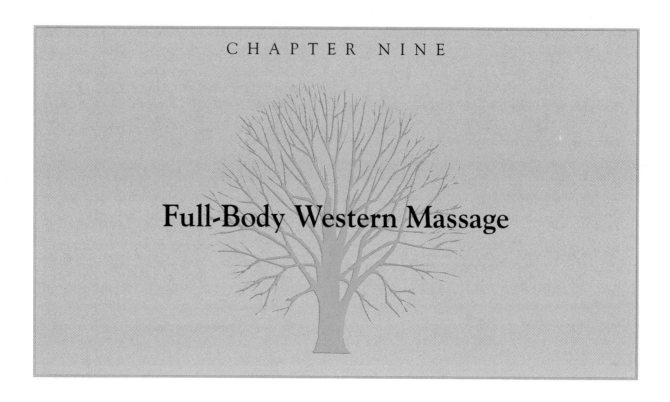

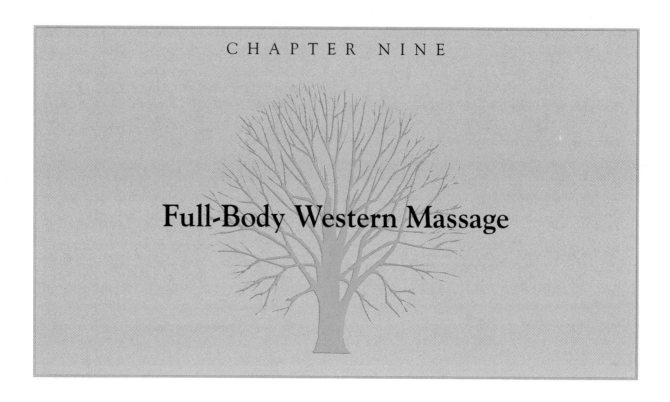
CHAPTER NINE

Full-Body Western Massage

LEARNING OUTCOMES

After studying this chapter, the student will have information to:

1. Discuss the form and intent of a full-body Western massage.
2. Plan the sequence of the massage session from region to region.
3. Apply techniques in appropriate order within each body region.
4. Choose opening, warm-up, transition and finishing techniques appropriately.
5. Apply the principles of continuity, rhythm, pacing, and specificity.
6. Perform a one-hour full-body Western massage for health promotion.

KEY TERMS/CONCEPTS

Continuity	Opening technique	Specificity
Draping	Order of techniques	Technique combination
Eclectic	Pacing	Transition technique
Finishing technique	Rhythm	Warming technique
Flow	Routine	
Full-body Western massage	Sequence of body regions	

 MEDIALINK

A companion CD-ROM, included free with each new copy of this book, supplements the techniques presented in this chapter. Insert the CD-ROM to watch video clips of massage techniques being demonstrated. This multimedia feature is designed to help you add a new dimension to your learning.

OVERVIEW

Full-body Western massage is typically given in sessions lasting from 30 to 90 minutes. Performed from a wellness perspective, these sessions focus on general health and wellbeing as well as meeting the therapeutic needs of the recipient. The goals for health promotion include improving circulation, relaxing the muscles, improving joint mobility, inducing the relaxation response, promoting healthy skin, and creating a general sense of wellbeing.

A full-body session usually includes techniques from all seven of the basic Western massage technique categories. Oil, lotion, or other lubricant is typically used to enhance sliding over the skin and to prevent chaffing. Types of topical substances and their properties are described in Chapter 6.

Although each practitioner combines and blends various massage techniques in different ways, there are some general guidelines for giving a full-body massage. These guidelines address draping, sequence of body parts, order of techniques, continuity, rhythm, pacing, and specificity. Table 9–1 summarizes the guidelines for performing full-body massage.

Table 9–1   SUMMARY OF THE ELEMENTS OF A FULL-BODY WESTERN MASSAGE ROUTINE

Goals	General health promotion
	    Improved circulation, relaxed muscles, improved joint mobility,
	    relaxation response, healthy skin, sense of wellbeing
	Therapeutic needs (e.g., reduce muscle stiffness and soreness, relieve trigger
	points, injury recovery)

Length of Time	30–90 minutes (typically 60 minutes)
Draping	Full sheet or large towel Body regions uncovered for massage and then recovered Genitals and women's breasts covered at all times

Sequence of Body Regions	Starting point
	Direction (e.g., clockwise)
	Ending point
	
	Starting prone (example)
	    Start on back
	    Buttocks, legs
	    Turn to supine
	    Legs/feet, arms/shoulders, neck, chest, abdomen
	    End with head and face
	
	Starting supine (example)
	    Start on head and face
	    Neck, arms/shoulders, chest, abdomen, legs/feet
	    Turn to prone
	    Legs, buttocks
	    End with back

Order of Techniques on a Specific Body Region	Opening technique (e.g., effleurage to apply oil or compressions)
	Warming techniques (e.g., effleurage or compressions)
	Combination of techniques
	    For general health (e.g., effleurage, petrissage, superficial warming
	    friction, joint movements
	        Specific therapeutic goals (e.g., deep friction, vibration, direct pressure)
	Transition techniques (e.g., effleurage, tapotement)
	Finishing techniques (e.g., effleurage, tapotement)

(continued)

Table 9–1   (Cont.)

Continuity	Sense of continuous touch throughout the session Avoid abrupt removal of touch
Flow	Orderly sequence and smooth transitions Skillful draping
Rhythm	Smooth and even rhythm
Pacing	Moderate speed
Specificity	For attention to specific muscle or small area Shorter length session = less specificity in full-body massage

GUIDELINES FOR FULL-BODY MASSAGE

Draping

Draping is done with a sheet or large towel, and body parts skillfully uncovered and recovered as needed. Genitals are covered at all times. Women's breasts are always covered, except when breast massage is performed by a practitioner with special training and then only with informed consent of the recipient. Breast massage will not be included in the general full-body routine described in this chapter.

Sequence of Body Regions

In a full-body session, the practitioner massages each region of the body (e.g., back, arm, and leg) in a particular **sequence.** The sequence usually includes supine and prone positions, and has a starting point, direction (e.g., clockwise), and an ending point. This establishes a routine way of working as discussed further below.

Recipients generally lie prone or supine for the first part of the massage, and then turn over for the second part. Whether they start prone or supine is a matter of preference for the practitioner and the recipient. Sometimes the side-lying position is used, for example, with pregnant women.

There are no hard and fast rules for sequence, but it should facilitate a smooth flow from one region of the body to the next. Some advocate moving clockwise around the table. The following are two suggestions for sequences in a full-body routine.

- If a session starts with the recipient in the prone position, a commonly used sequence of body sections would be the back, buttocks, and legs. The neck and feet are sometimes addressed prone, but are more easily accessed supine. Then turn over to the supine position with a sequence moving from legs and feet, to arms and hands, and then to shoulders, neck, chest and abdomen, and ending with the head and face.
- If the session starts with the recipient in the supine position, a commonly used sequence of body sections would be head and face, neck and shoulders, arms and hands, chest and abdomen, legs and feet. Then turn over to the prone position with a sequence moving from legs to buttocks and ending on the back.

The advantages of starting in the prone position include that it may feel safer to a recipient new to massage, back massage triggers the relaxation response sooner, and it allows those who need to be more alert at the end of the session to finish face-up. An advantage of starting in the supine position is that the practitioner can massage the head, face, and neck right away, which is good for recipients who do a lot of desk or computer work.

Order of Techniques

The general **order of techniques** for each region of the body is similar. Once a part is undraped, opening and warming techniques are applied. These are followed by a combination of techniques for general health promotion, as well as techniques for specific therapeutic effects. Finishing and transition techniques complete work on the region.

The most common **opening** and **warming technique** for each area to be massaged is effleurage. It is used to apply oil or other lubricant, to warm the area, and to facilitate circulation. It is applied first using lighter and then deeper pressure. Effleurage on the limbs should always be performed moving distal to proximal, unless the pressure used is very light. Compressions may also serve as an opening or warming technique.

The opening is followed by a combination of techniques to improve circulation, relax muscles, improve joint mobility, and other health promotion goals. **Technique combinations** at this stage usually include effleurage, petrissage, warming friction, and joint movements. Deep friction, vibration, and direct pressure are applied as appropriate for more specific work. Finish work on the area with effleurage and/or tapotement.

Transition techniques serve to provide continuity and flow from one section to another (see discussion below). For example, when moving from massage of the upper leg to the lower leg, a few effleurage strokes to the entire leg help tie the regions together kinesthetically for the recipient.

When ending work on a specific part of the body, the prone or supine side, or the entire session, some thought should be given to **finishing techniques.** Finishing techniques may be used to reconnect parts of the body that have been worked on more specifically or to further sedate or stimulate the recipient. Effleurage and tapotement are the usual finishing techniques that can be used to create a sense of wholeness. Light effleurage, sometimes called nerve strokes, is more soothing, while tapotement is more stimulating. Passive touch in the form of simple holding at the head or feet is calming and is sometimes used to end a session.

Continuity and Flow

A full-body session should have a sense of **continuity** and flow. Take care when establishing touch at the beginning of a session, and then create a sense of continuous touch throughout the session. Establishment or removal of touch should never be abrupt. This does not mean that you may never take your hands off a recipient during a session, but that doing so should be kept to a minimum and be done as imperceptibly as possible. A sense of **flow** is achieved through an orderly sequence and smooth transitions from one part of the body to the next. Skill in draping, including uncovering and recovering can add to the sense of smooth transitions.

Rhythm, Pacing, and Specificity

The **rhythm** of a classic full-body massage session may be described as smooth and even, and the **pacing** as moderate in speed. Trying to perform a full-body session in half an hour will necessitate a faster pace with less attention to detail. A session focusing on general relaxation will be slower paced and usually minimize or eliminate stimulating techniques such as tapotement. **Specificity** is required for attention to a specific muscle or small area. If the recipient requests more attention to certain parts of the body such as the back and neck, then those areas would receive more time and specific techniques, while the rest of the body would receive less specific massage.

FULL-BODY WESTERN MASSAGE ROUTINE

There is no one best way to perform a full-body Western massage. Practitioners usually develop their own styles and routine ways of performing a massage session. **Routines** generally involve a regular starting point and opening techniques, a specific sequence of body regions, a certain order of techniques in each body region, and a regular way of ending the session. These routines typically change with further training and experience, and are modified to meet the needs of the recipient on the table. Today's **eclectic** practitioners may use a full-body Western routine as a starting point and then integrate contemporary techniques as appropriate to accomplish the therapeutic goals of the session.

The following is an example of a one-hour full-body routine that may be used to practice the basic Western massage techniques on different parts of the body. By having a routine as a framework, the learner is free to focus on specific skills, including good body mechanics, draping, specific techniques, smooth transitions, continuity, rhythm, and pacing.

It is impossible to describe every single movement of a routine in writing. Use the routine described below as a framework but feel free to add variations of techniques as you become more attuned to the work. Experiment with what feels right to you. Most of the techniques described are illustrated in Chapters 7–10. To lengthen the routine you may repeat techniques or insert additional techniques as appropriate.

Prone Position (25 minutes)

Before leaving recipients alone to undress in private, request that when you return they be covered with the drape and lying face down on the table. Show them how the face cradle works, and position a bolster approximately where their ankles will be. Before you start the session, adjust the position of the face cradle and the bolster for safety and comfort.

Back (15 minutes).   Uncover the back down to the waist. Standing at the head, begin applying oil or lotion on the back. Bilateral tree stroking is a good technique to use to apply oil (Figure 7–6). The movement should be smooth, and cover the entire back and sides. Use light to moderate pressure. Repeat the technique three or four times.

Without losing contact, move to the recipient's right side. Stand at the hip and face the head. Work this side of the back entirely before moving to the other side. Perform the "shingles" effleurage technique along the near side of the spine (Figure 7–5). Fingers point toward the head. Use moderate to deep pressure. Fully warm the erector muscles of the spine. Perform deep friction with the fingertips along the erector muscles moving from the sacrum to the neck (Figure 7–21). To apply deeper pressure, use both hands, placing one hand on top of the other, as shown in Figure 9–1.

Perform deep effleurage with the thumbs on the lower back between the iliac crest and the last three ribs to massage the quadratus lumborum. Be sure that the thumbs are in proper alignment. (Warming friction using the knuckles may be substituted as easier on the hands; Figure 7–18.) Repeat this technique in two or three strips moving out laterally from the spine. Use moderate to deep pressure.

Reconnect the lower back with the shoulder with a few light "shingles" effleurage strokes. Then perform a deeper effleurage over the upper back and shoulder. Place one hand over the other to apply greater pressure, and use a circular movement around the shoulder, as shown in Figure 9–2.

Perform circular two-handed petrissage over the entire upper back (Figure 7–14). Follow with basic kneading to relax the upper trapezius. Kneading with one hand works better with smaller recipients, as shown in Figure 9–3. Begin finishing this side of the back with three-count stroking of the trapezius (Figure 7–7). Follow with horizontal stroking of the back moving from lower back to shoulders.

Transition to the other side by performing light effleurage from waist to shoulders as you walk around the head of the table. Repeat the entire sequence on the other side, beginning with shingles effleurage.

When both sides of the back have been massaged, redrape the back. Finish the entire back with rapping or some other form of tapotement using moderate force (Figure 7–25).

Lower Limbs and Buttocks (10 minutes).   Undrape the right leg up to the waist, being careful not to expose the natal cleft. Tuck the drape securely under the leg and at the waist (Figure 6–10).

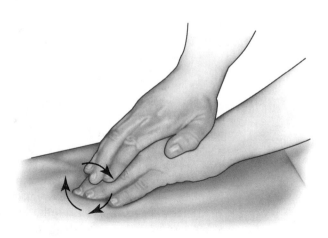

FIGURE 9–1. Circular friction with fingertips on erector muscles along side of the spine.

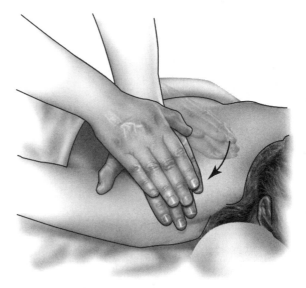

FIGURE 9–2. Deep effleurage over the upper back and shoulder.

Stand at the side of the table facing the head. Apply oil or lotion to the entire leg and hip with basic sliding effleurage using light to moderate pressure. Follow the curves of the leg in a continuous motion from foot to hip. Be sure to touch both sides of the leg, and not just the back of the leg. The inside hand will slide onto the back of the leg below the muscle attachments and follow the outside hand around the hip. Coordinate the movements of your hands so that as the outside hand starts to return down the leg, it is followed by the inside hand (see Figure 9–4). Both hands return to the ankle with a light sliding motion.

Note: Your hands should never touch or come unreasonably close to the genital area. Care should be taken when working on the inside of the leg to maintain ethical and comfortable boundaries. Skillful draping in this area will help to create a feeling of safety for both the recipient and the practitioner.

The lower limb and hip are massaged in this order: buttocks, upper leg, lower leg. Warm up the buttocks muscles using deep circular effleurage, one hand on top reinforcing the other as shown in Figure 9–5. Follow with compressions using the fist to reach deep gluteal muscles. Moderate to deep pressure may be used on these large muscles. Be sure to work the attachments along the iliac crest. Finish with circular effleurage as you started, using either the hand-over-hand position or the fist.

Two or three basic sliding effleurage strokes to the entire leg and hip help create a smooth transition to the upper leg. Perform deep effleurage with alternating fists on the hamstrings, from above the popliteal fossa to the attachments on the ilium, as shown in Figure 9–6. Continuing with one fist, perform effleurage along the iliotibial band and the tensor fascia lata muscle moving from the hip to the knee. This broad band of fascia and muscle can accept moderate to deep pressure.

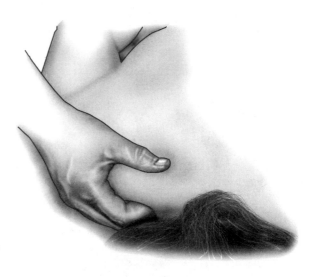

FIGURE 9–3. Basic one-hand kneading of the upper trapezius.

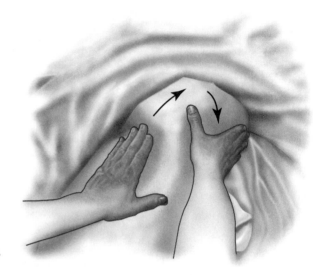

FIGURE 9–4. Applying oil to the entire leg, recipient in prone position.

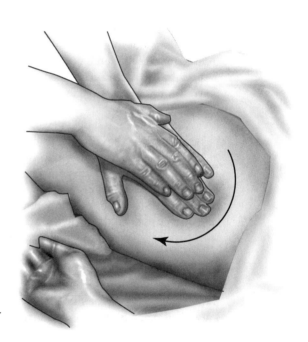

FIGURE 9–5. Deep effleurage to the gluteal muscles using reinforced fingertips.

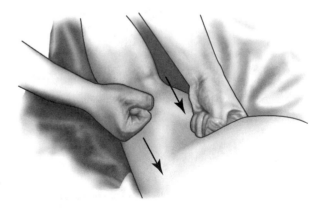

FIGURE 9–6. Deep effleurage to hamstring muscles using fists.

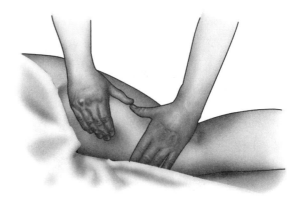

FIGURE 9–7. Two-handed kneading to adductors of the thigh.

Warm up the adductors with basic sliding effleurage using the palms. Reach to the medial side of the thigh, and then pull up and around to the back of the thigh in a smooth sliding motion. Alternating hands, move from the knee to just below the attachments of the adductors. Be mindful of boundaries as mentioned above when working the inside of the leg.

Perform basic two-handed kneading on the upper leg, including the back and both sides. Figure 9–7 shows kneading the adductors of the upper leg. Finish with basic sliding effleurage distal to proximal, first to the upper and then to the entire leg.

Use two-handed kneading to massage the lower leg. Finish with basic sliding effleurage to the lower leg, following the gastrocnemius to the attachments on either side of the knee (Figure 7–1). Perform horizontal stroking to the upper and lower legs, starting on the upper leg (Figure 7–8). Finish with a few basic effleurage strokes from ankle to hip. Redrape the leg. Finish this leg with nerve strokes from the buttocks to the ankle.

Move to the left side and repeat the entire leg sequence. Finish the back side of the body with the recipient fully draped. Place one hand on the back and the other hand on a lower leg, and gently rock the body. Switch hands from one leg to the other leg. This should take only 5–10 seconds. Perform 2–3 light effleurage stokes from shoulders to feet as a connecting maneuver, and to signal the end of the massage on the back side of the body.

Turning Over

Ask the recipient to turn over. Assist by anchoring the drape with your leg against the side of the table and holding the other side of the drape up. This is called tenting (Figure 6–12). Have the recipient roll away from you. This will prevent the drape from getting wrapped up around the recipient during the turnover. Lower the drape.

Note that the recipient was out of your sight as he or she turned over under the tent. If there is more than one session going on in the room, be sure that you do not expose the recipient to others.

Supine Position (35 minutes)

Lower Limbs (10 minutes).   Uncover left leg and tuck the drape securely (Figure 6–9). Apply oil to the entire limb using basic sliding effleurage.

Perform deep effleurage to the thigh using both hands. Follow this with two-handed kneading. Jostle the thigh muscles, causing passive movement in the hip and knee joints as shown in Figure 9–8. Use horizontal stroking to lift and compress the thigh muscles. Finish massage of the thigh with effleurage using both hands, distal to proximal.

Perform effleurage with moderate pressure to the entire limb as a transition, followed by effleurage from the ankle to the knee. Apply circular friction around the knee using the heels of the hands as shown in Figure 9–9.

Apply thumb stripping to the tibialis anterior as shown in Figure 9–10. Perform this technique on the lateral side of the lower leg from just above the ankle to the attachment on the lateral condyle of the tibia. You will complete two to four strips, depending on the size of the muscle. Follow the thumb

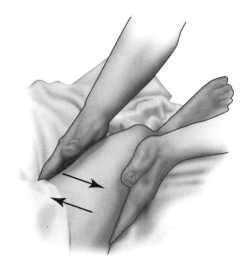

FIGURE 9–8. Jostling the thigh muscles, recipient in supine position.

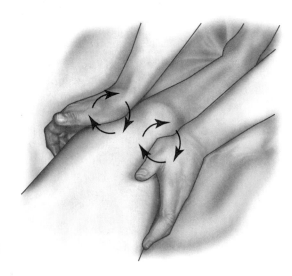

FIGURE 9–9. Circular friction around knee using the heels of the hands.

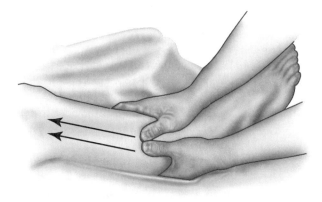

FIGURE 9–10. Thumb stripping along tibialis anterior.

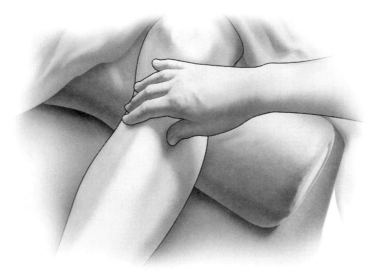

FIGURE 9–11. Direct pressure along tibialis anterior.

stripping with direct pressure along the tibialis anterior, moving about one inch at a time proximal to distal. Keep thumb and wrist in alignment as shown in Figure 9–11.

Slide down the lower leg and perform circular friction around the ankle with the fingertips. Then mobilize the ankle using the heels of the hands. The foot will wiggle back and forth as shown in Figure 9–12.

Perform effleurage between the metatarsals using the thumb or fingers (Figure 7–2). Slide along the bottom of the foot with the fist from the ball of the foot to the heel, as shown in Figure 9–13, using moderate to deep pressure. Finish with slapping tapotement on the bottom of the foot using the back of the hand.

Finish the entire limb with light effleurage moving distal to proximal, followed by nerve strokes moving proximal to distal. Redrape the leg.

Uncover the right leg, and repeat the entire sequence. After both legs have been massaged, and before moving to the upper body, some nerve strokes over the redraped legs may be used as a finishing and transition technique.

Arms and Shoulders (10 minutes).   Uncover the right arm and shoulder (Figure 6–8). Apply lubricant to entire upper limb using basic sliding effleurage, moving distal to proximal. The movement should flow from the hand to the shoulder, including around the deltoid muscle.

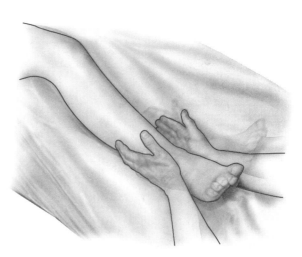

FIGURE 9–12. Ankle mobilizing technique using the heels of the hands. The foot moves from side to side.

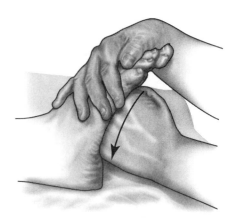

FIGURE 9–13. Effleurage to bottom of the foot using the fist.

Perform alternating one-hand petrissage to the upper arm. Squeeze the biceps side, then the triceps side, alternating in a rhythmical motion (Figure 7–13). Be sure to petrissage the entire upper arm from the shoulder to the elbow.

Mobilize the shoulder by grasping the upper arm with both hands just below the shoulder and moving the joint in a circle. This is a passive shoulder roll, in which the shoulders are brought forward, elevated, rolled back, and then depressed. Move both clockwise and counterclockwise (Figure 8–5).

After a few light effleurage strokes to the entire limb as a transition, perform one-hand effleurage to the lower arm as an additional warm-up using moderate to deep pressure. Knead the muscles of the lower arm, particularly near the elbow. Follow with thumb stripping to the flexor and extensor muscles on the lower arm, from the wrist to their attachments near the elbow. See Figure 9–14.

Interlock your fingers with the recipient's and press gently with your fingers to the back of his or her hand to mobilize the joints at the knuckle. Keeping the fingers interlocked, mobilize the wrist taking it through its normal range of motion. Apply effleurage to the back of the hand between metacarpals using your thumbs. Then lightly squeeze along each finger, moving proximal to distal. Turn the hand over so that it is palm up. Apply effleurage to the palm of the hand moving distal to proximal as shown in Figure 9–15. Grip the hand on the little finger and thumb sides, palm down, and gently squeeze the hand while broadening the palm and separating the metacarpals.

Use basic sliding effleurage from hand to shoulder to kinesthetically reconnect the arm. Lift the arm, holding just below the wrist, and perform effleurage on the pectoral muscles with a loose fist moving lateral to medial, and stopping at the breast tissue. See Figure 9–16.

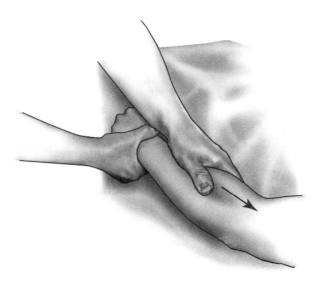

FIGURE 9–14. Thumb stripping along extensor muscles of the forearm.

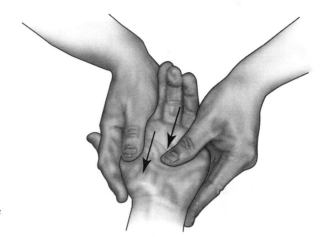

FIGURE 9–15. Effleurage to palm of the hand using thumbs.

A basic sliding effleurage stroke may be performed over the sternum as shown in Figure 9–17. Use good judgment in applying this stroke with women. It may be advisable to omit the technique if the woman has large breasts or if she might feel it as an invasion of her boundaries. Err on the side of omission, and ask permission if in doubt.

Finish with basic sliding effleurage to the entire upper limb using moderate pressure. Redrape the arm and shoulder. Repeat the entire sequence on the other arm.

Abdomen (5 minutes).   The abdomen is a vulnerable area for many people. If the recipient is new to massage, or new to you, ask permission to work in this area. Explain to women that the breasts will be draped. You might also want to explain the purpose of massaging the abdomen. Find out if they have eaten within the past hour, and skip the area if that is the case. People experiencing constipation or gas in the bowels may be sensitive to pressure; however, massage of the abdomen may help relieve those conditions.

Cover a woman's breasts with an additional drape before you pull back the larger drape to the iliac crest exposing the abdomen (Figure 6–11). Do not expose the pubic area.

Begin by gently laying a hand on the abdomen to establish contact. Perform effleurage moving clockwise in a circular pattern. Use the fingertips of one hand, while the other hand rests on top. See Figure 9–18. Move in a large circle along the bottom of the ribs and around the outline of the pelvis, followed by smaller, then even smaller concentric circles. Check with the recipient to make sure the pressure is comfortable.

Perform vibration to the area with the fingertips moving from place to place in a clockwise pattern (Figure 7–31). Take care in areas that recipients report as feeling sore. Petrissage the abdomen

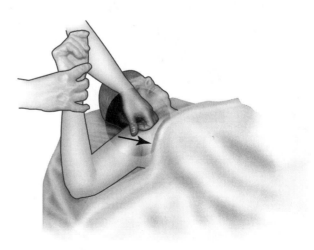

FIGURE 9–16. Effleurage to pectoral muscles using a loose fist.

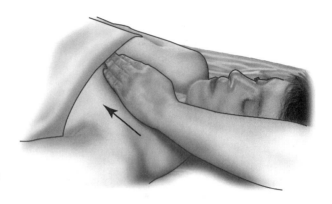

FIGURE 9–17. Basic sliding effleurage over sternum using palm of the hand.

with a flat hand, palm down, using an undulating or wavelike motion. Push in first with the heel of the hand, and then roll onto the fingertips. The soft tissues of the viscera are stimulated with the rhythmic compression. Move from place to place on the abdomen.

Repeat circular effleurage moving clockwise as a transition. Follow with horizontal stroking of the abdomen. Finish the area with passive touch in the center of the abdomen. Remove your hand and recover the recipient to the shoulders with the larger drape. The breast drape may remain in place for warmth or may be removed at this time.

Neck and Shoulders (5 minutes).   You may sit at the head of the recipient to work on the head and shoulders. Maintain good body mechanics for sitting, as in Figure 6–21. Establish contact by mobilizing the shoulders with a "cat paw" movement, alternating pushing one side and then the other as shown in Figure 9–19.

Apply lubricant to both sides of the neck (one hand on each side), performing effleurage along the trapezius from the shoulder tips to the occipital ridge. Turn the head slightly to the right side, exposing the left side of the neck. Perform effleurage with the fist on the upper trapezius from the occipital ridge to the shoulder as shown in Figure 9–20. The upper trapezius will stretch mildly.

Continuing on the left side, use circular friction along the occipital ridge and the neck to warm the deeper muscles of the region. Start with the suboccipitals (medial to lateral) and then down the cervicals to the base of the neck. Follow this with stripping using fingertips or a knuckle, to the posterior cervicals from the occiput to the base of the neck. Finish the left side with effleurage with the palm of the hand, moving back and forth from the tip of the shoulder to the occiput. Turn the head slightly to the left, and repeat the sequence to the right side.

Create a wavelike neck mobilization. Place the hands palms up at the base of the neck, one on either side of the spine, with fingertips pressing up on the cervical muscles. Draw the fingers toward the occiput, maintaining pressure upward. The cervical vertebrae will rise and fall as the

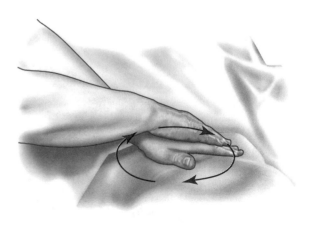

FIGURE 9–18. Effleurage in circular pattern applied to the abdomen.

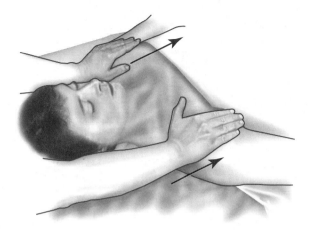

FIGURE 9-19. "Cat paw" motion to gently mobilize shoulders. Alternate hands pushing on shoulders.

fingers pass underneath. If the muscles are relaxed, this will create a wavelike motion in the neck. See Figure 9–21.

Finish with effleurage to both sides of the shoulders and neck. Start the movement at the tips of the shoulders and draw the hands toward the base of the neck and up to the occiput. Mobilize one shoulder at a time, holding the head with one hand and pushing on the tip of the shoulder with the other hand. Cradle the head briefly in both hands to end this section.

Face and Head (5 minutes). Use very little or no lubricant on the face. Ask the recipient what he or she prefers. Lotion may offer an acceptable solution; however, the entire face and head sequence can usually be performed quite well without using lubricant.

Place the hands gently on the face with fingertips at the jaw. Draw the hands toward the temples in an effleurage stroke using the full palm-side of the hands as shown in Figure 9–22. Repeat two or three times. Perform circular friction with the fingertips over the masseter and then the temporalis muscles. Stroke the muscles of the forehead using effleurage with the thumbs moving medial to lateral.

Petrissage the forehead using a circular motion of the thumbs. The movement is timed so that the tissues are lifted and pressed as the thumbs move by one another. This is similar to the two-handed circular petrissage described in Figure 7–14.

Stroke alongside of the nose and continue the effleurage movement along the cheekbones. Press up under the cheekbones with the fingertips using light to moderate pressure. Loosen the scalp with circular friction over the entire hair area. A relaxed scalp will have a greater degree of movement than a "tight" scalp. Loosening the area will improve blood supply to the skin and hair follicles.

Finish the entire session by holding the head without movement as shown in Figure 9–23. Hold for a few seconds until you can feel the recipient completely relax.

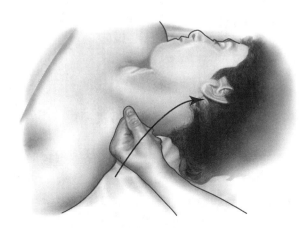

FIGURE 9-20. Effleurage to upper trapezius using fist.

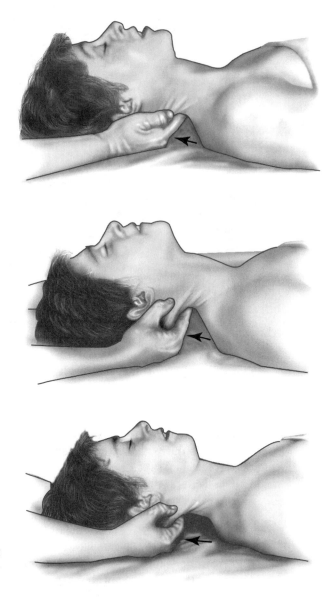

FIGURE 9–21. Wavelike neck mobilizing technique. Draw the fingers toward the occiput while maintaining pressure upwards.

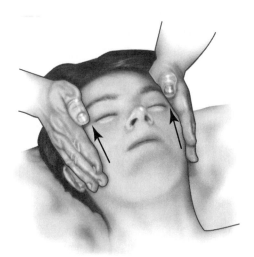

FIGURE 9–22. Effleurage to the face using palms.

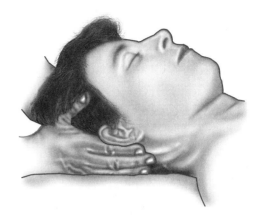

FIGURE 9–23. Cradling the head to finish the session.

SUMMARY

A full-body Western massage lasts from 30 to 90 minutes, and includes massage of the back, legs, abdomen, chest, arms, neck, and head. Performed from a wellness perspective, these sessions focus on general health and wellbeing as well as meeting the therapeutic needs of the recipient. Practitioners develop their own styles and routine ways of performing a massage session; however, some general guidelines apply.

The recipient is typically unclothed and draped with a sheet for modesty. The practitioner blends the seven basic Western massage techniques into a sequence to create a routine. The sequence usually includes both supine and prone positions, and has a starting point, a direction (e.g., clockwise), and an ending point. Oil or lotion is used to enhance movement over the skin and to prevent chafing.

The order of techniques for each part of the body includes opening and warming techniques like effleurage or compressions, followed by technique combinations for general health and specific therapeutic effects. Work on a particular area is concluded with finishing techniques to reconnect, smooth out, and gradually lighten touch. Finishing techniques typically include light effleurage, tapotement, or passive touch such as holding.

A full-body massage should have a sense of continuity and flow. Touch is established at the beginning of a session and maintained continuously throughout, with minimal interruption. A sense of flow is achieved through an orderly sequence and smooth transitions from one part of the body to the next.

The rhythm of a full-body massage is smooth and even, and the pacing is moderate in speed. Specificity is required when giving attention to small areas, or applying techniques for specific therapeutic purposes. Eclectic practitioners may use full-body Western massage as a starting point, and then integrate other massage forms as appropriate to meet the client's needs.

A look ahead . . .

A client will oftentimes need more specific attention to certain areas of the body, for example, the neck and shoulders, or legs and feet. Chapter 9 describes technique combinations for more specific therapeutic results in different areas of the body.

ADDITIONAL RESOURCES

Video

"Body massage for the day spa." (1997) Erica Miller Professional Education Series. Mile Ranch, British Columbia: Spa Expertise Canada LTD.

"Therapeutic Massage." Santa Barbara, CA: Real Bodywork. (*www.deeptissue.com*)

STUDY GUIDE

LEARNING OUTCOMES

Use the learning outcomes at the beginning of the chapter as a guide to your studies. Perform the task given in each outcome, either in writing or verbally into a tape recorder or to a study partner. This may start as an "open book" exercise, and then later from memory.

KEY TERMS/CONCEPTS

To study key words and concepts listed at the beginning of this chapter, choose one or more of the following exercises. Writing or talking about ideas helps you remember them better, and explaining them helps deepen your understanding.

1. Write a one- or two-sentence explanation of each key word and concept.

2. Make study cards by writing the explanation from problem 1 on one side of a 3 × 5 card, and the key word or concept on the other. Shuffle the cards and read one side, trying to recite either the explanation or word on the other side.

3. Pick out two or three key words or concepts and explain how they are related.

4. With a study partner, take turns explaining key words and concepts verbally.

5. Make up sentences using one or more key words or concepts.

6. Read your sentences to a study partner, who will ask you to clarify your meaning.

STUDY OUTLINE

The following questions test your memory of the main concepts in this chapter. Locate the answers in the text using the page number given for each question.

Guidelines for Full-Body Western Massage

1. From a wellness perspective, a full-body Western massage focuses on general _____, as well as meeting the _____ needs of the recipient. (p. 175)

2. Goals for general health promotion include to _____, _____, _____, _____, _____, and create a general sense of _____. (p. 175)

3. A full-body massage typically lasts from _____ minutes to _____ minutes. (p. 175)

4. Full-body includes massage of the general body regions of the back, legs, _____, _____, _____, and _____. (p. 176)

5. The practitioner blends the _____ techniques into logical sequence or routine. (p. 175)

6. The recipient is typically _____ with a sheet for modesty. (p. 176)

7. 7. Oil or lotion is used to enhance _____ over the skin and to prevent _____. (p. 175)

Draping

1. Recipients should be draped with a sheet or _____, and body parts skillfully uncovered and _____ as needed. (p. 176)

2. Genitals should be _____ at all times. (p. 176)

3. Women's breasts are always _____, except when breast massage is performed by a practitioner with _____ and then only with _____ from the recipient. (p. 176)

Sequence of Body Regions

1. A massage sequence has a _____ point, a _____, and an _____ point. (p. 176)

2. If the session starts in <u>prone position</u>, an effective sequence is back, _____, _____, turn to supine, and proceed with legs, _____, _____, _____, _____, and ending with head and _____. (p. 176)

3. If the session starts in <u>supine position</u>, an effective sequence is head and face, _____, shoulders and _____, chest and _____, legs and _____, turn to prone, and proceed to legs, buttocks, and ending on the _____. (p. 176)

4. Advantages of starting <u>prone</u> are that it often feels _____ to those new to massage, starting on the back seems to lead to _____ sooner, and ending supine helps the client be more _____ at the end of the session. (p. 176)

5. An advantage of starting <u>supine</u> is that beginning with massage of the head, face, and neck is relaxing for many who work at _____. (p. 176)

Order of Techniques

1. Massage of each region of the body begins with _____ techniques such as _____ and _____. (p. 177)

2. _____ of techniques are then applied for their general health promotion and specific _____ effects. (p. 177)

3. Work on a particular area is concluded with _____ techniques to reconnect, smooth out, and gradually lighten touch. (p. 177)

4. Common finishing techniques include light _____, _____, or _____. (p. 177)

5. _____ techniques serve to provide continuity and flow from one section to another. (p. 177)

Continuity and Flow

1. Establishment or removal of touch should never be _____. (p. 177)

2. A sense of flow is achieved through an orderly _____, and _____ transitions from one region of the body to the next. (p. 177)

Rhythm, Pacing, and Specificity

1. Full-body Western massage is usually performed with a _____ rhythm at _____ pace. (p. 177)

2. The shorter the session (e.g., 30 minutes), the less _____ is possible on any one region. (p. 177)

3. The more need for specific attention to a particular body region, the less specificity is possible _____. (p. 177)

Full-Body Western Massage Routine

1. Practitioners develop their own _____ and _____ ways of performing a massage session. These routines typically change with further _____ and _____. (p. 177)

2. Routines are modified to meet the _____ of the recipient on the table. (p. 177)

3. Today's _____ practitioners often use Western massage as a starting point and integrate other forms of massage and bodywork as desired to meet the goals of the session. (p. 177)

4. Practitioners use routines as a general _____, but vary actual techniques according to the needs and goals of the client at the time of the massage. (p. 177)

FOR GREATER UNDERSTANDING

The following exercises are designed to take you from the realm of theory into the real world. They will help give you a deeper understanding of the subjects covered in this chapter. Action words are underlined to emphasize the variety of activities presented to address different learning styles, and to encourage deeper thinking. Keeping a journal of your experiences can help make the lessons more valuable and accessible for review later.

1. <u>Receive</u> professional full-body massages from two different practitioners. <u>Compare</u> and <u>contrast</u> the two experiences. Notice the sequence used, the techniques chosen, and other elements of a session.

2. <u>Receive</u> two professional massages from the same person. <u>Compare</u> and <u>contrast</u> the two experiences. Did you notice a routine way of working, favorite techniques, and other similarities? Were there differences in the two sessions? If yes, what were they and why do you think there were differences?

3. <u>Receive</u> a 60-minute full-body massage and, at a later time, a 30-minute full-body massage from the same

practitioner. <u>Analyze</u> how the practitioner shortened the second session. How did the two experiences compare?

4. <u>Write</u> out an ideal 60-minute full-body massage routine noting sequence, and techniques to be used on each region of the body. <u>Plan</u> how much time to spend on each region of the body, opening techniques, finishing techniques and other elements of a session. <u>Perform</u> your routine. <u>Analyze</u> your experience. Did you stick to the plan? Why or why not?

5. <u>Videotape</u> the first 15 minutes of a full-body routine. <u>Watch</u> the videotape and <u>analyze</u> the elements of the routine with particular attention to the techniques chosen, and the continuity and flow. Discuss with a study partner or group.

6. Repeat problem 5 for the last 15 minutes of a routine.

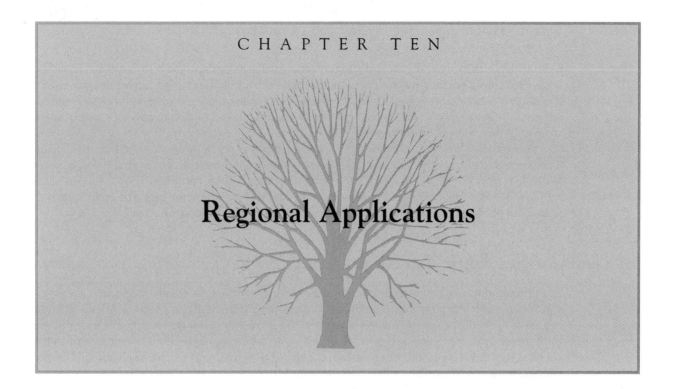

CHAPTER TEN

Regional Applications

LEARNING OUTCOMES

After studying this chapter, the student will have information to:

1. Discuss the "wholeness" of the human body.
2. Describe the human meaning of different regions of the body.
3. Describe the general anatomy of different regions of the body.
4. Explain the applications of massage for different regions of the body.
5. Perform massage technique variations for different regions of the body.

KEY TERMS/CONCEPTS

Human meaning   Regions of the body   Wholeness

 MEDIALINK

A companion CD-ROM, included free with each new copy of this book, supplements the techniques presented in this chapter. Insert the CD-ROM to watch video clips of massage techniques being demonstrated. This multimedia feature is designed to help you add a new dimension to your learning.

Practitioners may focus more time and attention on a particular region of the body, for example, on the back, neck or feet. Extended massage sessions on a smaller body area provide an opportunity for greater specificity. Added attention might result from a recipient request, or practitioner observation and assessment. Information on a health history form, or referral from a health care provider, could prompt more focus on a particular body region.

Advanced techniques and routines for specific **regions of the body** are described in this chapter. The face and head, neck, back, buttocks, lower extremities, upper extremities, chest, and abdomen are the regions represented. A discussion of the meaning of each specific part of the body in human terms is followed by the applications of massage, anatomy, and technique descriptions. The techniques presented can be integrated into the full-body Western massage described in Chapter 9.

WHOLENESS AND MEANING

Even though the body is massaged region by region during a session, its interconnectedness should always be kept in mind. Note that even though the following sections of this chapter focus on different regions of the body, a real body is not so easily divided. It has **wholeness** or integrity. For example, the upper trapezius is in the cervical region, while the whole trapezius extends down the spine through the thoracic region. For someone with rounded shoulders, you would want to address all anterior muscle shortening, as well as in the pectorals. More than just the most obvious muscles may be involved. You cannot isolate a region entirely and be effective. Work in a specific area will necessarily flow into the surrounding regions, and sometimes to the entire body.

Another consideration is that different regions of the body have special significance in human terms. Their **human meaning** is determined by what they allow us to do and to be in this world, their social and emotional associations, and their specific use in a particular person's life (e.g., a musician's hands or a runner's legs). Practitioners should keep in mind that they are not just working on body parts such as shoulders or legs, but that they are in relationship with human beings, who give meaning to their bodies and body regions. As you interact with a client, be aware that you are not just touching a body, you are touching a person.

HEAD AND FACE

Much of human consciousness is focused in the head and face. The head is the center for thinking and processing information. Our senses of sight, hearing, taste, and smell are housed here. The structures for bringing food into our bodies are here. We communicate with others through the structures of speech, and our faces convey our feelings and emotional states through facial expression. The muscles of the face are part of the process of thinking, as seen in furrowed brows and frowns of concentration. Relaxing the muscles of the head and face helps bring clarity of mind and release of mental and emotional stress.

Applications of Massage

Massage can help release tensions in the face and head acquired in daily living. This may be an area of tension for people whose jobs involve a lot of thinking or require extensive use of the eyes. Reading, writing, looking at a computer monitor, and doing activities that require fine hand–eye coordination such as needlework or drawing put strain on the muscles of the face, especially around the eyes. People who wear eyeglasses may feel strain from the weight of the glasses on the nose and ears.

Emotional distress may also lead to tension in the face and head. Worry and anxiety may create tension in the forehead and temporal area. Habitual clenching of the jaw can cause tension in the masseter and temporalis muscles and lead to TMJ pain syndrome. While crying can lead to a healthy release of emotions, it can also create strain around the eyes. Holding back emotions, and holding back tears, is accomplished by tension in the face, throat, and diaphragm.

The muscles of the face and head may also be affected by certain pathologies, such as stroke and Bell's palsy. Face and head massage can help relieve muscle tension from these conditions.

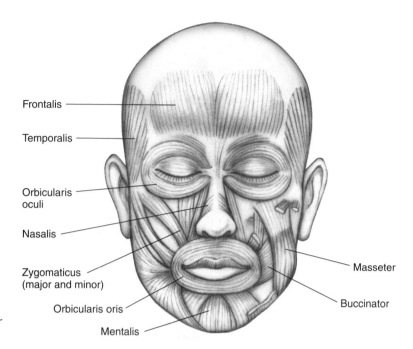

FIGURE 10–1. Major muscles of facial expression.

Labels: Frontalis, Temporalis, Orbicularis oculi, Nasalis, Zygomaticus (major and minor), Orbicularis oris, Mentalis, Masseter, Buccinator

Anatomy

The musculature of the face and head is complex and includes muscles of expression, mastication, and movement. Some muscles are skeletal muscles that create movement, such as the masseter. The muscles of expression in the face are embedded in the cutaneous tissue and move the skin itself, such as in wrinkling the forehead, frowning, and smiling. These muscles are relatively thin and more delicate than skeletal muscles. Some of the major muscles of facial expression are pictured in Figure 10–1.

Techniques

The following techniques may be integrated into a basic face and head massage. They provide more specific attention to the facial muscles, skin, and scalp.

Always ask the recipient if they are wearing contact lenses, since some of these techniques may dislodge them. A general rule is to avoid movements around the orbit, or over the eyes, if a person is wearing contact lenses.

Squeeze to Eyebrows.   The tissues in the eyebrow area become tense in people who squint, are sensitive to light, or use their eyes a lot in their work (e.g., computer work, reading, or activities that require fine hand–eye coordination). Congestion in this area often accompanies tension headache. The corrugator supercilii muscle, which draws the eyebrow downward and medially, is located there.

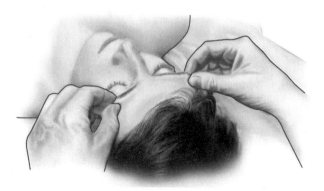

FIGURE 10–2. Gentle squeezing of tissues along the eyebrow line.

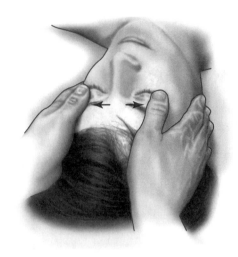

FIGURE 10–3. Very light effleurage over eyelids with the thumbs.

Gently squeeze the tissues between the thumb and the forefinger, beginning at the nose and moving laterally to the outside edge of the eye orbit. See Figure 10–2. Pressure should be light to moderate.

Effleurage over the Eyelids.   This technique is similar to the common gesture of rubbing the eyes when tired. It massages orbicularis oculi, the sphincter muscle of the eyelids. Gently, using very light pressure, stroke the closed eyelids with your thumbs as shown in Figure 10–3. The movement is medial to lateral. Stroke once near the top, once in the middle, and once near the bottom of the eyelid.

Thumb Slides along the Nose.   People who wear glasses often rub or squeeze the tissues between the eyebrows at the bridge of the nose to relieve pressure where the glasses sit. Procerus, a small muscle located there, draws the medial angles of the eyebrows downward and produces transverse wrinkles over the bridge of the nose. Those with sinus congestion may also feel tenderness in the external tissues of the upper nose area.

Using light to moderate pressure, slide a thumb over the procerus muscle, and then use both thumbs to slide along the outline of the nose from the eyes to the little depression at the base. See Figure 10–4.

Direct Pressure along the Zygomatic Arch.   Pressure to the zygomatic or cheekbone area will sometimes help relieve congestion there. Perform effleurage with the fingertips along the underside of the zygomatic arch starting at the base of the nose and moving laterally. Apply direct pressure to the little depression at the base of the nose, and then moving laterally as before, press up and under the zygomatic arch with the index and third fingers. See Figure 10–5. Use light to moderate pressure. The area will be tender if the sinuses are congested.

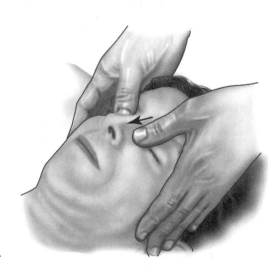

FIGURE 10–4. Thumb slides along the side of the nose.

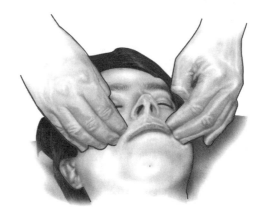

FIGURE 10–5. Direct pressure under zygomatic arch with the fingertips.

Massage Around the Mouth and Jaw.   There are a number of muscles around the mouth and jaw, which create movement for eating, speaking, and expression. For example, chewing, sipping, whispering, singing, smiling, frowning, and sneering all involve muscles around the mouth and jaw. Muscles that aid in mastication include the masseter, pterygoid muscles, and the temporalis.

Begin specific work around the mouth and jaw with effleurage using the thumbs to outline the upper lip (i.e., moustache area) and then the lower lip as shown in Figure 10–6. Knead the tissues on the chin and along the jawline with the thumb and first two fingers. Deep circular friction is effective on the strong jaw muscles such as the masseter.

Massaging the Ears.   The ears are made of soft cartilage and have many curves and folds. People who wear glasses, clip-on earrings, or any heavy earrings usually enjoy massage to the ears. Take care around hearing aids.

The ears may be massaged between the thumb and index finger. Follow the curves to rub the entire ear, including the ear lobes. As you approach the outer edges of the ear while rubbing, give a gentle pull to stimulate the area as shown in Figure 10–7. Perform circular friction all around the base of the ears to massage the small auricular muscles attached there. See Figure 10–8.

Mobilizing the Scalp.   The skin that covers the top of the head (i.e., the scalp) moves freely on most people. Stress can lead to tension in the muscles of the head, causing the scalp to be less mobile. Mobilizing the scalp has similar effects to skin rolling, which frees the underlying fascia and increases superficial circulation. Since circulation to hair follicles is increased, this helps promote healthy hair.

The scalp can be mobilized using a friction-like technique in which fingers placed on the scalp move the skin over the underlying muscle and bone. As the skin moves, the fingers stay in place on the skin surface. See Figure 10–9. Mobilize the entire scalp, including the back of the head. The pressure used is much lighter than deep friction, since the object is simply to move the scalp.

The hair may also be used to move the scalp. Grasp the hair close to the skin and use it as a handle to move the scalp back and forth. This works best with thick hair. It will not work if the recipient has hair that is too thin or too short to grasp.

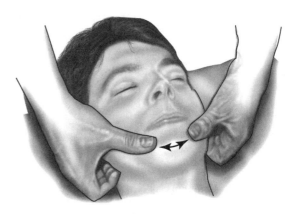

FIGURE 10–6. Thumbs outline the lower lip with effleurage.

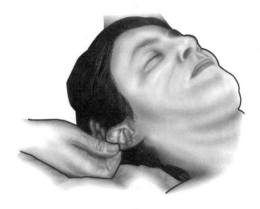

FIGURE 10–7. Gentle pull on the ear.

Muscles on the Head.   There are several broad thin muscles on the head. Some of these move the scalp, for example, the occipitofrontalis and temporoparietalis. The large temporalis muscle, found above the ears, elevates the mandible and aids in mastication. These muscles are massaged somewhat in the process of mobilizing the scalp as described above. Moderate pressure may be applied using circular friction with the fingers.

Passive Touch over the Eyes.   Placing the hands gently on the face with palms over the eyes can be soothing. It is similar to the self-comforting gesture of holding your face in your hands. See Figure 10–10. Pressure should be very light.

Pressing or Holding the Sides of the Head.   Pressing the sides of the head near the top as shown in Figure 10–11 can help relieve tension. Use the full hand, and press in with moderate to heavy pressure depending on the recipient. Slowly release the pressure. It is the sensation of compression, and then letting go, that is relaxing.

Simply holding the head as in Figure 9–23 can be relaxing and is a good finishing technique. Pressure should be light, since the idea is to give the impression of holding, not pressing.

NECK

The cervical or neck region is "pivotal" in many senses of the word. It links the head with the torso and houses the delicate spinal cord. Nerves and blood vessels going to the brain pass through the neck. It contains the muscles that hold the head in position during upright posture and movement in different planes. It is the pivot point for the head and provides the structure and musculature that allows us to access sensation as we turn our heads to look, listen, smell, and taste.

For some, the neck and throat are areas to be protected from touch by others. People who have experienced choking, near suffocation or drowning, neck trauma, or who fear such occurrences may respond negatively to touching the neck, especially the anterior neck, in any way. Protective responses

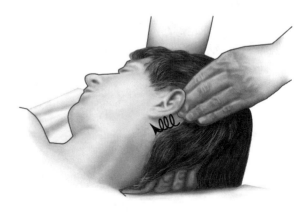

FIGURE 10–8. Circular friction around the base of the ear.

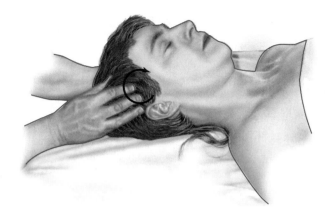

FIGURE 10–9. Mobilizing the scalp with the fingertips. The skin moves over underlying muscle and bone.

may include tightening the shoulder and neck muscles, raising the shoulders, lowering the chin, covering the throat with the hands, or even pulling the practitioner's hands from the neck.

Applications of Massage

Poor posture and body mechanics can lead to excessive tension in the neck. The *head forward* posture and poor sitting posture at workstations are two common sources of chronic neck tension. A cold draft on the back of the neck or sleeping in a cramped position can sometimes cause neck stiffness. Long airplane or automobile rides can also leave neck muscles painful and stiff.

Stressful life situations may aggravate cervical tension and may literally be a "pain in the neck." A major cause of tension headache is hypertonicity of the cervical muscles, which refer pain into the head. Trigger point work on the cervical and upper back muscles may be integrated into a Western massage routine for effective relief of a tension headache. The contraction of muscles and pain in the neck region from whiplash or wryneck (torticollis) may be relieved with massage.

Anatomy

The major muscles in the neck include the upper trapezius, splenius capitis and cervicis, semispinalis capitis and cervicis, longissimus capitis, levator scapulae, sternocleidomastoid (SCM); and the deeper smaller muscles of the suboccipitals (rectus capitis posterior major and minor, oblique capitis superior and inferior), multifidi and rotatores. Generally speaking, the more superficial muscles are larger and thicker, and the deeper ones are smaller and thinner. Some of the deeper muscles of the posterior neck are shown in Figure 10–12.

Cautions.   Endangerment sites in the cervical region include the anterior neck and throat, and the arteries and veins that supply the brain. The carotid artery and jugular vein are located on the sides of

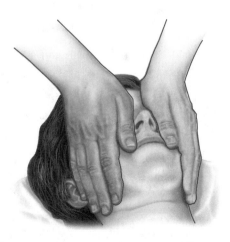

FIGURE 10–10. Passive touch over the eyes with the palms of the hands.

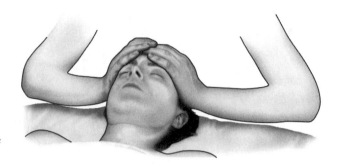

FIGURE 10–11. Pressing the sides of the head with the palms of the hands.

the neck. These areas should be avoided, especially in the elderly or anyone with a history of atherosclerosis, i.e., hardening of the arteries.

Techniques

The following techniques may be integrated into a basic massage of the neck. When working in the cervical area, attention should be given first to relaxing the superficial muscles, allowing better access to the deeper muscles. The area should be thoroughly warmed up before deeper techniques are performed.

Direct Pressure to the Cervical Muscles. With the recipient in the supine position, direct pressure may easily be applied to the cervical muscles on either side of the spine. Use the index finger to apply moderate pressure upward as shown in Figure 10–13. Apply pressure to both sides at the same time, or alternating back and forth from one side to the other. Start at the base of the neck and apply the direct pressure to one spot then the next, moving toward the suboccipital area. A slight movement of the neck will occur.

Deep Pressure to the Suboccipitals. With the recipient in the supine position, apply direct pressure to the suboccipital muscles using all of the fingers. Place the fingers along the suboccipitals and simply apply pressure upward. The chin will elevate, and the head will fall back slightly into a mild hyperextension.

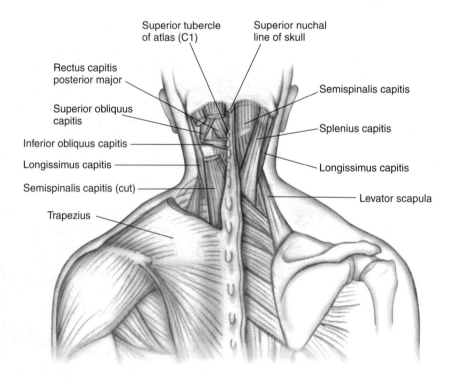

FIGURE 10–12. Deep muscles of the posterior neck.

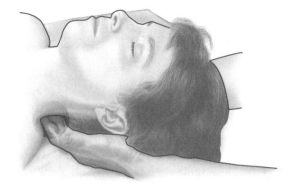

FIGURE 10–13. Direct pressure to posterior cervical muscles using fingertips with recipient supine.

Deeper pressure may be applied to the suboccipital muscles with the thumb. This is a useful technique when working with stiff or tense neck muscles. Cradle the head in one hand and rotate it away from the side you are working on. With the thumb of the other hand, slowly apply pressure into the suboccipital space. You can deepen the pressure by carefully accentuating the natural extension of the head. Instruct the recipient to take slow deep breaths to enhance relaxation. Hold the pressure for 1–2 breath cycles and then slowly release. Do not hold too long or press so deep that more pain is elicited. See Figure 10–14.

Direct pressure may be alternated with cross-fiber friction for a thorough and deep massage of the suboccipitals. This should be followed by gentle stretching for more lasting effects.

Direct Pressure to Thoracic Attachments—Supine.   Some of the muscles of the neck attach to the thoracic spine or ribs. Direct pressure to these attachments can help improve flexibility of the neck. When performing passive forward flexion of the neck, you can sometimes feel a resistance at the lower attachments of the cervical muscles. These attachments are affected during upper back massage, but may also receive attention with the recipient in the supine position.

Reach under the trunk, palms up, to about the fourth thoracic vertebra, and place the fingers on both sides of the spine. Press up at one spot, and then the next, moving upward toward the base of the neck. The weight of the trunk will offer resistance and allow deep pressure to be applied.

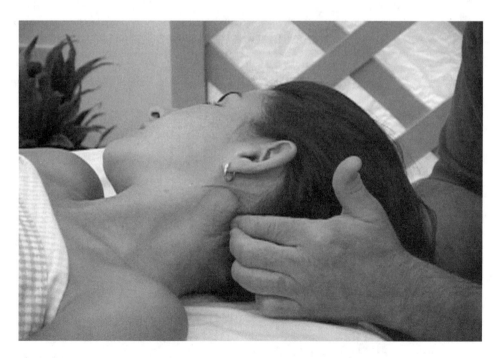

FIGURE 10–14. Direct pressure to suboccipital muscles with the thumb with recipient supine.

A variation of this technique is to use the same hand placement, but slide the fingers along the spine using deep pressure. The slide will help stretch tissues. Note that these techniques applied with the receiver supine take considerable strength on the part of the practitioner and should be performed only by those with strong flexors in the hands and wrists.

Neck Massage in the Prone Position.   The cervical muscles may be massaged when the recipient is in the prone or seated position. If using an adjustable face cradle, tilt it down so that the neck is slightly stretched. This creates more space.

Effleurage with the thumb or fingertips can be used to warm the cervical muscles. Perform effleurage from the base of the neck to the suboccipitals. Follow this with kneading using one hand as shown in Figure 10–15.

Once the muscles are warmed up, the thumb or the fingers may be used to apply direct pressure at an angle into the suboccipital space and toward the top of the head. Care should be taken not to apply so much pressure that the recipient's face feels smashed into the face cradle. Direct pressure may be applied with the thumbs or elbow over the thoracic attachments of the cervical muscles.

BACK

"Spend more time on my back" is a frequent request from recipients of massage. The back is the core area for maintaining upright posture, and the place of attachment for muscles that move the arms and legs. It is a heavily muscled area that works hard and is prone to tension, aches, and stiffness. Poor body mechanics when sitting, lifting, playing sports, or during physical activities such as gardening can cause backache.

The back is a common place where worry and anxiety are held, which is sometimes experienced as Atlas carrying the weight of the world on his shoulders. A bent-over posture evokes the image of weakness, discouragement, and defeat; a straight back presents the image of strength, self-confidence, and vigor.

Applications of Massage

Soothing back massage is associated with the qualities of nurturing, sympathy, and deep relaxation. Perhaps because the nerves of the parasympathetic nervous system exit the posterior vertebrae, the relaxation response is easily triggered during massage of the back. Back massage is often used to help people go to sleep.

Deep massage of the back muscles can help release tension held there and relieves the stiffness and soreness that accompanies heavy physical labor. Joint movements improve the mobility of the scapulae (i.e., shoulder blades), enhancing movement in the shoulder girdle. Tension in the upper trapezius can refer pain into the head. Massage of the shoulders can help relieve tension headache.

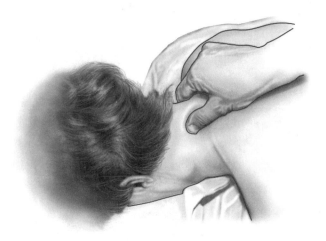

FIGURE 10–15. One hand kneading to posterior cervical muscles, recipient prone.

Anatomy

It is important for practitioners to develop a three-dimensional concept of the back. This includes the recognition that the "back" is the posterior portion of the torso, which also has sides. The back is thick with layers from large broad superficial muscles to the tiny deep muscles of the spine. The scapulae, or shoulder blades, located on the upper back are an integral part of the shoulder girdle. They glide over the posterior ribs and have numerous muscular attachments, which generate the free movement of the shoulder complex. Practitioners work at various depths of penetration during massage of the back.

The large superficial muscles of the back include the trapezius and latissimus dorsi. Spinal muscles include the erector spinae (iliocostalis, longissimus, spinalis), the deep posterior spinal muscles (multifidi, rotatores, interspinales, intertransversarii, and levatores costarum), and the semispinalis thoracis. Muscles surrounding the scapulae include subscapularis, upper trapezius, posterior deltoid, supraspinatus, infraspinatus, serratus anterior, teres major and minor, levator scapulae, and the rhomboids on the medial border. The quadratus lumborum is in the lower back, with attachments on the last rib, the transverse processes of the upper four lumbar vertebrae, and the iliac crest.

Techniques

The following techniques may be integrated into a basic back massage. They focus on muscles that move the spine and techniques for the back overall. Massage and movements for the shoulders are covered in more detail in the section on the upper extremities.

Skin Rolling.   Skin rolling is an excellent technique to help relieve tension in the back. It helps restore elasticity to the subcutaneous connective tissues and improves superficial circulation.

First perform a general warm-up of the area with effleurage or compression. Skin rolling is performed by lifting the cutaneous tissues from the underlying muscles. It may be applied sequentially by lifting the tissues in one place and then the next, eventually covering the entire back. It may also be performed in strips using a continuous motion, by lifting the tissues and, without letting go, sliding the hands along in a line. The tissues are lifted as the hands slide along by the pressure between the thumbs and fingers. Skin rolling is also described in Chapter 7, Figure 7–16.

Warming Friction of the Back.   Warming friction may be used to create heat in any relatively flat area. It is effective over the erector muscles on either side of the spine, over the rhomboids, and on the muscles covering the scapulae. Lubricant will reduce the effect of the friction and so should be used sparingly or wiped off before performing warming friction.

Sawing friction is performed with the ulnar side of the hands, palms facing each other. The hands are moved back and forth in a sawing motion, sliding over the skin and creating friction on the skin. Deeper pressure will create friction in deeper tissues. The skin will appear red as the superficial blood vessels dilate. Sawing friction is also described in Chapter 7, Figure 7–19.

Warming friction may also be performed with the knuckles. Figure 7–18 in Chapter 7 shows knuckling friction over the erector muscles of the thoracic region.

Effleurage Between the Ribs.   Effleurage of the intercostal muscles with the fingertips helps relax these tiny muscles. This facilitates easier and deeper breathing by allowing the rib cage to expand more. Find the intercostal spaces using palpation skills, and slide the fingers in the spaces moving from the spine laterally and around the sides of the rib cage. See Figure 10–16.

Therapeutic Sequence for the Lower Back.   The muscles of the lower back can get stiff and sore from sitting for long periods of time, especially in chairs or car seats with poor lumbar support. The following sequence of techniques helps relax the muscles of the lower back and relieve general fatigue of the area. A summary of the technique sequence for the lower back can be found in Table 10–1.

Warm up the entire back with effleurage and circular friction as described in the full-body Western massage. For the lower back portion of the routine, insert the following five-part combination of techniques. Position yourself at the client's hip, facing the head of the table for techniques applied inferior to superior, or at that lower back facing the side of the table for direct pressure, rocking, and horizontal stroking techniques.

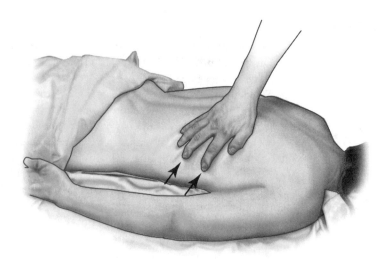

FIGURE 10–16. Effleurage of intercostal muscles using fingertips, recipient prone.

Once the lower back is warmed up, apply stripping in the space between the iliac crest and the twelfth rib (i.e., quadratus lumborum) using moderate to deep pressure. The first strip is applied just laterally to the spinous processes. Each strip is performed just laterally to the one before. See Figure 10–17. Stripping lengthens and broadens the muscle fibers.

Follow this with circular friction to the paraspinal muscles using the fingertips. Then apply direct pressure with the thumbs to the paraspinal muscles using moderate to heavy pressure. Begin at the 12th rib and press in at about one-inch intervals along the muscles, up to and along the iliac crest. See Figure 10–18.

Apply knuckle friction to the muscles in the region to further warm and bring blood to the lower back. Joint movement may be applied to the lower back by placing the thumb on one side of the spine and the fingers on the other, and gently rocking the spine from side to side. Apply rocking for a few seconds.

Table 10–1 THERAPEUTIC SEQUENCE FOR THE LOWER BACK*

General Description:
Massage to relieve tension and fatigue in the muscles of the lower back. Goals include relaxation and lengthening muscles in the lumbar region.

Note: Figures cited below illustrate the technique, but it may be performed on a different part of the body in the picture.

Warming Techniques
1. Effleurage to entire back (Figure 7–6, 7–7)
2. Effleurage to right side of spine, hips to shoulders (Figure 7–5)
3. Circular friction to paraspinal muscles on right side of spine (Figure 9–1)

Therapeutic Combination—Lower Back
4. Stripping between the 12th rib and the iliac crest (quadratus lumborum) (Figure 10–17)
5. Cross-fiber friction over paraspinal muscles (Figure 7–21)
6. Direct pressure along paraspinal muscles and iliac crest at 1-inch intervals (Figure 10–18)
7. Knuckle friction over lumbar region (Figure 7–18)
8. Gentle rocking of lower back

Finishing and Transition Technique
9. Horizontal stroking across lumbar region (Figure 7–8)
10. Effleurage from hips to shoulders to reconnect the back kinesthetically (Figure 7–5)

*This is an example of a therapeutic sequence for the lower back. It can be altered to meet the needs of an individual recipient. There are many variations of this sequence, and many more techniques that can be incorporated to achieve the overall goal of relieving tension and fatigue in the lower back.

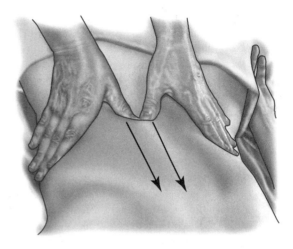

FIGURE 10–17. Thumb stripping along the lower back on quadratus lumborum.

To finish massage of the lower back and transition to the next phase of the session, apply horizontal stroking across the lower back. Follow with effleurage to the entire back to reconnect the lower back kinesthetically to the rest of the body.

Back Massage for Relaxation.   If the purpose of back massage is general relaxation, either avoid specific painful work on the back altogether, or spend at least five to seven minutes after painful work on lighter, soothing techniques. Use long flowing effleurage strokes with oil, maintaining full contact with the palm of the hand throughout the stroking. Use moderate to slow continuous motion. The movement should feel "seamless."

Vary the pattern to avoid boredom. Mix up vertical, circular, and horizontal patterns of effleurage. Some petrissage of the shoulder may be integrated for variety. Avoid tapotement, and finish either with nerve strokes or passive touch over the scapulae.

Sedating Effleurage of the Back.   Back massage is sometimes used in hospitals and nursing homes for those having trouble falling asleep. Sedating effleurage may be performed without oil or lotion. It is very effective for evoking the relaxation response, and promoting sleep. The movement consists of long gliding strokes directly over the spine that start at the base of the skull and go all the way to the coccyx. Hands alternate. As one hand is about to complete its motion near the coccyx, the other hand begins the next stroke starting at the base of the skull. Pressure must be light but firm and the rhythm monotonous. Pressure that is too light might stimulate rather than sedate. This gives the recipient the feeling of continuous contact, with one hand beginning the next stroke before the other

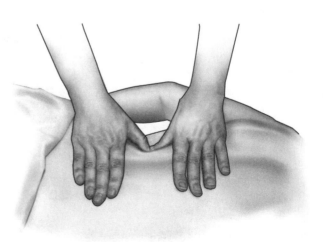

FIGURE 10–18. Direct pressure to muscles in the lower back using the thumbs.

hand finishes. Keep the motion going for a minute or two to help the recipient relax completely. A tingling sensation may be felt in the arms and legs as relaxation occurs. If this technique is applied for more than two or three minutes, it tends to stimulate rather than relax, so it should not be continued for too long.

BUTTOCKS

The large muscles of the hip region help support the entire body and provide the power for locomotion. They are the most important and the most stressed muscles in many sports. They are also the perch points for sitting.

The hips and buttocks are associated with sexual appeal. They may also be a source of poor self-image and embarrassment, particularly in women. For those physically or sexually abused as children, it is often a region of remembered pain and suffering. Practitioners should take great care when working in this region to create a feeling of safety and modesty.

Applications of Massage

Sports and fitness participants are often stiff and sore in the hip area from the strain of physical activity. On the other hand, those who are more sedentary may also experience stiffness from lack of movement. Tight buttock muscles can impinge on the sciatic nerve and cause leg pain. Soft-tissue manipulation and joint movements improve circulation to the area, relax muscles, and improve mobility at the hip joint. The elderly may especially benefit from improved hip mobility and, therefore, improved locomotion.

Anatomy

The more superficial muscles of the hip region are the large gluteals (maximus, medius, minimus), which run superior and inferior. The smaller, deeper hip rotators include the piriformis, gemelli, quadratus femoris, and obturator internus and externus. The deeper muscles run medial to lateral as shown in Figure 10–19.

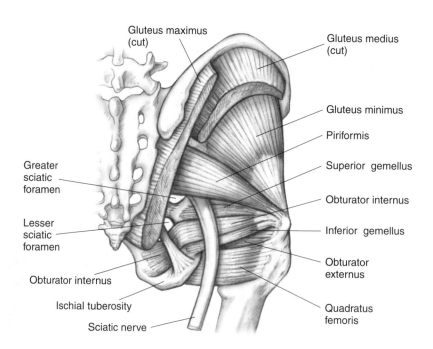

FIGURE 10–19. Deep muscles of the buttocks.

Techniques

The following techniques may be integrated into the basic massage of the lower limbs and buttocks. Some practitioners massage the buttocks as part of a back routine, while others include the buttocks in a lower limb sequence. Since most of the attachments are on the ilium and femur and create movement in the thigh, it may make more sense to treat the buttocks when massaging the lower limbs.

Use of the Elbow and Forearm.   Because you must work through the large superficial muscles to reach the smaller deeper muscles, it is useful to use the elbow or forearm to apply some techniques to the buttocks. You can apply more pressure and avoid straining the hands. However, care should be taken not to use too much pressure, especially around the sciatic nerve outlet in the buttocks. Palpatory sensitivity should be developed so that you can feel the condition of the tissues as you would with your hands. The elbow or forearm is not used to "muscle through" the tissues, but to apply more pressure skillfully.

The elbow or forearm may be used for broad strokes, and the point of the elbow (olecranon process) for more specific techniques such as direct pressure to a spot. The elbow or forearm may be used to apply effleurage, direct pressure, and circular or transverse friction. Figure 10–20 shows direct pressure to the deep buttock muscles using the elbow.

Use of the Fist.   The fist is useful for applying deep pressure during compressions or effleurage on the large muscles of the buttocks. Figure 10–21 shows compressions applied to the gluteal muscles using the fist. One advantage of this technique over using the palms is that the wrist can be kept straight, thus avoiding potential wrist damage when applying deep pressure.

Direct Pressure to Gluteal Attachments.   Direct pressure to the gluteal attachments helps relax the muscles and facilitates a better stretch. Use the thumbs, knuckles, or elbow to press along the attachments along the iliac crest and sacroiliac junction. Follow with effleurage to the area using the fist.

Mobilizations and Stretching.   A thorough treatment of the muscles of the buttocks should include both massage and joint movements. Mobilizing techniques and stretching help condition the deep rotators of the hip joint, which are difficult to reach directly with massage. While massage of the buttocks is necessarily performed with the recipient prone, most joint movements are done supine. If one of the major goals of the session addresses mobility in the hips, it may be useful to begin prone to warm up the muscles, and finish supine for the joint movements described in Chapter 8.

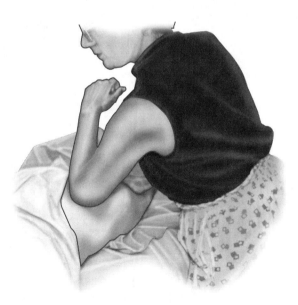

FIGURE 10–20. Use of the elbow to apply direct pressure to deep buttocks muscles.

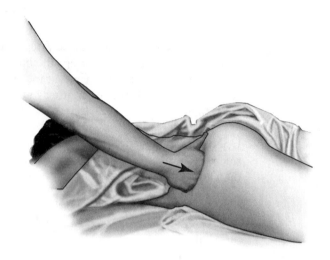

FIGURE 10–21. Compression to the gluteal muscles using the fist. Note the wrist alignment.

LOWER EXTREMITIES

The lower extremities are the principal means of locomotion for bipedal human beings. They afford us a great degree of independence as we can get from one place to another on "our own power." Loss or diminished use of the legs, through disease, accident, or old age, can result in greater dependence and loss of freedom. Having "a spring in your step" is a sign of vitality and positive outlook. Athletes depend on their legs to play their sports, and walking has become the premier fitness activity today.

In Western culture, shoes are worn for protection, and also confine the feet. It feels good to free the feet and kick off your shoes after wearing them all day. Going barefoot or wearing sandals is a sign of leisure and relaxation. If your feet hurt, you hurt all over. Foot massage is valued as a pleasurable treat.

Applications of Massage

People who stand long hours in their jobs often experience stress and pain in the legs and feet. Women especially tend to wear shoes with little support, and often wear high heels, which puts the feet and legs in a strained position. Those who sit a lot typically have problems with loss of leg strength, muscle shortening, and poor circulation. With age there is loss of strength, flexibility, and "spring," and muscles are more frequently stiff and sore. Massage and stretching can help the legs and feet feel and function better by improving circulation, joint mobility, and muscle relaxation.

Anatomy

For purposes of massage, the lower extremities may be thought of in three sections, that is, thigh, lower leg, and feet. In the prone position, the buttocks are often included with the lower extremities. There are three large joints in the lower extremities (i.e., hip, knee, and ankle), and several small joints within the feet.

Thigh.   The major muscles of the anterior thigh include the quadriceps (rectus femoris, vastus intermedius, vastus lateralis, vastus medialis), and sartorius. Muscles found on the medial thigh include the adductors, that is, adductor brevis, adductor longus, adductor magnus, gracilis, pectineus. High on the lateral thigh is tensor fasciae latae. The posterior thigh includes the hamstrings (i.e., biceps femoris, semimembranosus, semitendinosus). The iliopsoas (i.e., psoas and iliacus muscles), act on the hip joint, but, for the purposes of massage, are palpated in the abdomen. See Figure 10–22.

Lower Leg.   The muscles of the lower leg act largely on the ankle joint and include the anterior muscles (tibialis anterior, peroneus tertius, and the extensors), the lateral muscles (peroneus longus and brevis), and the posterior muscles (gastrocnemius, soleus, tibialis posterior, and the flexors).

Feet.   There are many small muscles intrinsic to the feet, most of which are on the plantar side or bottom. The plantar muscles include a superficial layer (abductor hallucis, flexor hallucis longus, flexor dig-

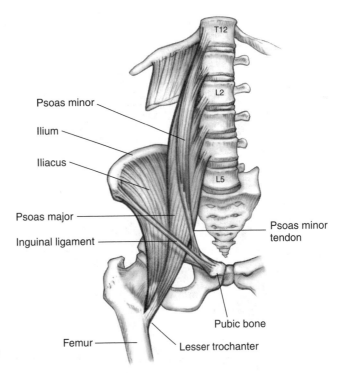

FIGURE 10–22. Components of the iliopsoas muscle.

itorum brevis, abductor digiti minimi brevis), a middle layer (lumbricales, flexor digiti minimi brevis, quadratus, flexor digitorum longus), and a deep layer (adductor hallucis, interossei plantares, flexor hallucis brevis, ligamentum plantarum longum). The plantar aponeurosis is a superficial strong fibrous band of fascia that runs from the heel to the ball of the foot and binds the longitudinal arch. It is the central part of a broad band of fascia that covers the muscles on the plantar side of the foot. The dorsal surface of the foot is fairly bony. The extensor digitorum brevis and the dorsal interossei are accessible to massage.

Cautions.   One of the major endangerment sites in the lower extremities is the popliteal fossa located behind the knee. Care should be taken not to apply pressure in this area. However, attachments of muscles may be followed around the area.

   Avoid deep pressure over varicose veins, which are common in older adults. Do not massage the legs if blood clotting or phlebitis is present.

   Avoid irritating bunions found at the base of the great toe. Watch for athlete's foot and other fungal infections that may be spread through touch. Avoid massaging feet with active infections.

Techniques

The following techniques can be integrated into the basic massage of the lower extremities. Detailed attention is given to the feet, lower leg, and thigh.

Foot Massage.   A thorough foot massage can make you feel good all over. It touches all of the small intrinsic muscles of the feet, as well as attachments of muscles of the lower leg, and mobilizes the many joints found there. It relaxes the muscles, improves circulation, and restores feeling to a part of the body encased in shoes most of the time.

   The following foot massage routine uses techniques described in more detail in Chapters 8 and 9. The sequence includes soft-tissue manipulation and joint movements for the complex musculoskeletal structure of the foot. A summary of the therapeutic sequence for foot massage can be found in Table 10–2.

   Begin by applying lubricant to the foot and ankle. Special lubricants are available for the feet that contain cooling substances such as peppermint and menthol. Be sure to cover the whole foot and each toe.

Table 10–2   THERAPEUTIC FOOT MASSAGE SEQUENCE*

General Description:
Massage to relieve sore tired feet, and improve mobility to joints in the feet. Relaxes muscles, improves local circulation, and restores feeling to the feet.

Note: Figures cited below illustrate the technique, but it may be performed on a different part of the body in the picture.

Warming Techniques
1. Apply lubricant to the entire foot with effleurage

Therapeutic Combination
Joint Movements (Caution: Do not snap or pull toes)
2. Mobilize the ankle using the heels of the hands (Figure 9–12)
3. Basic sliding effleurage on dorsal surface of the foot between metatarsals (Figure 7–2)
4. Scissoring movement between metatarsals (Figure 8–14)
5. Figure 8s on metatarsal-phalangeal joints (Figure 8–13)
6. Squeeze along each toe gently (proximal to distal)—top/bottom, sides
7. Thumb strokes to underside of each toe to "unflex" the toe
8. Pull on sides of the foot or interlock fingers and recipient's toes to create space between metatarsals (Figure 8–26, 8–27)

Soft Tissues
9. Broad pressure to foot bottom with fist (Figure 9–13)
10. Basic sliding effleurage with fist (Figure 9–13)
11. Direct pressure to points on foot bottom (Figure 10–23)
12. Repeat basic sliding effleurage with fist (Figure 9–13)

Finishing and Transition Techniques
13. Slapping foot bottom with back of hand
14. Holding the foot for a few seconds

*This is an example of a therapeutic sequence for the feet. It can be altered to meet the needs of an individual recipient. There are many variations of this sequence, and many more techniques that can be incorporated to achieve the overall goal of relieving sore and tired feet.

Mobilize the ankle using the heels of the hands. Using your thumb, apply basic sliding effleurage between the metatarsals on the dorsal surface of the foot, and then mobilize the space between metatarsals with a scissoring action. Mobilize each metatarsal-phalangeal joint with figure eights, and then gently petrissage each toe with a gentle squeezing action along the length of the toe moving proximal to distal. Do one length squeezing top and bottom, and then another squeezing the sides. Do not snap or pull the toes.

The toes are sometimes curled under into flexion. You may spend a little time straightening the toes with effleurage using thumb strokes to the underside of the toe while bracing the dorsal surface. Or you may prefer thumb on dorsal surface and index finger on the underside.

Use the fist to apply broad pressure to the bottom of the foot. Hold the dorsal surface of the foot with one hand while the other applies the pressure. You may shape the foot around the fist, stretching the top of the foot and accentuating the longitudinal and transverse arches. Basic sliding effleurage may also be applied to the bottom of the foot with the fist (Figure 9–13).

More specific pressure may be applied to the bottom of the foot with fingertips, knuckle or thumb. Pressing points on the bottom of the foot is thought to improve energy flow to the rest of the body (acupressure theory), and stimulate and increase circulation to corresponding body parts (reflexology theory). It also helps relax the small muscles found there. Figure 10–23 shows some areas on the bottom of the feet to press to stimulate healthy function of different regions of the body. Also see Chapter 15.

Space can be created between metatarsals by holding on to the sides of the foot and pulling the hands away from each other or by interlocking your fingers with the recipient's toes (Figures 8–26, 8–27). These techniques help relieve the feeling of the feet being squeezed inside of shoes.

Finish by slapping the bottom of the foot with the back of your hand. This should create a pleasant stimulating sensation. To finish, hold the feet. Repeat the entire sequence on the other foot.

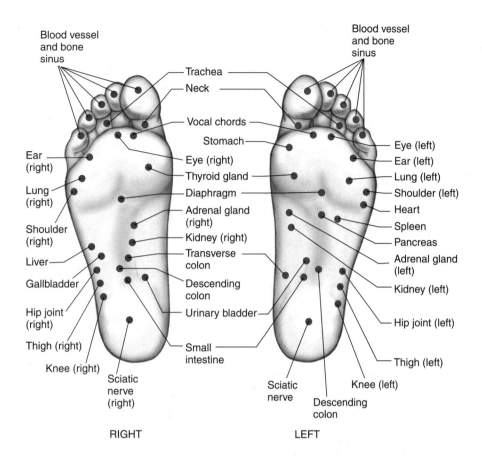

FIGURE 10–23. Areas to press on the bottoms of the feet to stimulate healthy function of different parts of the body.

Enhancing Mobility in the Lower Extremities. Mobility in the lower extremities may be restricted for a number of reasons. Overuse and shortening of muscles in athletes and physical workers, underuse and aging, recuperation from an extended illness or injury, or a sedentary lifestyle can all contribute to stiff joints and lack of fluid movement in the lower limbs.

For best results, all the muscles of the hips, thighs, lower legs, and feet should be thoroughly massaged with effleurage and petrissage and lengthened with stretching; major tendons should be loosened with friction to the point of attachment; and joints should be taken through their full range of motion. Direct pressure along muscles and tendons is used to help loosen them. The following techniques may be added to the basic full-body massage to further enhance mobility in the lower extremities. A technique sequence for enhancing mobility in the lower extremities can be found in Table 10–3.

Hips. After general massage of the buttocks, mobility at the hip joint may be further enhanced by pressing specific pressure points along the sacroiliac joint, the iliac crest, and around the trochanter at the hip joint. This may be done with the thumbs, an extended knuckle, or the elbow. Figure 10–24 shows some points to be pressed.

When the recipient is supine, take the upper leg through a full range of motion. The hip may be stretched by bringing the knee to the chest, out to the side in abduction, and across the body in adduction (Figures 8–18 to 8–21).

Thighs. After general massage of the thigh, perform deep effleurage along each major muscle, including the adductors, to the point of proximal attachment. Figure 10–25 shows the technique for reaching the proximal adductor attachments. You may perform cross-fiber friction near the point of attachment for further effect. Get the recipient's consent to work the attachments in the groin area, and provide secure draping of the genitals.

Table 10–3 THERAPEUTIC SEQUENCE FOR ENHANCING MOBILITY IN THE LOWER EXTREMITIES*

General Description:
Massage to relax muscles and restore mobility in the hips and legs. Relieves tension, increases circulation, and improves flexibility in the lower extremities.

Note: Figures cited below illustrate the technique, but it may be performed on a different part of the body in the picture.

Warming Techniques
1. Effleurage of the entire leg and hip

Therapeutic Combination
Prone

Hip
2. Effleurage of buttocks (Figure 9–5)
3. Petrissage of gluteal muscles (Figure 10–21)
4. Direct pressure to points along sacroiliac joint, iliac crest, and around the trochanter at the hip joint (Figure 10–24)

Thigh
5. Effleurage of hamstrings, adductors, abductors (Figure 7–3, Figure 9–6)
6. Petrissage to thigh (Figure 9–7)
7. Friction to muscle attachments
8. Stretch bringing heel of foot to buttocks (Figure 8–23)

Lower Leg
9. Effleurage to lower leg (Figure 7–1)
10. Petrissage to lower leg (Figure 7–11)
11. Dorsiflexion at ankle with direct pressure to foot bottom (Figure 8–24)

Supine
Thigh
12. Effleurage to quadriceps muscles, adductors, abductors (Figure 7–1)
13. Petrissage of thigh muscles (Figure 7–11)
14. Friction to muscle attachments at knee (Figure 7–20)
15. Friction to iliotibial band (Figure 7–22)

Lower Leg
16. Effleurage to lower leg (Figure 7–1)
17. Friction along tibialis anterior (Figure 7–18)
18. Direct pressure along tibialis anterior (Figure 9–11)

Foot
19. Foot massage sequence in Table 10–2

Joint Movements
20. Move hip through its full range of motion (Figure 8–18)
21. Knee to chest stretch (Figure 8–19)
22. Straight leg stretch in flexion (Figure 8–20)
23. Move ankle through full range of motion
24. Stretches at ankle in dorsiflexion and plantarflexion.

Finishing and Transition Techniques
25. Effleurage to reconnect the leg kinesthetically
26. Rocking the leg (Figure 8–17)

*This is an example of a therapeutic sequence for the lower extremities. It can be altered to meet the needs of an individual recipient. There are many variations of this sequence, and many more techniques that can be incorporated to achieve the overall goal of enhancing mobility in the lower extremities.

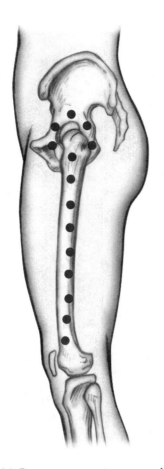
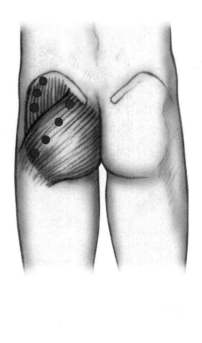

FIGURE 10–24. Points to press to improve mobility of the hip joint.

Perform circular friction over the muscle attachments at the knee, first with the heels of the hands, and then with the fingertips (Figure 9–9). These attachments are frequently sore to the touch. Cross-fiber friction may be performed over areas in which the tissues are adhering.

Lower Legs.   Perform general massage of the lower leg in the prone position. Loosen the Achilles tendon using direct pressure along its length, especially at the point of juncture with the muscle. See Figure 10–26. The tendon may be further loosened by moving it back and forth with the fingers after creating slack in it by slightly plantar flexing the foot. Perform mobilizing techniques at the ankle and stretch the muscles of the lower leg.

Feet.   The foot massage described previously will provide a nice finish to a thorough leg massage.

UPPER EXTREMITIES

Upright posture is thought to be an adaptation in the evolution of human beings to free us to use our hands for grasping and manipulating objects. Everyday activities such as cooking and eating, personal grooming, cleaning the house, and gardening are performed using the arms and hands. Hobbies and sports and most work activities also depend on the upper extremities.

The upper extremities are also important in communication. Some ethnic groups are known for using their hands to augment verbal expression. The hearing impaired use their hands for sign language. To be friendly or affectionate we shake hands, give pats on the back, and hug. Loss of the use of the arms or hands can be personally and socially devastating.

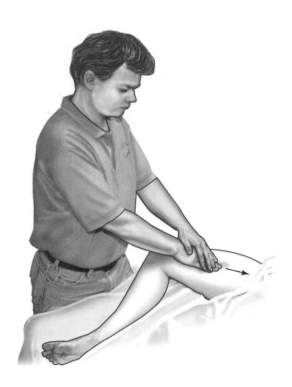

FIGURE 10–25. Position for reaching proximal adductor attachments. Be sure draping is secure.

Applications of Massage

People who work at computer terminals, or who perform other repetitive movements with the arms and hands often experience tightness and soreness in the upper extremities. Tennis elbow and golf elbow are repetitive strain injuries (RSI) common in those sports, and also in activities requiring similar movements of the arms. Massage and stretching can help keep muscles of the arms and hands relaxed and in good condition and help prevent overuse injuries. Massage is used with ice and rest to treat tennis and golf elbow.

Massage and joint movements can also help maintain shoulder flexibility. They can help restore mobility lost by poor posture, overuse, aging, or accident. The hands can be massaged and mobilized to help retain their function in old age.

Anatomy

For purposes of massage, the upper extremities may be thought of in four sections, that is, the shoulders, upper arms, forearms, and hands. The shoulders may be addressed as part of the upper back during massage, since the shoulder blades are located there. Functionally, however, the shoulder blades are part of the shoulder girdle and designed to facilitate use of the arms and hands. The joints of the upper extremities include the complex shoulder girdle, the elbows, wrists, and several small joints in the hands.

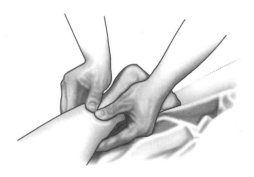

FIGURE 10–26. Direct pressure to Achilles tendon.

Shoulders. The muscles that move the shoulder include pectoralis major and minor, deltoid, subscapularis, supraspinatus, infraspinatis, teres major and minor, serratus anterior, levator scapulae, rhomboid major and minor, and trapezius. Latissimus dorsi is located on the back, but functions primarily to move the upper arm.

Arms and Hands. Muscles of the upper arm and forearms include the biceps brachii, triceps brachii, brachialis, the smaller muscles of pronation and supination (pronator teres, pronator quadratus, supinator), anconeus, coracobrachialis, and brachioradialis. The anterior forearm also contains the wrist flexors and palmaris longus, while the posterior forearm contains the wrist extensors. There are many small muscles intrinsic to the hand, which move the fingers and thumbs.

Techniques

The following techniques may be used to supplement a general massage of the upper extremities. The primary movers of the scapulae are located on the back and are best addressed as part of a back massage when the recipient is prone. The upper arms, forearms, and hands are most easily accessed and mobilized when the recipient is supine.

Enhancing Mobility of the Shoulder Girdle. Mobility of the shoulder girdle may be restricted for a number of reasons. Overuse and shortening of muscles in athletes and physical workers, underuse, aging, and recuperation from a shoulder injury can all contribute to loss of mobility in the shoulder.

A general approach to enhancing shoulder mobility would include warming of the superficial and deeper muscles of the upper back and upper arm with effleurage and petrissage, followed by deep

Table 10–4 THERAPEUTIC SEQUENCE FOR ENHANCING MOBILITY IN THE SHOULDER*

General Description:
Massage to relax muscles and restore mobility in the muscles of the upper back and shoulders. Relieves tension, increases circulation, and restores mobility in the shoulder.

Note: Figures cited below illustrate the technique, but it may be performed on a different part of the body in the picture.

Warming Techniques
  1. Effleurage and petrissage of the entire shoulder (Figures 9–2, 9–3)
  2. Circular friction along paraspinal muscles (Figure 9–1)

Therapeutic Combination
Prone
  3. Knuckle or sawing friction between and over the shoulder blades (Figure 7–18)
  4. Deep effleurage over upper trapezius and levator scapula
  5. Direct pressure along upper trapezius and medial scapula border (Figure 10–27)
  6. Swinging pendulum movement of arm
  7. Scapula mobilizing technique (Figures 8–6, 10–28)

Supine
  8. Direct pressure to subscapularis (Figure 10–29)
  9. Deep effleurage and compressions to pectoral muscles and anterior deltoid (Figure 10–31)
  10. Direct pressure to pectoral muscles (Figure 10–32)
  11. Passive shoulder roll (Figure 8–5)
  12. Arm stretches across the body and overhead (Figures 8–7, 8–8)

Finishing and Transition Technique
  13. Effleurage over entire arm and shoulder

*This is an example of a therapeutic sequence for the shoulder. It can be altered to meet the needs of an individual recipient. There are many variations of this sequence, and many more techniques that can be incorporated to achieve the overall goal of enhancing mobility in the shoulder.

friction on muscles, on tendons, and at attachments. Direct pressure on muscles and tendons, particularly at tender or trigger points, helps muscles to relax and lengthen.

The shoulders and upper arms should be mobilized and taken through their full range of motion. Care should be taken not to force movement, potentially damaging tissues. Mobility that has been restricted for some time will take time to regain. The following techniques may be added to the basic full-body routine described in Chapter 9 to further enhance mobility of the shoulder girdle. A technique sequence for enhancing mobility in the shoulder is summarized in Table 10–4.

Prone.   After general massage of the upper back, create a deeper warming by knuckling or sawing friction between and over the shoulder blades. How much pressure to use will be determined by the size and sensitivity of the recipient. The more heavily muscled the receiver, the more pressure you will use to affect deeper tissues.

Deep effleurage along upper trapezius and over the levator scapula will help loosen those muscles further. It may be useful then to apply vibration to the upper trapezius with an electric vibrator.

Direct pressure along the upper trapezius, and along the medial border of the scapula, will help relax these muscles. Apply pressure slowly, meeting the resistance offered by the tissue, then move along to another spot at about one-inch intervals. The reinforced thumb-over-thumb technique may be used for the large upper trapezius as shown in Figure 10–27.

With the receiver in the prone position, a gentle mobilization of the shoulder may be created by simply lifting the upper arm above the elbow, letting the forearm hang down toward the floor, and then swinging the forearm back and forth like a pendulum. This creates movement in the glenohumeral joint, as well as in the scapula. To create a larger and more controlled movement, place the recipient's arm alongside the body on the table. Grasp the upper arm just below the glenohumeral joint and move the shoulder superior and inferior, and then in a circle in a passive shoulder roll (Figure 8–5).

The scapula may be isolated for movement by placing the recipient's hand behind the back, which causes the scapula to lift away from the rib cage. Take care not to force this position, which may cause some discomfort. See Figure 10–28. You may modify this position by placing the hand next to the body with the elbow bent as shown in Figure 8–6. In either position, the scapula may be mobilized by placing a hand near the tip and on top of the shoulder and pressing lightly toward the feet. The other hand is placed at the inferior border of the scapula, assisting in the movement. The scapula will lift and move if the attached muscles are relaxed.

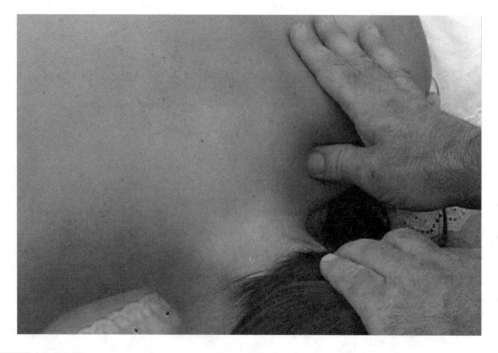

FIGURE 10–27. Direct pressure along upper trapezius with thumbs, recipient prone.

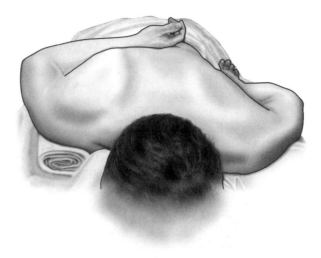

FIGURE 10–28. Mobilizing the scapula. Placing the recipient's hand behind the back causes the scapula to lift up.

Supine.   The subscapularis muscle may be accessed with the recipient supine. Stand at the side near the shoulder and face the table. Bring the recipient's lower arm across the chest with the upper arm perpendicular to the table. This will expose the underside of the scapula somewhat. Locate the subscapularis in the axilla (i.e., armpit) and press into the subscapularis muscle with the fingertips as shown in Figure 10–29. This is usually very tender, so proceed gently.

Teres major and latissimus dorsi may be located by passively extending the recipient's arm overhead. Grasp the lateral edge of these muscles near the armpit. Gently knead the muscles, and then pull along their length for a gentle stretch.

Mobility in the shoulder girdle may be restricted anteriorly by the pectoral muscles and the anterior deltoid. After general warming, apply deep effleurage to these muscles. Direct pressure along the length of the pectorals at half-inch intervals may help to loosen them further. Care should be taken, since the pectorals will likely be sore if hypertonic. Follow the more specific massage with stretches of the upper arm across the body and overhead.

Preventing Forearm Strain.   The muscles of the forearms create movement at the wrist and the hands. Certain occupations and activities tend to stress these muscles and produce chronic tension in them. Regular specific massage of the hands and forearms can help prevent overuse injuries in this area. A complete prevention program would also include regular resting time, stretching and self-massage, and biomechanically safe performance of the movements. Massage therapists themselves are prone to such overuse.

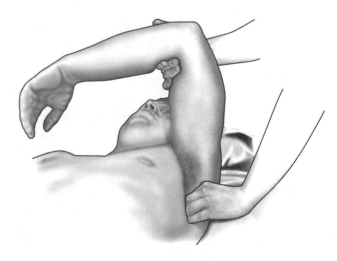

FIGURE 10–29. Accessing the subscapularis, recipient supine.

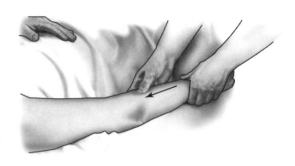

FIGURE 10–30. Deep stripping effleurage to the forearm muscles.

Warm the forearms and hands with general massage. Skin rolling over the wrist and forearm improves circulation to the area.

Add deep thumb stripping to the anterior and posterior forearms, following the long muscles from the wrist to their attachments at the elbow. See Figure 10–30. Apply deep circular friction to the attachments at the elbow. Direct pressure along the belly of the muscles of the forearms may help them relax. Mobilize the wrist joint and stretch the forearm muscles by passive flexion and hyperextension at the wrist.

To finish, perform the hand massage and joint movements described in Chapters 8 and 9. This will affect the forearm muscles that attach on the hand as well as muscles intrinsic to the hand itself.

CHEST AND ABDOMEN

The front of the body includes the chest and the abdomen. These areas are usually addressed separately during massage. However, they are connected for certain functions such as respiration and movements involving forward trunk flexion.

The expansion and contraction of the chest for breathing is evidence of life itself. Because it is the location of women's breasts, the chest is associated with both nurturing and sexual appeal. The chest is also associated with strength and power, as when the pectorals are more developed in men.

In the United States, women's breasts are kept covered in public and, therefore, should be draped to maintain modesty and proper professional boundaries. Practitioners can access the pectoral muscles and intercostals of women working around a small drape. When working on women with large breasts, it may be difficult to get to the muscles underneath.

Massage of the breast tissue itself is becoming more common as both a general health measure, and for certain clinical applications. Breast massage can be a valuable complementary therapy for women in treatment for breast cancer. It should be performed only after special training and with informed consent. (For further information, refer to *Breast Massage* by Debra Curties, 1999.)

The abdomen is a relatively vulnerable area extending from the diaphragm to the pubis. It contains the viscera, that is, the internal organs of digestion, elimination, and reproduction. It lacks the bony protection afforded the lungs and heart in the chest. The abdomen is contained and supported principally by the abdominal muscles. It is the soft belly exposed in humans because of our upright posture.

The word "visceral" has come to mean deeply felt, instinctive, or having to do with elemental emotions. This area is sensitive for many people and should be approached with care.

Applications of Massage

Poor posture, long periods of sitting at a desk, and carrying objects in the arms can all lead to shortening of the muscles of the chest and abdomen. A chronic slumped posture can inhibit the functions of the visceral organs, lead to back and neck tension and fatigue, and restrict breathing. Massage can help stretch and lengthen shortened anterior muscles that are the result of and contribute to chronic slumped posture. Along with proper strengthening exercises for the back and abdominal muscles, massage can help one maintain good postural alignment.

The chest cavity expands to accommodate expansion of the lungs during inhalation. Therefore, any muscular restriction in the area can adversely affect breathing. The major muscles of respiration are the diaphragm and intercostals. Forced inhalation and exhalation also involve the abdominal muscles, and muscles that move the rib cage such as pectoralis minor, serratus anterior, scalenes, and sternocleidomastoid. Massage can help maintain the muscles of respiration in optimal condition and relieve tension caused by poor posture or stress.

Breast massage is a specialized technique performed as a wellness measure for female breast health, and to address discomforts associated with the menstrual cycle, pregnancy and nursing. (Refer to *Breast Massage* by Debra Curties, 1999.)

Anatomy

The chest is defined by the rib cage, sternum, and muscles of the shoulder girdle that attach to them. The prominent muscles of the chest are pectoralis major and minor. Muscles located on the chest with the primary function of respiration include the diaphragm (separates the chest from the abdomen) and intercostals.

The breast structure sits over the muscles of the chest wall. It is "a specialized gland structure which evolves essentially as an appendage of the skin." The female breast is made up of fat tissue, and mammary glands and ducts with supporting connective tissue (i.e., fascia and ligaments). Breast tissue lies beyond the obvious contour of the breast, and extends inferior and laterally on the chest (Curties, 1999, p.19).

The abdomen lies between the thorax or chest and the pelvis. The abdominal cavity contains the stomach, liver, spleen, pancreas, small and large intestines, kidneys, bladder, reproductive organs in females, and other visceral organs. The abdominal muscles surrounding and supporting the viscera include the rectus abdominus and internal and external obliques.

Techniques

Rounded Shoulders.   When the pectoral and anterior deltoid muscles shorten, the effect is rounded or forward shoulders. A program of stretching the muscles of the chest and shoulders, while strengthening the muscles of the upper back, is needed to truly correct rounded shoulders. During a massage session, rounded shoulders may be addressed by relaxing and stretching the pectorals and anterior deltoid.

Warm up the anterior deltoid with effleurage and petrissage. Apply compression over the anterior deltoid with a loose fist as shown in Figure 10–31. Warm up the pectorals using effleurage with the fist. Start superficially and gradually deepen the pressure. Once the muscles are warmed up, you may apply circular friction along the sternal and clavicular attachments of pectoralis major. Apply deep effleurage with the thumbs along the length of pectoralis minor, pausing to hold static pressure over the attachment on the third, fourth, and fifth ribs. See Figure 10–32.

Stretch the arm overhead to lengthen pectoral muscles. At the end of the session, have the recipient sit on the edge of the table with his hands behind his head. Get up onto the table behind the

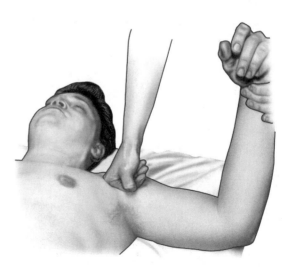

FIGURE 10–31. Compressions over anterior deltoid with loose fist.

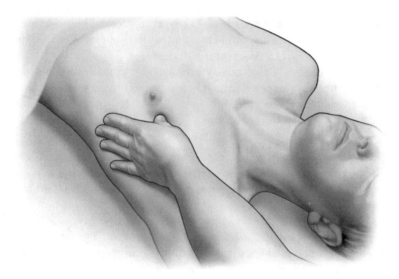

FIGURE 10–32. Direct pressure on attachments of pectoralis minor.

recipient and brace his back with your hip. Pull back on the elbows for a stretch of the pectorals as shown in Figure 10–33. Have the recipient inhale as you pull back and expand the chest.

Enhancing Respiration.   Breathing is easier when muscles of respiration are relaxed. Muscular tension in the diaphragm, intercostals, abdominals, scalenes, and levator scapulae can inhibit proper expansion and lifting of the chest during inhalation. A therapeutic sequence for enhancing respiration is described in Table 10–5.

During massage of the cervicals, perform effleurage specifically over the scalenes with the thumb or fingertips to help relax them. When the recipient is prone, perform thumb stripping along the

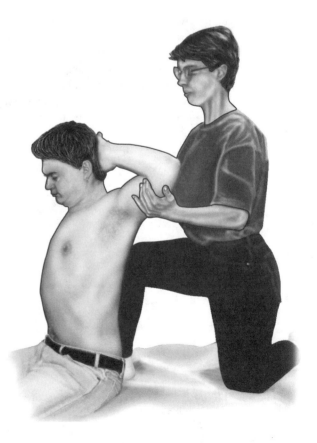

FIGURE 10–33. Stretching the pectorals with recipient in sitting position. Also used to enhance inhalation during deep breathing.

Table 10–5   THERAPEUTIC SEQUENCE FOR ENHANCING RESPIRATION*

General Description:

Massage to relieve muscular tension in the muscles of respiration to allow for greater expansion of the rib cage. General relaxation to encourage deep diaphragmatic breathing.

Note: Figures cited below illustrate the technique, but it may be performed on a different part of the body in the picture.

Warming Techniques
  1. Effleurage and petrissage to the cervical muscles and upper trapezius (Figure 9–2, 9–3)

Therapeutic Technique Combination
Prone
  2. Kneading of upper trapezius (Figure 9–3)
  3. Direct pressure to points along upper trapezius (Figure 7–37)
  4. Deep effleurage to levator scapula muscle moving superior to inferior
  5. Friction of levator scapula muscle and attachments
  6. "Cat paw" mobilizing technique to shoulders (prone version of Figure 9–19)
  7. Effleurage of intercostal muscles (Figure 10–16)

Supine
  8. Effleurage to upper trapezius using fist (Figure 9–20)
  9. Effleurage with thumb or fingertips over scalene muscles, moving superior to inferior
  10. Deep effleurage over pectoral muscles, moving superior to inferior (Figure 9–16)
  11. Direct pressure on pectoral muscle attachments (Figure 10–32)
  12. "Cat paw" mobilizing of shoulders (Figure 9–19)
  13. Effleurage to intercostal muscles (supine version of Figure 10–16)
  14. Rocking the rib cage (Figures 8–15, 8–16)
  15. Slide along diaphragm attachment and lift side (Figures 10–34, 10–35)

Finishing and Transition Technique
  16. Effleurage over shoulders and neck
  17. Cradle head to encourage relaxation and deep diaphragmatic breathing (Figure 9–23)

---

*This is an example of a therapeutic sequence to enhance respiration. It can be altered to meet the needs of an individual recipient. There are many variations of this sequence, and many more techniques that can be incorporated to achieve the overall goal of improving breathing.

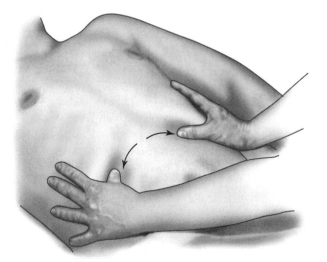

FIGURE 10–34. Sliding the thumbs along the attachment of the diaphragm.

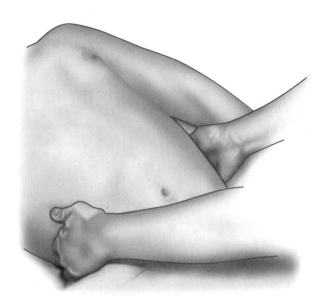

FIGURE 10–35. Lifting the abdominal muscles around the waist.

levator scapula to its point of attachment on the superior medial border of the scapula, lengthening the muscle. These are the muscles that elevate the shoulders and help expand the chest. They may be tense in people who are stressed and are breathing shallowly from the shoulders.

When the recipient is supine, lengthen the pectorals as described above to create space across the chest. Then perform effleurage over the rib cage from the opposite side of the table. Reach around as far as you can and pull up and over the rib cage with spread fingers. Try to find the spaces between the ribs to massage the intercostals. Rock the rib cage to further relax the area.

Stand at the waist of the recipient facing the head. Place your thumbs just beneath the sternum and have the recipient take a deep breath in. As he exhales, press in and slide your thumbs along the attachment of the diaphragm along the outline of the rib cage as shown in Figure 10–34. Be careful to avoid pressure on the xiphoid process. Finish by lifting up and around the sides of the abdominals. See Figure 10–35.

You may want to spend some time with the recipient practicing diaphragmatic breathing, or taking a full breath beginning with the diaphragm and expanding the chest. The stretching exercise shown in Figure 10–33 can also be used to help the recipient feel the expansion of the chest during inhalation.

Abdominal Massage.   Abdominal massage is described in Chapter 9 as part of full-body massage. Techniques include effleurage in a circular pattern moving clockwise around the abdomen, fingertip vibration in the same pattern, and gentle undulating compression of the area, followed by effluerage, horizontal stroking, and finishing with passive touch. These techniques help stimulate movement of the contents of the lower digestive tract.

SUMMARY

Practitioners may want to focus more time and attention on a particular region of the body. This could stem from a request from the recipient, the practitioner's own judgment, information on a health history form, or referral from a health care provider.

Even though the body is massaged region by region during a session, its interconnectedness should always be kept in mind. Also, different body regions may have significance or human meaning to an individual person. Practitioners need to be aware that they are not just touching body regions, but are touching a person.

The body regions addressed in a massage session are usually divided into head and face, neck, back, buttocks, lower extremities, upper extremities, chest and abdomen. The scapula is commonly massaged as part of the back. Knowledge of each region in terms of its human meaning, anatomy, cautions, and relevant massage applications and techniques is essential for meeting the recipient's needs.

The head and face region is the center for thinking and communication. The senses of sight, hearing, taste, and smell are housed there. Massage can release tension caused by job-related activities, by emotional distress, and by pathologies that affect the facial muscles. Specific techniques that can be integrated into a head and face massage include: squeeze to eyebrows, effleurage over eyelids, thumb slide along nose, direct pressure to zygomatic arch, massage around mouth and jaw, massage to ears, mobilizing the scalp, massage of head, passive touch over eyes, and holding the sides of the head.

The neck region links the head and torso, and contains the muscles that hold head in upright posture. Muscle tension in the neck may result from poor posture, stress, or injury. Endangerment sites in the region include the anterior neck, and arteries and veins to the brain. Specific techniques that can be integrated into massage of the neck include direct pressure to cervical muscles, deep pressure to suboccipitals, direct pressure to thoracic attachments, and neck massage in prone position.

The back region is the core area for maintaining upright posture, and the place of attachment for arms and legs. Soothing back massage helps elicit the relaxation response. Tension in the back may result from heavy labor, sports, poor posture, or stress. Specific techniques that can be integrated into back massage include skin rolling, warming friction, effleurage between the ribs, lower back massage, and back massage for relaxation.

The buttocks, or large muscles of the hip region, support the entire body and provide the power for locomotion. They can be a source of sexual appeal, as well as of embarrassment. Specific techniques that can be integrated into massage of the buttocks include use of elbow, forearm and fist, direct pressure to gluteal attachments, and mobilizing techniques and stretching.

The lower extremities are the principal means of bipedal locomotion. Stress and pain in the legs and feet may be the result of accident, old age, sports, or job requirements. Foot massage involves massage of intrinsic muscles of the feet and attachments of leg muscles, and mobilizing of joints. Mobility in lower extremities can be enhanced with massage of the hips, thighs, lower leg, and feet.

The upper extremities allow us to use our hands and manipulate objects. They are important for everyday and work activities, and for communication. Problems in the upper extremities can result from repetitive motion, poor posture, old age, or accident. Mobility of the shoulder girdle can be enhanced with massage.

The front of the body includes the chest and abdomen. The chest is the location of pectoral muscles and breasts, and is associated with both nurturing and sexual appeal in women and with strength in men. The abdomen is a relatively vulnerable region containing the viscera or internal organs. Applications of massage in the chest region include addressing poor posture, rounded shoulders, and enhancing respiration. Massage techniques performed on the abdomen help stimulate movement of the contents of the lower digestive tract.

A look ahead . . .

The effects of massage can be enhanced by hot and cold applications such as hot packs, ice packs, and by thermal facilities such as steam rooms. Chapter 11 provides information and guidelines for the safe and effective use of these adjuncts to massage.

REFERENCES

Curties, D. (1999) *Breast massage*. Moncton, New Brunswick, Canada: Curties-Overzet Publications.

ADDITIONAL REFERENCES

Videos

"Classical and innovative European facial massage." (1988). Erica Miller Professional Education Series. Mile Ranch, British Columbia, Canada: Spa Expertise Canada LTD.

"Head, Neck & Shoulder Massage." (2003). Massage Master Class™ Series. Riverside, CT: At Peace Media. (*www.atpeacemedia.com*).

"Japanese hand massage." (2001). With Shogo Mochizuki. Boulder, CO: Kotobuki Publications.

"Zoku shin do™, Volume 1: The art of Japanese foot massage." (1999). With Shogo Mochizuki. Boulder, CO: Kotobuki Publications.

STUDY GUIDE

LEARNING OUTCOMES

Use the learning outcomes at the beginning of the chapter as a guide to your studies. Perform the task given in each outcome, either in writing or verbally into a tape recorder or to a study partner. This may start as an "open book" exercise, and then later from memory.

KEY TERMS/CONCEPTS

To study key words and concepts listed at the beginning of this chapter, choose one or more of the following exercises. Writing or talking about ideas helps you remember them better, and explaining them helps deepen your understanding.

1. Write a one- or two-sentence explanation of each key word and concept.

2. With a study partner, take turns explaining key words and concepts verbally.

STUDY OUTLINE

The following questions test your memory of the main concepts in this chapter. Locate the answers in the text using the page number given for each question.

Wholeness and Meaning

1. Practitioners may want to focus more time and attention on a particular part of the body as the result of _____, _____, _____, or _____. (p. 194)

2. Even though the body is massaged region by region during a session, its _____ should always be kept in mind. (p. 194)

3. The human meaning of a particular body region is determined by _____, _____, _____. (p. 194)

4. As you interact with a client, be aware that you are not just touching a body, you are touching a _____. (p. 194)

Head and Face

1. The head is the center for _____ and _____. (p. 194)

2. Tension in the head and face may be caused by _____, and _____. (p. 194)

3. Worry and anxiety can lead to tension in the _____ and _____. (p. 194)

4. Pathologies that affect the face include _____ and _____. (p. 194)

5. The musculature of the head and face is complex and includes muscles of _____, _____, and _____ (p. 195)

6. Always ask a client if they are wearing _____ to avoid damage to the eyes. (p. 195)

7. Two types of muscles in the face are _____ and _____. (p. 195)

8. Squeeze to the tissues along the eyebrow feels good to people who _____, _____, or _____. (p. 195)

9. When performing effluerage over the eyelids, keep pressure _____. (p. 196)

10. Muscles that perform mastication (chewing) are _____, _____, and _____. (p. 197)

11. The ears are massaged between the _____, and the _____. (p. 197)

12. The scalp is massaged using _____ techniques. (p. 197)

13. A technique similar to the self-comforting gesture of holding your face in your hands is _____. (p. 198)

Neck

1. The neck is a _____ region that links the head with the torso, and facilitates movement of the head for _____, _____, _____, and _____. (p. 198)

2. Massage can help relieve tension in the neck caused by _____, _____, or long periods of _____. (p. 199)

3. _____ headaches can be relieved with massage. (p. 199)

4. A useful technique for specific massage of the neck is _____. (p. 200)

Back

1. The back is the core area for maintaining _____, and a place of attachment for muscles that _____. (p. 202)

2. Soothing back massage is associated with the qualities of _____, _____, and _____. (p. 202)

3. Tension in the upper trapezius can refer pain to the _____. (p. 202)

4. It is important for practitioners to develop a _____ dimensional concept of the back. (p. 203)

5. A technique in which superficial tissues are lifted from the underlying muscles is called _____. (p. 203)

6. Warming friction for the back can be performed with _____. (p. 203)

7. Effleurage between the ribs affects the _____ muscles. (p. 203)

8. Back massage for relaxation avoids causing _____ and includes long flowing _____ with oil performed with full firm contact with the palms. (p. 205)

9. Sedating effleurage of the back is performed with the fingertips lightly stroking the skin from _____ to _____. Hands alternate stroking for a _____ movement. (p. 205)

Buttocks

1. The large muscles of the buttocks region help support _____ and provide power for _____. (p. 206)

2. Positive associations with this region include _____. (p. 206)

3. Negative associations with this region include _____. (p. 206)

4. Take great care in this region to create a feeling of _____ and _____. (p. 206)

5. Populations that can benefit greatly from massage of this region include _____, _____, and _____. (p. 206)

6. Use of the _____, _____ and _____ to apply techniques can help with massage of the large muscles of this region. (p. 207)

Lower Extremities

1. The lower extremities are the principal means of _____ for bipedal human beings. (p. 208)

2. Massage of the feet is especially appreciated by those who _____ for long periods of time. (p. 208)

3. The lower extremities are generally massaged in three sections, i.e., _____, _____, and _____. (p. 208)

4. Caution is in order when massaging the legs of people with _____ veins. (p. 209)

Upper Extremities

1. Upper extremities are used for everyday activities, as well as _____, _____, and _____. (p. 213)

2. Tennis and golf elbow are categorized as _____ (RSI). (p. 214)

3. Loss of shoulder mobility may be caused by _____, _____, _____, or _____. (p. 214)

4. For the purposes of massage, the upper extremities may be thought of in four sections: _____, _____, _____, _____. (p. 214)

Chest and Abdomen

1. Expansion and contraction of the chest for _____ is evidence of life itself. (p. 218)

2. Women's chests and breasts are associated with _____, while well developed chests in men signify _____ and _____. (p. 218)

3. In the United States, women's breasts are kept _____ in public and should therefore be draped to maintain _____ and proper _____. (p. 218)

4. Breast massage for wellness and clinical applications is becoming more accepted in the United States and may be performed after special _____ and with _____. (p. 218)

5. The abdomen is associated with deep feeling and _____, and is _____ for many people. (p. 218)

6. Massage and stretching of the muscles of the chest and abdomen can help correct poor _____. (p. 218)

FOR GREATER UNDERSTANDING

The following exercises are designed to take you from the realm of theory into the real world. They will help give you a deeper understanding of the subjects covered in this chapter. Action words are underlined to emphasize the variety of activities presented to address different learning styles, and to encourage deeper thinking.

1. Write a description of the human meaning of your own body and body regions. Explain the meaning of regions with special significance, and how that might affect how you experience touch and massage there. Report verbally to a study partner or group.

2. Sketch your body on a piece of paper using different colors to represent different regions and their significance to you. Explain your drawing to a study partner or group.

3. Interview someone else about the meaning of their body regions as described in problems 1 and 2. Discuss findings with a study partner or group.

4. Interview someone who has received massage recently. Ask if massage of any particular body region was uncomfortable for them, and if so, ask them to explain why. Report your findings to a study partner or group, and discuss.

5. Interview two or more people who have received massage recently. Ask them to identify their favorite part of the massage, and explain their choice. Report your findings to a study partner or group, noting similarities and differences.

6. Receive a massage from a professional practitioner. Ask for special attention to a particular body region. Note how they address the request, and their approach to massage of the region. Report on their performance to a study partner or group.

7. Perform the therapeutic sequences in Tables 10–1 to 10–5 exactly as written. Then create variations identifying warming, therapeutic combinations, and finishing and transition techniques. Develop a routine way of approaching each body region that is well thought out.

8. Choose one of the following body regions for your focus: arm, leg, foot, back, head and face. Create a 30-minute massage for the region including warming, therapeutic combinations, and finishing and transition techniques. Perform your sequence, noting how you achieved specificity, avoided monotony, and made transitions.

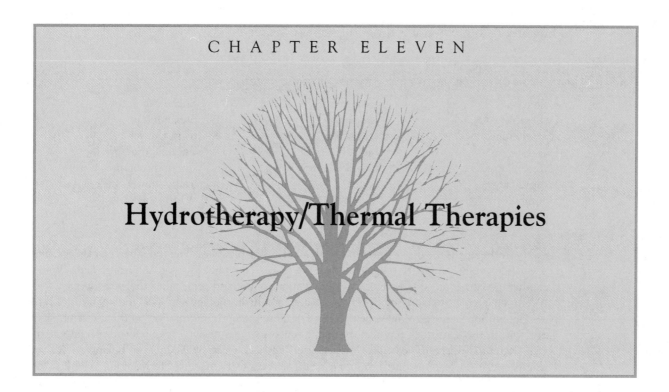

Hydrotherapy/Thermal Therapies

LEARNING OUTCOMES

After studying this chapter, the student will have information to:

1. Discuss the history of hydrotherapy.
2. Describe the healing properties of water.
3. Describe hydrotherapy facilities found in spas and health clubs.
4. Use hot packs within the scope of massage therapy.
5. Use cold and ice packs, and ice massage within the scope of massage therapy.
6. Compare the temperature ranges for different thermo- and cryo-hydrotherapy methods.
7. Observe the contraindications for hydro- and thermal therapies.
8. Use hydrotherapy facilities effectively and safely.
9. Use hot and cold applications effectively and safely.

HISTORICAL PEOPLE AND DEVELOPMENTS

Ancient Greek gymnasium
Battle Creek Sanitarium
European spas
Finnish sauna
Hippocrates
Hot springs

Kellogg, J. Harvey
Kneipp, Sebastian
Maya sweatbaths
Mineral springs
Mineral water hospitals
Natural healers

Naturopaths
Physical therapists
Priessnitz, Vincent
Roman baths
Turkish baths
Winternitz of Vienna

KEY TERMS/CONCEPTS

Cold pack	Ice cup	Steam cabinet
Cold shower	Ice massage	Steam room
Cryo-therapy	Ice pack	Swiss shower
Facial steam	Moist hot pack	Thermal therapy
Hydrocollator	Neutro-therapy	Thermo-therapy
Hydrotherapy	Sauna	Vichy shower
Hot tub	Shower	Whirlpool bath

Hydrotherapy is the use of water in health and healing practices. The trio of water, massage, and exercise is a natural combination found all over the globe in bath houses, spas, and health clubs. Water and other modalities are also used for local applications of hot and cold, called **thermal therapy.**

This chapter will explore some of the more common hydrotherapy methods, and hot and cold applications within the scope of massage therapy. For more in-depth information on the use of physical agents within the context of physical therapy, a much more extensive topic, refer to specialty textbooks. (Refer to *Evidence-Based Guide to Therapeutic Physical Agents* by Alain-Yvan Belanger, 2002, or *Physical Agents: A Comprehensive Text for Physical Therapists* by Bernadette Hecox et al., 1994.)

HISTORY OF HYDROTHERAPY

The use of water for bathing, relaxation and recreation is found all over the world. Wherever **mineral and hot springs** come to the earth's surface, people from time immemorial have enjoyed their soothing and cleansing properties. Hot, sometimes bubbling, mineral waters are collected in pools for bathers. People come to these spas and hot springs for relaxation and healing. Native Americans are said to have frequented natural springs for their healing effects. Later, in places like Saratoga Springs, New York; Hot Springs, Arkansas; and Calistoga, California, resorts were built where the hot and cold mineral waters were taken internally as well as used for bathing. (Refer to *Taking the Waters* by Alev Lytle Croutier, 1992.)

Archeologists studying the ancient Maya and Aztec civilizations have found the ruins of sweat baths throughout Central America. The oldest of the sweat baths date from about 1350 BCE. These structures called *temezcalli* are described in the first history of Mexico, written by Friar Diego Duran in 1567. Most were small buildings that had low ceilings and a small entranceway, and held about 10 people. Steam was created by pouring water over hot rocks. Herbs were used with the steam for their healing effects. Sweating was thought to purify the body. It was used for a variety of illnesses, and by women after childbirth. **Maya sweat baths** are the antecedents of today's *temescal* or sweat houses still found in Central America, and are reminiscent of sweat lodges common among North American natives (Benjamin 2004).

The **Finnish sauna** was developed as a health practice centuries ago. After sitting in the superheated rooms, hardy Finns would jump into cold rivers and snow banks to cool off. It is a practice that many believe builds stamina, energy, and strength.

Today's spas and health club facilities like whirlpool baths, showers, steam rooms, and sauna can be traced in Western civilization to the **ancient Greek gymnasium** and **Roman baths. Turkish baths** followed, becoming popular in Europe and the United States in the latter 19th century. Baths were also popular in ancient Asia—India, China, Korea and Japan. Massage and bodywork was and still is an integral part of the bath house experience.

Water-Based Therapies

The healing effects of water applications were known in ancient Greece. The famous Greek physician **Hippocrates** used compresses, spongings, bathing, and drinking water in his treatments (c. 460 BCE).

Water therapies of various kinds were among the natural healing methods that blossomed in the 1800s. **Vincent Priessnitz,** a farmer in the Austro-Hungarian Empire, was famous for the methods of water therapy he developed from 1829 to 1849. Priessnitz developed an entire system of baths, compresses, and other hot and cold applications to treat various diseases.

Sebastian Kneipp, born in 1821 in Bavaria, is perhaps the most famous water cure practitioner of his era. Kneipp was a priest who built on Priessnitz water-based therapies, and his own knowledge of herbal remedies, to become the foremost authority on the subject. His little book, *My Water Cure* (1889), was translated into many languages over the years. People flocked to him from all over Europe to be cured from a variety of ailments.

European spas, which cater to people seeking healing as well as relaxation, adopted the methods of Priessnitz and Kneipp. An example of a Kneipp treatment given at the Biltz Sanitarium in Weisbaden, Germany 1898 is shown in Figure 11–1. The great spas at Baden-Baden and Weisbaden in Germany, Montecatini Terme in Italy, and Evian-les-Bains and Eugenie-les-Bains in France, as well as many smaller hydrotherapy establishments, carry on the tradition of the water cure.

The idea of the natural healing resort was imported to the United States in places like the **Battle Creek Sanitarium** in Michigan. **J. Harvey Kellogg** wrote *Home Handbook of Domestic Hygiene and Rational Medicine* (1880), which covered hydrotherapy, electrotherapy, and Swedish remedial gymnastics. His book *Rational Hydrotherapy* (1900) described 200 water treatments.

Hydrotherapy in Medicine

Sir John Floyer, a physician in Lichfield, England wrote a treatise in 1702 titled *The History of Cold Bathing to the Ancient and Modern*. Later that century Dr. Currie of Liverpool, England wrote *Medical Reports on the Effects of Water, both Warm and Cold, as a Remedy in Fevers and Other Diseases* (1797). The use of water as a therapeutic agent was being recognized within the developing field of biomedicine by the 18th century.

Almost a century later, **Winternitz of Vienna** experimented with various forms of external water applications to treat a variety of diseases. He used the shower, spray, alternating hot and cold baths, along with manipulations and massage. He varied the temperature of the water and the force with which it was applied for his results (Graham 1923).

Mineral water hospitals were opened in England starting with Bath in 1738, Harrogate in 1824, Droitwich in 1836, and Buxton in 1858. Physicians controlled the larger spas, but had competition from lay natural healers whom they considered quacks. The medical-versus-lay split widened, although each side adopted methods of the other.

By the 1890s hydropathy had two main branches. At places like Nauheim, Bath and Malvern where the medical influence was strong, it became "hydrotherapy," a rational system of baths, exercises, and electricity. At continental mountain resorts, on the other hand, hydropathy tended toward "barefoot back-to-nature cults" masterminded by lay philosophers . . ." (Barclay 1994, p. 3).

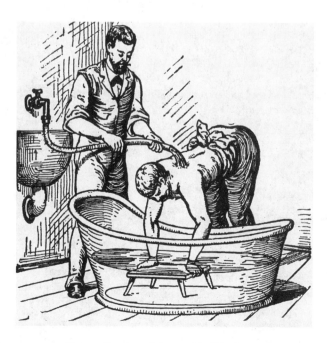

FIGURE 11–1. Kneipp treatment: Upper affusion with hose at the Biltz Sanitarium in Weisbaden, Germany, 1898.

Methods of natural healing and those of modern biomedicine were diverging into separate paths by the turn of the 19th century. Biomedicine opted largely for treatments with drugs and surgery. The old hydrotherapy became the province of **naturopaths** and other **natural healers.** Hydrotherapy retained its association with massage and movement therapies.

Physical Therapy

Members of the Chartered Society of Trained Masseuses (later Physiotherapy) in England treated injured servicemen during World War I (1914–1918) with hydrotherapy, massage, and related therapies (Barclay 1994). This idea was imported to the United States at about the same time, and the profession of physical therapy as we know it here was born. **Physical therapists** continue to research the therapeutic uses of water as a science.

HEALING PROPERTIES OF WATER

Water is relaxing to look at in rivers, lakes and ponds, and to listen to by the seashore, waterfall, or in a desk top water fountain. Flowing water feels pleasurable on the skin.

Taken internally and externally, water is the basis of many natural healing methods. The therapeutic use of water taken internally is outside of the scope of massage therapy, aside from encouraging clients to drink plenty of water, and perhaps filtering water to rid it of unhealthy contaminants. However, external applications of water in various forms, and immersion in water, have an association with massage that goes back to ancient times. Hydrotherapy and thermal therapy may be roughly divided into thermo-, neutro-, and cryo-. **Thermo-therapy** involves methods above normal body temperature. **Neutro-therapy** uses methods at about body temperature. **Cryo-therapy** involves methods below body temperature. Table 11–1 outlines the temperature sensations for these thermal ranges.

Methods within the scope of massage therapy include types of hydrotherapy used for health promotion such as those found in health clubs and spas. It also includes therapeutic uses of hot and cold applications in the forms of hot and cold packs, and ice. The general temperature ranges for these methods are listed in Table 11–2.

Healing properties of water are related to its use in cleansing the body, and its ability to raise and lower the core body temperature or the temperature of specific body tissues. Water can assume different forms—liquid, steam, and ice—each with its own contribution to healing. Water pressure from a shower, hose, or water jets is also used for a type of massage of the soft tissues.

Table 11–1   TEMPERATURE SENSATIONS FOR THERMO-, NEUTRO-, AND CRYO-HYDROTHERAPY

Descriptions are based on perception of temperature on the skin. These perceptions are subjective and vary from person to person.

Type	Description	Fahrenheit	Celsius[*]
Thermo	Very hot	111° to 120°	44° to 49°
	Hot	101° to 110°	38° to 43°
	Warm	94° to 100°	34° to 38°
Neutro	Neutral	90° to 93°	32° to 34°
Cryo	Tepid	80° to 92°	27° to 33°
	Cool	70° to 79°	21° to 26°
	Cold	55° to 69°	13° to 21°
	Very cold	31° to 54°	1° to 12°
	Freezing	32° and below	0° and below

[*]Temperature conversion Fahrenheit (°F) to Celsius (°C): °C = (°F − 32°)/1.8

Source: Adapted from *Day Spa Techniques* by Erica Miller (1996), Albany, NY: Milady Publishers; *Evidenced-Based Guide to Therapeutic Physical Agents* by Alain-Yvan Belanger (2002), Philadelphia: Lippincott Williams & Wilkins.

Table 11–2 TEMPERATURE RANGES FOR HYDROTHERAPY AND THERMAL THERAPY METHODS FROM COLD TO HOT APPLICATIONS

Method	Temperature range
Ice	23° to 32°F (−5° to 0°C)
Cold pack	33° to 50°F (1° to 10°C)
Cold water	50° to 80°F (10° to 27°C)
Bath—cool/cold	70° to 80°F (21° to 27°C)
Whirlpool bath—warm	95° to 104°F (35° to 40°C)
Whirlpool bath—hot	105° to 110° (41° to 43°C)
Steam room[*]	105° to 130° (41° to 54°C)
Sauna[**]	160° to 180° (71° to 82°C)
Hot pack—wet	165° − 170°F (74°−77°C)

[*] Wet heat with 100% humidity
[**] Dry heat with 6–8% humidity

Source: Adapted from *Day Spa Techniques* by Erica Miller (1996), Albany, NY: Milady Publishers; *Evidenced-Based Guide to Therapeutic Physical Agents* by Alain-Yvan Belanger (2002), Philadelphia: Lippincott Williams & Wilkins.

WHIRLPOOL BATHS, SHOWERS, STEAM ROOM, SAUNA

Typical spa and health club settings offer whirlpool baths, showers, steam rooms, and/or sauna in addition to massage services. Hot tubs and Esalen massage have been part of the California scene since the 1970s. Massage practitioners should know something about these facilities to be able to give their clients guidance, and to suggest their safe and effective use in relation to massage.

The benefits of warm to hot forms of hydrotherapy include raising the body temperature, producing sweating, cleansing skin pores, increasing superficial circulation, and general relaxation. These are best used before receiving massage.

The benefits of cool to cold forms of hydrotherapy include lowering body temperature, closing skin pores, decreasing superficial circulation, and general invigoration or stimulation. The cold shower is the most common form of cryo-hydrotherapy in the spa setting. Cold showers, or a contrasting hot to cold shower, are best taken after massage. See Table 11–3 for major effects of hot and cold hydrotherapy.

A **whirlpool bath** consists of a tub filled with water that has air or water jets causing movement or churning of the water. Private whirlpool bathtubs are deep enough that a person can lie down. In the spa, health club, or bath house, whirlpools are usually communal baths, where people sit on benches and are immersed with just their heads above water. Whirlpool baths within the context of physiotherapy may be smaller to accommodate an arm or a leg, and are made out of stainless steel.

The temperature of the water in a whirlpool bath is generally hot, but may vary considerably depending on the purpose of the bath, and the health of the patron. The recommended water temperature for relaxation ranges from about 95° to 105° (Miller, 1996).

The healing effects of the whirlpool bath stem from the water heat, and from the pressure of the water coming out of the jets and hitting the body. The churning of the water helps sustain the heat of the water on the skin, and stimulates the touch receptors of the skin.

A **hot tub** is a barrel-shaped tub made with wood slats, and a rubber or plastic liner. Hot tubs have water heaters, and may have whirlpool jets. They are especially popular on the West Coast. The guidelines for whirlpool baths apply also to hot tubs.

Showers are created by water streaming out of showerheads mounted on the wall. Showers may have no added pressure, i.e., falling like rain, or may have added pressure or pulsing pressure. Showers may be hot or cold. Hot showers have a similar effect as whirlpool baths, i.e., relaxation and increased superficial circulation.

Cold showers are stimulating and help reduce general body heat. They may be taken as a cool down after thermo-hydrotherapy or exercise.

Variations of the shower found in spas include the **Swiss shower** in which showerheads surround the bather at different levels from head to toe. The **Vichy shower** is given with the patron lying down

Table 11–3 GENERAL EFFECTS OF HYDROTHERAPY COMPARING THERMO-HYDROTHERAPY AND CRYO-HYDROTHERAPY*

Hydrotherapy refers here to methods that are applied to the whole body, e.g., whirlpool, shower, steam room, and sauna.

Thermo-hydrotherapy
- Increase core body temperature
- Increase pulse rate
- Decrease blood pressure
- Increase respiratory rate
- Decrease muscle tone
- Induce sweating
- Relaxing/sedative effect

Cryo-hydrotherapy
- Decrease core body temperature
- Decrease pulse rate
- Increase blood pressure
- Decrease respiratory rate
- Increase muscle tone
- Induce shivering
- Invigorating/stimulating effect

*The actual effects of specific hydrotherapy methods depend on the health of the client, the actual temperature of the water or room, and the length of time a person is exposed to the heat or cold.

Source: Adapted from Table 14–4, Body Systemic Effects Generally Associated with Cryo-, Thermo-, and Neutro-hydrotherapy, in *Evidenced-Based Guide to Therapeutic Physical Agents* by Alain-Yvan Belanger (2002), Philadelphia: Lippincott Williams & Wilkins.

on a table with water showering down from about 4 feet above. The Vichy shower can be varied with pulsating water, with alternating hot and cold water, or with a salt or shampoo scrub. An attendant controls the water pressure and temperature from a panel (Miller 1996).

Steam rooms are generally tiled spaces from floor to ceiling with benches for sitting. Steam comes out from jets in the wall and fills the space with wet heat from 105° to 130°F (41° to 54°C) with 100% humidity. Patrons in the steam room inhale the steam, which helps clear sinuses and relieve respiratory congestion. Steam also raises the body temperature and causes sweating. It is a relaxing, cleansing experience.

A variation of the stream room is the **steam cabinet.** The patron sits on a stool in an enclosed box with the head sticking out. Steam is pumped into the box, raising core body temperature, and causing sweating. Since the head is out of the box, the steam is not inhaled. A cold shower following a steam room or cabinet experience can help wash off sweat and bring body temperature down to normal.

When raising the core body temperature is contraindicated or undesirable, **facial steam** may be beneficial. Facial steam devices focus steam to the face and are used in skin care as well as to improve respiration.

The **sauna** is a practice that originated in Finland, and involves sitting in a room with dry heat from 160° to 180°F (71° to 82°C) with 6 to 8% humidity. The sauna is typically a wood-lined room heated without steam, and the air is very dry. Patrons sit on wooden benches. Occasionally, water may be poured over hot rocks to produce steam, adding some moisture to the air. A cold shower or a plunge into a swimming pool or lake (or snow bank) after sitting in a sauna is stimulating, closes the skin pores, and helps reduce body temperature.

Contraindications for thermo-hydrotherapy are listed in Table 11-4. The most serious contraindications are related to heart, circulatory, and other systemic diseases. People with skin rashes should also avoid the increase in superficial circulation that results from immersing in hot water. Of course, people using public facilities should be careful not to spread contagious disease of any kind.

Although it is possible to overdo cryo-hydrotherapy causing adverse reactions, it is more common for people to stay too long in the hot hydrotherapy baths and rooms. First-time bathers should only stay

Table 11-4 CONTRAINDICATIONS FOR THERMO-HYDROTHERAPY

These contraindications apply to hydrotherapy methods that raise the core body temperature. In some cases, using water with lower temperature and/or limiting the time in the hot water or steam may make their use safer.

- High or low blood pressure
- Heart or circulatory problems
- Pregnancy
- Systemic diseases such as hepatitis
- Seizures
- Multiple sclerosis
- Infection or inflammatory condition
- Vascular problems associated with phlebitis, varicose veins, diabetes
- Skin rashes
- Allergies to water additives
- Contagious conditions
- Some cancers and cancer treatments

Certain medications may make hydrotherapy unsafe for a client. These include drugs that:

- Alter how blood vessels react to hot and cold
- Change skin sensitivity to hot and cold
- Alter the body's temperature control or cooling mechanisms

Source: Adapted from *Day Spa Techniques* by Erica Miller (1996), Albany, NY: Milady Publishers; *Massage Therapy and Medications* by Randall S. Persad (2001), Toronto: Curties-Overzet Publications; *Evidenced-Based Guide to Therapeutic Physical Agents* by Alain-Yvan Belanger (2002), Philadelphia: Lippincott Williams & Wilkins.

5–15 minutes in hot water, while healthy experienced bathers may stay up to 30 minutes. People who are weak or over 60 years old should limit their exposure to hot baths and steam to 5–15 minutes (Miller 1996).

If a client reports feeling lightheaded or dizzy, is nauseous, or develops a headache, they probably stayed immersed too long in hot water or steam. Take measures to reduce the body temperature gradually such as sitting or lying in a neutral temperature environment, and sipping tepid to cool water. If symptoms persist or get worse, consider medical evaluation. Guidelines for safe use of thermo-hydrotherapy facilities are listed in Table 11–5.

Table 11-5 GUIDELINES FOR SAFE USE OF THERMO-HYDROTHERAPY FACILITIES: WHIRLPOOL, SHOWER, STEAM ROOM, AND SAUNA

1. Check to make sure that no contraindications are present before using thermo-facilities. See Table 11–4.
2. Wait for at least one hour after eating before using thermo-facilities.
3. Avoid alcohol before or during use of thermo-facilities.
4. Wear sandals or shoes with non-slip bottoms to avoid slipping and falling.
5. Check temperature of the water or room (steam and sauna) for therapeutic range (Table 11–2), and for individual tolerance.
6. Limit use according to experience in thermo-facilities, and factors such as general health and age. In general less experienced, less healthy, weaker, or over age 60 limit use to 15 minutes, and otherwise 15–30 minutes.
7. Drink plenty of water or other fluids during and after thermo-hydrotherapy to replace loss through sweating.
8. Always have someone to call for help if needed.
9. Monitor how you feel, and if weak, dizzy, or nauseous get out of the water or room. Lie or sit down in a cooler place, and replace fluids by sipping a cool drink.
10. If reaction to heat is severe or lasts a long time, consider seeking medical evaluation.

Use <u>before massage</u> is beneficial for initiating general relaxation, muscle relaxation, and increased superficial circulation and connective tissue pliability.

Use <u>after massage</u> may continue benefits described above. Be sure to wash off oil and lubricant thoroughly before entering thermo-facilities. Lubricants can contaminate water, and leave slippery films on benches and floors.

The most commonly used methods of thermal therapy within the scope of massage therapy are hot packs, ice, cold packs, and ice massage. The focus of the following section is on local applications of thermal therapy.

HOT APPLICATIONS — THERMO-THERAPY

Healing Effects of Heat

Heat applied locally to muscles and related soft tissues not only feels good, but also helps muscles relax, increases local circulation, and makes connective tissues more pliable. Sore stiff muscles benefit from the increased circulation and heat.

Raising tissue temperature to between 104° and 113°F (40°–45°C) increases cell metabolism and blood flow for various therapeutic results. Lower temperatures have little therapeutic effect, and higher temperatures will damage cells (Belanger 2002).

Although heat is applied locally, use of hot packs can raise core body temperature. In that case, contraindications for thermo-hydrotherapy also apply. See Table 11–4. Local contraindications for the use of hot packs include burns, wounds, swelling, inflammation, and skin conditions (e.g., rashes) that could be made worse by heat. Check the area visually and/or by palpation for evidence of contraindications before deciding to use hot packs.

Hot Packs and Massage

The application of hot packs *prior* to massage can help begin muscle relaxation, enhance circulation locally, and prepare the area for deeper massage techniques. *After* massage of an area, hot packs can enhance muscle relaxation and prolong increased local circulation.

Heat sources may be from moist hot packs, or dry hot packs or pads. Moist hot packs are more penetrating. However, some newer types of dry hot packs heated in microwave ovens can be good heat sources, are generally easier to use, and can be used with warm, damp cloths to create moist heat.

Typical **moist hot packs** come in various sizes and shapes, and are heated in hot water. **Hydrocollator** units are metal containers with electrical heating elements used to keep the water within a constant range: 158°–168°F (51°–54°C). Hot packs are suspended in the hot water to a therapeutic temperature, and then applied to the client.

Table 11–6 SUMMARY OF GUIDELINES FOR SAFE USE OF MOIST HOT PACKS BEFORE AND DURING MASSAGE

1. Be clear about your goals for using hot packs in association with massage.
2. Check to make sure that no contraindications are present and that the client is not taking medications that reduce sensation or alter circulation.
3. Get informed consent from the client to apply hot packs.
4. Instruct the client on the need for feedback about how the hot pack feels to them, especially if it feels too hot.
5. Check hot pack to make sure it is correct temperature. Touch to own skin (e.g., wrist) to judge if it is hot enough or too hot, and how many layers of towels to use.
6. Apply layers of towels between the client's skin and the hot pack to help avoid burns. Use more layers for more sensitive skin and for clients over 60 years old.
7. Apply a towel over the hot pack to help keep heat from escaping.
8. Ask for feedback from client every 5 to 7 minutes or more if needed. Heat of tissues increases the longer the hot pack is applied.
9. Add additional towels beneath the hot pack if the client complains of too much heat.
10. Remove hot pack immediately if you judge potential for damage to skin or if client is having negative reaction to heat (e.g., dizziness, nausea).
11. Maximum time for hot pack use on a local area is about 20 minutes.

Always check how the hot pack feels on your own skin, e.g., at the wrist, prior to applying it to a client. Packs that have been sitting in the hydrocollator for a long time (i.e., over 60 minutes) will be hotter than packs that are used often, or that have been heating for only a few minutes.

Care must be taken not to burn the client's skin. This is accomplished by placing towels between the hot pack and the skin. Ask the client for feedback every 5 to 7 minutes about how the pack feels, i.e., if it feels too hot. A visual and tactile check is also a good idea. Clients taking medications that reduce skin sensation, or alter the reaction of blood vessels to heat, or reduce their body heat control mechanisms, are not good candidates for hot packs. See Table 11–6 for guidelines for the use of moist hot packs with massage.

COLD APPLICATIONS—CRYOTHERAPY

Healing Effects of Cold

Cold applied locally to muscles and related soft tissues causes vasoconstriction and decreased local circulation. There is also decrease in cell metabolism, nerve conduction velocity, pain, muscle spindle activity, and spasm in the cold area. After about 20 to 30 minutes of continuous application, cold-induced vasodilation is thought to occur. This may lead to increased circulation, but it is doubtful that circulation rises to a baseline of before the cold was applied. Cold applied locally can also act eventually to lower core body temperature (Belanger 2002; pp. 267–270).

Cold applications to tissues after trauma or injury can decrease secondary cell and tissue damage. This limits worsening of soft tissue injury, and prevents further swelling of tissues and edema.

First aid for a strain or sprain, or a blow to soft tissues, includes immediate application of cold, preferably as cold as ice. This limits hemorrhaging, swelling, and secondary cell hypoxia or damage. If a limb is involved, the R.I.C.E.S. first aid principle applies, i.e., rest, ice, compression, elevation, and stabilization.

Cryotherapy is used most often with massage in settings where clients are likely to have soft tissue injury or pain. These include sports medicine and rehabilitation settings, and chiropractic offices. However, any client may have had a recent injury or have muscle spasms, so knowledge of the use of cold applications can be useful. (Refer to *Cryotherapy in Sport Injury Management* by Kenneth L. Knight, 1995.)

Table 11–7   CONTRAINDICATIONS FOR CRYO-HYDROTHERAPY AND COLD APPLICATIONS

These contraindications apply to hydrotherapy methods that lower the core body temperature.

- Circulatory insufficiency or vasospastic disorders (e.g., Raynaud's disease, diabetes)
- Cardiac disorder
- Allergy to cold
- Cold hypersensitivity or chilling
- Multiple sclerosis
- Asthma
- Rheumatoid arthritis
- Osteoarthritis
- Some cancers and cancer treatments
- Infection
- Depression
- Pregnancy

Certain medications may make hydrotherapy unsafe for a client. These include drugs that:

- Alter how blood vessels react to hot and cold
- Change skin sensitivity to hot and cold
- Alter the body's temperature control or cooling mechanisms

Source: Adapted from *Cryotherapy in Sports Injury Management* by Kenneth L. Knight (1995), Champaign, IL: Human Kinetics; *Evidenced-Based Guide to Therapeutic Physical Agents* by Alain-Yvan Belanger (2002), Philadelphia: Lippincott Williams & Wilkins; *Massage Therapy and Medications* by Randall S. Persad (2001), Toronto: Curties-Overzet Publications.

Contraindications to local cold applications include circulatory insufficiency such as with Raynaud's disease and diabetes, allergic reaction to cold, cold sensitivity, or chilling. Clients with multiple sclerosis or asthma may not react well to cold. Take special care with clients taking medications that reduce skin sensation, alter the reaction of blood vessels to heat and cold, or reduce their body temperature control mechanisms. See Table 11–7 for a summary of contraindications for cryo-hydrotherapy and cold applications.

Cold Packs, Ice, Ice Massage

Cold packs of various kinds are commercially available. They are usually made of materials that hold cold over a period of time and stay pliable even when near freezing. They have coverings for comfortable contact with skin.

Ice packs are made with ice cubes or crushed ice inside plastic bags that can be sealed. A disadvantage of ice is that it melts over time, and plastic bags can leak water. Ice, water below 32°F (0°C), is also hard to the touch and may be less comfortable over injuries. However, ice is readily available, and generally stays cold longer than cold packs. Ice can be replaced in bags as needed to hold a freezing temperature.

Cold packs are used as adjuncts to massage to reduce muscle spasm or muscle pain, or if a client has swelling from a recent injury like a sprained ankle. Cold may be applied to reduce spasm and pain so that the area can be massaged. It can also be used instead of massage if massage would further aggravate the injury or spasm. Cold or ice may be applied to an area for up to 30 minutes at a time, during massage of other parts of the body.

Ice massage involves rubbing ice directly on the skin using an ice cube or ice cup. **Ice cups** are made by filling paper cups with water, and putting them in the freezer to harden. The paper is peeled back to expose the ice, and some paper left on for holding the cup.

Ice massage is usually performed in a circular motion over a small area for about 5–10 minutes, until the area becomes numb. Ice massage may be used to numb an area before performing deep transverse friction such as in a case of tendinitis. It allows the therapist to work deep enough without causing severe pain. Ice is also used after this treatment to continue to numb the area.

The person receiving the cold application will normally feel the following: (1) a sensation of cold, (2) tingling or itching, (3) pain, aching or burning, and (4) numbing or analgesia. It is good to inform the client about what they will feel, since some of the sensations can be uncomfortable.

Be careful not to apply very cold applications for too long (a one-hour maximum) to avoid tissue damage and frostbite. Guidelines for cold applications are found in Table 11-8.

Table 11–8 SUMMARY OF GUIDELINES FOR SAFE USE OF COLD AND ICE PACKS BEFORE AND DURING MASSAGE

1. Be clear about your goals for using cold applications in association with massage.
2. Check to make sure that no contraindications are present and that the client is not taking medications that reduce sensation or alter circulation.
3. Get informed consent from client to apply cold packs.
4. Instruct the client on the need for feedback about how the cold application feels to them.
5. Inform them of the stages of sensation to expect with cold applications, i.e., (1) cold sensation, (2) tingling or itching, (3) aching or burning, and (4) numbness or analgesia.
6. Apply the cold or ice pack directly to the desired area.
7. Do not apply cold-gel packs under a compression bandage, since it may cause frostbite.
8. Use the R.I.C.E.S. principle if injury on a limb, i.e., rest, ice, compression, elevation, stabilization.
9. Ask for feedback on the cold application every 5 to 7 minutes.
10. Remove cold pack immediately if it causes an adverse reaction, e.g., skin rash, chilling.
11. Maximum time for continuous cold application is one hour; 15 minutes is sufficient in the context of a massage session.

SUMMARY

Hydrotherapy is the use of water in health and healing practices. Water is also a medium for local applications of hot and cold called thermal therapies.

The history of the use of water in health and healing can be traced to ancient times in all parts of the globe. The European and Western traditions of water-based therapies include the names of Priessnitz, Kneipp, Winternitz, Kellogg, and the Chartered Society of Trained Masseuses in England.

Hydrotherapy and thermal therapy can be roughly divided into thermo-, neutro-, and cryo-therapy based on the temperature of the water or other medium. Water is used in form of liquid, steam, and ice. Water pressure from shower, hose, or water jets serves as a type of massage of the soft tissues.

Hot forms of hydrotherapy include whirlpool baths, showers, steam rooms, and sauna. Effects of hot hydrotherapy include raising the body temperature, producing sweating, cleansing skin pores, increasing superficial circulation, and general relaxation. These are best used before a massage session. Guidelines should be observed for safe use of these facilities.

Heat applied locally to muscles and related soft tissues feels good, helps muscles relax, increases local circulation, and makes tissues more pliable. Moist hot packs are typically used for thermo-therapy. Measures to avoid burning the client's skin include using towels as a safety barrier, and limiting the time the hot pack is applied.

Cold applications or cryotherapy causes vasoconstriction and decreased local circulation, cell metabolism, nerve conduction, and reduced pain and spasm. Cold applications are used in first aid for trauma and injury. Cryotherapy methods include cold and ice packs, and ice massage.

Contraindications and safety guidelines for all forms of hydrotherapy and thermal therapies should be observed to avoid harm to the client.

A look ahead . . .

A variety of contemporary massage and bodywork approaches have been developed to address specific body tissues and systems. Chapter 12 describes specialized techniques used to improve the health of the body's myofascial tissues.

REFERENCES

Barclay, J. (1994). *In good hands: The history of the chartered society of physiotherapy 1894–1994.* London: Butterworth-Heinemann.

Belanger, A.-Y. (2002). *Evidenced-based guide to therapeutic physical agents.* Philadelphia: Lippincott Williams & Wilkins.

Benjamin, P. J. (2004). "Massage and sweatbaths among the ancient Maya." *Massage Therapy Journal,* Spring, pp. 148–154.

Croutier, A. L. (1992). *Taking the waters: Spirit, art, sensuality.* New York: Abbeyville Press.

Graham, R. L. (1923). *Hydro-hygiene: The science of curing by water.* New York: The Thompson-Barlow Company.

Hecox, B., Mehreteab, T. A., & Weisberg, J. (1994). *Physical agents: A comprehensive text for physical therapists.* Norwalk, CT: Appleton & Lange.

Knight, K. L. (1995). *Cryotherapy in sport injury management.* Champaign, IL: Human Kinetics.

Miller, E. T. (1996). *Day spa techniques.* Albany, NY: Milady Publications.

Monastersky, R. (2002). "Plumbing ancient rituals: Sweatbaths in Maya cities provide a window into lives long ago." *The Chronicle of Higher Education.* 17 May 2002, pp. A22–23.

Persad, R. S. (2001). Massage therapy & medications: General treatment principles. Toronto: Curties-Overzet.

ADDITIONAL REFERENCES

Videos

"Day Spa 1: Hydrotherapy Treatments." (1997) Erica Miller Professional Education Series. Mile Ranch, British Columbia, Canada: Spa Expertise Canada LTD.

S T U D Y   G U I D E

LEARNING OUTCOMES

Use the learning outcomes at the beginning of the chapter as a guide to your studies. Perform the task given in each outcome using the information in the chapter. This may start as an "open book" exercise, and then later from memory.

KEY TERMS/CONCEPTS

To study the key concept and terminology listed at the beginning of this chapter, choose one or more of the following exercises. Writing or talking about ideas helps you remember them better, and explaining them helps deepen your understanding.

1. Match historical people, places, and modalities that are related in some way. Explain your choices and their relationship to a study partner or group.

2. Research the biography of an important person in the history of hydrotherapy. Write a report or make a verbal report to a study group.

3. Write out the definition of key terms and concepts.

4. With a study partner, take turns defining key terms and concepts verbally from memory.

5. Group key terms and concepts that are related in some way. Explain your choices and their relationship to a study partner or group.

6. Explain your choices and their relationship to a study partner or group.

STUDY OUTLINE

The following questions test your memory of the main concepts in this chapter. Locate the answers in the text using the page number given for each question.

1. Hydrotherapy is the use of _____ in health and healing practices. (p. 228)

2. Therapeutic use of local hot and cold applications is called _____ therapy. (p. 228)

History of Hydrotherapy

1. Native Americans visited _____ and _____ springs for their healing effects for centuries. (p. 228)

2. Resorts were later built at the sites of mineral springs in places like _____ Springs, NY; _____ Spring, Arkansas, and _____, CA. (p. 228)

3. Archeologists studying ancient _____ and _____ civilizations have found the ruins of _____ throughout Central America. (p. 228)

4. The sauna was developed in _____. (p. 228)

5. A tradition of bathhouses is found all over the world, i.e., the ancient Greek _____, _____ and _____ baths, and in ancient India, China, _____ and _____. (p. 228)

6. The Greek physician _____ (c. 460 BCE) used compresses, sponging, and bathing to treat disease. (p. 228)

7. Vincent _____ of the Austro-Hungarian Empire developed an entire system of hot and cold water therapy (c. 1840). (p. 228)

8. Sebastian _____ from Bavaria further developed therapeutic use of water adding his knowledge of herbs (c. 1880). (p. 229)

9. European spas adopted the methods of Kneipp in places like Baden-_____, Germany; Montecatini, Italy; and Evian-les-_____, France. (p. 229)

10. At the natural healing resort, the _____ Creek Sanitarium in Michigan, _____ offered hydrotherapy and wrote two books on the subject (c.1900). (p. 229)

11. _____ hospitals controlled by physicians were opened in England in the 1700–1800s at Bath, Harrogate, Droitwich, and Buxton. (p. 229)

12. By the early 20th century, the old water therapies were largely the province of naturopaths, _____, and _____ practitioners. (p. 230)

13. Injured soldiers in World War I (1914–1918) were treated with hydrotherapy, massage, and related therapies, thus beginning the evolution of today's profession of _____. (p. 230)

Healing Properties of Water

1. Therapeutic use of water taken _____ is outside the scope of massage therapy except for encouraging clients to drink plenty of clean pure water. (p. 230)

2. _____ applications of water, and _____ in water have been associated with massage since ancient times. (p. 230)

3. Hydro- and thermal therapies can be roughly divided into temperature ranges called _____ (above body temperature), _____ (at body temperature), and _____ (below body temperature). (p. 230)

4. Healing properties of water are related to its uses in _____ the body, and its effects for raising or lowering core _____ and the temperature of specific _____. (p. 230)

5. Water _____ acts as a form of massage. (p. 230)

Whirlpool Baths, Showers, Steam Room, Sauna

1. Temperatures for hydrotherapy and thermal therapy methods range from _____ cold to hot and _____ heat. (Table 11–1)

2. Massage practitioners should know something about hydrotherapy facilities to be able to give their clients _____, and to suggest their _____ and _____ use in relation to massage. (p. 231)

3. Benefits of warm/hot hydrotherapy include _____ the body temperature, causing _____, cleansing _____, increase in _____ circulation, and general relaxation. They are best taken (choose one: before or after) massage. (p. 231)

4. Benefits of cool/cold hydrotherapy include _____ body temperature, _____ pores, _____ superficial circulation, and general stimulation. They are best taken (choose one: before or after) massage. (p. 231)

5. Thermo- or heat therapy (choose one: increases or decreases) body temperature, pulse rate, and respiratory rate; (choose one: increases or decreases) blood pressure and muscle tone; and has a (choose one: sedating or invigorating) effect. (Table 11–3)

6. Cryo- or cold therapy (choose one: increases or decreases) body temperature, pulse rate, and respiratory rate; (choose one: increases or decreases) blood pressure and muscle tone; and has a (choose one: sedating or invigorating) effect. (Table 11–3)

7. The _____ bath consists of a water tub with air or water jets that cause water movement or churning. Healing effects are from water _____ and the pressure from _____ as a massage. (p. 231)

8. _____ showers are relaxing and increase superficial circulation. (p. 231)

9. _____ showers are stimulating and reduce overall body temperature. (p. 231)

10. _____ showers surround the bather from head to toe. (p. 231)

11. _____ showers are taken lying down on a table, and may include a salt or shampoo scrub. (p. 231)

12. Steam rooms provide _____ heat from 105° to 130°F (41° to 54°C) with 100% humidity. (p. 232)

13. Steam _____ apply steam to the body, but not the head. (p. 232)

14. _____ steam devices are used in skin care and to improve respiration. (p. 232)

15. Steam can help clear sinuses and _____ congestion, (choose one: raise or lower) body temperature, and induce sweating. (p. 232)

16. _____ provide dry heat from 160° to 180°F (71° to 82°C) with 6 to 8% humidity. (p. 232)

17. A cold shower or plunge into a pool following a sauna helps return _____ to normal. (p. 232)

18. General _____ for thermo- (hot) hydrotherapy include circulatory diseases, pregnancy, some systemic diseases, seizures, multiple sclerosis, skins rashes, certain allergies, contagious conditions. (p. 232)

19. _____ that alter skin sensation, how blood vessels react to heat, or the body's temperature control mechanisms are contraindications for hot and cold hydrotherapies. (Table 11–4)

Hot Applications—Thermo-Therapy
Healing Effects of Heat

1. Heat applied locally feels good, helps muscles _____, increases _____ circulation, makes connective tissue more _____, and _____ core body temperature slightly. (p. 234)

2. Raising temperature of tissues to 104° to 113°F (40° to 45°C) increases cell _____ and _____ flow for certain therapeutic effects. (p. 234)

3. General contraindications for _____ hydrotherapy may also apply to hot applications. (p. 234)

4. Local _____ for heat applications include burns, wounds, swelling, and skin conditions that could be made worse with heat. (p. 234)

Hot Packs and Massage

1. Hot packs applied prior to massage can begin muscle _____, increase circulation _____, and prepare area for _____ massage techniques. (p. 234)

2. Moist hot packs come in various shapes and sizes, and are heated in electrical units called _____. (p. 234)

3. _____ are placed between the hot pack and the client's skin to prevent burns. (p. 235)

Cold Applications—Cryotherapy

Healing Effects of Cold

1. Cold applied locally causes vasoconstriction; and (choose one: increased or decreased) local circulation, cell metabolism, _____ conduction velocity, pain, muscle spindle activity, and spasm. It can also act to (choose one: raise or lower) core body temperature slightly. (p. 235)

2. Cold applied for over _____ minutes may induce vasodilation. (p. 235)

3. Cold applied to tissues after trauma or injury can (choose one: increase or decrease) secondary cell or tissue damage, and prevent further _____. (p. 235)

4. Cold applications are part of first aid for trauma to limbs, i.e., R.I.C.E.S. (_____, _____, _____, _____, _____). (p. 235)

5. Contraindications to local cold applications include _____ and heart problems, allergy to _____ cold hypersensitivity, chilling, multiple _____, asthma, arthritis, infection, depression, and pregnancy. (Table 11–7)

6. Medications that alter skin _____, how blood vessels react to _____, or the body's _____ control mechanisms are contraindications for hot and cold hydrotherapy. (Table 11–7)

Cold Packs, Ice, Ice Massage

1. Cold packs are commercially available, or may be made from _____ or _____ in plastic bags. (p. 236)

2. Cold or ice packs may be used as adjunct to massage to reduce muscle _____, muscle _____, or tissue _____. (p. 236)

3. Cold may be applied for up to _____ hour at a time. (p. 236)

4. _____ involves rubbing ice directly on a small area in a circular motion using an ice cube or ice cup. (p. 236)

5. Ice massage is performed for 5 to 10 minutes until the area is _____. It is sometimes used with _____ friction to an injury site. (p. 236)

6. Stages of sensation when applying ice are (1) _____, (2) _____, (3) _____, (4) _____. (p. 236)

FOR GREATER UNDERSTANDING

The following exercises are designed to take you from the realm of theory into practical applications. They will help give you a deeper understanding of the information covered in this chapter. Action words are underlined to emphasize the variety of activities presented to address different learning styles, and to encourage deeper thinking. *Do not do any exercise if it is a contraindication for you or your practice partner.*

1. Visit a spa or health club with hydrotherapy facilities. Experience as many facilities or treatments as you can. Write about which ones you enjoyed or didn't enjoy, and which were beneficial and why you think so. Report your findings to a study partner or group.

2. Visit a spa or health club with hydrotherapy facilities. Observe how other people use the facilities. Was there anything you thought they needed instruction about, for example, contraindications or how best to enjoy the experience? Were there any signs or people to

instruct patrons on how to use the facilities? <u>Report</u> your observations to a study partner or group.

3. <u>Practice applying</u> hot packs to a study partner. <u>Observe</u> all of the guidelines in Table 11–6.

4. Repeat problem 3, applying hot packs to the back. <u>Apply</u> moist heat for 10 minutes. Remove the hot packs and <u>perform</u> a 10-minute back massage. Note the effects of the heat on the massage. <u>Discuss</u> your observations with the practice partner.

5. <u>Practice</u> applying cold or ice packs to a study partner. Observe all of the guidelines in Table 11–8.

6. <u>Immerse</u> your foot or hand into a bucket of ice water. <u>Notice</u> the phases of sensation you experience. Say them out loud to a study partner as you experience them. (Variation: Apply cold pack instead.)

7. <u>Practice</u> ice massage on yourself or a practice partner. <u>Discuss</u> the effects you see and feel with a study partner.

8. <u>Visit</u> a training room with a certified athletic trainer. <u>Observe</u> how they use hydro- and thermal therapy in treatment of athletes. <u>Report</u> your observations to a study partner or group.

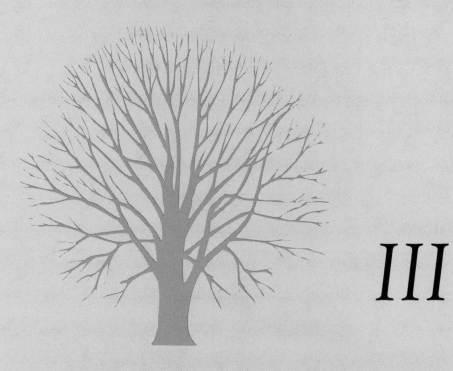

III

Contemporary Massage
and Bodywork

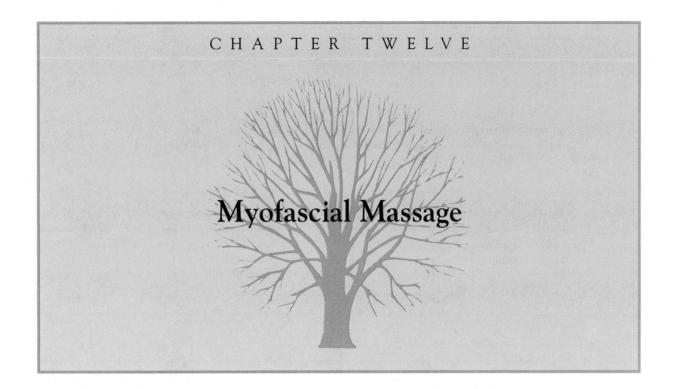

CHAPTER TWELVE

Myofascial Massage

LEARNING OUTCOMES

After studying this chapter, the student will have information to:

1. Identify people important in the history of myofascial massage.
2. Explain the effects of myofascial massage.
3. Describe the nature of fascia and fascial anatomy.
4. Perform basic myofascial techniques effectively.
5. Follow the basic principles of myofascial massage.

HISTORICAL PEOPLE AND DEVELOPMENTS

Barnes, John
Bindegewebsmassage
Connective Tissue Massage
  (CTM)

Dicke, Elizabeth
Myofascial Release (MFR)
Rolf, Ida
Rolfing

Ward, Robert

KEY TERMS/CONCEPTS

Arm and leg pulls
Collagen

Cross-handed stretches
Deep fascia

Deepest fascia
Elastin

MEDIALINK

A companion CD-ROM, included free with each new copy of this book, supplements the techniques presented in this chapter. Insert the CD-ROM to watch video clips of massage techniques being demonstrated. This multimedia feature is designed to help you add a new dimension to your learning.

Fascia	Myofascial massage	Skin lifting
Fascial anatomy	Myofascial mobilization	Skin rolling
Fascial restrictions	Myofascial release	Subcutaneous fascia
Fascial sheath	Myofascial spread	Subserous fascia
Fascial structure	Myofascial techniques	Thixotropy
Melting	Myofascial unwinding	Transverse plane stretches

Myofascial massage addresses the body's **fascial anatomy,** i.e., the fibrous connective tissue that holds the body together and gives it shape. The general intent of myofascial massage is to release restrictions in superficial fascia, deep fascia surrounding muscles, and fascia related to overall body alignment. **Myofascial techniques** stretch fascial sheets, break fascial adhesions, and leave tissues softer and more pliable. These techniques release **fascial restrictions** that limit mobility and cause postural distortion, poor cellular nutrition, pain, and a variety of other dysfunctions.

HISTORY OF MYOFASCIAL MASSAGE

There have been several manual techniques or systems of treatment that have focused on the fascia of the body. **Connective Tissue Massage (CTM),** sometimes known as **Bindegewebsmassage,** was developed by **Elizabeth Dicke** of Germany in the late 1920s and 1930s. CTM, as Dicke taught it, is the systematic application of light strokes without oil to various areas of the skin. CTM is thought to improve circulation in subcutaneous connective tissue, which results in reflex actions to other parts of the body including the visceral organs.

Structural integration, or **Rolfing,** was developed by **Ida Rolf** (1896–1979) and taught at the Esalen Institute in California in the 1960s. Rolfing seeks to re-establish proper vertical alignment in the body by manipulating the myofascial tissue so that the fascia elongates and glides, rather than shortens and adheres. Rolf's work spawned a number of other systems of bodywork that address realignment of the structure of the body through manipulation of the deep fascia.

An osteopath named **Robert Ward** coined the term **myofascial release** in the 1960s to describe his system of treating the body's myofascial anatomy. In the 1980s, the term myofascial release **(MFR)** was adopted by a physical therapist named **John Barnes** as the designation for his method of freeing restrictions in the myofascial tissues. The overall intention of MFR according to Barnes is to relieve pain, resolve structural dysfunction, restore function and mobility, and release emotional trauma (Knaster, 1996).

Variations of myofascial techniques continue to be developed and are known variously as myofascial release, myofascial unwinding, myofascial manipulation, and myofascial massage. They all view a healthy myofascial system as integral to good health.

THE NATURE OF FASCIA

Fascia is loose irregular connective tissue found throughout the body. Fascia surrounds every muscle, nerve, blood vessel, and organ. It holds structures together giving them their characteristic shapes, offers support, and connects the body as a whole. It can be thought of as winding through the body in a continuous sheet.

Fascia is composed of three primary elements: gel-like ground substance, collagen, and elastin. Ground substance is a mucopolysaccharide, the same liquid that forms interstitial or intercellular fluid. Fascia displays an intriguing characteristic called **thixotropy,** that is, it can change from a more solid to a more liquid gel consistency. It becomes more pliable with movement, stretching, and increase in temperature (Juhan, 1987).

Fascia is described by Cantu and Grodin as sparse, with a loose arrangement of **collagen** fibers and with greater amounts of **elastin** than the dense regular connective tissue found in ligaments and tendons (1992). Sheets of fascia are formed by hydrogen bonds between collagen fibers. Figure 12–1 illustrates the multi-directionality and low density of fibers in typical fascia.

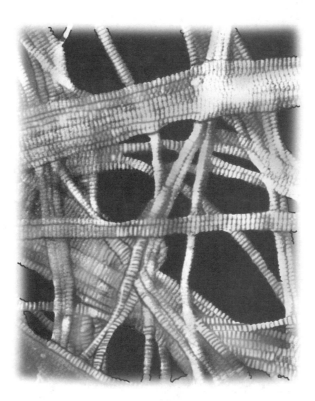

FIGURE 12–1. Illustration of multi-directionality and low density of fibers in typical fascia, that is, loose irregular connective tissue.

Fascia has a greater amount of ground substance than other types of connective tissue and is the immediate environment of every cell in the body. It forms the interstitial spaces and has important functions in support, protection, separation, cellular respiration, elimination, metabolism, fluid flow, and immune-system function. Any restriction or dysfunction of the fascia can lead to a variety of problems, including poor exchange of cellular nutrients and wastes, pain, and poor mobility.

Fascia is distinguished as lying at three different depths in the body, i.e., subcutaneous fascia, deep fascia, and subserous fascia. **Subcutaneous fascia** is a continuous layer of connective tissue over the entire body between the skin and the deep fascia. **Deep fascia** is an intricate series of dense connective sheets and bands that hold the muscles and other structures in place throughout the body. **Subserous fascia** lies between the deep fascia and the serous membranes lining the body cavities in much the same manner as the subcutaneous fascia lies between the skin and the deep fascia (Anderson & Anderson, 1990). Myofascial massage focuses on the subcutaneous and deep fascia related to the musculature.

John Barnes defines another layer of fascia that he calls **deepest fascia,** which is within the dura mater of the craniosacral system (cranium, spine, and sacrum) (1987). It is interesting to note that a researcher reported finding cerebrospinal fluid inside collagen fibrils, which suggests that the connective tissue framework may function as a circulatory system carrying chemical messages throughout the body (Juhan, 1987). There is clearly much more to learn about this important system of the body.

The study of fascial anatomy includes identifying **fascial structures** that shape the body such as the body straps or retinaculae that give the body contour, and **fascial sheaths** that surround muscles and link muscle groups. For example, Figure 12–2 shows the fascial anatomy of the large muscles of the back of the body. Knowledge of fascial structures helps practitioners locate and release restrictions. (Refer to *The Endless Web: Fascial Anatomy and Physical Reality* by R. Louis Schultz and Rosemary Feitis, 1996.)

The pervasiveness and interconnectedness of fascia throughout the body creates a situation in which restriction in one part of the body can affect other parts as well. A metaphor often used to describe the fascia is a knitted sweater. Because all of the threads of yarn are connected, a pull in one section of the sweater may cause a pull in a spot distant from the original, or distortion of the shape of the entire sweater.

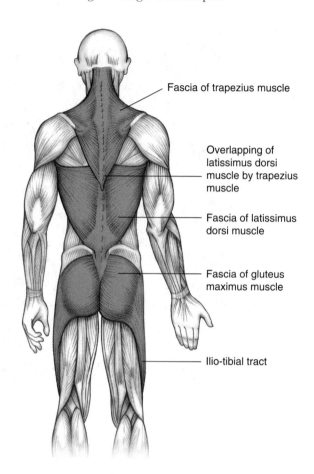

Fascia of trapezius muscle

Overlapping of latissimus dorsi muscle by trapezius muscle

Fascia of latissimus dorsi muscle

Fascia of gluteus maximus muscle

Ilio-tibial tract

FIGURE 12–2. Fascial sheaths surrounding and linking the muscles of the back of the body.

In addition, fascia surrounding muscle can prevent full relaxation and elongation of muscle tissue, thus restricting movement. As Scheumann relates: "However, a muscle cannot regain its resting length even when contracted fibers are relaxed if the surrounding fascial membranes are binding it . . .Techniques that address the unique characteristics of fascia must be applied to liberate contracted myofascial tissue fully" (Scheumann 2002, p. 45).

MYOFASCIAL TECHNIQUES

Myofascial techniques may be categorized in different ways. Reihl identifies four broad categories. First is **skin rolling,** which addresses superficial fascia. Second are **arm and leg pulls,** or full-body stretches that help release restrictions in the fascial web from head to toe. Third are **cross-handed stretches** that affect the skin, and release of local lines of restriction. Fourth are **transverse plane releases** that work on the restrictions in the pelvic floor, respiratory diaphgram, and thoracic area (Reihl, 2001).

Scheumann describes three types of connective tissue techniques: fascial (skin) lift and roll, myofascial spread, and myofascial mobilization. In the **myofascial spread** hands engage the skin side-by-side and then pull apart, spreading the tissues until resistance is felt. Resistance eventually yields and hands slide further apart. In **myofascial mobilization,** tissues are rolled against underlying muscle and bone in a back-and-forth or circular motion to free up adhesions. This is similar to cross-fiber and circular friction in Western massage (Scheumann, 2002).

A simple technique used to free subcutaneous fascia is **skin lifting** or **skin rolling,** a type of petrissage using Western massage terminology. The skin is gently picked up and slowly pulled away from underlying structures as shown in Figure 12–3. This technique stretches the subcutaneous fascia, breaks cross-links, and makes the tissue more pliable. Increase in local circulation is evidenced by increased redness in the area.

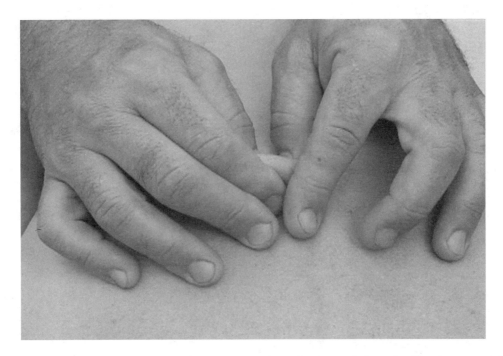

FIGURE 12–3. Skin lifting or rolling stretches subcutaneous fascia, breaks cross-links, and makes tissues more pliable.

Cross-handed stretches involve a sustained pull of fascial tissues. Figure 12–4 shows a horizontal stretch of the fascia of the back. While one hand anchors the skin near the sacrum, the other hand slowly pushes the skin and underlying tissue horizontally and superior, that is, toward the head. The stretch is held at the point of resistance. You may feel a subtle release of tissues after a few minutes. Then move to a different spot, working your way along the back toward the shoulders. Figure 12–5 shows a cross-handed stretch of superficial tissues across the back and perpendicular to the spine.

Fingertips can be used to engage and elongate superficial fascial tissues. Sensitive fingers can feel restrictions in the fascia as shown in Figure 12–6. Fingertips stretch the tissues horizontally to the point of resistance, and then wait until "melting" or release is felt.

The forearm may be used to release restrictions in deep fascia in areas like the upper back. See Figure 12–7. The forearm applies enough pressure to engage deeper fascia and then slowly stretches the tissues horizontally. Little if any lubricant is used to prevent the arm from sliding over the skin superficially. Stretching helps elongate deep fascial tissues and release cross-links within the tissues.

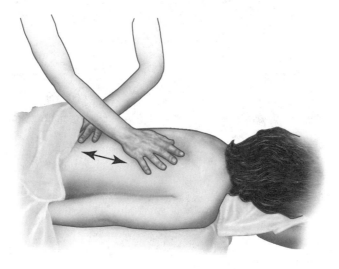

FIGURE 12–4. Cross-hand stretch parallel to the spine for elongation of the superficial fascia of the back.

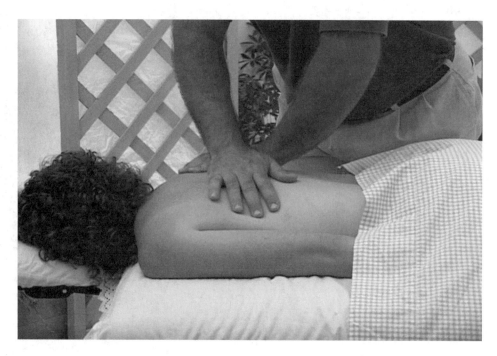

FIGURE 12–5. Cross-hand stretch perpendicular to the spine for elongation of the superficial fascia of the back.

In addition to the mechanical effects of stretching the tissues, techniques applied with the practitioner's hand or arm also impart heat to the area. Stretching and heat together produce a softer consistency of fascial tissue and free restrictions, an example of thixotropy.

Myofascial techniques can be integrated into a standard Western massage, or may be applied systematically in a session or series of sessions focused on myofascial release. Special training is available for gaining proficiency in myofascial massage. (For further information refer to *The Balanced Body*, 2nd Edition, by Donald W. Scheumann; Physical therapists refer to *The Myofascial Release Manual*, 3rd Edition, by Carol Manheim, P.T.)

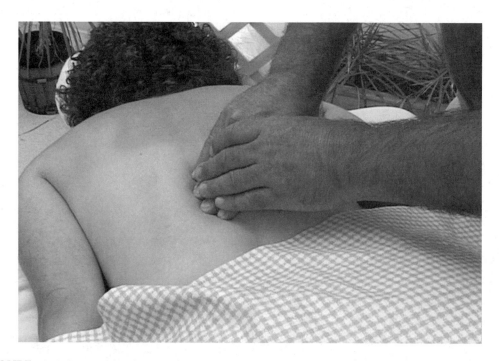

FIGURE 12–6. Fingertips used to stretch fascial tissues.

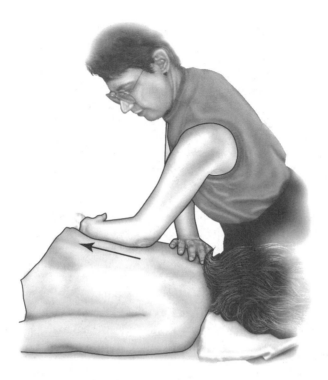

FIGURE 12–7. Use of forearm for release of deeper fascial tissues.

GUIDELINES FOR PERFORMING MYOFASCIAL MASSAGE

Several different approaches to myofascial massage have been developed by experts in the field. While approaches differ in some respects, common useful principles can be identified. Table 12–1 summarizes guidelines for myofascial massage gleaned from sources cited in this chapter.

Fascial restrictions may be located by visual analysis of the client's posture. Areas of fascial shortening that cause postural distortion can be observed. Restrictions may also be detected through palpation of tissues, or feeling where tissues seem to "stick together" or resist lengthening. Once restrictions are located, they are released by applying a gentle horizontal stretch until the tissues elongate or "give."

Table 12–1   GUIDELINES FOR MYOFASCIAL MASSAGE

This list of myofascial massage guidelines summarizes instructions from many sources cited in this chapter.

1. Use observation of posture, palpation skills, and knowledge of fascial anatomy to identify areas of fascial restriction.
2. Choose myofascial massage techniques suitable for the area, and for the depth at which you are working.
3. Use no or very little lubricant so that you can feel fascial restrictions, and apply techniques without sliding over the skin.
4. Make gentle contact and enter tissues slowly until a point or area of resistance is felt.
5. Shift tissues horizontally once you are at the depth you wish to affect.
   - Avoid compressing tissues into bone.
6. Hold a stretch of fascial tissues until they release, usually in 2 to 5 minutes.
   - Maintain a continuous stretch.
   - Release feels like "melting," softening, or "giving" in tissues.
7. Flow with the tissues. Let the direction of the stretch be determined by which way the tissues seem to want to release.
8. Exit tissues with as much care and awareness as when you melted into them.
9. Let fascial tissues rest and integrate after a stretch.

Myofascial techniques are generally applied using very little, if any, lubricant. Practitioners must be able to feel subtle restrictions in the movement of fascial tissues and the letting go or melting that occurs as the fascia elongates and becomes more pliable. Such palpation is hindered by sliding over the skin, which tends to happen when oil is used. Myofascial techniques also require traction on the skin as tissues are slowly and gently pushed, pulled, and stretched.

Instructions for myofascial release outlined by Reihl include (1) hold a stretch for 2–5 minutes; (2) maintain a continuous stretch; (3) use light pressure; (4) flow with the tissues (2001).

Schultz and Feitis (1996) recommend lifting the tissues, and moving them in a direction that avoids compression into a bone. Awareness of fascial anatomy and fiber direction provides information about the depth of tissue being influenced. Finally, let fascial tissues rest and integrate after a stretch to avoid overworking them (p. 125).

In his *Myofascial Massage Therapy* training manual, Robert King (1996) recommends that the practitioner make gentle contact, enter slowly until a point or area of resistance is felt, and wait for a feeling of **melting** (i.e., softening or "giving") in tissues. He advises to shift tissues horizontally and that "pressure should be used to get you to the layer you need to work on. Once you're there, direction is what's most important." When finished, exit the tissues with as much care and awareness as when you melted into them.

Barnes (1987) describes the process as follows: "At first the elastic component of the fascia will release, and at some point in time the collagenous barrier will be engaged. This barrier cannot be forced (it is too strong). One waits with gentle pressure, and as the collagenous aspect releases, the therapist follows the motion of the tissue, barrier upon barrier until freedom is felt."

Myofascial unwinding refers to the unwinding of abnormal twists and turns of the fascia from a three-dimensional view of the body. Unwinding restores structural integrity and proper alignment and promotes improved functioning of tissues and organs.

Myofascial techniques may be integrated into a general full-body massage or may be used as the primary approach in a session or treatment. For best results, myofascial release techniques are often combined with soft-tissue manipulation, trigger point therapy, and craniosacral manipulation. Proper exercise, nutrition, relaxation, and psychotherapy may also be involved for a complete approach to a problem for which myofascial release is indicated.

SUMMARY

Myofascial massage addresses the body's fascial anatomy with the intent of releasing restrictions in the superficial fascia, deep fascia surrounding the musculature, and fascia related to body alignment. Myofascial techniques release restrictions that limit mobility, cause postural distortion, poor cellular nutrition, pain, and a variety of other dysfunctions.

The history of massage that addresses connective tissue and fascia specifically includes the work of Elizabeth Dicke and Bindegewebsmassage (1920s), and Ida Rolf and Rolfing (1960s). The term myofascial release was coined by an osteopath named Robert Ward in the 1960s, and adopted by John Barnes as MFR in the 1980s. Systems of myofascial massage continue to be developed under terms like myofascial release, myofascial unwinding, and myofascial manipulation.

Fascia is loose irregular connective tissue found throughout the body. It surrounds muscles, nerves, blood vessels, and organs, giving them their shapes. It winds through the body in a continuous sheet, and supports and connects the body as a whole. Fascia is composed of ground substance, collagen and elastin. Sheets of fascia are formed by hydrogen bonds between collagen fibers. Functions of fascia include support, protection, cellular respiration, elimination, metabolism, fluid flow, and immune system function. Fascia has a characteristic called thixotropy, that is, it becomes more pliable with movement, stretching, and increased temperature.

Fascia lies at three different depths in the body as subcutaneous fascia, deep fascia, and subserous fascia. Barnes defines another layer called deepest fascia in the craniosacral system. Fascial anatomy includes structures like horizontal straps that give the body contour, and sheaths surrounding and linking muscles.

Restrictions in the fascial web can cause distortion in other parts of the body, and restrict movement. Myofascial massage focuses on subcutaneous and deep fascia.

Myofascial techniques promoted by Reihl include skin rolling, arm and leg pulls, cross-hand stretches, and transverse plane releases. Scheumann describes connective tissue techniques of fascial lift and roll, myofascial spread, and myofascial mobilization. Myofascial techniques are applied with full palm, fingertips, and forearm.

Guidelines for performing myofascial techniques include location of restrictions by visual analysis of posture, and palpation. Myofascial techniques are chosen based on the area and depth of application. Little to no lubricant is used to allow the practitioner to feel fascial restrictions and to get sufficient skin traction. Movement is gentle and slow and proceeds until a point of resistance is felt in the tissues. Tissues are shifted horizontally to provide a stretch and release restrictions. Stretch is held until restrictions release (i.e., melt, soften, give), usually in 2 to 5 minutes. Movement flows with the tissues. Exit the stretch with care and awareness. Tissues should rest after the stretch.

A look ahead . . .

Trigger points are taut bands of muscle tissue that are painful when pressed, restrict movement, and refer pain to other parts of the body. Neuromuscular therapy (NMT) is a form of massage that deactivates trigger points and brings relief from the pain they cause. Chapter 13 explains the theory and describes the techniques of NMT.

REFERENCES

Anderson, K. N., & Anderson, L. E. (1990). *Mosby's pocket dictionary of medicine, nursing, & allied health*. St. Louis: C.V. Mosby.

Barnes, J. F. (1987). Myofascial release. *Physical Therapy Forum*, September 16.

Cantu, R. I., & Grodin, A. J. (1992). *Myofascial manipulation: Theory and clinical application*. Gaithersburg, MD: Aspen Publishers.

Juhan, D. (1987). *Job's body*. Barrytown, NY: Station Hill Press.

King, R. K. (1996). *Myofascial massage therapy: Towards postural balance*. Self-published training manual by Bobkat Productions, Chicago.

Knaster, M. (1996). *Discovering the body's wisdom*. New York: Bantam Books.

Manheim, C. (2001). *The myofascial release manual*, 3rd ed. Thorofare, NJ: Slack Inc.

Reihl, S. (2001). "Beginning myofascial release." Instructional video produced by Real Bodywork.

Scheumann, D. W. (2002). *The balanced body: A guide to deep tissue and neuromuscular therapy*. 2nd edition. Philadelphia: Lippincott, Williams & Wilkins.

Schultz, R. L. and R. Feitis (1996). *The endless web: Fascial anatomy and physical reality*. Berkeley, CA: North Atlantic Press.

WEBSITES

The Rolf Institute of Structural Integration (*www.rolf.org*)
Myofascial Release. Com (*www.myofascial-release.com*)

ADDITIONAL RESOURCES

Videos

"Advanced myofascial release." (2000). Santa Barbara, CA: Real Bodywork. (*www.deeptissue.com*)

"Beginning myofascial release." (2001). Santa Barbara, CA: Real Bodywork. (*www.deeptissue.com*)

"Deep tissue massage and myofascial release: A video guide to techniques." (2003). Seven Volumes. Art Riggs. (*www.deeptissuemassagemanual.com*)

"Myofascial release: Lumbar region." (2002). Halifax, Nova Scotia, Canada: Jenings. (*www.jenings.com*)

"Myofascial release: Cervical Region." (2003). Halifax, Nova Scotia, Canada: Jenings. (*www.jenings.com*)

STUDY GUIDE

LEARNING OUTCOMES

Use the learning outcomes at the beginning of the chapter as a guide to your studies. Perform the task given in each outcome, either in writing or verbally into a tape recorder or to a study partner. This may start as an "open book" exercise, and then later from memory.

KEY TERMS/CONCEPTS

To study key words and concepts listed at the beginning of this chapter, choose one or more of the following exercises. Writing or talking about ideas helps you remember them better, and explaining helps deepen your understanding.

1. Write a one or two sentence explanation of each key word and concept.

2. Make study cards by writing the explanation from problem 1 on one side of a 3 × 5 card, and the key word or concept on the other. Shuffle the cards and read one side, trying to recite either the explanation or word on the other side.

3. Make study cards as in problem 2, this time writing a historical figure's name on one side and their contribution to the development of myofascial massage on the other.

4. Pick out two or three key words or concepts and explain how they are related.

5. With a study partner, take turns explaining key words and concepts verbally.

STUDY OUTLINE

The following questions test your memory of the main concepts in this chapter. Locate the answers in the text using the page number given for each question.

1. Myofascial massage addresses the body's _____ anatomy. (p. 246)

2. The general intent of myofascial massage is to release restriction in _____ fascia, and fascia related to the _____, and overall body _____. (p. 246)

3. Myofascial techniques release fascial restrictions that cause limited _____, postural _____, poor cellular _____, _____, and other dysfunctions. (p. 246)

History of Myofascial Massage (p. 246)

1. A system of _____ massage (CTM) called Bindegewebsmassage was developed by _____ of Germany in the 1920–30s. Light strokes without oil to various areas of the skin are thought to have _____ effects to other parts of the body and to visceral organs. (p. 246)

2. Structural integration, or Rolfing, was developed by _____ and taught at the Esalen Institute in the 1960s. Rolfing seeks to reestablish proper _____ alignment by manipulating _____ tissues. (p. 246)

3. The term myofascial release was coined by osteopath _____ in the 1960s to describe his system of treating the body's fascial anatomy. (p. 246)

4. The term myofascial release (MFR) was adopted by John _____ in the 1980s to designate his system of freeing restrictions in the myofascial anatomy. (p. 246)

5. Myofascial techniques continue to evolve and are known variously as myofascial _____, myofascial _____, myofascial _____, and myofascial _____. (p. 246)

The Nature of Fascia

1. Fascia is loose irregular _____ tissue found throughout the body. (p. 246)

2. Fascia fills the interstitial spaces, and _____ every muscle, nerve, blood vessel, and organ. (p. 246)

3. Fascia has important functions including _____, _____, _____, _____, _____, _____, and _____. (p. 247)

4. Fascial restrictions lead to a variety of problems including poor exchange of cellular _____ and _____, _____, and _____ mobility. (p. 247)

5. Fascia has a characteristic called _____, i.e., it can change from a more solid to a more gel consistency with _____ and _____. (p. 246)

6. Three depths of fascia have been distinguished: (1) _____ fascia, a continuous layer of connective tissue over the entire body between skin and deep fascia; (2) _____ fascia, sheets and bands of connective tissue that hold muscles and other anatomical structures in place; (3) _____ fascia, connective tissue between deep fascia and serous membranes lining body cavities. (p. 247)

7. Deepest fascia is a concept defined by John Barnes as a layer within the dura mater of the _____ system. (p. 246)

8. The study of fascial anatomy includes identifying fascial structures that shape the body and give it _____, and fascial _____ that surround muscles and _____ muscle groups. (p. 247)

9. A metaphor often used to describe fascia is a _____. A pull in one section may cause a pull in a spot distant from the original, or distortion in the shape of the entire thing. (p. 247)

10. Scheumann states that a muscle cannot regain its resting length if surrounding fascial _____ are binding it. (p. 248)

Myofascial Techniques

1. Reihl's four broad categories of myofascial techniques are 1. skin _____, 2. arm and leg _____, 3. _____-handed stretches, 4. _____ plane releases. (p. 248)

2. Scheumann describes three types of fascial techniques: (1) fascial _____ and _____; (2) myofascial _____; and (3) myofascial _____. (p. 248)

3. In a technique called _____, the skin is gently picked up and slowly pulled away from underlying structures. (p. 248)

4. Cross-hand stretches provide a gentle release of _____ fascia. (p. 249)

5. Fingertips can be used to _____ and _____ superficial fascial tissues. (p. 249)

6. The forearm can be used to release restrictions in _____ fascia. (p. 249)

Guidelines for Performing Myofascial Massage

1. Fascial restrictions can be located through _____, as well as _____. (p. 251)

2. Little if any lubricant is used to apply myofascial techniques so that practitioners can feel _____ in fascia, and so that hands do not _____ as tissues are slowly and gently pushed, pulled, and stretched. (p. 252)

3. Four guidelines from Reihl are (1) hold a stretch for _____ minutes; (2) maintain a _____ stretch; (3) use _____ pressure; (4) _____ with the tissues. (p. 252)

4. Schultz and Feitis recommend avoiding compressing tissues into _____, and letting the tissues _____ after stretching to prevent overworking them. (p. 252)

5. Knowledge of _____ and _____ direction can provide valuable information about the depth of tissues being influenced when applying techniques. (p. 252)

6. _____ is a term sometimes used to describe the release (i.e., softening or giving) of a myofascial restriction. (p. 252)

7. Barnes recommends being patient since the _____ component of fascia releases first, and the _____ barriers release later. (p. 252)

8. Myofascial _____ is a term sometimes used to describe the release of abnormal twists and turns of fascia from a three-dimensional view of the body. (p. 252)

FOR GREATER UNDERSTANDING

The following exercises are designed to take you from the realm of theory into the real world. They will help give you a deeper understanding of the subjects covered in this chapter. Action words are underlined to emphasize the variety of activities presented to address different learning styles, and to encourage deeper thinking.

1. Visit the Web sites mentioned as additional resources for this chapter. Read the information they offer on their style of myofascial massage. Describe what you find with a study partner.

2. Locate a practitioner with special training in a form of myofascial massage. Receive a myofascial session or series of sessions. Write down your experience or verbally describe it to a study partner.

3. After completing problem 2, compare your experience with that of a study partner who also received a myofascial session. Discuss similarities and differences, and your reactions to the sessions.

4. Observe a session with a practitioner with advanced training in myofascial massage. Verbally, or in writing, describe the techniques they use, and their overall approach. Explain their intent in applying techniques, and how tissues seemed to respond.

5. Interview someone who has received a series of myofascial massage sessions from a specially trained practitioner. Ask them to describe their reason for receiving the sessions, how the sessions were conducted, and how they think they benefited.

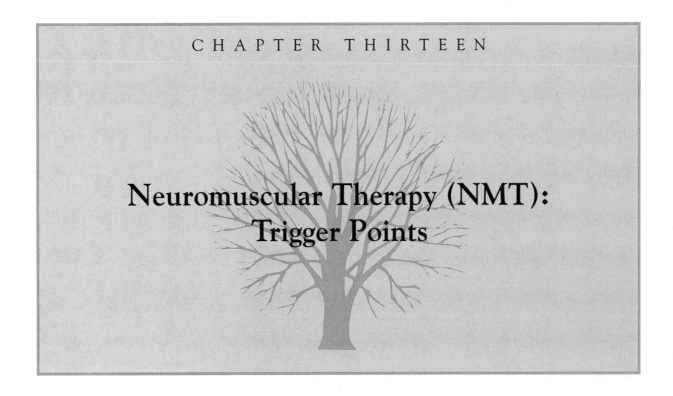

Neuromuscular Therapy (NMT): Trigger Points

LEARNING OUTCOMES

After studying this chapter, the student will have information to:

1. Discuss the origins of neuromuscular therapy, and the roles of important people in its history.
2. Define trigger point, and describe the different types.
3. Explain trigger point referral patterns.
4. Identify the origin of trigger points.
5. Locate trigger points by palpation.
6. Perform trigger point deactivation techniques.

HISTORICAL PEOPLE

Lief, Stanley   Prudden, Bonnie   Travell, Janet

KEY TERMS/CONCEPTS

Active TrP   Local pain   Referred pain
Associated TrP   Neuromuscular therapy (NMT)   Satellite TrP
Hand tools   Pincer technique   Secondary TrP
Ischemic compression   Primary TrP   Trigger points
  techniques   Reference zone
Latent TrP   Referral pattern

 MEDIALINK

A companion CD-ROM, included free with each new copy of this book, supplements the techniques presented in this chapter. Insert the CD-ROM to watch video clips of massage techniques being demonstrated. This multimedia feature is designed to help you add a new dimension to your learning.

Neuromuscular therapy (NMT) is performed to deactivate tender spots called trigger points (TrP) in muscle and related connective tissues. Trigger points may develop as a result of trauma, poor posture, repetitive strain, or overwork of muscles. TrPs cause pain, weakness, and limited flexibility, and can refer pain to other areas.

HISTORY OF NEUROMUSCULAR THERAPY

The origins of **neuromuscular therapy (NMT)** can be traced in Europe to a natural healer named **Stanley Lief,** who was born in Latvia in the 1890s. Lief studied physical culture with Bernarr Macfadden in the United States and was trained in chiropractic and naturopathy. He established a world-famous natural healing resort in 1925 in Champneys in Hertfordshire, England. There he developed soft tissue manipulative methods that closely resemble what is known in the United States today as neuromuscular therapy. NMT was part of a holistic approach to healing, incorporating diet, emotional health, and hydrotherapy, as well as soft tissue manipulation (Chaitow, 1996).

Janet Travell, MD, who pioneered trigger point therapy in the Unites States, published her first work on the subject in 1952. Dr. Travell is credited with relieving the debilitating pain of the young Senator John F. Kennedy, who was injured in World War II. Dr. Travell was later appointed White House physician to both Presidents Kennedy and Johnson in the 1960s. These appointments brought Dr. Travell's work to the attention of the public (Claire, 1995, p. 42). Travell, along with David Simons, MD, has written the definitive work on trigger point therapy in two volumes (1999, 1992).

A systematic approach to addressing trigger points was developed and made popular by **Bonnie Prudden** in the 1970–1980s. Prudden's two books, *Pain Erasure* (1980) and *Myotherapy* (1984), offer practical descriptions of how to locate and relieve common trigger points in different parts of the body. Prudden helped make NMT accessible within the developing field of massage therapy, and to the general public.

Other systems of relieving trigger points have been promoted by their developers and have various names. Neuromuscular therapy (NMT) is a common generic designation for trigger point therapy.

TRIGGER POINTS (TrP)

Massage practitioners will often find small spots in muscles that are sore or radiate pain when pressed. In the absence of other obvious causes (e.g., bruising) trigger points should be suspected. These points of tenderness may be palpated as tense bands of tissue in muscles and tendons, and are relieved through a variety of methods. A **trigger point** (TrP) is defined by Travell and Simons as "a focus of hyperirritability in a tissue that, when compressed, is locally tender and, if sufficiently hypersensitive, gives rise to referred pain and tenderness, and sometimes to referred autonomic phenomena and distortion of proprioception" (1999, p. 4).

Two criteria for a trigger point are that it be an "exquisitely tender spot in a taut band of the muscle." A microscopic view of the muscle would reveal tiny contraction knots along the muscle fibers. This probably accounts for why TrPs feel nodular and taut (Mense, Simons 2001, pp. 250–251).

REFERRAL PATTERNS

Trigger points cause **local pain,** and may also cause **referred pain** in their **reference zone.** For example, TrPs in the trapezius and muscles of the neck can result in referred pain experienced as a tension headache. The referred pain of myofascial trigger points is described as "dull and aching, often deep, with intensity varying from low-grade discomfort to severe and incapacitating torture. It may occur at rest or only in motion" (Travell and Simons, 1999, p. 13).

Trigger points may elicit pain on being pressed or may be tender and radiate pain without pressure. Pressing on an active TrP usually intensifies pain in the reference zone of the trigger point. The involved muscle may be stiff and weak and may be restricted in range of motion. Attempts to stretch the muscle, either actively or passively, usually increase the pain felt. Muscles in the immediate area of a TrP often feel tense and ropelike.

Other sensory, motor, and autonomic phenomena may be "triggered" by active TrPs. These include pain, tenderness, increased motor unit activity (spasm), vasoconstriction (blanching), coldness, sweating, pilomotor response (goose bumps), vasodilation (increased local circulation), and hypersecretion (increased gland secretions). These effects can occur at a distance from the trigger point, but within the general area to which a specific TrP refers pain (Travell and Simons, 1992, p. 5).

Figure 13–1 shows some of the common trigger point locations. While trigger point charts are useful for confirming common locations and referral patterns, you may find points and patterns unique to each receiver.

VARIETIES OF TRIGGER POINTS

Trigger points may be described as latent or active, primary or secondary, satellite, or associated. **Latent trigger points** are painful only when pressed. **Active trigger points** are always tender, prevent full lengthening, weaken the muscle, and refer pain on direct compression. **Primary trigger points** are activated by acute or chronic overload of a muscle, while **secondary TrPs** become active because of their reaction to a muscle containing a primary trigger point. A **satellite trigger point** becomes active because

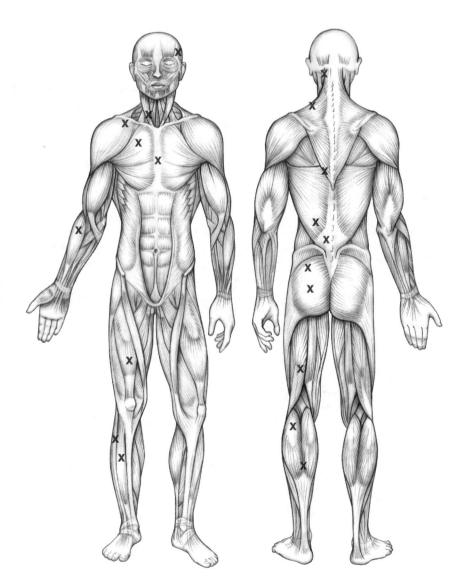

FIGURE 13–1. Common trigger point locations, anterior and posterior.

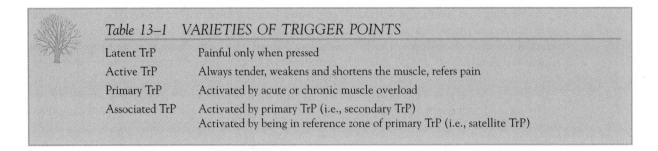

Table 13-1	VARIETIES OF TRIGGER POINTS
Latent TrP	Painful only when pressed
Active TrP	Always tender, weakens and shortens the muscle, refers pain
Primary TrP	Activated by acute or chronic muscle overload
Associated TrP	Activated by primary TrP (i.e., secondary TrP)
	Activated by being in reference zone of primary TrP (i.e., satellite TrP)

the muscle is in a zone of reference of another TrP. **Associated trigger points** refer to secondary or satellite TrPs (Travell & Simons 1983, pp. 1–4). Table 13–1 summarizes the varieties of trigger points.

ORIGIN OF TRIGGER POINTS

Trigger points may be activated by direct stimuli such as acute overload or overwork of a muscle, chilling, or gross trauma. Indirect stimuli may also activate trigger points, e.g., arthritic joints, emotional distress, certain visceral diseases, and other TrPs (Travell and Simons, 1999, p. 16).

People who perform repetitive stressful tasks, such as athletes, musicians, artists, and physical laborers, are prone to trigger points. Poor posture during daily activities such as sitting at a desk or driving a car may also elicit TrPs. Forward head posture, which places the upper body in a round-shouldered slumped forward position, is known to produce TrPs in the pectoral and posterior cervical muscles (Travell & Simons, 1992, p. 20). Something as simple as carrying a heavy purse or briefcase on the same side all the time can cause the muscle overload that leads to trigger points.

LOCATING TRIGGER POINTS

Suspect myofascial trigger points when clients complain of muscle tension causing pain or localized muscle soreness and shortening, or when they describe one of the common pain patterns associated with TrPs. Self-reports of when and how the pain developed may also give clues as to its origin. For example, reports of a fall or blow to a muscle, a repetitive motion, or sustained immobile posture such as in driving or sitting at a workstation all point to the possibility of trigger points.

It is useful to have recipients map out areas of pain on a blank chart, which can help the practitioner locate probable active trigger point sites. The more knowledgeable the practitioner is about TrPs and their predictable referral patterns, the more easily the exact points may be located.

Ultimately, precise trigger point locations are discovered by palpation. You may locate points from clues given from verbal reports or charts, or you may happen upon latent TrPs in the course of a massage session. The taut bands of tissue characterizing trigger points can be felt. Recipients can give feedback on the exact location of the TrP, the degree of pain experienced, the referral pattern upon pressure, and the diminishing pain upon deactivation.

Recipients will often say something like "you're almost on it, but not quite." A slight change in location or angle of pressure is often enough to get the exact point. The pain reported is frequently out of proportion to the pressure applied. Pressure elicits a "jump sign" or outcry from the recipient. With pressure directly on the TrP, recipients may report increased pain in the same area or pain referred to another area.

DEACTIVATION TECHNIQUES

It is important to locate and deactivate primary trigger points whether latent or active. For total relief from pain and to restore full function to a muscle, associated points (i.e., secondary and satellite) must also be relieved once they are activated.

Trigger points may be deactivated by a variety of non-manual methods, including spray and stretch, saline injection, dry needling and anesthetics. Manual techniques found to be effective in deactivating TrPs include ischemic compression using the hands or a tool, deep stroking massage (stripping), deep friction at the TrP site, and vibration. These techniques are typically followed by a stretch of the affected muscles.

The stretch of the affected muscles seems to be especially important to complete the deactivation of the trigger point and return the affected tissues to a normal state. Other deactivation methods that focus on stretching, and are mentioned by Travell and Simons (1992), include contract–relax, reciprocal inhibition, relaxation during exhalation, percussion and stretch, muscle energy technique, and myofascial release.

Ischemic Compression Techniques

Ischemic compression techniques are those methods in which compression of the tissues at the trigger point site causes blanching with hypoxia, followed by a reactive hyperemia (Travell and Simons 1999 p. 27). In other words, the compressed tissues become white from lack of blood and oxygen, followed by an increase in blood flow to the area once pressure is released. Ischemic compression may be created with sustained digital pressure, with a tool, or with a pincer technique. Travell and Simons recommended application of pressure for about 20 seconds to 1 minute.

Pressure is gradually increased as the sensitivity of the TrP wanes and the tension in its taut band fades. Pressure is released when the clinician feels the TrP tension subside or when the TrP is no longer tender to pressure. Sustained pressure should not be applied to blood vessels or a nerve or when it induces numbness and tingling. Ischemic compression should be followed by lengthening of the muscle, except when stretching is contraindicated (e.g., with hypermobile or unstable joints) (1992, p. 9).

The thumbs are commonly used to provide the sustained digital pressure in deactivating trigger points. Figures 13–2 and 13–3 illustrate the use of the thumb in applying direct pressure to TrPs. Note the hand mechanics with thumb and wrist joints in alignment. Avoid pressure while the thumb is abducted.

To relieve the thumbs, other parts of the hands may be used to apply pressure, for example, the fingertips as in Figure 13–4. For more heavily muscled areas, the elbow may be used. Figure 13–5 shows the use of the elbow with the recipient in the seated position to deactivate TrPs in the large trapezius muscle. The elbow is also useful when working through larger muscles to affect deeper muscles in an area, for example, to reach the deeper muscles of the buttocks as shown in Figure 10–20.

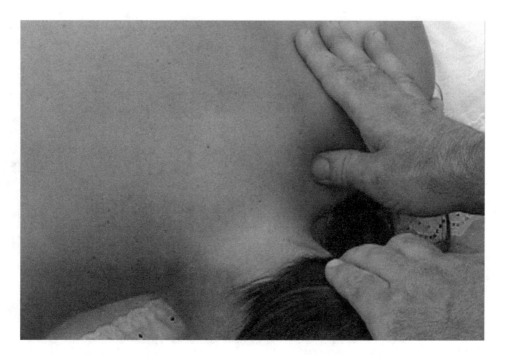

FIGURE 13–2. Ischemic compression to trigger point with thumb.

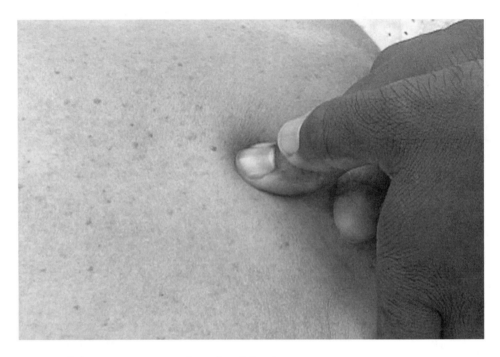

FIGURE 13–3. Ischemic compression with reinforced thumb.

To protect the small joints of the hands from overuse, small **hand tools** may be used effectively for applying pressure. Find trigger points through palpation with the fingertips, and then place the tip of the tool on the point to apply pressure. If used with sensitivity, the quality of touch with the tool may be indistinguishable from using the hand directly. It is important to keep the wrists straight when using tools. Figure 13–6 demonstrates the use of a wooden hand tool to apply pressure to trigger points.

In the above examples, the tissue containing the TrP is compressed between the practitioner's hand or hand tool, and tissues underneath the point. In the **pincer technique,** the tissue at the TrP site

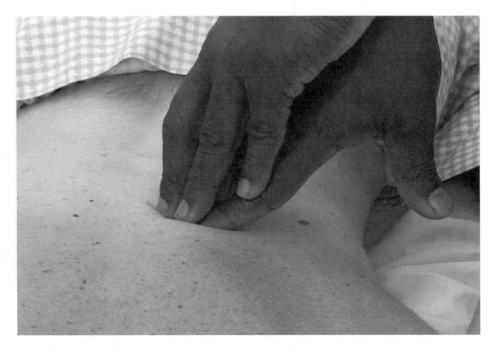

FIGURE 13–4. Finger pressure to trigger point.

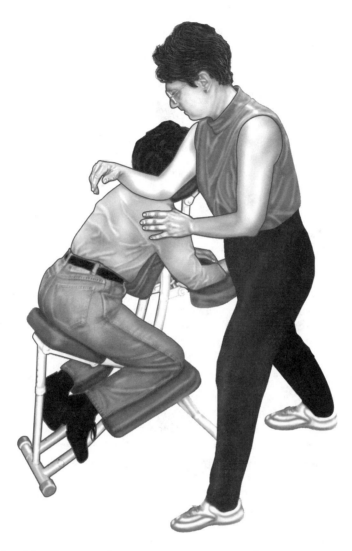

FIGURE 13–5. Use of the elbow to apply pressure to trigger points in the trapezius, receiver in sitting position.

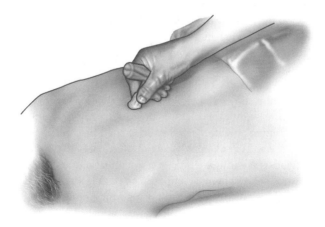

FIGURE 13–6. Use of a hand tool called a "T-bar" to apply pressure to a trigger point.

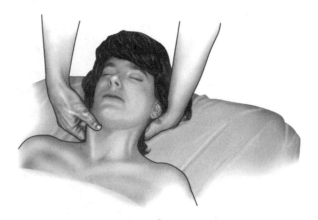

FIGURE 13–7. Squeezing the sternocleidomastoid (SCM) with a pincer technique.

is compressed between the fingers and thumb of the practitioner. For example, TrPs in the sternocleidomastoid (SCM) may be compressed using the pincer technique as shown in Figure 13–7. Take care to avoid the carotid artery located anterior to the SCM.

Other Manual Techniques

Deep friction, deep stroking or stripping, vibration, and stretching are other manual techniques used in deactivating TrPs. These techniques are applied in conjunction with ischemic compression for best results.

A combination of techniques can be applied to deactivate trigger points, separate tissues that are adhering, and improve circulation to the area. Since muscle shortening is often a result of TrPs, stretching is an important finishing technique to help bring affected muscles back to full length.

SUMMARY

Neuromuscular therapy (NMT) is performed to deactivate tender spots called trigger points (TrP) in muscle and related connective tissues. Trigger points may develop as a result of trauma, poor posture, repetitive strain, or overwork of muscles. NMT techniques deactivate TrPs that cause pain, weakness, and limited flexibility.

In the early 1900s, a European natural healer named Stanley Lief developed soft tissue methods that closely resemble NMT. Janet Travell, MD pioneered trigger point therapy in the United States in the 1950s. Travell and David Simons wrote the definitive trigger point manuals. Bonnie Prudden developed a popular system of trigger point therapy in the 1980s, which she called *myotherapy*. Neuromuscular Therapy (NMT) is the generic term for manual therapy that addresses trigger points.

Trigger points (TrPs) are taut bands of tissue in muscles and tendons. TrPs are tender locally and may also refer or radiate pain to their reference zones. TrPs cause muscles to be sore, stiff, weak, and less flexible, and may trigger sensory, motor, and autonomic phenomena. TrPs are classified as latent, active, primary, secondary, satellite and associated.

Trigger points may be caused by muscle overload or overwork, trauma, chilling, arthritis, emotional stress, disease, or other TrPs. People prone to TrPs include athletes, musicians, artists, laborers, and those with poor posture. TrPs can be located from self-reports of pain by recipients, and by palpation of the taut bands in muscles. Recipient feedback helps practitioners find exact locations of points.

Deactivation techniques include nonmanual methods like saline injection and dry needling, and manual methods like ischemic compression, muscle stripping, deep friction, vibration, and stretching. Ischemic compression includes methods in which compression of the tissues at the trigger point site causes blanching with hypoxia, followed by a reactive hyperemia. Pressure is applied directly to the TrP with the thumb, fingers, elbow, or small hand tool, and held for 20–60 seconds. Compression is followed by a stretch of the affected muscle.

A look ahead . . .

Special soft tissue manipulation techniques have been developed to enhance the flow of lymph fluid and improve function of the body's lymphatic system. Chapter 14 explains the theory and describes the gentle techniques of lymphatic drainage massage.

REFERENCES

Chaitow, L. (1996). *Modern neuromuscular techniques.* London: Churchill Livingston.

Claire, T. (1995). *Bodywork: What type of massage to get and how to make the most of it.* New York: William Morrow.

Mense, S. and D. G. Simons (2001). "Myofascial pain caused by trigger points." Chapter 9 in *Muscle pain: Understanding its nature, diagnosis, and treatment.* Philadelphia: Lippincott, Williams & Wilkins.

Prudden, B. (1980). *Pain erasure: The Bonnie Prudden way.* New York: M. Evans.

Prudden, B. (1984). *Myotherapy: Bonnie Prudden's complete guide to pain-free living.* New York: Ballantine Books.

Travell, J. G., & Rinzler, S. H. (1952). The myofascial genesis of pain. *Postgraduate Medicine,* 11, 425–434.

Travell, J. G., & Simons, D. G. (1999). *Myofascial pain and dysfunction: The trigger point manual, Volume 1—Upper half of the body,* 2nd ed. Baltimore: Williams & Wilkins.

Travell, J. G., & Simons, D. G. (1992). *Myofascial pain and dysfunction: The trigger point manual, Volume 2—The lower extremities.* Baltimore: Williams & Wilkins.

ADDITIONAL RESOURCES

Videos

"Deep tissue and neuromuscular therapy: The torso." Santa Barbara, CA: Real Bodywork. (*www.deeptissue.com*)

"Deep tissue and neuromuscular therapy: The extremities." Santa Barbara, CA: Real Bodywork. (*www.deeptissue.com*)

STUDY GUIDE

LEARNING OUTCOMES

Use the learning outcomes at the beginning of the chapter as a guide to your studies. Perform the task given in each outcome, either in writing or verbally into a tape recorder or to a study partner. This may start as an "open book" exercise, and then later from memory.

KEY TERMS/CONCEPTS

To study key words and concepts listed at the beginning of this chapter, choose one or more of the following exercises. Writing or talking about ideas helps you remember them better, and explaining them helps deepen your understanding.

1. Write a one- or two-sentence explanation of each key word and concept.

2. Make study cards by writing the explanation from problem 1 on one side of a 3 × 5 card, and the key word or concept on the other. Shuffle the cards and read one side, trying to recite either the explanation or word on the other side.

3. Make study cards as in problem 2, this time writing a historical figure's name on one side and their contri-

bution to the development of neuromuscular therapy on the other.

4. Pick out two or three key words or concepts and explain how they are related.

5. With a study partner, take turns explaining key words and concepts verbally.

STUDY OUTLINE

The following questions test your memory of the main concepts in this chapter. Locate the answers in the text using the page number given for each question.

1. Neuromuscular therapy (NMT) is performed to deactivate _____ spots called trigger points in _____. (p. 258)

HISTORY OF NEUROMUSCULAR THERAPY

1. In the 1920s, a European natural healer named _____ developed soft tissue manipulation methods that resemble today's NMT. (p. 258)

2. _____, MD poineered trigger point therapy in the United States in the 1950s. Her work got the attention of the public when she treated a number of U.S. presidents, including John Kennedy. (p. 258)

3. _____ popularized trigger point therapy in the 1980s with her own system called myotherapy. (p. 258)

Trigger Points (TrP)

1. Trigger points are tender spots in muscles and tendons that radiate _____ when pressed. (p. 258)

2. Two criteria for TrPs are exquisite pain upon _____ and a _____ band of tissue. (p. 258)

3. A microscopic view of TrPs reveals nodules or tiny _____ knots in muscle tissue, which probably accounts for the nodular _____ feel of the tissue on palpation. (p. 258)

Referral Patterns

1. TrPs cause _____ pain and can refer pain to _____. (p. 258)

2. Referred pain of TrPs is described as dull and _____, often deep, with intensity varying from low-grade discomfort to _____. (p. 258)

3. Muscles with TrPs may be stiff and weak, and _____ in length. Muscles in the immediate area may feel tense and _____-like. (p. 258)

4. Other phenomena that may be caused by active TrPs are muscle _____, vaso-_____ and _____, coldness, sweating, _____ response, and _____-secretion. (p. 259)

Varieties of Trigger Points

1. _____ TrPs are painful only when pressed. (p. 259)

2. _____ TrPs are always tender, weaken and shorten the muscle, and refer pain upon direct compression. (p. 259)

3. _____ TrPs are activated by acute or chronic overload of a muscle. (p. 259)

4. _____ TrPs become active because of their reaction to a muscle with a primary TrP. (p. 259)

5. _____ TrPs become active because a muscle in their zone of reference contains an active TrP. (pp. 257–260)

Origin of Trigger Points

1. Direct stimuli that activate TrPs include muscle _____ or _____, chilling, and _____. (p. 260)

2. Indirect stimuli that activate TrPs include _____, emotional _____, _____, and other _____. (p. 260)

3. Sports, playing a musical instrument, poor posture, and carrying heavy objects are examples of _____. (p. 260)

Locating Trigger Points

1. Suspect myofascial TrPs when clients complain of _____. (p. 260)

2. Precise TrP locations are discovered by palpation of _____ and _____ in muscle tissue, along with client feedback regarding pain, especially if the pain reported seems _____. (p. 260)

3. Pressure directly on the TrP may cause pain at _____, or may refer pain to the entire _____ area. (p. 260)

Deactivation Techniques

1. For total relief from pain and to restore full function, _____ TrPs must be treated or deactivated. (p. 260)

2. Non-manual methods of deactivating TrPs include spray and _____, _____ injection, _____ needling, and anesthetics. (p. 261)

3. Manual techniques effective for deactivating TrPs include _____ compression with hands or small tools, muscle _____, deep _____ at the TrP site, and vibration. (p. 261)

4. It is important to follow manual techniques with _____ to help restore the muscle to its normal length. (p. 261)

Ischemic Compression Techniques

1. Ischemic compression involves pressing into the TrP site with enough pressure to cause _____ (i.e., cutting off blood to the spot), followed by increased blood flow to the area upon release. (p. 261)

2. Ischemic compression may be performed with the _____, _____, _____, or small _____. (pp. 261–262)

3. A _____ technique in which the TrP is squeezed between the thumb and fingers may be used for muscles that can be accessed, e.g., sternocleidomastoid. (p. 262–263)

FOR GREATER UNDERSTANDING

The following exercises are designed to take you from the realm of theory into the real world. They will help give you a deeper understanding of the subjects covered in this chapter. Action words are underlined to emphasize the variety of activities presented to address different learning styles, and to encourage deeper thinking.

1. Locate a practitioner with special training in neuromuscular therapy. Receive a NMT session or series of sessions. Write down your experience or verbally describe it to study partner.

2. After completing problem 1, compare your experience with that of a study partner who also received NMT. Discuss similarities and differences, and your reactions to the sessions.

3. Observe a session with a practitioner with advanced training in NMT. Verbally, or in writing, describe the techniques they use, and their overall approach. Explain their intent in applying techniques, and how tissues seemed to respond.

4. Interview someone who has received NMT from a trained practitioner (e.g., athlete, artist, musician, physical worker). Ask them to describe their reason for receiving NMT, how the sessions were conducted, and how they think they benefited.

5. Practice locating and deactivating trigger points on a study partner. Solicit feedback about their experience.

6. During problem 5, compare your partner's feedback on TrP pain referral patterns to a commercial chart. Did the zones on the chart match your partner's experience? Did you find TrPs not on the chart? Discuss with your study partner.

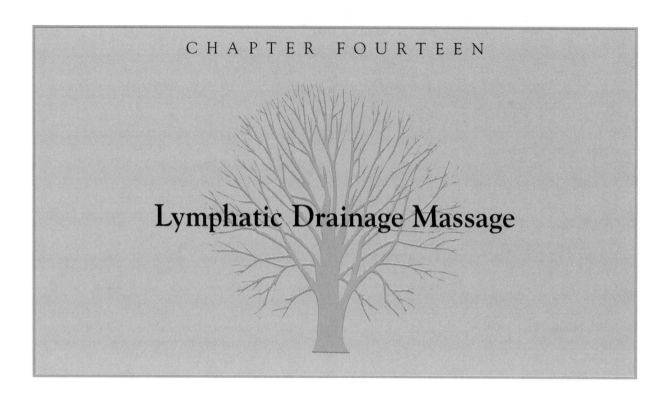

CHAPTER FOURTEEN

Lymphatic Drainage Massage

LEARNING OUTCOMES

After studying this chapter, the student will have information to:

1. Discuss the history of lymphatic drainage massage.
2. Explain the general anatomy and physiology of the lymphatic system.
3. Identify indications and contraindications for LDM.
4. Perform four basic LDM techniques.
5. Follow basic principles for performing LDM.
6. Discuss important considerations in the application of LDM.

HISTORICAL PEOPLE AND DEVELOPMENTS

Complete Decongestive
  Therapy (CDT)
Foldi, Michael and Ethel

Manual Lymph Drainage
  (MLD)
Vodder, Emil and Astid

Vodder's MLD
Von Winiwarter, Alexander

KEY TERMS/CONCEPTS

Collector vessels
Initial lymphatics

Lymph
Lymphangions

Lymphatic drainage massage
  (LDM)

MEDIALINK

A companion CD-ROM, included free with each new copy of this book, supplements the techniques presented in this chapter. Insert the CD-ROM to watch video clips of massage techniques being demonstrated. This multimedia feature is designed to help you add a new dimension to your learning.

Lymphatic system vessels   Pre-collector vessels   Scoop technique
Lymphedema   Pump technique   Stationary circles
Lymph nodes   Rotary technique

Lymphatic drainage massage (LDM) refers to systems of soft tissue manipulation designed to assist the function of the lymphatic system. LDM techniques consist of gentle, slow, repetitive strokes performed in a specific direction and sequence to improve lymph circulation. It is a precise and rhythmic massage used for general wellness, to enhance healing, and to treat lymphedema.

HISTORY OF LYMPHATIC DRAINAGE MASSAGE

The use of soft tissue manipulation to increase the movement of lymph fluid is an old practice found in many parts of the world. As early as 1894, Western scientific studies examined the use of massage and exercise as methods of increasing lymph flow. **Alexander von Winiwarter,** a German surgeon, treated lymphedema in the 1890s with a combination of methods including cleanliness, compression, exercise, and massage (Kurz et al., 1978; Kelly 2002).

In the 1930s, Danish physiotherapists **Emil and Astid Vodder** developed their system of **manual lymph drainage** (MLD), which has become the prototype for lymphatic drainage massage in Western medicine. **Vodder's MLD,** originally developed in France, is widely used today in Europe and North America. Many of the principles and techniques described in this chapter are derivatives of Vodder's MLD.

In the 1970s, Hungarian physicians **Michael and Ethel Foldi,** combined Vodder's MLD with other therapies into a comprehensive treatment for lymphedema called **Complete Decongestive Therapy (CDT).** CDT includes skin care, bandaging, exercise and massage. The Foldi Clinic in Germany trains practitioners from around the world in CDT. The first treatment centers offering CDT in North America were opened in the 1980s, and from that time there has been an increasing interest in CDT, including the LDM component.

Although LDM has always held potential as a wellness measure, the increase in the incidence of lymphedema in recent years has raised awareness of its health benefits. Reasons for the increase in lymphedema patients include improved survivorship from cancer, debilitating effects of certain cancer treatments, improved diagnosis of lymphedema, patient advocacy, and increase in information about the condition and its treatment (Kelly 2002).

In the 1990s and 2000s, applications of lymphatic drainage massage broadened to include use in injury rehabilitation and sports massage. Spas and salons offer LDM as a relaxation and beauty treatment, particularly for the facial area.

LYMPHATIC SYSTEM AND LDM

Knowledge of the structure and function of the lymphatic system helps in understanding LDM techniques, as well as the precise sequence in which they are applied. Some of the basics are outlined below, and references at the end of the chapter may be studied for greater detail.

The lymphatic and cardiovascular systems function together to ensure healthy circulation of fluids in the body. Uninterrupted movement of lymph and blood is necessary for the proper functioning of the immune system, tissue repair, and maintenance of a proper fluid and chemical environment for body cells. About 90 percent of interstitial fluid is reabsorbed into the blood capillaries, while about 10 percent flows into lymphatic vessels for eventual return to the cardiovascular system.

Lymph is a clear, colorless fluid that contains water, protein molecules, cellular components, and fatty acids that need to be transported back into blood circulation. Molecules and particles from intercellular spaces too large to enter blood capillaries are absorbed through the walls of the lymphatic capillaries called **initial lymphatics.**

Lymphatic system vessels are responsible for the absorption, collection, and transport of lymph fluid. Seventy percent of lymphatic vessels are located in the skin. The smallest vessels are the initial lymphatics. They are located in almost all tissues and organs. The initial lymphatic walls are only one cell thick with openings between cells to allow fluid and large solutes such as protein molecules to enter the tiny vessels. A schematic representation of the initial lymphatics is shown in Figure 14–1.

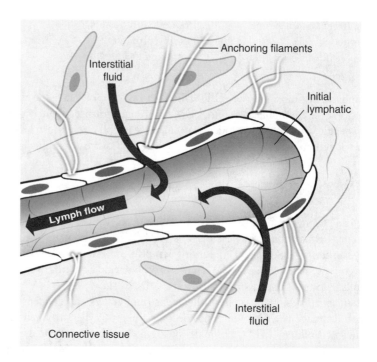

FIGURE 14–1. Schematic drawing of initial lymphatics. One cell thick walls with overflaps where lymph fluid enters the lymphatic system. Location in superficial skin.

The overlapping design of cell junctions creates one-way valves to prevent backflow of fluid into the interstitial spaces. It is at the site of the initial lymphatics that lymphatic drainage massage has its greatest effect.

> Opening of the *flaps* or *overlaps* is stimulated by several mechanisms, including variations of tissue pressure . . . and contraction of *fibrils* or *anchoring filaments* attached to the exterior cells walls and surrounding connective tissue . . . An increase in interstitial fluid will cause a pull on the fibrils, which will open the flaps. External, mechanical stimulation to superficial connective tissue, such as gentle skin tractioning, may contribute to flap opening by pulling on the anchoring filaments (Kelly, 2002, p. 5).

Heavy pressure (e.g., with deep massage) closes the flaps, and slows or stops the flow of lymph into the initial lymphatics. This is the reason that lymphatic drainage massage is applied with only enough pressure to create traction and movement in the superficial layers of the skin.

Fluid from the initial lymphatics flows into intermediate or **pre-collector vessels,** and finally into valved vessels called **collectors.** The walls of these deep collector vessels contain contractile smooth muscle in segments called **lymphangions.** The lymphangions contract in sequence like tiny heartbeats to move lymph fluid along. They are stimulated by the nervous system, contraction of adjacent muscles, changes in pressure from breathing, lower blood pressure in deep veins, increased volume of fluid in lymph vessels, and mechanical stimulation or traction (Kelly 2002).

Lymphatic flow occurs in an asymmetrical pattern in the body. Lymph from both legs and the left side of the body flows into the thoracic (left lymphatic) duct where it empties into the left subclavian vein. Lymph vessels from the right side of the head, neck, upper chest, and right arm flow into the right thoracic duct. This normal pattern of lymph flow, as shown in Figure 14–2, helps determine the sequence in LDM. The goal of LDM is to direct the lymph fluid through the system of vessels and eventually into its proper duct.

Lymph nodes are distributed throughout the lymphatic system at strategic points. They facilitate the immune response helping to protect the body from infection and disease. Major lymph node clusters are located in the head, neck, chest, abdomen, and groin. Lymph passes through the nodes as it circulates. There, *macrophages* act as a waste disposal site by removing bacteria, cell debris, and foreign

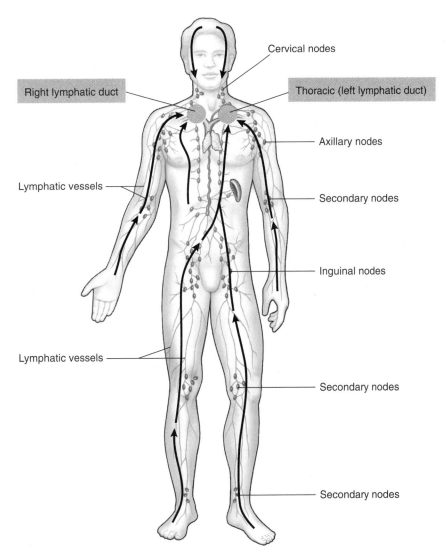

FIGURE 14–2. Schematic drawing showing the lymph system, and the general direction of flow of lymphatic fluid into the right and left thoracic ducts.

material. Lymphocytes are produced in nodes and released to process infectious material. Superficial drainage pathways leading to lymph nodes are shown in Figure 14–3.

INDICATIONS AND CONTRAINDICATIONS

LDM is used to treat a number of common conditions that involve lymphatic blockages, and that improve through better lymph drainage. These include allergy symptoms, arthritis, colds, colitis, edema, sinus congestion, and psoriasis. Healing of musculo-skeletal injuries may also be enhanced with LDM (Berube 1988).

LDM is also used in treatment of a chronic disorder called **lymphedema.** Lymphedema is characterized by an abnormal accumulation of lymph fluid in tissues of an arm, leg, or other body region. It is most often due to a mechanical insufficiency of the lymphatic system. Its symptoms include swelling, pain, numbness, sensation of pressure, increased susceptibility to infection, loss of mobility, and impaired wound healing.

Anything that disrupts the free flow of lymph in the vessels and nodes of the system may cause lymphedema. Common causes of secondary lymphedema include surgery, radiation therapy, trauma,

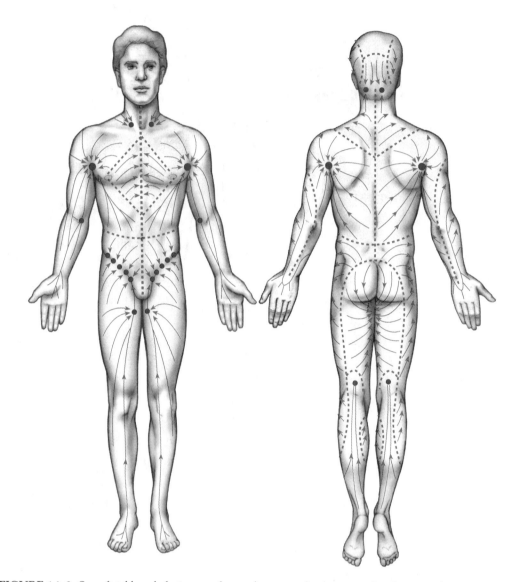

FIGURE 14–3. Superficial lymph drainage pathways determine the direction of application of LDM techniques. (Adapted from Vodder, E., *Die manuelle lymph drainage ad modum Vodder.*)

tumors, scarring, and chronic infections. Many of the treatments for cancer result in lymphedema (Kelly 2002).

Several organizations have missions related to the improvement and cure of diseases of the lymphatic system. (Refer to the National Lymphedema Network at www.lymphnet.org, and the Lymphatic Research Foundation at www.lymphaticresearch.org. Also see Chapter 4 for further discussion of massage for treatment of lymphedema.)

Contraindications to LDM include infection, malignant tumors, thrombosis, phlebitis, and major heart problems. Any conditions that may be worsened by increased fluid circulation warrant caution when applying LDM. This includes people with kidney problems, asthma, thyroid conditions, those receiving chemotherapy, and menstruating women.

NATURE OF LDM

Lymphatic drainage massage (LDM) is a specialized form of Western massage. To the casual observer, LDM techniques resemble the milder manipulations of classic Western massage, especially light effluerage. However, closer examination reveals that LDM is considerably more exact, following a specific sequence of application and using techniques specially designed to improve lymph drainage (Wittinger & Wittinger 1986).

Application of Techniques

Reihl (2000) lists five things that a practitioner should know before applying LDM techniques: correct pressure, direction, rhythm, sequence, and contraindications.

Pressure is very light, and only enough to cause traction so that the superficial surface of the skin moves over the underlying tissues. That is about 1–4 ounces of pressure. Pressure is applied as the hand moves toward the node, and then released as the hand returns to its original spot before repeating the movement.

Direction of the active part of the stroke is toward the targeted lymph node. The skin is stretched in the desired direction and then released so that it "snaps back" to its original spot. There is a rest (i.e., zero pressure) phase after each stroke to let lymph move through the vessels.

There is a certain **rhythm** to LDM movements as lymph is pushed along in the vessel. It is created by alternating an active (pressure) phase and a passive (no pressure) phase in a repetitive rhythm. Each stroke is repeated 6–8 times in a rhythmic pattern.

LDM sessions proceed in a specific **sequence** to ensure optimal drainage of lymphatic vessels. Figures 14–2 and 14–3 illustrate the body's overall and superficial lymph drainage pathways. A general description of the process is provided by Kurz et al. (1978):

> The massage starts at the left supraclavicular space, draining the ductus thoracicus into the venae axillaris and subclavia. Next the stagnation created at the regional lymph nodes, either inguinal or subaxillar, is gently alleviated. Finally, the proximal, then the distal parts of the limbs are massaged (p. 767).

LDM TECHNIQUES

Specific techniques used to effect the movement of lymph are described in more detail below. The CD ROM included with this text, and instructional videos listed at the end of the chapter in "additional resources" offer visual demonstration of LDM techniques which are difficult to describe in words.

Note that lymphatic drainage massage is best learned from qualified people in special training programs. Demonstrations and supervised practice of techniques will assure that the student has acquired the skill to perform LDM techniques safely. Only properly trained practitioners should use LDM to address serious medical conditions such as lymphedema. Websites for information regarding training programs is provided at the end of the chapter.

Four examples of LDM techniques will be described here. They are based on classic techniques of the Vodder method. The techniques are used to gently move lymph fluid into and through the initial lymphatic vessels. These techniques are performed in combinations of round or oval, small or large, deep or shallow circular movements. The techniques described here are stationary circles, the pump, scoop, and rotary techniques.

Stationary Circles

The fingertip pads are placed flat on the skin using just enough pressure to create traction and move superficial skin layers. Fingertips move in "stationary circles," meaning that fingertips return to the starting place once a circular movement has been completed, and repeat the circles 6–8 times in the same place before moving on. They may also be applied as expanding spirals. Stationary circles are commonly applied to the neck, face, and lymph nodes.

Stationary circles may also be performed on the body and extremities by making circles hand on hand or with eight fingers placed next to each other. In the latter case, the fingers move the skin circularly in one direction working together as shown in Figure 14–4. The direction of movement is determined by the lymph drainage direction desired. The fingers lie flat. Each of these circles is executed with a gentle pressure on the tissue to create traction, movement in the direction desired, and a release of pressure as the fingers move back to their original position.

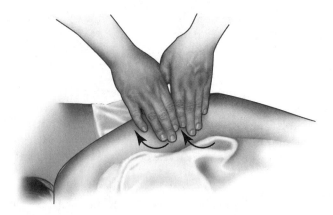

FIGURE 14–4. Stationary circles, lymphatic drainage massage technique.

Scoop Technique

The **scoop technique** is designed for the extremities. It is performed on the arm in Figure 14–5. The scoop is described as a "giving motion" since the practitioner gently moves the skin toward the recipient (distal to proximal). The flexion and extension of the wrist effects a corkscrew movement of the wrist–hand unit. The fingers are outstretched and swing toward the body, moving the skin in the direction of the axillary lymph nodes for the arm, and the inguinal nodes for the leg.

Pump Technique

The **pump technique** is designed for rounded surfaces like the anterior thigh. The thumb is abducted and the skin contacted in the "V" formed between the thumb and index finger, as well as with flats of the fingers. In the pump technique, the thumb and fingers move forward together stretching the skin, and then release pressure as the hand moves to the next spot. The technique is performed with exaggerated movements of the wrist, which acts like a hinge. The fingers are outstretched; the fingertips have no function in this technique. The forward motion of the fingers is carried out under pressure, the hinge motion of the wrist without pressure.

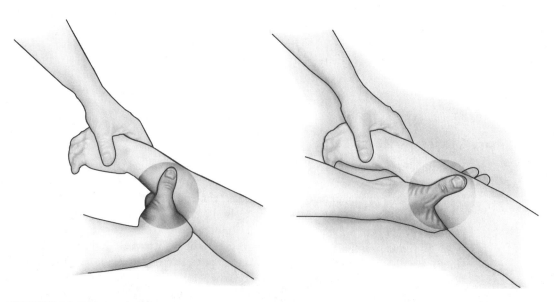

FIGURE 14–5. Scoop, lymphatic drainage massage technique.

Rotary Technique

The rotary technique is used on relatively broad areas of the body such as the back. Palms and fingers lie flat on the skin. The wrists move up and down in various degrees of extension during the application. As they press downward, the fingers swing from the outside toward the inside (i.e., lateral to medial) applying light pressure to the skin. The thumb also makes circular movements in the direction of the lymph drainage. In the pressureless phase the wrist is raised, and the four outstretched fingers move back into position to repeat the movement.

Other Vodder techniques are described in *Compendium of Dr. Vodder's Manual Lymph Drainage.* These include special techniques like the long journey, the rabbit technique, seven technique, colon treatment and panniculose technique (Kasseroller 1998).

BASIC PRINCIPLES OF LDM

The following are some basic principles to keep in mind when performing lymphatic drainage massage. (Adapted from Kurz (1986, 1990), and Reihl (2000).)

- Lymph is pushed toward the nodes in a specific sequence.
- The area proximal to a node is treated before the distal area so that the proximal area is emptied to make room for the fluid flowing in from the distal end.
- Pressure is limited to just enough to move the skin, about 1–4 ounces.
- With each movement the skin is stretched with enough intensity that it "snaps back" when released.
- There is a rest or zero pressure phase after each stroke to let lymph move through the vessels.
- The techniques and variations are repeated rhythmically, usually six to eight times, either at the same location in stationary circles or in expanding spirals. The inertial mass of the tissue fluid needs time and repetition before it responds.
- The pressure phase of a circle lasts longer than the relaxation phase.
- As a rule, reddening of the skin should <u>not</u> appear.
- Techniques should <u>not</u> elicit pain.

APPLICATION OF LDM

The effect of LDM is largely derived from the mechanical displacement of fluids and the substances they carry. It is important that the manual techniques be executed precisely, with sensitivity in palpation of tissues, and following the superficial lymph pathways. Experience shows that the more exact the technique, the better the results.

The amount of pressure to use when applying LDM techniques depends largely on the condition of tissues to be treated. One could say the softer the tissue, the softer the massage.

There are only general rules about the length of time to spend on a particular body part, the amount of pressure to use, and the pace of movements. Theoretical lessons are meant to explain the effect of LDM and providing background for an understanding of its value and use. However, in practice, no two clients are identical. Ultimately, the dosage of LDM is best determined by practitioners using their knowledge, skill, experience, and intuition. Any description of LMD must be read and understood with this in mind.

SUMMARY

Lymphatic drainage massage (LDM) refers to systems of soft tissue manipulation designed to assist the function of the lymphatic system. LDM techniques consist of gentle, slow, repetitive strokes performed in a specific direction and sequence to enhance lymph circulation. It is a precise and rhythmic massage used for general wellness, to enhance healing, and to treat lymphedema.

The history of lymphatic drainage massage includes the work of several people who developed treatments for lymphedema including Alexander von Winiwarter, a German surgeon (1890); Emil and Astid Vodder who developed Manual Lymph Drainage (MLD) in the 1930s; and Michael and Ethel Foldi, who developed Complete Decongestive Therapy (CDT) in the 1970s.

Today, LDM is also used to enhance soft tissue healing, in sports massage, and is offered in spas as a beauty aid.

Lymph fluid movement is essential for proper immune function, tissue repair, and cellular health. About 10 percent of interstitial fluid is returned to circulation via the lymph vessels. Lymph fluid contains various molecules and particles that enter the system through lymphatic capillaries called initial lymphatics. Initial lymphatic walls are one cell thick, and particles enter these tiny vessels through overflaps that open upon movement in superficial layers of the skin. This is the basis of LDM techniques. Lymph then flows to pre-collector vessels, and collectors where it is pushed along in lymphangions or smooth muscle segments, and through lymph nodes. Major lymph node clusters are found in the head, neck, chest, abdomen, axillary (armpit), and groin.

Indications for LDM include allergies, arthritis, colds, colitis, edema, sinus congestion, psoriasis, and lymphedema. Contraindications include infection, malignant tumors, thrombosis, phlebitis, and heart disease. Caution should be used with people with kidney disease, asthma, thyroid conditions, those receiving chemotherapy, and menstruating women.

LDM techniques should be applied with correct pressure, direction, rhythm, and sequence. Examples of classic lymphatic techniques include stationary circles, scoop, pump, and rotary. Basic principles for technique application include using just enough pressure to cause traction and move the skin, letting the skin "snap back" after stretching, repeating each movement 6–8 times in a rhythmic manner, and allowing a brief rest phase between movements. Lymph is moved in a specific sequence toward a lymph node, and application is proximal to distal in relation to the node. There should not be reddening in the area or pain.

LDM is best learned from qualified teachers who can supervise practice, and practitioners should receive special training before applying LDM on patients with lymphedema. Exact application and dosage of LDM is best determined by knowledge, skill, experience, and intuition.

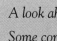

A look ahead . . .

Some contemporary systems of massage and bodywork are based on theories outside of standard bioscience. Although these systems are difficult to explain in scientific terms, many people have found them to have therapeutic value. Chapter 15 takes a look at one such system that combines a theory called zone therapy and compression massage of the feet.

REFERENCES

Berube, R. (1988). *Evolutionary traditions: Unique approaches to lymphatic drainage & circulatory massage techniques.* Hudson, NH: Robert Berube.

Kasseroller, R. (1998). *Compendium of Dr. Vodder's manual lymph drainage.* Heidelberg: Karl F. Haug Verlag.

Kelly, D. G. (2002). *A primer on lymphedema.* Upper Saddle River, NJ: Prentice Hall.

Kurz, W., Wittlinger, G., Litmanovitch, Y. I., et al. (1978). Effect of manual lymph drainage massage on urinary excretion of neurohormones and minerals in chronic lymphedema. *Angiology, 29,* 64–72.

Kurz, I. (1986). *Introduction to Dr. Vodder's manual lymphatic drainage.* Vol. 2, Therapy 1. Heidelberg: Haug Publishers.

Kurz, I. (1990). *Introduction to Dr. Vodder's manual lymphatic drainage.* Vol. 3, Therapy 2. Heidelberg: Haug Publishers.

Reihl, S. (2000). "Lymphatic drainage massage." An instructional video by Sean Reihl. Real Bodywork.

Wittinger, H., & Wittinger, G. (1986). *Introduction to Dr. Vodder's manual lymphatic drainage.* Vol. 1, 3rd rev. ed. Heidelberg: Haug Publishers.

ADDITIONAL RESOURCES

Instructional Videos

"Lymphatic drainage massage." (2000). Santa Barbara, CA: Real Bodywork. (*www.deeptissue.com*)

WEBSITES

Academy of Lymphatic Studies in Sebastian, Florida (*www.acols.com*)
Dr. Vodder School North America in Victoria, BC, Canada (*www.vodderschool.com*)
Lymphatic Research Foundation (*www.lymphaticresearch.org*)
National Lymphedema Network (*www.lymphnet.org*)

STUDY GUIDE

LEARNING OUTCOMES

Use the learning outcomes at the beginning of the chapter as a guide to your studies. Perform the task given in each outcome using the information in the chapter. This may start as an "open book" exercise, and then later from memory.

KEY TERMS/CONCEPTS

To study the key concept and terminology listed at the beginning of this chapter, choose one or more of the following exercises. Writing or talking about ideas helps you remember them better, and explaining them helps deepen your understanding.

1. Write a one- or two-sentence definition of each key work or concept.

2. Choose two or three key words that are related and explain the relationship.

3. Explain to a study partner the structure and function of initial lymphatics (Figure 14–1), lymph system vessels (Figure 14–2), and lymph node clusters (Figure 14–3) and their significance in lymphatic drainage massage.

4. Tell a study partner about the historical background of lymphatic drainage massage, and the important people in its development. Who were von Winiwarter, the Vodders, the Foldis? When and where did they work?

STUDY OUTLINE

The following questions test your memory of the main concepts in this chapter. Locate the answers in the text using the page number given for each question.

1. Lymphatic drainage massage (LDM) is a system of soft tissue manipulation designed to assist the function of the _____. (p. 269)

2. LDM techniques consist of _____, _____, and _____ strokes performed in a specific sequence that enhances _____ circulation. (p. 269)

3. LDM is a precise and rhythmic massage used for general _____, to enhance _____, and to treat _____. (p. 269)

History of Lymphatic Drainage Massage

1. As early as 18_____, research on the effects of massage showed its benefits for increasing lymph flow. (p. 269)

2. In the 1890s _____ of Germany treated lymphedema with cleanliness, compression, exercise and massage. (p. 269)

3. In 1930s, Danish physiotherapists _____ developed a precise method of _____ (MLD) while living and working in France. (p. 269)

4. Most modern systems of lymphatic drainage massage are based on _____. (p. 269)

5. In the 1970s Hungarian physicians _____ developed a comprehensive system for treating lymphedema called _____ (CDT). (p. 269)

6. Recent increase in _____ patients has led to a renewed interest in CDT and lymphatic drainage massage. (p. 269)

7. Recently the use of LDM has broadened to include _____ healing, _____ massage, and as a _____ aid in spas. (p. 269)

Lymphatic System and LDM

1. About _____ percent of interstitial fluid is reabsorbed through the blood capillaries, and _____ percent through lymphatic vessels. (p. 269)

2. Lymph is a clear colorless fluid that contains water, _____ molecules, cellular _____, and _____ acids. (p. 269)

3. Lymphatic vessels are responsible for the _____, _____, and _____ of lymph fluid. (p. 269)

4. Initial lymphatic vessel walls are _____ thick with openings between cells to allow fluids and large molecules to enter. Their cell junctions overlap to create one-way _____ to prevent _____. (p. 269)

5. Opening of initial lymphatic flaps can be caused by increase in _____ fluid, and aided by mechanical stimulation such as gentle skin _____ that tugs on the anchoring filaments. (p. 270)

6. _____ pressure closes the flaps and slows or stops the flow of lymph; therefore, LDM techniques are applied with very _____ pressure. (p. 270)

7. Lymph fluid continues to move to larger and larger vessels called _____ and _____ vessels. (p. 270)

8. Lymph is moved along in collector vessels by _____ that act like little heartbeats contracting sequentially. (p. 270)

9. Lymphangions may be stimulated to contract by the _____ action of LDM. (p. 270)

10. Lymph nodes facilitate the _____ response, and are designed for _____ production and circulation. (p. 270)

Indications and Contraindications

1. LDM is used to treat a number of conditions that improve with better lymph drainage, e.g., allergy symptoms, _____, colds, _____, edema, sinus _____, _____, and lymphedema. (p. 271)

2. LDM can enhance healing of _____ injuries. (p. 271)

3. _____ is the abnormal accumulation of lymph fluid in tissues. (p. 271)

4. Contraindications to LDM include _____, _____, _____, _____, _____. (p. 272)

LDM TECHNIQUES

1. LDM requires special training to perform safely and effectively, especially with _____ patients. (p. 273)

2. Classic LDM techniques include stationary _____, _____, _____, and _____ techniques. (p. 273)

3. Stationary circles are performed with _____ pads. (p. 273)

4. The scoop technique is described as a _____ motion, with rotating movement from the wrist. (p. 274)

5. In the pump technique, the wrist moves like a hinge to push the fingers forward _____ the skin. (p. 274)

6. The rotary technique is used on relatively _____ areas of the body, and is performed primarily with the palms and thumbs moving along with up-and-down wrist motion. (p. 275)

Basic Principles of LDM

1. Lymph is pushed toward the nodes in a specific _____. (p. 275)

2. Proximal body areas are treated before _____ areas in relation to lymph nodes. (p. 275)

3. Pressure is limited to just enough to _____. (p. 275)

4. LDM techniques are applied with enough pressure that the skin _____ when released. (p. 275)

5. There is a zero _____ phase after each stroke. (p. 275)

6. Techniques are repeated _____ for _____ to _____ times. (p. 275)

7. _____ of the skin should not appear. (p. 275)

8. Techniques should not elicit _____. (p. 275)

Application of LDM

1. The effects of LDM are largely derived from the mechanical displacements of _____ and _____. (p. 275)

2. In applying techniques, the softer the tissues, the _____ the pressure should be. (p. 275)

3. There are theoretical general rules for application of LDM, but in real practice practitioners use their _____, _____, _____, and _____ to determine the length of time to spend on a particular body region, the amount of pressure to use, and the pace of the movements. (p. 275)

FOR GREATER UNDERSTANDING

The following exercises are designed to take you from the realm of theory into practical applications. They will help give you a deeper understanding of the techniques covered in this chapter. Action words are underlined to emphasize the variety o activities presented to address different learning styles, and to encourage deeper thinking.

1. After reading this chapter, review an instructional video demonstrating LDM techniques. Describe the application of techniques to a study partner. Did the system shown follow the general guidelines outlined in the chapter?

2. Receive an LDM session from a specially trained practitioner. Describe your experience to a study partner, comparing it to what you expected after reading this chapter. Be specific regarding similarities and differences.

3. Look through a magazine or journal targeted for massage therapists. Are there any ads for LDM training? How do they describe LDM? If they give Web sites, visit the site for more information about the system and the training.

4. Search the Web for LDM systems and training. List and describe what you discovered.

5. Interview an LDM practitioner. Ask them what system they studied, the name of their teacher, and where they got their training and how long it was. Ask them how they like the work, and how it differs from performing other kinds of massage. How do they incorporate LDM into their practice? How do clients benefit from receiving LDM?

6. Take an introductory training in an LDM system. Practice techniques learned on a partner. Describe your experience learning the techniques.

7. Interview someone who receives LDM for a medical condition. Ask them about benefits they experience from the LDM sessions.

8. Search a research database for studies related to lymphatic drainage massage. Make a list of studies and their findings, and report to a study partner or group.

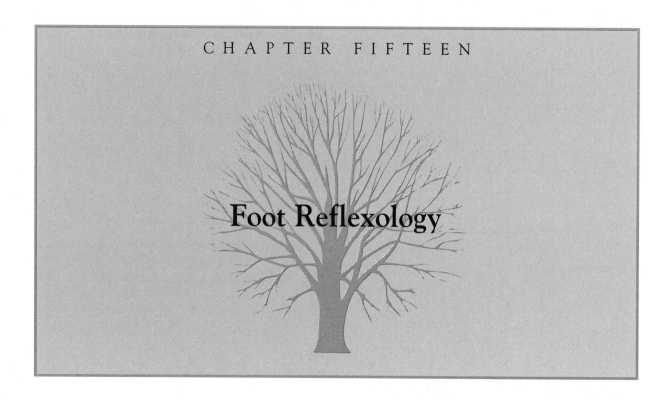

CHAPTER FIFTEEN

Foot Reflexology

LEARNING OUTCOMES

After studying this chapter, the student will have information to:

1. Discuss the history of reflexology including the contributions of Eunice Ingham.
2. Explain various theories about how reflexology works including zone therapy.
3. Relate areas of the feet to their corresponding parts of the body.
4. Position the client to receive a reflexology session.
5. Use good body mechanics when performing foot reflexology.
6. Perform basic reflexology techniques.

HISTORICAL PEOPLE AND DEVELOPMENTS

Egyptian	Ingham, Eunice	Riley, Joseph
Fitzgerald, William		

KEY TERMS/CONCEPTS

Direct finger pressure	Hook and backup	Squeezing
Finger walking	Reflexology charts	Thumb walking
Foot reflexology	Semi-reclining	Zone therapy

 MEDIALINK

A companion CD-ROM, included free with each new copy of this book, supplements the techniques presented in this chapter. Insert the CD-ROM to watch video clips of massage techniques being demonstrated. This multimedia feature is designed to help you add a new dimension to your learning.

Foot reflexology is based on the theory that pressure applied to specific spots on the feet stimulates corresponding areas in other parts of the body. For example, pressing the center of the big toe is believed to stimulate the pituitary gland, and pressing the ball of the foot affects the lungs. The stimulation is thought to help normalize function and increase circulation in the part of the body targeted.

Maps of the feet, like the one in Figure 15–1, help practitioners identify which part of the body is being stimulated as they press different spots on the foot. Practitioners use reflexology as part of a full-body or foot massage, or may perform an entire session using the theory and techniques of foot reflexology.

HISTORY OF REFLEXOLOGY

Massaging or pressing into the soft tissues of the feet is an ancient health practice found in many parts of the world, including India and China. A wall painting found in an ancient **Egyptian** tomb depicts two seated men receiving foot massage. The painting is from the tomb of an Egyptian priest named Ankhmahor in about 2200 BCE (Calvert 2002, p. 28).

Modern foot reflexology has its origin in the work of **Eunice Ingham** (1889–1974) and her system combining zone therapy with compression massage of the feet. Ingham was a physiotherapist who lived in Rochester, New York and wintered in St. Petersburg, Florida. When in Florida, she worked for an eclectic natural healer named **Joseph Shelby Riley,** who introduced her to zone therapy. Zone therapy was popularized in the early 1900s by **William Fitzgerald,** a respected physician and prominent nose and throat surgeon at St. Francis Hospital in Hartford, Connecticut. His book, *Zone Therapy,* was published in 1917. The theory of zone therapy is explained below.

Ingham is credited with taking the theory of zone therapy and combining it with compression of the soft tissues of the feet to develop the prototype for systems of reflexology practiced today. Through clinical experience, she was able to make a detailed map of the feet and chart the areas of the body affected at each spot.

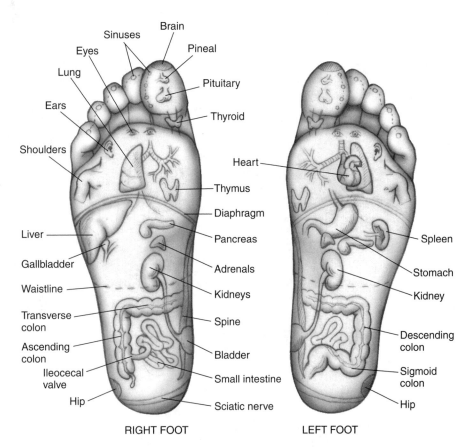

RIGHT FOOT   LEFT FOOT

FIGURE 15–1. Reflexology chart showing location of spots with corresponding anatomical structures and organs affected.

Ingham developed her method of reflexology in the 1930–1940s before World War II. In the 1950–1960s, she traveled across the United States by car, teaching her methods in workshops. Her primary audience in those early days was from the ranks of natural healers, and masseurs and masseuses (Benjamin 1989 a,b).

By the end of the 20th century, reflexology had spread to countries all over the world. Links to Web sites for reflexology organizations in different parts of the globe can be found at www.reflexology.org. Reflexology has also been adopted by massage and bodywork practitioners, who use it as an adjunct to standard Western massage.

THEORIES OF REFLEXOLOGY

Explanations of how reflexology works are generally outside of the realm of biomedicine, and are speculation at this point. However, some controlled studies have been done and citations for them can be found on the Internet (www.reflexology-research.com). The following are historical and alternative ways of looking at reflexology.

Modern foot reflexology was derived from the theory of **zone therapy.** According to this theory, the body can be thought of as divided lengthwise into 10 zones, 5 on each side of the body. See Figure 15–2. The longitudinal zones have endpoints in the feet, hands, and top of the head.

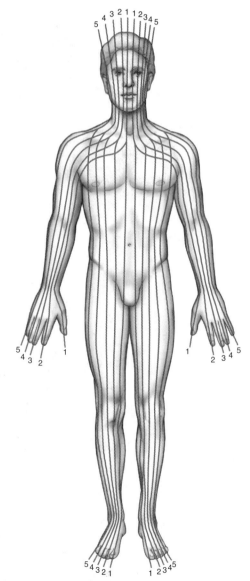

FIGURE 15–2. Longitudinal zones of the body according to Dr. W. Fitzgerald, writing on zone therapy in 1917. There are 10 zones, 5 on each side of the body.

The theory is that pressure applied anywhere in the zone affects the entire zone. Direct pressure on the endpoints will produce reflex actions along the whole length of their corresponding zones. Therefore, pressure applied to the feet can affect structures and organs in other parts of the body. The feet have proven an especially sensitive and easily accessed place to apply pressure for zone therapy.

Reflexology charts of the feet are derived from zone therapy, and show which spots on the feet to press to affect specific structures and organs in the zones. These maps provide a useful reference tool for practitioners (Figure 15–1).

Eunice Ingham believed that the techniques of reflexology dissolved crystalline deposits in the feet. These deposits were thought to interfere with nerve and blood supplies (Ingham, 1938).

Another view holds that the feet are a "mirror image of the body, [which] reflects any disturbances in the body's equilibrium in the form of blockages of the zones" (Kunz and Kunz 1991, p. 18). According to this theory, zonal blockages manifest as either internal or external blockages, e.g., pooling of lymph fluid. Reflexology restores balance to the body as described below:

> Reflexology is aimed at restoring lost balance. This is achieved through stimulating the reflexes in the feet to cause a relaxation in the corresponding body part. Improved circulation brings in the needed elements to repair and equalize the environment. The glands and organs in turn seek their equilibrium. The chain is completed . . . Reflexology acts on the body to release it to do its complex job of maintaining its many operations (Kunz and Kunz, 1982, p. 17).

Some believe that zones are more like the energy meridians of Chinese medicine, and that reflexology helps keep energy flowing freely. According to these theories, "stimulation to specific points activates the movement of energy to corresponding parts of the body to clear out congestion and restore normal functioning" (Knaster, 1996, p. 310).

Regardless of the theory used to explain the mechanism behind reflexology, many find it to be effective for improving good health and as a complementary treatment for certain pathologies.

POSITIONING THE RECEIVER

Foot reflexology can be given with the recipient lying supine like during standard Western massage. If the session is devoted entirely to reflexology, the receiver might be more comfortable in a **semi-reclining** position propped up with pillows on the massage table. Some massage tables have hinged tops that can be adjusted to create a back rest for a semi-reclining client. Recliner chairs that tilt back and lift the legs can also be used for reflexology.

A bolster placed under the knees will take the pressure off of knee joints. It can also raise the receiver's legs for better body mechanics for the practitioner.

BODY MECHANICS

Regardless of the position of the receiver, the practitioner should observe proper body mechanics, including good head, neck and back alignment. Sitting on a chair is preferred when performing reflexology. Avoid bending the back and neck to reach the recipient's feet. Adjust table height, bolsters under the legs, and practitioner chair or stool height to achieve proper alignment. Review good body mechanics for sitting, as shown in Figure 6–21.

TECHNIQUES

The basic technique of foot reflexology is **direct pressure.** A special technique called **thumb walking** is used to apply pressure quickly and systematically to points along the bottom of the feet.

To practice thumb walking, hold the back of the foot with one hand while the other hand performs the technique. An alternative is to bend the toes back with one hand while thumb

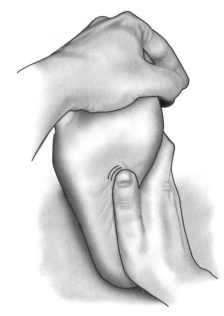

FIGURE 15–3. Thumb walking.

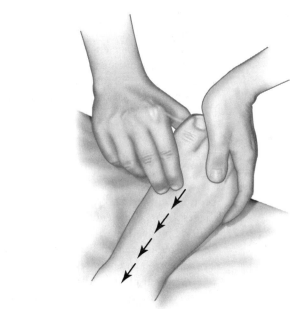

FIGURE 15–4. Finger walking.

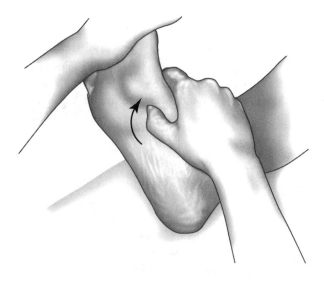

FIGURE 15–5. Hook and backup technique.

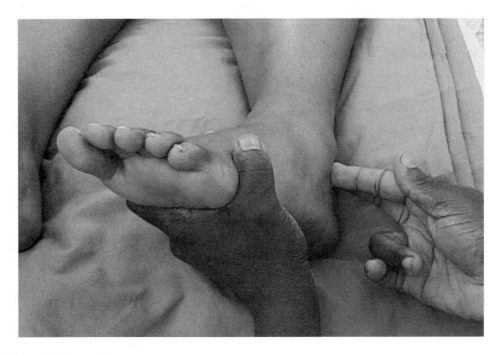

FIGURE 15–6. Direct fingertip pressure.

walking with the other hand. Starting at the heel of the foot on the lateral side, "walk" your thumb up the foot to the toes. To do this bend the thumb at the first joint, press into the tissues, then straighten the thumb and move to the next spot. This action is repeated as the thumb "walks" in line along the foot. Pressure is applied with the edge of the thumb just to the side of the nail. See Figure 15–3.

Thumb walking is rhythmical and steady. The application of pressure is enhanced by using the four fingers of the working hand in opposition to the thumb. The holding hand can also assist by pressing the foot into the thumb as the thumb is "walking." Thumb walk in parallel lines from heel to toes covering the entire foot bottom, and also up the sides and across the ball of the foot.

The walking technique can also be applied with the fingers. **Finger walking** is useful for applying pressure to the top of the foot between the metatarsals as shown in Figure 15–4.

The **hook and backup** technique is used to apply deep pressure to a specific spot. Locate the spot you wish to press, place your thumb directly on the spot, and bend the first joint to apply pressure. Then pull the thumb to the side across the spot to deepen the pressure as shown in Figure 15–5.

Spots around the ankle can be stimulated with direct pressure with the fingertips (Figure 15–6). The **squeezing** technique is effective for spots on the toes, for example, for stimulating the sinuses via the pads of the toes as demonstrated in Figure 15–7.

These basic reflexology techniques can be combined with foot massage and joint movements to stimulate reflex points and their corresponding zones. More detailed information on reflexology can be found in textbooks devoted to the subject. (Refer to *Better Health with Foot Reflexology* by Dwight Byers; *The Complete Guide to Foot Reflexology* by Kevin and Barbara Kunz; *Feet First: A Guide to Foot Reflexology* by Laura Norman and Thomas Cowan.)

SUMMARY

Foot reflexology is based on the theory that pressure applied to specific spots on the feet stimulate corresponding areas in other parts of the body. This stimulation is thought to normalize function and increase circulation in the part of the body targeted.

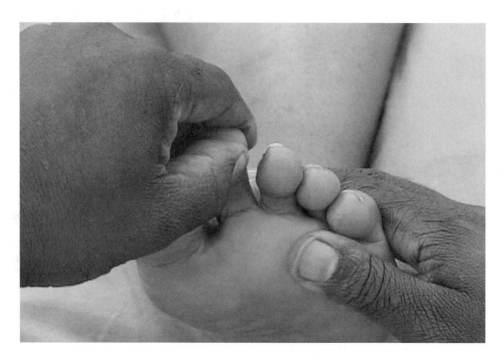

FIGURE 15–7. Squeezing the pads of the toes.

Ancient civilizations in India, China and Egypt all had some form of foot massage. Modern reflexology is derived from zone theory popularized by W. Fitzgerald in the early 1900s. Eunice Ingham combined zone theory with compression massage of the feet to develop reflexology and teach it throughout the United States in the 1950–1960s. Since that time, reflexology has spread to many different countries throughout the world.

Explanations of how reflexology works are generally outside of the realm of biomedicine, and are more historical and alternative in nature at this point. However, some controlled studies have been done. According to zone therapy theory, the body is divided into 10 longitudinal zones, and pressure in any zone stimulates the entire length of the zone. Therefore, direct pressure on the zone endpoints in the feet stimulates corresponding structures and organs throughout the body. Reflexology charts map out these relationships.

Eunice Ingham believed that reflexology dissolved crystals in the feet and restored good circulation. Others believe that reflexology balances zonal blockages, or that it balances energy as in Chinese medicine.

The recipient of reflexology may be lying in a supine position, or semi-reclining on a massage table, or sitting in a recliner chair. A bolster is placed under the knees.

Practitioners sit on chairs or stools, and practice good sitting body mechanics while performing reflexology. Adjustments are made in the table height, bolsters, and practitioner's chair to achieve proper alignment.

Reflexology techniques include thumb walking, finger walking, hook and backup, fingertip pressure, and squeezing. Basic techniques can be combined with foot massage and joint movements to stimulate reflex points and their corresponding zones.

A look ahead . . .

Some contemporary forms of massage and bodywork are based on theories of energy fields that are within and surround the physical body, and that affect health and wellbeing. Chapter 16 describes techniques used to balance the body's energy field according to polarity theory, developed by Randolph Stone in the early 20th century.

REFERENCES

Benjamin, P. J. (1989a). Eunice Ingham and the development of foot reflexology in the United States. Part one: The early years—to 1946. *Massage Therapy Journal*, Spring, pp. 38–44.

Benjamin, P. J. (1989b). Eunice Ingham and the development of foot reflexology in the United States. Part two: On the road 1946–1974. *Massage Therapy Journal*, Winter, pp. 49–55.

Byers, D. C. (1997). *Better health with foot reflexology*. Revised. St. Petersburg, FL: Ingham Publishing.

Calvert, R. N. (2002). *The history of massage*. Rochestor, VT: Healing Arts Press.

Fitzgerald, W. H. & Bowers, E. F. (1917). *Zone therapy*. Columbus, OH: I.W. Long.

Ingham, E. D. (1938). *Stories the feet can tell: Stepping to better health*. Rochester, NY, author.

Knaster, M. (1996). *Discovering the body's wisdom*. New York, NY: Bantam Books.

Kunz, K. and Kunz, B. (1982). *The complete guide to foot reflexology*. Englewood Cliffs, NJ: Prentice Hall.

Norman, L. and Cowan T. (1988). *Feet first: A guide to foot reflexology*. New York: Fireside.

ADDITIONAL RESOURCES

Instructional Video

"Reflexology for the feet and hands with Geri Riehl." (2001). Santa Barbara, CA: Real Bodywork. (*www.deeptissue.com*)

"Reflexology with Rhonda Funes, Volume 1: The feet." (2001). Massage Master Class[TM] Series. Riverside, CT: At Peace Media. (*www.atpeacemedia.com*)

WEB SITES

Reflexology Research Project (*www.reflexology-research.com*)

Home of Reflexology (*reflexology.org*)

International Institute of Reflexology (*www.reflexology-usa.net*)

STUDY GUIDE

LEARNING OUTCOMES

Use the learning outcomes at the beginning of the chapter as a guide to your studies. Perform the task given in each outcome using the information in the chapter. This may start as an "open book" exercise, and then later from memory.

KEY TERMS/CONCEPTS

To study the key concept and terminology listed at the beginning of this chapter, choose one or more of the following exercises. Writing or talking about ideas helps you remember them better, and explaining them helps deepen your understanding.

1. Write a one- or two-sentence definition of each key work or concept.

2. Choose two or three key words that are related and explain the relationship.

3. In your own words, tell a study partner about the historical development of foot reflexology. When was modern reflexology developed? How are zone therapy and reflexology related? Who was Eunice Ingham? How did knowledge of reflexology spread?

4. Explain the various theories about how reflexology works to a study partner.

5. Look at a reflexology chart, and relate the location of various body structures and organs to the zones of zone therapy. Explain the logic of the charts to a study partner.

6. Using a reflexology chart, draw the various organs and structures on a partner's feet. Then see if you can accurately locate and draw them without looking at the chart. Alternate: draw on paper.

STUDY OUTLINE

The following questions test your memory of the main concepts in this chapter. Locate the answers in the text using the page number given for each question.

1. Foot reflexology is based on the theory that _____ applied to specific spots on the feet stimulates corresponding areas in _____. (p. 281)

2. This action is thought to help normalize _____ and increase _____ in the part of the body targeted. (p. 281)

History of Reflexology

1. Massaging or pressing the feet for health and healing is an old practice found in many parts of the world including ancient _____, _____, and _____. (p. 281)

2. William Fitzgerald, MD popularized a treatment called _____ (1917) that served as the theoretical base for modern reflexology. (p. 281)

3. _____, a physiotherapist and natural healer, is credited with taking the theory of _____ therapy and combining it with _____ massage of the feet to develop the prototype for reflexology systems today. (p. 281)

4. Through _____ experience, she was able to make a detailed _____ of the feet and chart which areas of the body were affected by pressure on specific spots on the feet. (p. 281)

Theories of Reflexology

1. Theories of reflexology are generally outside of the realm of _____, and are more _____ at this point. (p. 282)

2. _____ studies about the effectiveness of reflexology have been conducted in recent years. (p. 282)

3. According to zone therapy theory, the body is divided _____ into _____ zones. (p. 282)

4. These zones have endpoints in the _____, _____, and _____. (p. 282)

5. Pressure applied anywhere in the zone affects the _____ zone. (p. 283)

6. Reflexology charts show which areas of the feet correspond to _____ (p. 283)

7. Ingham believed that reflexology dissolved _____ deposits in the feet. (p. 283)

8. Other believe that reflexology balances _____. (p. 283)

Positioning the Receiver

1. Recipients of reflexology can be lying _____ on a massage table, or propped up with pillows into a _____ position. (p. 283)

2. Recipients may also sit in a _____ chair. (p. 283)

3. A bolster is placed under _____ to take pressure off of the _____ joints. (p. 283)

Body Mechanics

1. The preferred position for the practitioner performing reflexology is _____. (p. 283)

2. Avoid bending the _____ and _____ to reach the recipient's feet. (p. 283)

3. To achieve good body alignment adjust the _____, _____, and _____. (p. 283)

Techniques

1. The basic technique of foot reflexology is _____. (p. 283)

2. Thumb _____ technique is used to apply pressure quickly and systematically to points along the bottoms of the feet. (p. 283)

3. Finger _____ is useful to apply pressure to the tops of the feet. (p. 285)

4. The _____ and _____ technique is used to apply deep pressure to a specific spot. (p. 285)

5. Spots around the ankles can be pressed using _____ pressure. (p. 285)

6. The _____ technique is used for the pads of the toes. (p. 285)

FOR GREATER UNDERSTANDING

The following exercises are designed to take you from the realm of theory into practical applications. They will help give you a deeper understanding of the information covered in this chapter. Action words are underlined to emphasize the variety of activities presented to address different learning styles, and to encourage deeper thinking.

1. Receive a reflexology session from a certified practitioner. Notice how they conduct the session. What did reflexology feel like? Did you notice any reaction to the techniques in the rest of your body? Write up or discuss your findings with a study partner.

2. Interview a certified reflexologist. Ask them about their training, their practice, and types of clients they work with. What kind of results do they experience?

3. Observe a certified practitioner perform reflexology. Notice their body mechanics, and the techniques they use. Describe what you saw to a study partner. (Alternative: Watch an instructional video.)

4. Review a clinical study(s) about reflexology. What was the study trying to find out? How was it conducted? What were the findings? Conclusions? Write a summary of the research.

5. Practice reflexology techniques on a partner. Ask for feedback about how it feels. Have an observer comment on your body mechanics and technique application.

6. Take an introductory course in reflexology from a qualified teacher.

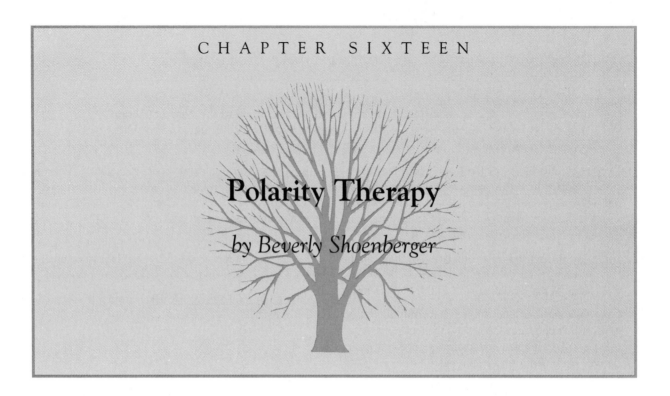

CHAPTER SIXTEEN

Polarity Therapy

by Beverly Shoenberger

LEARNING OUTCOMES

After studying this chapter, the student will have information to:

1. Trace the origins of polarity therapy, its connection to India and the work of Randolph Stone.
2. Describe the physiological effects of polarity therapy, and its benefits in terms of Western science.
3. Explain the basic principles of polarity therapy including energy, love, removing obstructions, understanding, and nutrition and exercise.
4. Perform basic polarity techniques and movements.

HISTORICAL PEOPLE AND DEVELOPMENTS

Ayurvedic medicine	Pannetier, Pierre	Stone, Randolph

KEY TERMS/CONCEPTS

Energy	Nutrition and exercise	Removing obstructions
Love	Polarity therapy	Understanding

 MEDIALINK

A companion CD-ROM, included free with each new copy of this book, supplements the techniques presented in this chapter. Insert the CD-ROM to watch video clips of massage techniques being demonstrated. This multimedia feature is designed to help you add a new dimension to your learning.

Polarity therapy is a holistic health practice involving exercises, nutrition, and love, as well as gentle bodywork techniques. Polarity techniques involve simple touching and gentle movements. The practitioner always has both hands on the receiver's body, either resting them in specific places, rocking the body, or rhythmically pressing in at various depths. These touches are designed to release obstructions to the free flow of energy through the body, so that the person is supported in returning to health.

HISTORY AND PHILOSOPHY

Polarity therapy was developed by **Randolph Stone** (1890–1981) in the mid-1900s. He was trained in the natural healing methods of chiropractic, naturopathy, and osteopathy. Stone was intrigued by the thought that there must be a basic principle underlying the effectiveness of diet change, manipulations, exercise, and other natural cures. Why did the same health problem respond positively to diet change in one person, spinal manipulation in another, and exercise in another? Why did some people seem predisposed to illness, whereas others seemed to have an innate vitality?

The search for this underlying principle led Stone to study Chinese acupuncture and herbal medicine, the Hermetic Kabalistic systems of the Middle East, and the ancient **Ayurvedic medicine** of India. In each of these traditions, he found two complementary elements, that is, the belief in a subtle form of life energy that permeates the body and gives it health, and the understanding that disease is a result of obstruction to that flow of energy. Stone theorized that all natural healing techniques are effective because they support the individual's innate capacity for health by stimulating the free and balanced flow of life energy. He combined his Western skills with techniques from all the Eastern traditions he had studied and explored them from the unique vantage point of their effect on the subtle life energy.

Stone then spent many years practicing methods for freeing energy flow and studying meditation in India. Indian philosophical framework permeates his writings on polarity therapy. The life energy is described in terms of longitudinal, horizontal, and diagonal lines of force, *chakras* (energy centers in the body), and the five elements (earth, water, fire, air, and ether). Foods, hands-on work, and exercises are discussed according to their effect on the balancing of these elements. This rather esoteric aspect of polarity therapy, along with the incorporation of chiropractic and osteopathic techniques, makes his writings difficult for the average reader. After Stone's retirement in 1973, **Pierre Pannetier** began to spread the practice of polarity therapy across the United States through seminars. Pannetier did much to systematize the series of physical mobilizations and make the more esoteric nature of Stone's work accessible to the lay practitioner. (For original writings of R. Stone, refer to *Dr. Randolph Stone's Polarity Therapy: The Complete Collected Works* by Randolph Stone, Harlan Tarbell [Illustrator], 1987; *Health Building: The Conscious Art of LivingWell* by Randolph Stone, 1991.)

However, the very eclectic nature of Stone's teaching makes it difficult to define polarity therapy. In its truest sense, polarity therapy includes anything that promotes life. Through the years, different practitioners have tended to incorporate whatever supplemental skills they might have, and rightly so, in order to best support the health of the client. Various schools of polarity therapy that have sprung up are very different from each other in style of hands-on work, amount of pressure used, emphasis on the esoteric, and supplemental skills such as training in Gestalt therapy.

Many polarity therapists emphasize the esoteric aspect of the tradition and may use this framework to explain or develop their sessions, "I am working with your fire current, as an imbalance in it is undermining the health of your sinuses." However, acceptance of the esoteric aspects is not at all essential to the practice of polarity. Pannetier often advised his students to forget their intellects, including all thoughts based on Ayurveda. He would instruct them to sense the obstructions with their hands and work intuitively in that present moment of touching, using Stone's manipulations as springboards and developing new methods as needed. There is a wealth of powerful and effective techniques in the system of polarity, and this attention to intuition is in no way meant to downplay or degrade the value of learning technique. It is simply that the practitioner must learn to go beyond the intellect's limitations into the direct experience of working with the subtle energies.

Studying polarity therapy is similar to studying music, where many scales are practiced, and new melodies and styles are learned in order to stretch the student's capacity and stimulate creativity. Theory can be a valuable aid, but is not essential. The desired end result is to play from one's heart in a responsive manner that is open to the needs of the present moment. (For further information on polarity therapy philosophy and training, visit the American Polarity Therapy Association website at www.polaritytherapy.org.

PHYSIOLOGICAL EFFECTS

Although we have yet to reach scientific understanding of what happens during polarity therapy, both givers and receivers report feeling something happening during a polarity session. There are subjective as well as objective indications that some principle not yet recognized by Western medicine is involved. For example:

- Subjectively, health is often equated with being full of energy, whereas the first sign of impending illness is often its absence.
- Subjectively, the therapist feels a definite tingling in his or her hands when doing the various movements. The degree and pattern of this tingling vary with the state of health of the area being worked, and change as the area is treated.
- Subjectively, the patient and therapist often note simultaneous changes in their sense of energy. The receiver feels freer, lighter, more relaxed; the therapist notes a balancing and strengthening of the tingling in his or her hands, and a sense of an overall increase in energy.

The polarity therapist views these changes as a response to unblocking the life energy by affecting muscular relaxation and structural change, and balancing the autonomic nervous system. Western medicine would probably say that the tingling is simply vasodilation in the hands; the talk of energy is pseudoscience; the positive health gains are a result of the placebo effect.

Yet Western science would also have to note that there are objective changes taking place. After just a few minutes of polarity therapy, signs of deep relaxation appear. Often, cheeks flush, blood pressure drops, salivation increases, the heart rate slows, the eyes may tear, and the stomach and intestines may grumble with the increase in peristalsis. These are objective signs of a relaxation response from the parasympathetic nervous system.

Closer examination reveals clear physiologic rationales for the effectiveness of many of the specific techniques. Many can be seen as stimulation to nerve centers. For example, one commonly given technique involves very light oscillating pressure over the pressure-sensitive baroreceptors in the carotid arteries along the sides of the neck. It is probable that, although the pressure is so slight as to cause no interference with the blood supply to the brain, it is sufficient to activate the neurologic reflex signal that slows the heart rate and lowers blood pressure. This same reflex is usually triggered by stretching of the baroreceptors from within when the blood pressure going to the brain is too high.

Polarity techniques often involve rocking motions of the limbs and trunk. These vary from small, gentle oscillations to large, vigorous oscillations that move the entire body. This rocking commonly induces relaxation, lowers muscle tone, reduces pain, and encourages an increase in the active range of motion afterward. Western medicine is just beginning to be aware of the tremendous benefits of this pain-free way of stimulating the joint mechanoreceptors, the nerve endings that receive messages about movements in the joints. It appears that when these receptors are gently stimulated, a reflex response will lower muscle tone, increase circulation, and stimulate endorphin release, which results in a decrease in pain sensation.

In addition, it appears that the alternating rhythmic manner with which the two hands are used and the style of touch often induce a light hypnotic state. Recipients frequently report experiencing an unusual mind state in which they feel as though every part of their body and mind were relaxed and even asleep, except for their simple awareness of sensory stimuli. This state of deepened relaxation lays the foundation for health and wellbeing by returning the body and mind to a state of balanced homeostasis. Even if only temporary, the moments of peace provided by a polarity session are a much needed experience in this stressful culture. In addition, this state of quiet awareness allows people to see their problems from a broader perspective, often seeing solutions that had previously been buried by the noisiness of the conscious mind. Hidden feelings may surface, making polarity therapy an excellent adjunct to psychotherapeutic work. Thus, although Western science does not view energy as a structurally existing entity, it would seem apparent that, functionally, the human body responds to the polarity touch in a manner that supports health of the body and mind.

It is interesting to note how many of the techniques are as easily set within the framework of modern medicine as they are within Ayurvedic philosophy. It is as though the basic principle Stone sought transcends all ideas, ancient or modern, and is instead embodied in the actual experience of the hands-on work, rather than in the particular theories used to explain it. Energy is simply an abstracted metaphor—one way of looking at the results obtained through polarity therapy. Neurologic reflex is another abstracted metaphor—a way of explaining a mechanism we cannot see, except in its effects.

PRINCIPLES OF POLARITY THERAPY

The basic principles of polarity therapy are related to the concepts of energy, love, working with obstructions, understanding, and nutrition and exercise. The following sections briefly explore these concepts in the context of polarity therapy and offer some experiential exercises.

Energy

Working with **energy** is a concept foreign to most Westerners. And yet it is not as difficult or unusual as we might expect. In Western culture, not much time or value is placed on subtle awareness of changes in the hands. A simple experiment can show how these sensations can be picked up and amplified.

Rub the palms of your hands together, waking the nerve endings and bringing your awareness to your palms. Then hold them about six inches apart; relax, and center your awareness, amplifying incoming sensory input by focusing. Experiment with moving your hands closer and farther apart to see if and how the feeling changes. Then move the hands so that the palms are no longer facing, and be aware of how they feel.

Many people find that when the palms are facing each other, there is a tingling sensation of relatedness, as though the hands were "plugging into" each other. Try the same sequence with your eyes closed; from the sensation or its absence you may know whether or not your palms are directly opposite each other.

Love

The foremost principle espoused in polarity therapy is the importance of working with love. Pannetier used to say that **love** was the most vital element of the whole session. He would say, "If you don't know what to do, just put your hands on the person and love them."

What is this love? Obviously it is not sloppy sentimentality or an overbearing affection. Beyond that, it is difficult to put into words. Trying to act in a loving manner, or matching an idea of what we think Pannetier is talking about, misses again. To really love is a matter quite different from holding an idea about love. This love of which he spoke has no objective, not even that of healing or helping someone. It is a caring so powerful that it carries with it no agenda, no end result that must be obtained.

The practitioner does his or her work simply, always responding to the felt need, and yet without attachment to healing. This love is serving life. The practitioner who "cares enough not to care," as Dylan Thomas once said, "can truly let go and trust in the universe." The seeds of this relaxation are then watered in the recipient's own being. This fosters an extremely deep state of relaxation and trust. It is in this relaxed state that healing occurs, if it is meant to be. Once the practitioner has begun to understand this principle, the rich wealth of polarity techniques can be explored, but always with the understanding that it is not the particular technique that heals. This attitude of surrender and openness, this simple "getting out of the way" of the body's inherent tendency to homeostasis allows healing on many levels. Muscles relax, digestion improves, circulation increases in areas where it is needed, hormone levels normalize, endorphins increase, breathing deepens, and so on.

A good place to begin exploring this quality of love is a simple "front-to-back" polarity technique. You will need a partner for this exercise.

Instruct your partner to sit on a stool or sideways in a chair so that the chest and thoracic area (upper back) are both easily accessible. Stand at the person's left side, and slowly and gently place your left palm over the person's heart and your right palm over the upper back between the shoulder blades. Move your hands slowly around until you feel a sensation of the palms "plugging into each other," as though they were connected by a flow of energy. See Figure 16–1. Simply hold your hands in place. Check your own posture to see that it is relaxed and that your breathing is natural and uncontrolled. After a bit, your

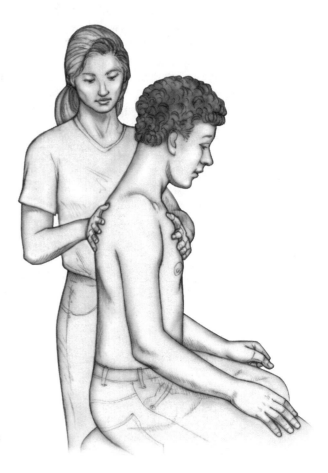

FIGURE 16–1. Feeling palms "plugging into each other."

palms may begin to tingle more or less strongly, or feel unusually warm. Some practitioners do not experience these signs, but feel an inner sense of rightness, an increasing sense of peace and completion. The experience is different for everyone. The recipient may sigh, visibly relax, and show a change in his or her breathing pattern. You may feel a change in your hands or in your mind state at about the same time. After a few minutes, very slowly withdraw your hands.

Many practitioners find that their discursive intellects are quite loud during this exercise and that they are unable to tune into their hands or their subtle feelings. They are so busy watching for results or criticizing their own efforts that awareness of subtle changes in their hands is impossible. It takes practice and a continual "letting go" on the part of the giver.

Removing Obstructions

Another principle in polarity is that obstructions to the free flow of energy must be removed for optimal results. An **obstruction** is an area of the body where there seems to be a stagnation or a holding pattern that interferes with a free flow of energy. For example, a person who is experiencing chronic anxiety may have abdominal tension, disturbed peristalsis, and nausea. Their posture may be somewhat caved in, as though they were trying to protect themselves from imminent danger. If you were to look at such a person, you might imagine that lines of energy trying to flow vertically through that person are disturbed in the abdominal-diaphragmatic area. The practitioner using polarity would respond to those obstructed areas with techniques that release tension and encourage a free flow of naturally organized and balanced energy.

An alert practitioner will begin assessing clients visually as soon as they walk in the door. They will be looking for areas that seem out of alignment, do not move with the rest of the body when the person walks, or seem held or protected. Further clues are found from the receiver's self-reports, and by palpation, as the bodywork session begins. The following exercise is designed to introduce you to the principle of finding and locating obstructions.

Have your partner lie supine, facing upward. Slowly and gently place your right palm on his or her abdomen between the navel and the pubic bone. You may sense tension or the opposite—flaccidity—in the musculature. Become alert to the breathing pattern. Does it seem restricted or unusually fast or slow? Does the breathing pattern change as you touch the person? You may sense irregularities in the skin temperature or tightness only in a certain area, as though there were a pocket of gas under your hand. Make certain that your hand, wrist, elbow, and shoulder muscles are completely relaxed, and that your own breathing is calm. The touch should be light. If you are able to relax, you can increase the pressure slightly, first with the heel of the hand and then the fingers, alternating in wavelike motion.

Leaving your right hand resting on the abdomen, place your left hand over your partner's forehead as shown in Figure 16–2. With practice, you will be able to sense whether the head is held rigidly by the neck muscles and whether the person is subtly moving toward or away from your hand. As you lightly touch, see if you can feel the sensation of your hands "plugging in" again. Feelings of warmth or tingling may begin in one or both hands. Gently rock the lower body a few minutes with the right hand, as though you were rocking a baby to sleep. The left hand should remain resting lightly on the forehead throughout, without rocking. As the sensation of being connected or tingling increases, you may see signs of an increased energy flow. Your partner's face may show more color, muscles may relax, and the breathing may deepen and become more regular. You have helped melt areas of tension, or obstructions, in the areas under and between your two hands.

Understanding

The principle of **understanding** invites the practitioner to be open to the recipient's experience and to the effects of polarity therapy. It calls for knowledge of the broader picture in terms of the physiological and psychological reactions happening in a session.

For example, in the above exercise, it is quite possible that your partner experienced the opposite of the relaxation response. At times, the muscular armoring has served an important function for the person, helping him or her to feel safer, for example. As these muscles release their tension, it is common for fear to arise. The person may be confused by this response, which can be of some magnitude. For this reason, many schools of polarity include basic counseling skills. Pannetier used a common-sense approach emphasizing a caring attitude, acceptance, and trust that whatever happens is from the "clearing of blocks" and is for the best.

Polarity is a gentle art. The giver invites the receiver to enter a deeply relaxed state and invites the muscles to relax. Nothing is ever forced. Pannetier would often say that no harm could come from polarity so long as the touch is gentle enough not to override the receiver's natural tendency to homeostasis. If the receiver wishes to enter into and pass through the feeling of obstruction, the practitioner

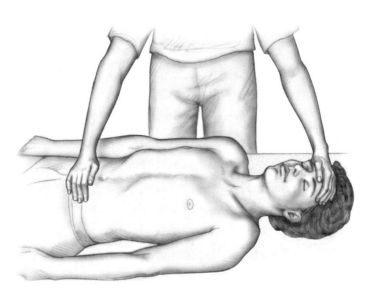

FIGURE 16–2. General position for releasing blocks in the torso and head.

will continue to work with areas of holding, deepening the relaxation, and allow the energy flow between the hands to build and balance. If the receiver wishes to pull away from the experience, reassurance can be given and alternate areas can be worked that are not threatening, perhaps building trust for work with the more tightly defended areas at a later time. It is often the case that as the receiver lets go in other areas, highly charged areas may release without his or her conscious awareness.

Thus, Pannetier would say, it is vital for the practitioner to have a proper understanding of personal responsibility. The recipient is reaping the effects of past actions and present decisions. The giver is not there to rescue the receiver, but to plant seeds of letting go and trusting, to be an accepting friend. This attitude protects the practitioner from taking on the recipient's ailments in a misguided attempt to heal.

Nutrition and Exercise

Both **nutrition and exercise** take a prominent part in the therapeutic regimen. Commonsense stretching and toning, sometimes with the addition of sounds to stimulate the flow of energy, are suggested. Their selection is again based on the Ayurvedic concepts of freeing and balancing the life energy. The specific system of exercise is loosely derived from yoga, but it has become more eclectic as teachers have incorporated their own experiences and viewpoints. The one basic stretch is the youthful pose, or squatting posture. In this position, it is said, all the currents are stimulated and the cosmic forces are attracted for health and rejuvenation.

Dietary suggestions are primarily based on Ayurvedic theory, that is, on the energetic qualities of various foods. Clients or patients are commonly led through a period of "cleansing," during which intake of certain foods is severely limited. Daily use of a liver flush, a drink made of garlic, olive oil, and lemon juice followed by specific herbal teas, is often recommended. A simple vegetarian diet is recommended for daily fare. It should be noted that the primary emphasis in polarity is on eating with a relaxed mind state, rather than on the particulars of what is eaten. Just as in hands-on work, the subtle mental aspects of diet are far more important than the material aspects and serve as a foundation for digesting and assimilation of whatever is eaten.

The emphasis on eating nutritious foods while in a relaxed state of mind and on exercising in a balanced manner is certainly basic to a Western view of health. However, the particulars are controversial, and unless one is approaching polarity in its entirety as an offshoot of Ayurvedic medicine, they are not essential to an appreciation of the hands-on technique. For this reason, the remaining section of this chapter will deal solely with the hands-on art of polarity.

BASIC POLARITY MOVEMENTS

Polarity students are typically taught a general session of 15–22 movements that serve to stimulate and balance the entire body. The gentle holding, rocking, and probing techniques form a generally relaxing session and also aid the practitioner in locating areas that appear to be obstructed and in need of further attention.

Some of these techniques are derived from osteopathy, craniopathy, and chiropractic of the 1930s and 1940s. Some were derived by Stone from observations made by psychics, from his study of acupuncture, and from Egyptian medicine. Some were derived from theories of harmonic resonance, that is, that certain parts of the body vibrate harmonically when other areas are worked. All in all, the techniques form a fascinating and rich array of moves that must be experienced in order to be appreciated.

ABBREVIATED GENERAL SESSION

What follows is an abbreviated version of a general session of polarity therapy. For simplicity, the receiver will be consistently referred to as "him." To begin, have the receiver lie on his back on the massage table, while you sit on a chair at his head.

1. **The tenth cranial (the cradle).** Overlap the last three fingers of your left hand on the last three fingers of your right hand, palms up, to form a cradle as shown in Figure 16–3. Rest your hands on the table, supporting the recipient's head in your palms. Your index fingers should extend

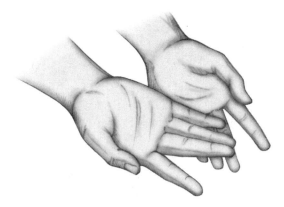

FIGURE 16-3. Hand position for the cradle.

along the grooves beside the sternocleidomastoid muscle (where the carotid artery and tenth cranial nerve travel). Rest your thumbs on your index fingers rather than over the receiver's ears. Hold 1 to 2 minutes, or until the current is strongly felt. See Figure 16-4.

2. **Neck stretch.** Rest the receiver's head on the palm of your right hand, so that your first or second finger and thumb can take a firm hold on the base of his skull. Your left hand rests lightly on his forehead with your left thumb on the anterior fontanel (the "soft spot" in an infant). With firm, steady pressure from the right hand only, apply gentle traction toward you. As the recipient exhales, slightly release; as he inhales, slightly increase the traction. This move is contraindicated if the receiver is know to be hypermobile or if there is any increase in pain in the arms, shoulders, neck, or head during the movement. See Figure 16-5.

3. **Tummy rock.** Standing on the recipient's right side, rest your left hand on his forehead and your right hand on his abdomen halfway between the navel and the pubic bone. Rock the abdomen gently, trying to tune into the person's natural "rocking rhythm." This movement was also described earlier, as a means of releasing blocks in the torso and head. See Figure 16-6.

4. **Leg pull.** Grasp both feet behind the heels and gently pull legs straight toward you several inches above the table. Rest the legs back on the table gently and place your hands over the feet for a few moments before proceeding.

5. **Inside ankle press.** You can sit on a stool at the receiver's feet if that is more comfortable for you than standing. Place the heel of your left hand on the ball of his right foot, with your fingers lightly grasping the toes. With the heel of his right foot resting in your right hand, gently press spots around the inner ankle bone (medial malleolus) with your thumb. Figure 16-7 shows performing the ankle press on the recipient's left foot, so please reverse for the right foot.

Apply rhythmic gentle compressions around the ankle bone until the points are pain free. Keeping your right hand in place, press on the ball of the foot with your left hand to flex the ankle forward (dorsiflexion). With practice, you will be able to alternate rhythmically between pressing an ankle point and flexing the ankle.

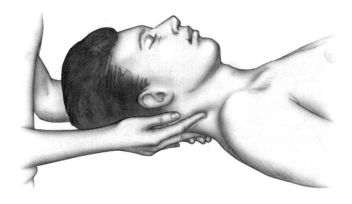

FIGURE 16-4. The cradle.

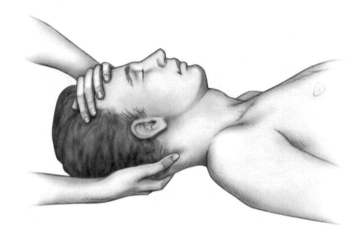

FIGURE 16–5. The neck stretch.

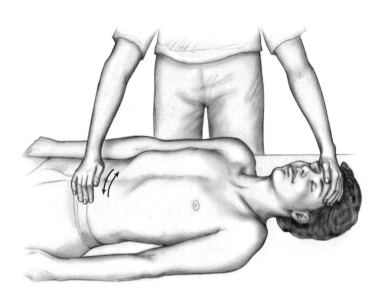

FIGURE 16–6. The tummy rock.

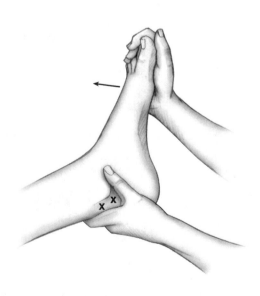

FIGURE 16–7. Inside ankle press on the left foot.

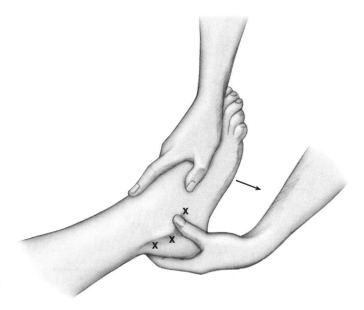

FIGURE 16–8. Outside ankle press on the right foot.

6. **Outside ankle press.** Now, support the heel of his right foot with your left hand. (If the receiver has a markedly externally rotated hip, you may need to lift the entire leg and rest it in your palm in a more neutral position in order to have the outside of the ankle accessible for work.) With your left thumb, find any tender areas along the area under the outside ankle bone (lateral malleolus). With your right hand, press the top of the foot downward (plantarflexion) giving a good stretch. Rhythmically alternate pressing and stretching the foot. See Figure 16–8.

   Note: Movements 7–11 are performed in sequence on the right side and are then repeated on the left side with instructions for left–right reversed, before moving on to movements 12–15.

7. **Pelvis and knee rock.** Hold the feet again for a moment, and move up to the person's right side. Place your left hand on his lower right abdomen, just above the thigh crease, with the fingers pointing down toward the feet. Place your right hand just above the knee. Very gently apply pressure with the right hand in a rhythmic fashion, gently rocking his leg. Continue for 10 to 30 seconds. Allow the leg to slow and then to be still. Continue holding for 30 seconds or so, again being aware of any sensations you feel. Carefully and slowly remove your hands. See Figure 16–9 for left pelvis and knee rock.

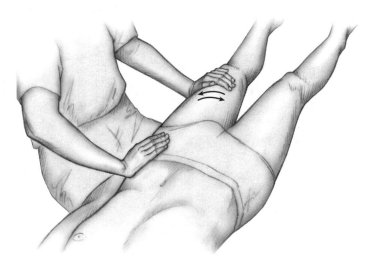

FIGURE 16–9. Left-side pelvis and knee rock.

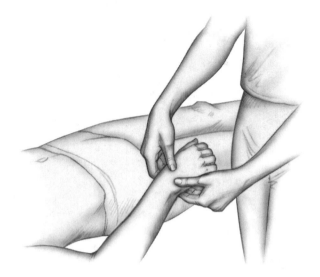

FIGURE 16–10. Arm–shoulder rotation.

8. **Arm–shoulder rotations.** Hold the receiver's right wrist as show in Figure 16–10. Controlling movement from the wrist, gently rotate the shoulder in a small circle, alternately compressing and distracting the shoulder point. Do this about 10 times toward you and 10 times away from you.
9. **Thumb web–forearm stimulation.** Using the thumb and finger of your left hand, squeeze the webbing between his thumb and finger, concentrating on any tender areas. Press the pad of your right thumb into a point one inch below the elbow crease and a half inch from the inside of his arm. Rhythmically alternate stimulation with each hand. See Figure 16–11.
10. **Elbow milk–abdomen rock.** Place your left hand under the recipient's right elbow and lay your thumb across the elbow crease. Milk upward with your thumb. Place your right hand lightly along the bottom edge of the rib cage, and gently rock the abdomen. Alternate milking and rocking, about 10 to 12 times each for about a minute. See Figure 16–12.
11. **Pelvic rock.** Place your right hand over the recipient's left hip bone (anterior superior iliac spine). Place your left hand over his right shoulder. Stabilizing the shoulder girdle with your left hand, gently rock the trunk with the right. Gradually increase the rocking movement for 20 seconds, and then gradually decrease. Hold for a moment before moving on. See Figure 16–13.

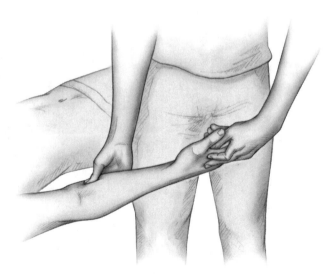

FIGURE 16–11. Forearm stimulation using the thumb.

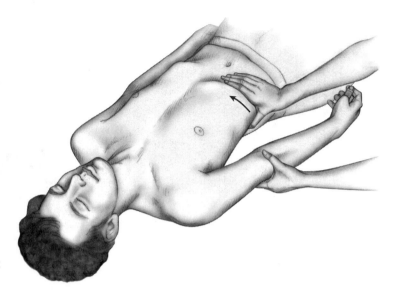

FIGURE 16–12. Elbow milk and abdomen rock.

12. **Occipital press.** Sitting at the recipient's head, turn his head slightly to the left. Using the second finger of your right hand, perform circular friction to the suboccipital muscles just under the base of the skull and to the right of the midline. Your left hand should be supporting his head by resting lightly on the left side of his forehead. Your index finger should rest gently on the spot known in India as the "third eye," the area between and just above the eyes. The hand on the back of the head should feel as though it were plugged into the palm of the hand on his forehead. Hold and feel for a sensation of tingling. When a steady gentle pulsation is felt in the hands, or a minute or so has passed, turn the head to the other side and repeat, switching hands. See Figure 16–14.

13. **Cranial polarization.** Lightly place both thumbs on the anterior fontanel, with both index fingers touching on the "third eye" and the remaining fingers across the forehead. If your hands are large enough, rest your little fingers on the temperomandibular joints, with the other fingers evenly spaced on the forehead. It is important that you relax your hands, arms, and shoulders as much as possible, and that your breathing is relaxed and your posture comfortable. Hold for about one minute, or until a steady gentle pulsation is felt. See Figure 16–15.

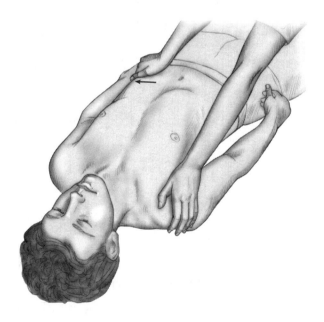

FIGURE 16–13. Pelvic rock.

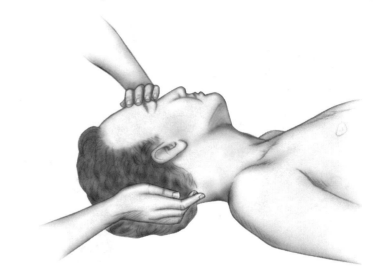

FIGURE 16–14. Occipital press.

14. **Navel–third eye.** Move to the recipient's right side. Lightly place your left thumb pad between his eyebrows and your right thumb in his navel, with the thumbs pointing toward each other. Hold one minute, and then lift hands very slowly, initiating movement from the thumbs, rather than the shoulders.

15. **Brushing off to finish.** Wait a few moments, and then in a quiet voice ask the person to sit up with his legs off the side of the table. Standing behind him, place your hands on his shoulders. With a sweeping motion, brush your hands across the spine then down to the sacrum, and out to the crest of the hips. Repeat several times. See Figure 16–16.

Standing in front of him, place his hands on his knees. Place your hands on his shoulders, and in a sweeping manner, brush down his arms to the knees and down his legs. Repeat several times. See Figure 16–17.

If you decide to explore these techniques, remember the primary principle of love. If you get confused, let yourself laugh. If you find the rhythm difficult, remember to let your breathing relax, your shoulders down. If you are relaxed and accept yourself, the receiver will benefit, regardless of your skill level. Do the best you can in a simple way, and be kind to yourself. Although you are not "the healer," you may find yourself being healed while giving polarity. You may find that in the circle of love and self-acceptance your own obstructions begin to disappear and you are no longer sure who is "giving" polarity to whom.

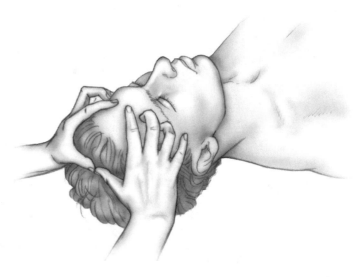

FIGURE 16–15. Cranial polarization.

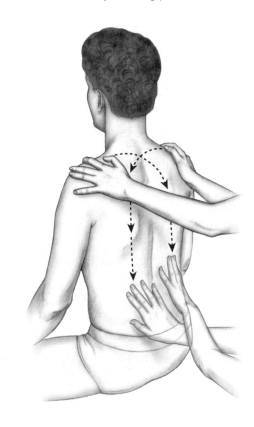

FIGURE 16–16. Brushing off the back.

You may integrate any of these movements into a Western full-body massage. You may find them useful for beginning or ending a session, or before the receiver turns over from prone to supine. During a full-body session, you may sense energy blockages and use one or more of these basic techniques to try to allow energy to flow freely again. Once you are familiar with them, you can insert them where it seems like the right thing to do.

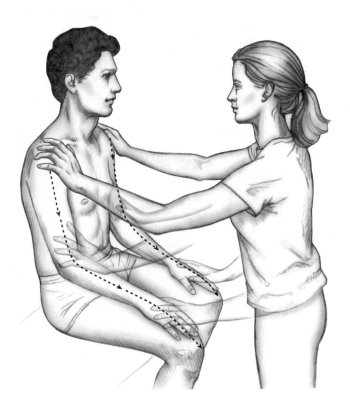

FIGURE 16–17. Brushing off the front.

SOME FINAL THOUGHTS

The unique gift of polarity therapy is its simplicity. Behind the techniques and esoterica is an opening and surrendering to life and to being at home with our natural energies. The ideal supplement to this brief introduction would be to receive a session from a professional polarity therapist, as it is very difficult to convey the experience of polarity in writing. Polarity therapy is truly an art form, requiring much study and dedicated practice to master the rhythm and quality of touch that are so important to the effects. In addition, the hands-on work is only a small part of the therapy, which usually includes basic nutritional guidance, exercise, and support for emotional balancing.

SUMMARY

Polarity therapy is a holistic bodywork approach that involves simple touching and gentle movements such as rocking and pressing. Polarity techniques are designed to release obstructions in the free flow of energy through the body, thus supporting health and healing.

Objective changes in the body observed during polarity sessions indicate deep relaxation and include flushed cheeks, drop in blood pressure, increased salivation, muscle relaxation, slower heart rate, and grumbling in the digestive system associated with the activity of peristalsis. Western science may find physiological reasons for some of these effects such as stimulation of nerve centers and mechanoreceptors in joints.

The basic principles of polarity therapy are related to the concepts of energy, love, working with obstructions, understanding, and nutrition and exercise. The techniques include gentle holding, rocking, and probing movements that are combined into relaxing sessions. Techniques also aid the practitioner in locating areas that appear to be obstructed and in need of further attention.

Polarity techniques may be used alone or integrated into a traditional Western massage. The unique gift of polarity is its simplicity.

A look ahead . . .

Traditional Chinese medicine is an ancient system of health and healing familiar in Western countries in the form of acupuncture and herbal medicine. Several forms of Asian bodywork therapy (ABT) apply these ancient theories using soft tissue manipulation. Part IV takes a look at some popular forms of ABT. Chapter 17 sets the stage with an overview of the theory of traditional Asian medicine.

REFERENCES

Stone, Randolph. (1987). *Dr. Randolph Stone's Polarity Therapy: The complete collected works*. Harlan Tarbell, Illustrator. Sebastopol, CA: CRCS Publications.
Stone, Randolph. (1991). *Health building: The conscious art of living well*. Sebastopol, CA: CRCS Publications.

ADDITIONAL RESOURCES

Books

Gordon, R. (1979). *Your healing hands: The polarity experience*. Santa Cruz, CA: Unity Press.
Siedman, M. (1982). *Like a hollow flute: A guide to polarity therapy*. Santa Cruz, CA: Elan Press.
Siegel, A. (1986). *Live energy: The power that heals*. Bridgeport, Dorset, England: Prism Press/Colin Spooner.
Sills, Franklin. (2002). *The polarity process: Energy as a healing art*. Berkeley, CA: North Atlantic Books.

WEB SITE

American Polarity Therapy Association (*www.polaritytherapy.org*)

INSTRUCTIONAL VIDEO

"Polarity therapy: Five elements." (2001). Santa Barbara, CA: Real Bodywork. (*www.deeptissue.com*)
"Polarity therapy: Three Principles." (2001). Santa Barbara, CA: Real Bodywork. (*www.deeptissue.com*)

S T U D Y   G U I D E

LEARNING OUTCOMES

Use the learning outcomes at the beginning of the chapter as a guide to your studies. Perform the task given in each outcome, either in writing or verbally into a tape recorder or to a study partner. This may start as an "open book" exercise, and then later from memory.

KEY TERMS AND CONCEPTS

To study key words and concepts listed at the beginning of this chapter, choose one or more of the following exercises. Writing or talking about ideas helps you remember them better, and explaining them helps deepen your understanding.

1. Write a one- or two-sentence explanation of each key word and concept as explained in the chapter.

2. With a study partner, take turns explaining key words and concepts verbally. Ask each other questions about the meaning of the terms.

3. Try to express in your own words what the author means by each principle of polarity therapy. Compare and contrast to other systems of massage and bodywork that you have studied.

4. Make study cards by writing the explanation from problem 1 on one side of a 3 × 5 card, and the key word or concept on the other. Shuffle the cards and read one side, trying to recite either the explanation or word on the other side.

STUDY OUTLINE

The following questions test your memory of the main concepts in this chapter. Locate the answers in the text, using the page number given for each question.

History and Philosophy

1. Polarity therapy was developed by _____ in the mid-1900s. He was trained in the natural healing methods of _____, _____, and _____. (p. 291)

2. Stone also studied a variety of healing systems from the East, including Chinese _____, Hermetic Kabalistic healing, and _____ medicine from India. (p. 291)

3. Combining the Western and Eastern healing methods, polarity therapy focuses on removing obstructions to the flow of _____. (p. 291)

4. When Stone retired in 1973, Pierre _____ assumed leadership in spreading the practice of polarity therapy throughout the United States. (p. 291)

Physiological Effects

1. There are subjective indications that some principle not yet recognized by Western medicine is at work in polarity therapy, i.e., equating of health with _____ and its absence with disease; _____ in the hands of the practitioner at work; client and practitioner feeling _____ in their energy during sessions. (p. 292)

2. Objective changes during polarity sessions include signs of deep _____. (p. 292)

3. Polarity techniques that may cause physiological changes include light _____ pressure over sensitive areas, gentle _____, and alternating _____ movement of hands. (p. 292)

4. The style of touch in polarity therapy may induce a light _____ state. (p. 292)

5. The principle behind polarity transcends all ancient and modern theories, and is instead embodied in the _____ of the _____. (p. 293)

6. Energy and physiological effects may be considered _____, or ways of explaining a mechanism we cannot see, except in its effects. (p. 293)

Principles of Polarity Therapy

1. Polarity therapy is a holistic bodywork approach that involves simple _____ and gentle movements such as _____ and _____. (p. 291)

2. Polarity techniques are designed to release _____ to the free flow of _____ through the body, thus supporting health and healing. (p. 291)

3. Energy is a concept foreign to most Westerners, but with awareness may be felt in the hands as _____. (p. 293)

4. Love refers to serving life, caring, and responding to the recipient's _____ without _____ to results. (p. 293)

5. Understanding the appropriate response to the recipient's _____ reactions during a polarity session is an important practitioner skill. Pannetier would say that the giver is not there to _____ the receiver, but to plant seeds of letting go and trusting, to be an _____ friend. (pp. 295–296)

6. Nutrition and exercise are part of the full approach to polarity therapy, and were originally derived from _____ practices. A more _____ approach to nutrition and exercise is followed by current practitioners. (p. 296)

Basic Polarity Movements

1. Polarity students are typically taught a general session of 15–22 movements that serve to _____ and _____ the entire body. (p. 296)

2. These gentle _____, _____, and _____ techniques form a generally relaxing session and also aid the practitioner in locating areas that appear to be obstructed and in need of further attention. (p. 296)

Some Final Thoughts

1. The unique gift of polarity therapy is its _____. Behind the techniques and theories is an opening and surrendering to life and being at home with our natural _____. (p. 304)

FOR GREATER UNDERSTANDING

The following exercises are practical applications of the guidelines presented in this chapter. Action words are underlined to emphasize the variety of activities presented, and to encourage advanced skill development. These exercises can be done with a study partner or group, or in class.

1. Receive a polarity therapy session from a certified practitioner. Be aware of any feeling of the movement of energy as the practitioner performs various techniques. Discuss your experience with the practitioner and later with a study partner.

2. Observe a trained polarity therapist give a session. Note how it is different from a Western massage session. Write your observations and/or discuss them with a study partner. [Alternative: watch a video of a polarity therapy demonstration.]

3. Practice the "front-to-back" polarity technique described in the chapter and illustrated in Figure 16–1. The purpose of the exercise is for the practitioner to practice being focused, to develop a sense of energetic connection, and to observe the recipient's response. Afterwards, discuss the exercise with your study partner.

4. Practice the torso and head polarity technique described in the chapter and illustrated in Figure 16–2. The purpose of the exercise is for the practitioner to practice sensing and releasing blocks to energy flow. Afterwards, discuss the exercise with your study partner.

5. Practice the polarity routine described in this chapter. Be aware of how your hands feel, and any movement of energy that you sense. Were you aware of energy flow or obstruction in any part of the body, or during

a specific technique? <u>Discuss</u> your and the recipient's experience afterwards.

6. <u>Take</u> an introduction to polarity therapy class for additional instruction and supervision.

7. <u>Watch</u> an instructional video or <u>read</u> one of the references mentioned at the end of the chapter, for deeper understanding of the theory of polarity therapy.

8. <u>Visit the Web site</u> of the American Polarity Therapy Association (*www.polarity therapy.org*). <u>Read</u> about polarity therapy, practitioner registration, and their Standards for Practice and Education and Code of Ethics. <u>Report</u> your findings to a study partner or group.

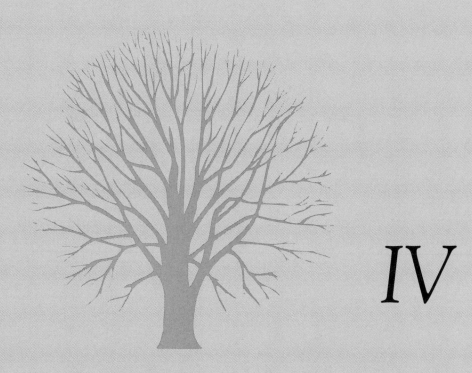

IV

Asian Bodywork Tradition

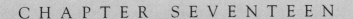

Asian Bodywork Therapy—Theory

by Barbra Esher and John J. Johnston

LEARNING OUTCOMES

After studying this chapter, the student will have information to:

1. Identify different forms of Asian Bodywork Therapy (ABT).
2. Trace the origins and history of ABT.
3. Compare the paradigms of Asian (Chinese) and Western medicine.
4. Discuss the principles of Yin and Yang.
5. Explain the concept of Qi and its functions.
6. Identify the Five Elements and their application to Asian medicine.
7. Describe the Shen and Ko cycle.
8. Use the Chinese body clock model to examine the peak flow of Qi within the energy channels.
9. Describe the Four Pillars of Assessment.
10. Locate important acupoints and name their applications.
11. Explain how Traditional Asian Medicine (TAM) theory is applied in different forms of ABT.

HISTORICAL PEOPLE AND DEVELOPMENTS

Anmo
Book of Changes

Classical Chinese medicine
(CCM)

Kampo
Namikoshi, Tokujiro

MEDIALINK

A companion CD-ROM, included free with each new copy of this book, supplements the techniques presented in this chapter. Insert the CD-ROM to watch video clips of Asian Bodywork Therapy techniques being demonstrated. This multimedia feature is designed to help you add a new dimension to your learning.

Naturalist school
Qi Bo
Soulie de Morant

Traditional Asian medicine
  (TAM)
Traditional Chinese medicine
  (TCM)

Yellow Emperor
Yellow Emperor's *Classic of
  Internal Medicine*

KEY TERMS/CONCEPTS

ABT techniques
Asian Bodywork Therapy
  (ABT)
American Organization for
  Bodywork Therapies of
  Asia (AOBTA®)
Chinese body clock
Earth

Fire
Five Elements
Ko cycle
Metal
National Certification
  Commission for
  Acupuncture and Oriental
  Medicine (NCCAOM)

Scope of practice
Qi
Sheng cycle
Water
Wood
Yang
Yin

ASIAN BODYWORK THERAPY

Asian Bodywork Therapy (ABT) is a term used to describe forms of bodywork with roots in Chinese medicine. Over the centuries, practitioners in Asian countries such as China, Japan, and Korea, and more recently in the West, have changed and developed these forms into separate and distinct approaches.

Specific forms of ABT described later in this text include Amma (Chapter 18), Zen Shiatsu (Chapter 19) and Jin Shin Do® (Chapter 20). Others recognized by the **American Organization for Bodywork Therapies of Asia (AOBTA®)** are: acupressure, AMMA Therapy®, Chi Nei Tsang, Nuad Bo' Ran (traditional Thai medical bodywork therapy), Tuina and five distinct forms of Shiatsu (Zen, integrative eclectic, Japanese/Namikoshi, macrobiotic/barefoot and five element).

> Asian Bodywork Therapy (ABT) is the treatment of the human body/mind/spirit, including the electromagnetic or energetic field, which surrounds, infuses and brings that body to life, by pressure and/or manipulation. Asian Bodywork is based upon traditional Chinese medical principles for assessing and evaluating the energetic system. It uses traditional Asian techniques and treatment strategies to primarily affect and balance the energetic system for the purpose of treating the human body, emotions, mind, energy field and spirit for the promotion, maintenance and restoration of health (AOBTA Web site, 5/27/03).

The **scope of practice** of ABT includes assessment and treatment of energetic imbalances according to Chinese medicine theory. Note that diagnosed Western medical conditions are not "treated" per se, but may be affected by correcting energetic imbalances. Assessments are based on Chinese medicine parameters related to the person's energetic balance.

ABT techniques include, but are not limited to, (1) touching, pressing or holding of the body along meridians and/or on acupoints, primarily with the hands; (2) stretching; (3) external application of medicinal plant foods; (4) application of heat or cold; (5) dietary and (6) exercise suggestions. Cupping, *gua sha*, moxibustion and other methods or modalities may also be used by properly trained practitioners (AOBTA Web site 5/27/03).

Asian bodywork therapy is one of the three branches of Chinese medicine for which the **National Certification Commission for Acupuncture and Oriental Medicine (NCCAOM)** certifies practitioners for entry-level practice. The others are acupuncture and Chinese herbology.

HISTORY OF ABT

Although the origin of Chinese medicine is lost in antiquity, it is assumed to have developed from Chinese folk remedies and thousands of years of empirical evidence. It has many aspects in common with other Asian healing traditions, such as medicinal herbs. However, the practice of acupuncture and its theories are unique to China and have spread into common usage to most of Asia.

The earliest known text on Chinese medicine is the Huang Di Nei Jing, or the ***Yellow Emperor's Classic of Internal Medicine.*** It is traditionally ascribed to the legendary Yellow Emperor, Huang Di, who is thought to have lived around 2500 BCE. Nei Jing includes two works: the Suwen, or Simple Questions; and the Lingshu, or Spiritual Pivot. In ancient times, the Lingshu was called the Acupuncture Treatise, and the Suwen was called the Nei Jing (Niuen, 1995).

Both books of the Nei Jing are written as a conversation between the **Yellow Emperor** and his minister, **Qi Bo.** It was once thought that there were more books in the Nei Jing on Chinese bodywork, but they were evidently destroyed during dynasties when touch was considered improper (Wang, 1994).

The earliest reference to Yin and Yang is thought to have been in the Yi Jing or ***Book of Changes,*** written in about 700 BCE. The Yin-Yang School of Philosophy dedicated itself to the study of Yin-Yang and the Five Elements. It is sometimes called the **naturalist school,** because it sought to find ways to live in harmony with nature rather than subdue it. One of its main exponents was Zou Yan (350–270 BCE) (Maciocia 1998).

These philosophies, along with the concept of Qi or *life energy*, channels of energy or *meridians*, and points of contact with Qi or *acupoints*, form the foundation of classical Chinese medicine. Different forms of Asian bodywork therapy (ABT), and movement practices such as qi gong and tai ji, are designed to maintain balance and harmony in the body, mind and spirit.

Early Development

Chinese medicine is thought to have originated in the barren lands north of the Huang Ho or Yellow River in China. The inhabitants of this area used acupuncture, moxibustion (burning the herb mugwort over or on an acupoint on the body), and **anmo** (manual or bodywork methods) to heal various ailments.

Over many years of experience and observation, the Chinese people came to identify the energy channels and points on the body where such therapy produces maximum effects. There is strong evidence to support the theory that the energy channels were discovered first, with knowledge of specific points coming later. Writings in a silk book discovered during the excavation of the Western Han Tomb Mawangdui support this sequence of events (Deadman, 1998). It was the sensations created when pressing the body, as well as awareness during meditation and qi gong practice, that led to the discovery of the 12 primary and other energy channels. This system of channels and points forms the basic energetic anatomy of Chinese medicine (Figure 17–1).

The early healing practices of northern China developed according to the prevailing beliefs about nature and the universe. In China, Taoist philosophy had a major impact on developing theories of medicine, as did the Yin-Yang or naturalist school of philosophy mentioned above. Practice and theory evolved over centuries into a unique approach to health and healing.

In the United States, Chinese medicine is sometimes referred to as **traditional Asian medicine (TAM)** to acknowledge the extent of its adoption throughout eastern Asia before coming to the West. TAM is a broad term used to classify many traditions based in Chinese medicine.

Classical Chinese medicine (CCM) refers to the systems of medicine from the ancient texts such as the Nei Jing and the Nan Jing. Some even include works from the Ming Dynasty (1500s) within CCM, but purists consider this era relatively modern and not "classical."

Spread Throughout Asia

Chinese medicine eventually spread throughout the territory known today as the People's Republic of China and north to the Korean peninsula. From Korea it made its way to Japan as **kampo,** the Chinese way, in about 600 CE. A map of East Asia where TAM developed is shown in Figure 17–2.

Religion and philosophy, martial arts, healing methods, and other practices from China were absorbed into indigenous cultures with modifications according to the local beliefs and practices. This accounts for some of the regional differences in how Chinese medicine is practiced. More information on the development of TAM in Japan can be found in Chapter 18.

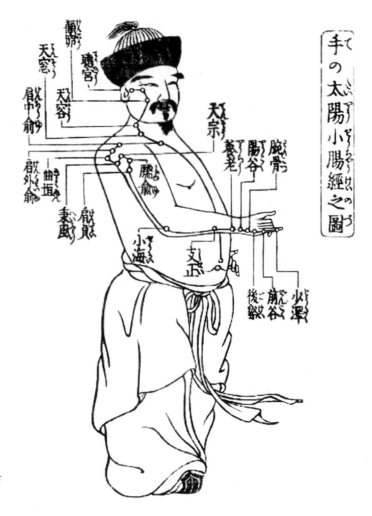

FIGURE 17–1. Ancient drawing of energy channels.

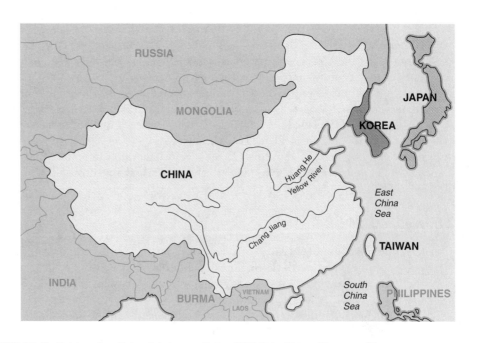

FIGURE 17–2. Origins of traditional Asian medicine (TAM) in China, Korea, and Japan.

East to West

Knowledge of East Asia was brought to Europe in the 13th century in a rare written account, *Travels of Marco Polo*. Later in the 17th century, Asian philosophies and healing practices were described by Jesuit missionaries returning from Imperial China.

This knowledge did not greatly impact Western healing practices until the mid-20th century, when the French diplomat **Soulie de Morant** published his voluminous writings on the subject of acupuncture. This led to acupuncture associations and study groups in Western countries. In the 1940s Morant's work was hailed in France, Italy, Britain, Germany, Russia, Eastern European nations, and Argentina in South America.

Furthermore, immigrants from Asia have brought knowledge of Chinese medicine wherever in the world they have traveled. In the United States this knowledge remained largely within the immigrant communities until the 1970s.

Asian bodywork forms from Japan have been especially popular in the United States. Tokujiro Namikoshi, famous shiatsu developer in post–World War II Japan, wrote a book published in 1969 in English titled *Shiatsu: Japanese Finger-Pressure Therapy*. His son, **Toru Namikoshi,** gave shiatsu demonstrations throughout the United States between 1953 and 1960. Asian bodywork was first welcomed in the United States by natural healers and alternative health practitioners.

In the 1970s, when trade between China and the United States was opened once again, interest in acupuncture and Chinese medicine was renewed in the West. This coincided with the Human Potential Movement in the United States, which opened Western minds to Asian philosophies and healing practices. That interest continues to this day.

Several systems of Asian bodywork therapy (ABT) were introduced in the West in the 1970s by people like DoAnn Kaneko (Anma Shiatsu); Shizuto Masunaga (Zen Shiatsu); Shizuko Yamamoto (Barefoot-Macrobiotic Shiatsu); Toshiko Phipps (Eclectic Shiatsu) and Takashi Nakamura (Amma). Some systems like Jin Shin Do® have been developed in modern times in the West, building on ancient Chinese practices.

West to East

In China and Japan, traditional healing practices have evolved over the centuries. During the Meiji Restoration (c. 1868), and especially after World War II, Western medicine was integrated with traditional practices in Japan. A similar integration happened in China during the Cultural Revolution in the 1980s (Tedeschi 2000).

Tuina, a vigorous form of bodywork based on Chinese medicine, is practiced today side by side with acupuncture, herbal medicine and Western therapies in many Chinese medical centers. Namikoshi's shiatsu uses Western anatomy to locate acupoints. These examples represent the flip side of what is happening with integrative medicine in the West, where Western medicine is beginning to integrate healing practices from other parts of the world.

More history of specific forms of Asian bodywork therapy can be found in Chapters 18–20. The following sections explain some of the principal theories of Traditional Asian Medicine in greater detail.

ASIAN AND WESTERN MEDICINE

Dynamically changing relationships form the basis of Asian medicine. This simple statement introduces a primary difference between Asian medicine and the Western medical paradigm.

In Western medicine, humans are considered separate from and largely unaffected by the phenomena of nature. The philosophical base of Western medicine is the Cartesian split, often identified as the mind/body disconnect. In the Cartesian model, humans essentially are composed of two very different aspects: the material substance or body, and the nonmaterial mind.

This duality creates a mechanized view of the body. The body and its functions can be measured, and thus, Western medical science can verify that it actually exists. The mind is not as accessible to measuring devices and as such is more nebulous and difficult to scrutinize.

Therefore, the focus of Western medicine has been on what can be reliably measured, predicted and controlled. In essence, each body system, each organ, each symptom is viewed as separate from others and from the individual as a whole. Humans are seen as machines with the heart working like a pump, lungs a bellows, the brain a computer without Internet access—yet subject to disabling viruses. As with machines, parts wear out and can be, to some extent, replaced. Emergency breakdown repair is where Western medicine excels, rather than on maintenance or wellness.

In contrast, at the core of Asian medicine is the concept that the universe is dynamic, that is, constantly moving and changing, yet still maintaining a unity, a oneness. Humans are a natural, integral aspect of the universe. Humans exist, or "stand out," from the background of the universe, yet nevertheless, humans exist in relationship to the fabric of the universe and are made of the same threads.

Consider this moving and changing universe as a vast ocean. Humans stand out as waves upon this ocean. Although waves are seen as literally standing out of the water, they are nevertheless an aspect of the water with the same composition and characteristics as the body of water from which they emerge. Humans stand out from the fabric of nature, yet are composed of naturally occurring materials and are subject to the same laws of nature that affect any other aspect of existence. Thus humans are related to and connected with all that exists.

YIN AND YANG

Yin and **Yang** illustrate this concept of relatedness and connection of all. The Yin/Yang symbol has been described as two comets chasing each other. The image is a circle composed of a large rounded white area that curves within the circle and becomes gradually thinner until it seems to blend into the outline of the circle. At the blending area is a large black area that curves around toward the white area, thinning just like the white until the black becomes part of the circle's edge. Within the largest part of the white is a small black circle. Likewise, within the largest area of the black is a small white circle. One can visualize the movement and change of the universe in this symbol, which is so meaningful in Asian medicine. The Yin/Yang symbol and Chinese characters are presented in Figure 17–3.

The Chinese character for Yin depicts the shady side of a hill or mountain. This is the dark part of the symbol described above. Yin, relatively speaking, is the dark, deep, dense aspect of the universe. It is characterized as feminine, interior, still, substantial, cool and contracting in contrast to Yang.

The Chinese character for Yang is also a hillside, but in full sun. In relationship to Yin, Yang is the light, energetic, and ethereal aspect of the universe. Yang is masculine, exterior, moving, nonsubstantial, warm and expanding, and opposing but also supporting Yin.

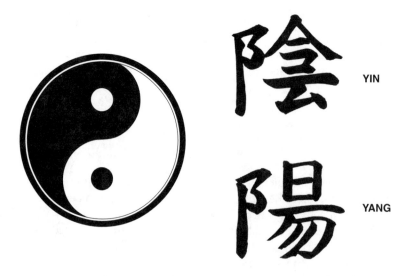

YIN

YANG

FIGURE 17–3. Yin / Yang in traditional Asian medicine. (Calligraphy by Rev. Zenko Okimura)

Principles

Consider a cold dark winter night with a welcoming, cozy fire in the fireplace. The warmth of the fire dispels the evening's chill. The light brightens the room as the dancing flames delight our eyes. This fireplace illustrates the five principles of Yin and Yang.

The first principle is **opposition.** Yin and Yang control and restrict each other. The Yang warmth of the fire is controlling the Yin cold of the room. Just as above, with seed of Yang within Yin, in the fire appears like a Yang spot within the larger dark Yin room.

The second principle is **interdependence.** Although opposite, Yin and Yang cannot exist in isolation; they are relative concepts totally dependent on each other. It is impossible for one to exist without the other. Indeed it is impossible to have a "jar of Yang," and vice versa. One could say that the fire is Yang in relationship to the room which is Yin. But relative to the outside cold night air, the room is Yang and outside is Yin. Yin and Yang are relative in that each requires the other and is known only in its relationship to the other.

The third principle is the mutual **consuming/supporting relationship** of Yin and Yang. In the fireplace, the flames are the Yang aspect of the fire. Yet, upon closer look, the dense dark Yin logs are nourishing the flames. The Yin substance (logs) must be present or there is no Yang energy (flame). Yin substance is creating the Yang energy. Both are essential for that fire to exist. Yin and Yang maintain a constant dynamic balance. There must be appropriate portions of each. If there is not enough fuel, the flames die. Should too many logs be dumped upon a fire, the flames could be smothered.

Intertransformation is the fourth principle. Intertransformation means that Yin and Yang are not static; they are constantly transforming into each other. The Yin logs transform into Yang flames and heat. Ultimately, the flames transform the logs into cool ashes. Indeed, as the night progresses later and gets darker, it eventually transforms into day at the break of dawn.

Lastly, Yin and Yang have an **infinite divisibility.** How "Yin" something is can be divided endlessly. The temperature of each log can be measured from the end furthest away from the fire at microscopic intervals until reaching the center of the hottest area of flame. The temperature will change from very cool (Yin) far from the flames to very hot (Yang) nearer the flames. Everything can be infinitely divided into Yin and Yang.

We find this same dynamic balance applying the Yin and Yang concept to the human body. Yang corresponds to the back, head, exterior, lateral (posterior) aspects of the limbs, the Yang organs and the functions of the organs. The Yang organs are organs that transform, digest and excrete "impure" products of food and fluids (Maciocia 1998).

The Yin aspects of humans are the front, interior, medial (interior) aspects of the limbs, the Yin organs and structure of the organs. The Yin organs are those that store the pure essences extracted from food by the Yang organs (Maciocia 1998).

THE CONCEPT OF QI

The concept of **Qi** has existed in China since the beginning of recorded history. Qi is pronounced "chee," also written as *Chi* or in Japanese, *Ki.* In a large sense, everything in the universe is Qi, sometimes called the Big Qi. Blending at the same moment the substantial and insubstantial, Qi is a continuous form of energy in material form when it condenses, and nonmaterial when it disperses.

This idea is depicted in the Chinese character for Qi, symbolizing rice cooking in a pot with the steam escaping (Figure 17–4). Qi is the rice *and* the steam, the material *and* the energy. As matter, Qi forms rocks, trees, rain drops, birds, and humans. Qi dispersed becomes energy, sunshine, starlight and the movement of wind. That is, more the movement, and less the wind itself.

This is not unlike the more modern idea of quantum physics. If only scientists would read the classical Chinese medical texts they could save themselves so much trouble! So often, modern "discoveries" are clearly outlined in the *Nei* and *Nan Jing,* written thousands of years ago in China. (Refer to *The Tao of Physics* by Fritjof Capra, 1983; and *The Dancing WuLi Masters* by Gary Zukav, 1979.)

Qi in the more narrow sense, the Little Qi, is being validated by Western science as well. Often translated as the *life force* or *life energy,* it is what makes people "go," much like the unseen wind propels a sailboat forward. The energy is extracted from the food we eat and the air we breathe, and then

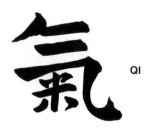

FIGURE 17–4. Chinese character for Qi or life energy. (Calligraphy by Rev. Zenko Okumura)

transformed further by our genetic essence into the useable Qi that circulates through a network of channels, also called meridians.

Traditional Asian medicine focuses on harmonizing the ease and flow of Qi along with the other fundamental substances: Shen, Jing, Blood, and Jin/Ye. If Qi is deficient, one tonifies it. If it is excess, one disperses it. If it is stagnant, one moves it. If it is sinking, one uplifts it. And if it is rebellious, one rectifies it. Included in ABT's techniques are those that tonify, disperse, move, uplift or rectify Qi.

Qi's functions are often summarized as follows: transforming, transporting, holding, protecting, and warming. If there are any disharmonies in the functions of Qi, disease will result.

Qi **transforms** the air Qi and the food Qi into Qi that can be used by the body. If the transforming function of Qi is not working properly, at best, one may feel tired after eating; at worst, one may feel absolutely exhausted all of the time. Fatigue is often due to a dysfunction of the Qi's transforming function; it is not able to extract the essential nutrients from the food and air.

Qi **transports** nutrients and blood throughout the body. It is even responsible for the ease and flow of the emotions. Qi can stagnate, causing stress, repressed anger and depression.

Qi **holds** everything together, keeping the organs in place and the blood in the vessels. If a person "just can't keep it together," it could be related to a lack of Qi's holding function. Bruising easily, prolapsed organs and hemorrhoids could also be related to a Qi deficiency.

Qi **protects** the body as well, energizing the immune system. If a person becomes sick easily and often, it relates to the quality and quantity of their defensive Qi.

Qi **warms** the body. If a person gets cold easily, it could be seen as a lack of the warming function of Qi. Metabolism relates to Qi's warming function as well. Food is cooked by the Qi heating it up, so the essential energy can be extracted from it for daily use.

FIVE ELEMENTS AND THEIR ORBS OF INFLUENCE

Traditional Asian medicine (TAM) looks *beyond* any Western diagnosis people may have, to see the energetic relationships within people and to the outside world. An excellent paradigm for doing this is the five elements. The **Five Elements** are a poetic but scientific way of using natural phenomenon like the changing of the seasons to explore and treat our psyche, spiritual state, anatomy, physiology and the dynamics of the disease process as a whole.

Qi flows through the body in daily cycles from dawn to night, yearly cycles from Spring to Winter and lifetime cycles from birth to death. Qi rises then falls; grows then decays, thus creating the circle of life envisioned as Five Elements. People are as inextricably connected to these cycles as the moon and sun. They are not considered merely part of nature. They *are* nature, with the same rhythmic flows as the entire cosmos.

The Five Elements in TAM are: **Wood, Fire, Earth, Metal** and **Water.** Each of the Five Elements has its own characteristics and correspondences within the body and to its environment. Also, each Element has its associated channels of energy. As discussed above, Asian medicine has its focus on *relationships*. The relationship of one Element to another, their natural balance and flow, is an essential aspect of understanding, using and living the Five Elements. The Five Elements and corresponding energy channels are listed in Table 17–1.

Wood

Wood is a Yang Element, though less Yang than Fire is. Wood energy is the most evident in spring, when seeds are germinating and pushing upward toward the sun. There is a similar feeling at sunrise, the start

Table 17–1 THE FIVE ELEMENTS AND CORRESPONDING CHANNELS

Element*	Yin Channel	Yang Channel
Fire	Heart (Ht)	Small Intestine (Si)
Fire	Pericardium (Pc)	Triple Burner (Tb)
Wood	Liver (Lv)	Gall Bladder (Gb)
Earth	Spleen (Sp)	Stomach (St)
Metal	Lung (Lu)	Large Intestine (Li)
Water	Kidney (Ki)	Bladder (Bl)

*Elements are arranged from most Yang (Fire) to most Yin (Water).

of a new day. Wood is heard in a shouting voice and felt in anger. Wood is associated with green, the wind, sour taste, tears (as fluid in the eyes, not crying), and the sense of sight.

One is able to see clearly into the future, make plans and decisively select a course of action through the power of Wood. A balanced Wood Element is seen in benevolence, discernment and patience. Individuals who are unbalanced in their Wood Element may be belligerent or timid, rigid or indecisive (Jarrett, 2000).

The **Liver** (Yin) and **Gall Bladder** (Yang) organs and channels are associated with the Wood Element. Each has a role in smooth effective decision making. The Liver functions as the strategy maker, much like an army general. The Gall Bladder functions like the tactician, making judgments and fostering the courage to be decisive. The Liver stores blood; assures the smooth flow of Qi, including emotional flexibility; dominates the sinews/tendons; opens to the eyes and manifests in the nails. The Gall Bladder also stores and excretes bile.

Fire

Fire is the most Yang Element. It is clearly evident in the season of summer and the heat of the day. It appears in our ability to feel warm, both physically and emotionally. Fire provides heat and light. It is heard in laughter, tasted in bitter, smelled in scorched, and felt with joy. Fire is associated with sweat, the tongue and the vessels.

Fire gives the capacity to be loving, passionate, joyful, self-realized and confident beings. Individuals manifest a balanced Fire Element in their constitution of propriety, insight and intimacy. Imbalance may appear as guardedness, vulnerability, excessive control or apathy (Jarrett, 2000).

The Fire Element is expressed in four channels: the **Heart** (Yin), **Small Intestine** (Yang), **Pericardium** (Yin), and **Triple Burner** (Yang). Each of these channels and organs has its own primary function.

The Heart governs the Blood and blood vessels; houses the Shen, opens to the tongue; governs sweating and manifests in the complexion. The Small Intestine separates pure from impure and is essential to sorting out options. It is also involved in the transportation of fluids. The Pericardium assists the heart in its function of governing the Blood and housing the Shen. Further, it protects the heart from pathogens.

The **Triple Burner** (also called Triple Warmer) regulates digestion and assimilation and elimination. It helps control water passages and the fluid metabolism. Yuan Qi/ Original Qi forms between the two kidneys and is circulated by the Triple Burner through the channels, surfacing at the Yuan/source points. By circulating Yuan Qi, the Triple Burner contributes to the strength of the defensive Qi, thus helping to protect the body.

Earth

Earth is felt the most in late summer when the weather is humid and damp and the seasons are in transition. In fact, the Earth Element is also felt as the change between all of the seasons, having mainly a transformative quality. Thus, the direction is centered as one must be clearly rooted, secure and centered to flow with changes. Earth is heard in singing, tasted in sweet, and smelled in fragrant.

In balance, the Earth energy is seen in those individuals who display integrity, altruism and adaptability. Without balance in the Earth element, individuals are selfish or martyrs, self-sufficient or needy, stubborn or compliant (Jarrett 2000).

The energy of the Earth element flows through the Spleen and Stomach channels. Their primary function is digesting food and drink which nourishes the body.

The **Spleen** channel is in charge of transformation and transportation of ingested liquid and solids. Therefore, it plays a major role in digestion and the production of Qi and Blood. It also controls the Blood, keeping it in its proper place. The Spleen dominates the muscles; the sense of taste; opens to the mouth and controls the raising of Qi. It further keeps intentions focused for mental activity, such as studying.

The **Stomach** channel controls rotting and ripening. It controls descending and the first stage of digesting fluids.

Metal

Metal is Yin, but not as Yin as the Water Element. Metal is felt most in autumn, when the trees let go of their leaves, the birds leave their nests and people let go of their gardens and other outdoor summer activities. It is also felt at dusk, in grief and heard in crying. Metal has a pungent taste and rank smell. Metal is associated with the sense of smell, the climate of dryness, and mucus, the body fluid most susceptible to that climate.

An individual who is balanced in the Metal Element appears inspired, balanced and receptive. Metal in excess or deficit produces behaviors such as vanity, self-deprecation, zealotry or despondency (Jarrett, 2000).

The Lung and Large Intestine are the two channels through which the Metal Element flows. The functions of both of these channels are holding on and letting go.

The Lung channel governs Qi and controls respiration, bringing Air Qi in for nourishment, then letting go of the waste. It also controls disseminating and descending, regulates the water passages, controls the skin and body hair and opens to the nose.

The **Large Intestine channel** salvages pure fluid from the impure matter passed from the Small Intestine. It holds waste material and lets go of it.

Water

Water is the most Yin element. It is felt in the cold, dark, quiet winter, northern direction and at night. It flows through us in our blood, perspiration, tears, saliva and urine. The Water Element is the most yielding. The Water Element is associated with hearing, fear, the sound of groaning. Other associations are a rotten smell and a salty taste. Bones are influenced by the Water Element, as are the ears, kidneys and bladder.

Individuals manifest a Water Element in their constitution in the virtues of wisdom, concentration, and contemplation. An imbalance, excess or deficiency in the Water Element may appear as extreme recklessness or scatteredness, or as someone profoundly conservative or physically or emotionally dormant (Jarrett, 2000).

The channels for the Water Element are the kidney and bladder. The **Kidney** channels store Essence (Jing); control birth, development and reproduction; produce marrow, and govern short-term memory. The **Bladder** channel temporarily stores and excretes impure fluids such as urine.

SHENG AND KO CYCLES

There are two important cycles that involve the Five Elements. These are the Sheng or generating cycle and the Ko or controlling cycle.

The **Sheng cycle** is also called the creation, generating, or promoting cycle. In the Sheng cycle, each Element supports the next. For example, Wood feeds Fire which creates ash residue which becomes Earth. Deep within the Earth, metals are developed which are then found in trace amounts in the Water which springs out from the ground. The waters nourish the trees or Wood and the cycle continues. In clinical practice it might be found that a Liver or Gall Bladder disorder, i.e., Wood disorder, may be due to the Water element found in the Bladder and Kidney channels not providing sufficient nourishment and support.

The control or acting cycle is called the **Ko cycle.** Each Element controls another and is also controlled by another Element. Metal, such as an ax, will control wood. Wood controls Earth, such as the trees covering the ground or the roots of trees holding the earth to prevent erosion. Earth can dam or channel Water. Water will control or extinguish Fire. Fire will melt the metal blade of the ax. The Ko cycle balances the Sheng cycle to avoid unrestrained growth.

One can see that certain Elements, if especially strong, can either nourish or control another Element. If especially weak, it will fail to nourish or can be easily overcome. The balanced cyclic relationship of the Elements maintaining one another is considered to foster the healthiest life.

THE PRIMARY CHANNELS

The channels (or meridians), collaterals, and vessels are as important to Asian medicine as anatomy is to Western medicine. Even though the ancient Chinese paid little attention to the physical structures inside the body, an intricate network of pathways is described in the texts using minute detail. Every part of the body inside and out is enlivened, nourished and warmed by Qi and Blood through this network, allowing the body to function as a single unit rather than separate parts.

> It is by virtue of the twelve channels that human life exists, that disease arises, that human beings can be treated and illness cured. The twelve channels are where beginners start and masters end. To beginners it seems easy; the masters know how difficult it is . . . Qi cannot travel without a path, just as water flows or the sun and moon orbit without rest. So do the Yin vessels nourish the zang and the Yang vessels nourish the fu (*Huang Di Nei Jing, Ling Shu,* 200 AD, quoted by Deadman, 1998).

The meridian charts on the inside back cover show the external pathways of the twelve primary channels. Two of the eight extraordinary vessels are pictured as well, traveling along the midline of the torso front and back. Not pictured are 16 luo collaterals, 12 cutaneous regions, minute collaterals, 12 sinew channels and 12 divergent channels. These more obscure channels are not covered in the scope of this chapter.

The complete name of each channel has three parts. The first is the limb where it starts or ends, like foot or hand. The second part is its six-channel relationship with another of the same polarity, i.e., Yin with Yin, Yang with Yang. The third is the organ the channel relates to, each channel having a Yin/Yang, exterior/interior relationship with another.

Even though most charts show only the external pathway of the primary channels, the descriptions that follow offer a description of the internal pathways as well. It is important to be aware of the deep channels since they can connect seemingly unrelated signs and symptoms. They can also help explain the actions of the acupoints. For example, PC 6 is used when the stomach Qi is rebellious, resulting in nausea. The external pathway primarily runs along the medial aspect of the arm, but internally, the pathway goes to the area of the stomach, called the Middle Burner.

CHINESE BODY CLOCK

The channels flow through the body according to a natural, rhythmic cycle. This cycle has been called the **Chinese body clock,** summarized in Table 17–2. Each channel has a peak flow when its Qi is at its maximum and a valley when its Qi is at its minimum, on the a.m. and p.m. sides of the clock.

From **3:00 to 5:00 a.m.,** the **Hand Taiyin Lung channel** energy is at its peak. Humans awaken, stretch and breathe deeply. The Lung is Yin compared to its Yang partner, the Large Intestine; they both relate to the Metal element. The Lung, being Hand Taiyin, also correlates to the Spleen, which is Foot Taiyin.

The Lung channel's general terrain is from the chest, where the exterior pathway of the Liver ends, to the hand, where the Large Intestine begins. It originates in the Middle Burner, runs down to the Large Intestine; up to the stomach; passes through the diaphragm, lungs and emerges at the first intercostal space, below the distal end of the clavicle. It runs along the anterior medial aspect of the arm, ending at the medial side of the thumb.

Next, from **5:00 to 7:00 a.m.,** the **hand Yangming Large Intestine channel** becomes strong and many individuals have a bowel movement. During the Metal time, one lets go of what one doesn't need. It connects with the Foot Yangming Stomach channel according to the six channel theory.

Table 17–2   CHINESE BODY CLOCK

	3:00–5:00 a.m.	Hand Taiyin Lung channel
	5:00–7:00 a.m.	Hand Yangming Large Intestine channel
	7:00–9:00 a.m.	Foot Yangming Stomach channel
	9:00–11:00 a.m.	Foot Taiyin Spleen channel
	11:00 a.m.–1:00 p.m.	Hand Shaoyin Heart channel
	1:00–3:00 p.m.	Hand Taiyang Small Intestine channel
	3:00–5:00 p.m.	Foot Taiyang Bladder channel
	5:00–7:00 p.m.	Foot Shaoyin Kidney channel
	7:00–9:00 p.m.	Hand Jueyin Pericardium channel
	9:00–11:00 p.m.	Hand Shaoyang Triple Burner channel
	11:00 p.m.–1:00 a.m.	Foot Shaoyang Gall Bladder channel
	1:00–3:00 a.m.	Foot Jueyin Liver channel

The Large Intestine channel starts close to where its partner, the Lung channel, ends, running generally from the hand to face. It starts at the tip of the index finger, up the lateral anterior part of the arm. At the shoulder, it goes to a point below C-7 and descends to the supraclavicular fossa, to the lung and then the large intestine. From the clavicle, it ascends to the lower gums and ends at the opposite side of the nose, where it connects to the Stomach channel.

The **foot Yangming Stomach channel** energy dominates **7:00 a.m. until 9:00 a.m.,** when many people take their first nourishment of the day, aiding digestion. It is Yang, its Yin pair being the Spleen channel, both relating to the Earth Element. Its six-channel theory partner is the hand Yangming Large Intestine.

The Stomach channel by and large runs from the head to the feet, starting from the lateral side of the nostril, ascending to meet the Bladder channel and descending to enter the upper gums. Its exterior pathway starts below the eye, runs down the face to the jaw, up to the corner of the head, down along the throat, entering the body at the supraclavicular fossa, passing through the diaphragm, entering the stomach and spleen. The superficial channel passes through the nipples, abdomen, inguinal area, veering laterally to follow the anterior lateral aspect of the leg to end at the lateral side of the second toe. It connects with the Spleen from the highest part of the dorsum of the foot to the big toe.

The **foot Taiyin Spleen channel** is strongest between **9:00 and 11:00 a.m.,** when the workday begins and individuals digest (transform) their food as well as adapt to the workday demands, transforming tasks into accomplishments. Its six-channel theory pair is the hand Taiyin Lung.

The Spleen channel runs from the feet to chest, starting at the big toe, running along the medial arch of the foot, in front of the medial malleolus, ascending along the medial anterior aspect of the leg, entering the abdomen at the inguinal area, ascending to the spleen, stomach, diaphragm, heart, esophagus and ending at the center of the tongue. Its exterior pathway passes through the lateral costal region, close to where the Heart channel begins.

The heart of the day finds the **hand Shaoyin Heart channel** energy at its strongest from **11:00 a.m. until 1:00 p.m.** It is Yin, with its Yang pair being the Small Intestine and both channels relating to the Fire Element. Its six-channel pair connects with the foot Shaoyin Kidney.

The Heart channel starts at the chest and flows to the arm, originating from the heart. It passes through the diaphragm, connects with the small intestine, enters the lung and emerges at the axilla. From there, the superficial channel runs along the anterior medial aspect of the arm to end at the medial side of the tip of the little finger.

The **hand Taiyang Small Intestine channel** is most active from **1:00 until 3:00 p.m.,** when one might get aching shoulders. It's paired with the Heart channel in its interior/exterior Fire relationship and the foot Taiyang Bladder channel with the six-channel theory.

Basically, the Small Intestine channel runs from the hand to the head, starting where the Heart channel leaves off from the ulnar side of the little finger. It follows the posterior lateral side of the arm to the shoulder joint then circling the scapula. It connects with the point below C-7, forward to the supraclavicular fossa and descends to the heart and small intestine. The superficial pathway from the clavicle ascends to the neck, cheek and ear. From there, a branch links to the Bladder channel between the eyes.

From **3:00 to 5:00 p.m.**, the **foot Taiyang Bladder channel** energy is strongest. It is Yang in relationship to its Water partner, the Kidney channel. Its six-channel partner is the hand Taiyang Small Intestine.

Mainly, the bladder channel is the longest channel and runs from the head to the feet. It starts where the Small Intestine leaves off at the inner canthus, ascends the forehead back to the nape of the neck, connecting internally to the Governing vessel, the temple, the vertex and entering the brain. Two branches run down the back, connecting internally with the Kidney and Bladder. It travels down the center of the back of the leg, through the popliteal fossa where it meets its second branch. It continues as one down the posterior of the leg, the lateral side of the foot, ending at the lateral side of the little toe. (Often remembered by Westerners as the little piggie that went "wee wee" all the way home!)

The **foot Shaoyin Kidney channel** energy peaks from **5:00 until 7:00 p.m.** Individuals with deficient Kidney Qi may find that they are troubled with low back pain and fatigue and want to stop to recharge artificially at a happy hour around this time of evening! It's coupled with the hand Shaoyin heart channel in the six-channel theory.

The Kidney channel runs from the feet to the chest, starting internally under the little toe where the bladder leaves off, surfacing on the sole of the foot. This makes it the only channel that doesn't start or end on a finger or toe. It circles the ankle, running up the posterior medial aspect of the leg. It goes inward toward the sacrum, up the lumbar spine to the kidneys and bladder, Liver, diaphragm, lung, and throat, terminating at the root of the tongue. Its external pathway emerges beside the pubic bone and ascends parallel to the midline to points below the sterno-clavicular joint. From its internal connection to the heart it flows to the chest to connect to the next channel in the circuit, the pericardium.

7:00 until 9:00 p.m. is the time for the **hand Jueyin Pericardium channel.** It's the best time to curl up and hug someone, which presses on the entire channel. Its Fire partner is the Yang Triple Burner channel and it's also paired with the foot Jueyin Liver.

Generally originating from the chest and running to the hand, it starts its internal pathway going from the chest, to the pericardium, diaphragm and abdomen, to communicate with the Upper, Middle and Lower burners. A branch from the chest emerges lateral to the nipple, runs in front of the axilla, down the middle of the arm to the middle finger. A branch from the middle of the palm connects the Pericardium channel to the next channel, the triple burner.

The **hand Shaoyang Triple Burner channel** dominates the next two hours, from **9:00 until 11:00 p.m.** A good way to press your own Triple Burner channel is to cross your arms and rub the top of your opposite arm as if to warm yourself up. The Triple Burner also pairs with the next channel, the foot Shaoyang Gall Bladder channel in a Yang/Yang relationship.

Running from the hand to the head, it starts from the ulnar side of the ring finger and runs laterally between the bones of the forearm, up to the shoulder joint, supraclavicular fossa, then descends to connect with the upper, middle, and lower burners. From the chest, a branch goes up to the clavicle, neck, around the back of the ear, ending in the infra-orbital region, above the beginning of the Gall Bladder channel.

The next cycle is the Wood cycle. This is thought of as the time when you can't decide, you "sleep on it." That's because the Wood element gives you the power to be decisive! The **foot Shaoyang Gall Bladder channel** flows from **11:00 p.m. until 1:00 a.m.** from the head to the feet. It may not be the longest channel, but it is the most convoluted and difficult to follow. An abbreviated look at its pathway starts from the outer canthus of the eye, going down to the ear, zigzagging on the side of the head, in, around and through the ear, to the forehead above the eye and back to the occiput. It descends to the shoulders, supraclavicular fossa, descending to the chest, diaphragm, liver and gall bladder. The main portion of the channel from the shoulder descends to the axilla, lateral side of the chest, hips, lateral aspect of the leg and thigh, ending at the lateral aspect of the fourth toe. A branch from the dorsum of the foot connects with the beginning of the Liver at the big toe.

The **foot Jueyin Liver channel** finishes this cycle from **1:00 to 3:00 a.m.**, flowing externally from feet to chest, connecting with the Lung channel. It starts its flow from the lateral aspect of the big toe, ascending along the dorsum of the foot, crossing the Spleen channel at the medial aspect of the leg, curving internally around the genitalia, to the lower abdomen, stomach, liver and gall bladder. It continues to ascend to the costal region, diaphragm, throat, then eyes, ending at the top of the head.

This 24-hour cycle occurs every day throughout an individual's life. Asian Bodywork therapists keep this in mind as an assessment tool. When a problem occurs at a certain time of day, one would look at the channel strongest at that time, to see if there could possibly be a relationship. For example, if back pain starts at around 4:00 pm everyday, one would investigate the possibility that the Bladder channel down the back might be involved.

The body clock can be utilized as a possible time to treat as well. Although not particularly convenient sometimes, it is preferable to treat the meridian during its two-hour cycle. Again, in the above example, it would probably not be a problem to schedule a client any time between 3 and 5 p.m. But someone with an imbalance in the Lung channel (3 to 5 a.m.) who wakes with breathing problems during that time might be difficult to see then. In that case, instruction to work on points given as homework can be helpful.

THE FOUR PILLARS OF ASSESSMENT

When an individual appears in the clinic of a practitioner of Asian medicine, that individual is assessed utilizing the theoretical viewpoint detailed above. An assessment is conducted according to the four pillars: looking, touching, listening/smelling and asking (See Figure 17–5).

To assess by **looking,** the clinician observes the physical appearance, demeanor, movement, hair, and face color such as pale or dark circles under the eyes. The eyes are also observed. The tongue is carefully considered in every assessment. The color, shape, and coating of the tongue offers much information on the condition of the client and his or her energy.

Touching assessment is another of the four pillars. Individuals may report discomfort in certain areas that may be palpated to assess rigidity or flaccidness. The pulses also give instrumental information on the flow of energy through the channels. Each of the twelve primary channels can be assessed utilizing the pulses on each hand.

Listening and smelling are related assessment tools. The client may have a **smell** about them that corresponds to the smells related to the elements. (Recall that Earth's smell is fragrant and Fire scorched.) **Listening** to the sound quality of the voice may also lead the practitioner to consider likely areas to investigate. A crying quality to the voice suggests some issues with Metal, while an individual who seems to shout is often someone with a Wood imbalance.

Asking or questioning the client is another assessment method. The practitioner inquires about the individual's psycho-spiritual-physical functioning. Questions are asked regarding appetite, diet, digestion, and elimination. Sleep patterns, dreaming, relationship concerns or conflicts, feelings of hot or cold, energy levels, are often explored. For women, questions regarding the menstrual cycle can help gain insights to the level of balance in their lives. Additionally, clients are quizzed about issues that they may want addressed in their treatment as well as any possible contraindications to treatment.

The practitioner synthesizes the information gathered from the four pillars, much like a jigsaw puzzle of numerous pieces, into a picture of the client's present life situation. From a careful scrutiny of the assessment picture, the treatment plan is developed.

An additional method of assessment is *hara diagnosis*. In hara diagnosis, the abdominal or Tanden region is palpated to detect energy flow and blockages. Chapter 19 explains more about hara diagnosis.

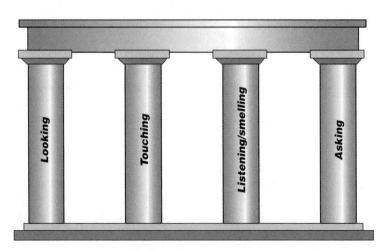

FIGURE 17–5. Four pillars of assessment.

ACUPOINTS

There are 365 classical pressure points or acupoints located along the major energy channels. Acupoints are places where Qi can collect, and can be accessed and influenced by applying pressure.

Acupoints are used for diagnosis as well as treatment of energy imbalances. Acupoint locations are identified by channel name and point number, e.g., Gall Bladder 20 (GB20). In acupuncture, needles are typically used to stimulate a point; however, ABT systems use pressure on the points with thumb, fingers, or elbow. The figures on the inside back cover show the major energy channels and important acupoint locations.

The effective use of acupoints is based in part on accurate Asian medical assessment and often will not work if used in a Western symptomatic fashion (i.e., seeking to eliminate specific symptoms). In China, the practitioner who treats based on symptoms that manifest *after* the person becomes ill is considered the lowliest unskilled practitioner.

Wellness and prevention is the strength and focus of traditional Asian medicine. The most accomplished and expert practitioner can prevent an illness by treating *before* a person becomes sick. In the ancient *Huang Di Nei Jing,* it states, "The sages don't treat people who are already sick, but treat before they become sick. The same as in organizing a country: taking medicine after becoming sick is like making regulations after turmoil, or just like starting to dig a well when you feel thirsty, or beginning to make new weapons when the enemy is approaching your border. Isn't it too late?"

That's why the focus of this chapter has been assessing the person in relationship to natural forces with an emphasis on bringing the individual back into balance. A human being's life should follow the Qi of heaven and earth. For example, in spring, Yang Qi is growing along with everything else and the Qi of the universe is rising. Therefore, people should go to bed early, get up early and have a relaxed walk in the cool, invigorating air. Wearing one's hair and clothes loosely, gently moving one's body as if you are the God of Spring who cares for everything helps the growing Qi inside rise as well. Respectively, Summer, Autumn and Winter have their corresponding action and mind in harmony with the nature (Wang, 1999).

Thus, there are no points that can be used on everyone at any time. One would not want to give a general "relaxing" session to someone who is deficient, just as one would not want to tonify someone with an excess condition. It is essential to look at that person's relative state of balance within the ebb and flow of Yin, Yang and the Five Elements. There is a tendency for people to want to sleep later and eat more in the Winter. Certainly, one's approach wouldn't be to tonify that person. More likely, as part of the session, the practitioner would encourage the client to live as much as possible in harmony with nature, resting more and eating warming foods. Therefore, acupoints are selected based on supporting an individual's movement into balance, based on the Four Pillars of Assessment.

There are 20 useful acupoints listed in Table 17–3. This table can be used as a reference, keeping in mind that its effectiveness as a resource will increase with accurate assessment. See Figures 17–6 to 17–10 for anatomical locations of these useful acupoints.

Caution: certain points are contraindicated when specific conditions are present. For example GB 21, LI 4, Sp6, and Bl 60 are not to be used on pregnant women unless it is to promote and ease the flow of labor.

Table 17–3 TWENTY USEFUL ACUPOINTS

Figures 17–6 to 17–10 show anatomical locations of the 20 useful acupoints.

Head and Face

GB 20 (Fengchi) Wind Pond

Location: Below the occiput, in the depression between the origins of the sternocleidomastoid muscle and the trapezius

Nature: Meeting point of these channels: GB, TB, Yang Wei Mai and Yang Qiao Mai

Action: dispels wind (exterior or interior); benefits head, ears and eyes; clears the brain; subdues Liver Yang

Indications: temporal, one-sided or occipital headaches; dizziness, vertigo or eye problems; stiffness of the neck and shoulders, common cold, insomnia

(continued)

Table 17–3   (Cont.)

Ex 1, Yintang (M-HN-3) Seal Hall

Location: On the midline between the eyebrows

Action: Dispels wind; clears heat; calms the mind

Indications: Relieves anxiety; insomnia; frontal headaches; sinus blockages; stops convulsions

EX 2, Taiyang, Supreme Yang (M-HN-9)

Location: At the temple, one cun (approximately the width of the thumb) posterior to the midpoint between the lateral end of the eyebrow and the outer corner of the eye

Action: Eliminates wind and clears heat; benefits the eyes

Indications: Hypertension due to Yang excess; one sided headaches due to Liver Yang or Liver Fire; dizziness; toothaches; eye problems due to heat

LI 20 (Yingxiang) Welcome Fragrance

Location: In the nasolabial groove, at the level of the midpoint of the lateral border of the nostril

Nature: Meeting point of St and LI channels

Action: Dispels exterior wind; clears heat

Indications: Nasal congestion, nosebleed, sneezing, facial paralysis, trigeminal neuralgia, tics

Shoulders and Arms

GB 21 (Jianjing) Shoulder Well

Location: Midway between C-7 and the acromion, at the highest point of the shoulder

Nature: Meeting point of GB, TB and Yang Wei Mai

Actions: Relaxes the sinews; regulates Qi; promotes lactation and delivery

Indications: Pain in the head, neck and/or shoulders; mastitis; difficult lactation; prolonged labor; *strong stimulation contraindicated during pregnancy!*

LI 15 (Jianyu) Shoulder Transport Point

Location: In the depression of the acromion in the center of the deltoid muscle when the arm is raised to 90 degrees

Nature: Point on LI and Yang Qiao Mai

Actions: Benefits sinews and promotes Qi circulation; stops pain and expels wind

Indications: Shoulder pain and inability to raise arm due to Bi syndrome

LI 11 (Quchi) Crooked Pool

Location: When the elbow is flexed, the point is in the depression at the lateral end of the transverse cubital crease, midway between the lung meridian and the lateral epicondyle of the humerus.

Nature: He-Sea and Earth point on LI channel

Actions: General heat clearing point; cools blood, drains dampness and stops itching; expels wind, activates channel and alleviates pain

Indication: Heat as in sore throat, skin eruptions (damp-heat), hypertension or febrile disease; elbow, shoulder and neck pain or atrophy

Pc 6 (Neiguan) Inner Gate

Location: 2 cun above the transverse crease of the wrist, between the palmaris longus and the flexor radialis tendons

Nature: Luo-connecting point of Pc channel; master point of Yin Wei Mai

Actions: Opens chest and regulates Qi; calms the spirit and regulates the Ht; harmonizes stomach

Indications: Nausea, vomiting, hiccups and stomachache; chest pain, stuffiness and palpitations; insomnia, agitation or irritation due to Qi stagnation or Ht patterns

(continued)

Table 17–3 (*Cont.*)

Lu 7 (Lieque) Broken Sequence

Location: Proximal to styloid process of radius, between the tendons of the brachioradialus and abductor pollicis longus

Nature: Luo-connecting point of Lu channel, master point of Ren Mai

Action: Stimulates the descending and dispersing action of Lung-Qi; releases exterior and dissipates wind; regulates the water passages; opens Ren Mai

Indications: Beginning stages of common cold; all types of asthma; emotional problems caused by worry and sadness; headache and stiffness of the neck; combined with Ki 6 for menstrual irregularities and dry throat and eyes (due to it being master point of the Ren Mai)

TW 5 (Waiguan) Outer Gate

Location: 2 cun above the wrist crease, on the dorsal aspect of the arm, between the radius and the ulna

Nature: Luo-connecting point of TB channel; master point of Yang Wei Mai

Actions: Expels, clears heat and releases exterior; benefits ear and head; subdues Liver-Yang

Indications: Febrile disease and alternating fever and chills; headache on the side of the head; tinnitus, deafness or other ear problems; red and swollen eyes; pain in the ribs; Bi-painful obstruction syndrome affecting arm, neck, shoulder or any pain caused by wind

LI 4 (Hegu) Union Valley or Tiger's Mouth

Location: On the dorsum of the hand, between the 1st and 2nd metacarpal bones, approximately in the middle of the 2nd metacarpal bone on the radial side

Nature: Source point of LI

Actions: Dispels exterior wind and releases the exterior; stops pain and removes obstructions from the channel; regulates defensive Qi and sweating; induces labor

Indications: *Contraindicated for pregnant women unless used to promote delivery; frontal headache, toothache, neck pain, nasal obstruction and hay fever symptoms due to its strong direct influence on the face and eyes; sweating problems

SI 3 (Houxi) Back Stream

Location: At the apex of the distal palmar crease on the ulnar side of a clenched fist, proximal to the head of the fifth metacarpal bone

Nature: Shu-stream and Wood point of SI channel; master point of Du Mai

Actions: Eliminates exterior wind and heat and interior wind from Du Mai; benefits sinews along occiput, neck and back; resolves dampness and jaundice; calms the spirit

Indications: Interior wind symptoms affecting Du Mai such as convulsions, tremors, stiff neck, shoulders and back (use with Bl 62); occipital headache; gives person "backbone" emotionally as well as strengthening the spine physically

Hips and Legs

GB 30 (Huantiao) Jumping Round

Location: At the junction of the lateral 1/3 and medial 2/3 of the distance between the greater trochanter and the hiatus of the sacrum

Nature: Meeting point of GB and Bl channels

Actions: Activates channel and alleviates pain; dispels wind-damp; clears heat

Indications: Sciatica; lumbar pain; frustration; atrophy syndrome and the sequelae of wind stroke

BL 40 (Weizhong) Entrusting Middle

Location: Midpoint on the transverse crease of the popliteal fossa, between the tendons of the biceps femoris and the semitendinosus

Nature: He-Sea and Earth point on the Bl channel; command point of lower back

Actions: Clears heat, summer-heat and cools blood; eliminates stasis of blood; resolves dampness and removes obstruction from channel

Indications: Lower back pain (more acute than chronic); hip problems; motor impairment of the lower extremities; abdominal pain; vomiting and or diarrhea; heat stroke or epilepsy; burning urination

(continued)

Table 17–3 *(Cont.)*

GB 34 (Yanglingquan) Yang Mound Spring or Sunny Side of the Mountain

Location: In the depression anterior and inferior to the head of the fibula

Nature: He-Sea and Earth point of GB channel; influential point of tendons

Actions: Promotes smooth flow of Liver-Qi; resolves damp-heat; relaxes sinews; activates channel and alleviates pain; clears Lv-GB damp-heat; subdues rebellious Qi

Indications: Tendon contractions, spasms or cramps; lateral costal pain; bitter taste in the mouth; numbness, weakness or pain in the lower extremities; Liver Qi stagnation symptoms such as frequent sighing and irritability.

BL 60 (Kunlun) Kunlun Mountain

Location: In the depression between the lateral malleolus and the calcaneal tendon

Nature: River and fire point of Bl channel

Actions: Pacifies wind and clears heat by lowering Yang; removes obstructions from Bl channel and alleviates pain; relaxes the sinews and strengthens the back

Indications: Occipital headache, chronic stiff neck, shoulders, back and/or heel pain; prolonged labor. *Contraindicated for pregnancy!

St 36 (Zusanli) Foot 3 Miles

Location: 3 cun below the knee cap, 1 cun lateral to the anterior crest of the tibia

Nature: He-Sea and Earth point of the St channel; command point of abdomen; sea of nourishment

Actions: Harmonizes stomach and spleen; tonifies Qi, Blood and Yin; clears pathogenic factors and calms the spirit; uplifts Yang and restores consciousness; alleviates pain in the channel

Indications: Use with moxa as a general tonic and energizing point for all deficiency patterns; stomach pain, indigestion, vomiting or belching; diarrhea or gas; insomnia due to stomach disorders; knee or wrist pain (possibly due to its connection with the LI channel on the arm or if the pain is due to cold-damp invasion); secures the fetus in threatened miscarriage and used for postpartum dizziness

St 40 (Fenglong) Abundant Bulge

Location: On the lower leg, midway between the popliteal crease and lateral malleolus, two finger widths from the crest of the tibia

Nature: St channel luo connecting point

Action: Resolves phlegm and damp; clears heat; calms and clears the mind; opens the chest and calms asthma

Indications: Used to eliminate phlegm in all parts of the body manifesting as asthma, lumps, a heavy feeling in the body or mental disturbances

Sp 6 (Sanyinjiao) 3 Yin Crossing

Location: 3 cun directly above the tip of the medial malleolus, on the posterior border of the medial aspect of the tibia

Nature: Intersecting point of Sp, Ki and Lv channel

Actions: Nourishes Blood and Yin; regulates, tonifies and strengthens spleen Qi and Yang; strengthens function of the Liver, particularly the smooth flow of Qi; tonifies Kidney Yin, Qi and Jing; resolves damp-heat or damp-cold; regulates the uterus, menstruation and induces labor; benefits urination and the genitals; calms the spirit; alleviates pain in the channel

Indications: *Contraindicated during pregnancy; prolonged labor; lower abdominal pain; insomnia due to blood or Yin deficiency; menstrual disorders; medial knee pain; diarrhea and edema due to Sp deficiency; sexual dysfunction due to Qi deficiency; urination problems

Lv 3 (Taichong) Great Surge

Location: On the dorsum of the foot, distal to the junction of the 1st and 2nd metatarsal bones

Nature: Yuen-source, shu-stream and Earth point of Lv channel

Actions: Regulates and tonifies Liver Qi, Yang, Yin and Blood; expels interior wind; calms the spirit; regulates menstruation and lower jiao; clears head and eyes

Indications: Uterine bleeding between periods or other menstrual irregularities; soothes the Liver, hernia, headache, hypertension or dizziness due to Lv Yang rising; depression, sighing, irritability or lateral costal distention due to Lv Qi stagnation; hangover, jetlag (combine with LI 4 for "4 Gates"), red, painful, itchy or swollen eyes; spasms, contractions or cramps in the muscles

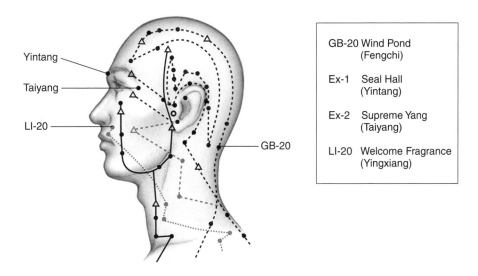

GB-20 Wind Pond
(Fengchi)

Ex-1 Seal Hall
(Yintang)

Ex-2 Supreme Yang
(Taiyang)

LI-20 Welcome Fragrance
(Yingxiang)

FIGURE 17–6. Useful acupoints on the head.

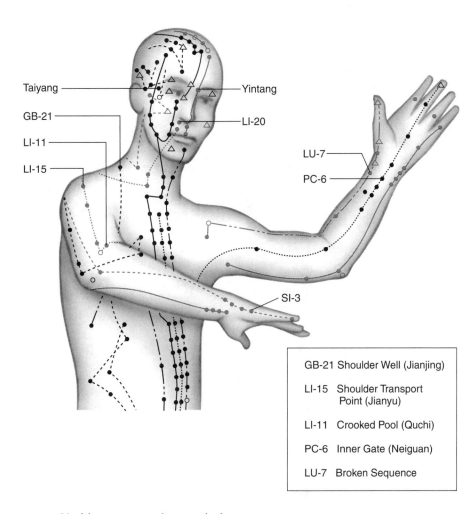

GB-21 Shoulder Well (Jianjing)

LI-15 Shoulder Transport
Point (Jianyu)

LI-11 Crooked Pool (Quchi)

PC-6 Inner Gate (Neiguan)

LU-7 Broken Sequence

FIGURE 17–7. Useful acupoints on the upper body.

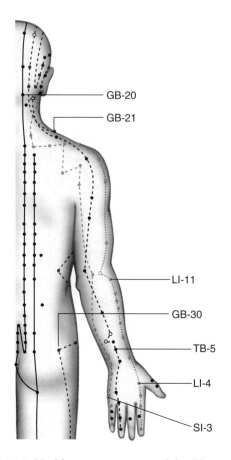
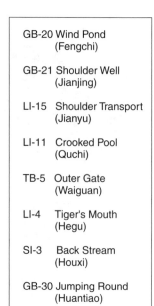

GB-20 Wind Pond
(Fengchi)

GB-21 Shoulder Well
(Jianjing)

LI-15 Shoulder Transport
(Jianyu)

LI-11 Crooked Pool
(Quchi)

TB-5 Outer Gate
(Waiguan)

LI-4 Tiger's Mouth
(Hegu)

SI-3 Back Stream
(Houxi)

GB-30 Jumping Round
(Huantiao)

FIGURE 17–8. Useful acupoints on arm and shoulder.

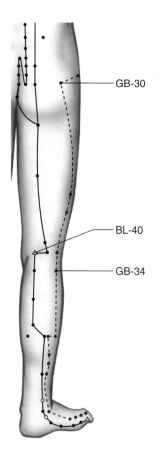

GB-30 Jumping Round
(Huantiao)

GB-34 Sunny Side of
Mountain
(Yanglingquan)

BL-40 Entrusting Middle
(Weizhong)

FIGURE 17–9. Useful acupoints on
the back of the leg and hip.

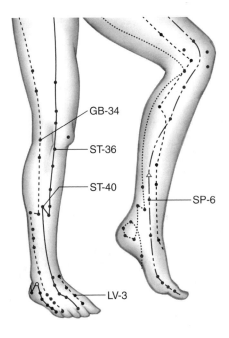

St-36	Foot 3 Miles (Zusanli)
GB-34	Sunny Side of Mountain (Yanglingquan)
St-40	Abundant Bulge (Fenglong)
Sp-6	3 Yin Crossing (Sanyinjiao)
Lv-3	Great Surge (Taichong)

FIGURE 17–10. Useful acupoints on the lower leg.

APPLICATION TO ABT PRACTICE

How the theories presented in this chapter are utilized depends on the form of ABT practiced and the preferences of the practitioner. For example, a Zen Shiatsu therapist focuses on the meridians, whereas one who does acupressure uses acupoints more. A tuina therapist applies techniques to balance Qi and blood circulation, while someone who does Jin Sin Do® will be more concerned with the Eight Extraordinary vessels. ABTs with training use moxa to warm the vessels when there are symptoms of cold or *guasha* to move Qi and Blood when there is stagnation.

The commonality that binds them all together as Asian bodywork therapists is the rich history, eloquent theories and years of evolution of Chinese medicine. Not only is it a masterpiece of beauty, harmony and intricacy, but centuries of successful applications are evidence that it works.

SUMMARY

Asian Bodywork Therapy (ABT) is a term used to describe forms of bodywork with roots in Chinese medicine. These forms come originally from East Asian countries of China, Korea, and Japan. Specific ABT systems described in this text include Amma, Zen Shiatsu, and Jin Shin Do®. Other forms are also recognized by the American Organization for Bodywork Therapies of Asia (AOBTA®).

The scope of practice of ABT includes assessment and treatment of energetic imbalances according to Chinese medicine theories. ABT techniques include touching, pressing, holding along meridians or on acupoints, stretching, application of medicinal plant foods, application of heat or cold, and dietary methods. ABT is one of the three branches of Chinese medicine, along with herbology and acupuncture, for which practitioners can receive certification from the National Certification Commission for Acupuncture and Oriental Medicine (NCCAOM).

Chinese medicine is assumed to have developed from Chinese folk remedies and thousands of years of empirical evidence. The earliest known text on Chinese medicine is the *Yellow Emperor's Classic of Internal Medicine*, written about 2500 BCE. The earliest reference to Yin and Yang is thought to have been in the *Book of Changes*, written about 700 BCE. The naturalist school of philosophy (c. 300 BCE) sought to find ways to live in harmony with nature, and further developed concepts of yin and yang, and the five elements. These ideas, plus the concept of Qi or life energy, are the foundation of classical Chinese medicine.

Chinese medicine originated in northern China near the Yellow River more than 5,000 years ago. The inhabitants there developed acupuncture, moxibustion, and *anmo* (manual methods) to heal various ailments. They also came to identify the energy channels and acupoints that form the basic energetic anatomy of Chinese medicine.

Chinese medicine spread throughout the territory of China, then to Korea, and from there to Japan in about 600 CE. The principles of Chinese medicine were absorbed into the indigenous cultures to which they spread with modifications according to local beliefs and practices. Thus Chinese medicine differs somewhat from area to area. Terms used for Chinese medicine include traditional Asian medicine (TAM), traditional Chinese medicine (TCM), and classical Chinese medicine (CCM).

Knowledge of Chinese medicine was brought to Europe in the 17th century by Jesuit missionaries returning from Imperial China. In the mid-20th century, the French diplomat Soulie de Morant wrote about acupuncture, which lead to study groups in many Western countries in the 1940s. Immigrants from Asia brought knowledge of Chinese medicine wherever in the world they settled. In the 1950s Toru Namikoshi brought shiatsu to the United States. In the 1970s, a number of teachers introduced different forms of ABT into the United States and other Western countries. In the past century, Western medicine has been integrated into the traditional medical practices in China, Japan, and other Asian countries.

The core of Asian medicine is the concept that the universe is dynamic while still maintaining a unity. According to TAM, humans exist in relationship to the fabric of the universe. They are related to and connected with all that exists.

Yin and Yang illustrate this connection, and the Yin/Yang symbol depicts movement and change in the universe. Yin is (relative to Yang) dark, deep, dense, feminine, interior, still, cool, and contracting. Yang is (relative to Yin) light, energetic, ethereal, masculine, exterior, moving, warm, and expanding. The principles of Yin and Yang are opposition, interdependence, consuming/supporting relationship, intertransformation, and infinite divisibility.

Qi is a continuous form of energy existing in material form when it condenses, and non-material form when it disperses. The Chinese character for Qi is rice cooking in a pot. Qi in a more narrow sense is the life energy that is extracted from the food we eat, and the air we breathe. It is then transformed as usable Qi that circulates through a network of channels in the body. ABT techniques tonify, disperse, move, uplift or rectify Qi. Functions of Qi are transforming, transporting, holding, protecting, and warming.

The Five Elements of Chinese medicine are Wood, Fire, Earth, Metal, and Water. Each element is associated with a degree of Yin or Yang, and has associated channels of energy. In the Shen or generating cycle, each element is seen as supporting the next, e.g., Wood feeds Fire, Fire creates ash (Earth), Earth develops Metals. In the Ko or controlling cycle, each element is seen as controlling the next, e.g., Metal as ax controls Wood, Wood as trees acts on Earth, Earth dams water. The balanced cyclic relationship of the elements within the individual fosters a healthy life.

Channels or meridians provide a path for Qi or energy to flow. There are twelve primary channels, eight extraordinary vessels, and other energy networks identified in Chinese medicine. A complete channel name has three parts: the place where it starts or ends, its six-channel relationship, and the organ that the channel relates to. There are both external and internal pathways to a channel, although most charts show only the external pathway. Knowledge of the internal pathway is useful to understand the action of the acupoints.

The channels flow through the body according to a natural rhythmic cycle referred to as the Chinese body clock. At different times of the day, the energy in one of the channels is at its peak. Knowing the Chinese body clock can help in assessment and treatment of energy imbalances.

The Four Pillars of Assessment of energy imbalance are looking, touching, smelling/listening and asking. Hara diagnosis is another assessment method. The practitioner synthesizes the information gathered from the four pillars to devise a treatment for any energy imbalance detected.

In an ABT session, acupoints are chosen and stimulated according to the energy assessment made by the practitioner. Although specific acupoints are commonly associated with certain symptoms, the effective application of ABT requires an accurate assessment of each recipient's situation. Specific points are contraindicated with pregnancy and certain medical conditions.

Different forms of ABT utilize the theories of Chinese medicine in different ways. For example, some focus on meridians, others on acupoints. But they all share its rich history, eloquent theories, and years of evolution.

A look ahead . . .

The next three chapters take a closer look at specific forms of Asian bodywork therapy, two from Japan and one from the contemporary United States. They illustrate the diversity of application of traditional Asian medicine, and the continuing evolution of these ancient practices. Chapter 18 examines Amma, traditional Japanese massage.

REFERENCES

American Organization for Bodywork Therapies of Asia, *www.AOBTA.org*. Accessed 5/27/2003.

Capra, F. (1999). *The Tao of Physics: An Exploration of the Parallels between Modern Physics and Eastern Mysteries*. Boston: Shambhala Publications.

Deadman, P. (1998). *A Manual of Acupuncture*, East Sussex, England: Journal of Chinese Medicine Publications.

Jarrett. L. (2000). *Nourishing Destiny: The Inner Tradition of Chinese Medicine*, Stockbridge, MA: Spirit Path Press.

Maciocia, G. (1998). *The Foundations of Chinese Medicine: A Comprehensive Text for Acupuncturists and Herbalists*. Edinburgh: Churchill Livingstone.

Namikoshi, Toru (1969). *Shiatsu: Japanese Finger-Pressure Therapy*. Tokyo: Japan Publications.

Ni, M. (1995). *The Yellow Emperor's Classic of Medicine: A new translation of the Nei Jing Suwen with commentary*. Boston: Shambhala.

Tedeschi, M. (2000). *Essential Anatomy for Healing and the Martial Arts*. Tokyo: Weatherwill.

Wang, J. (1994). *The History of Massage in Mainland China*. American Organization for Bodywork Therapies of Asia (AOBTA), Video 13, Boston, MA convention.

Wang, J. (1999). "To Treat Before Sick" from *Pulse*, Voorhees, NJ: AOBTA.

Yuen, J. (2001). *Light on the Essence of Chinese Medicine: The Nei Jing Su Wen*, New England School of Acupuncture, Boston, MA.

Zukav, G. (1980). *The Dancing WuLi Masters: An Overview of the New Physics*. New York: Bantam Books.

ADDITIONAL RESOURCES

Beresford-Cooke, C. (1999). *Shiatsu Theory and Practice*. Edinburgh: Churchill Livingstone.

Cheng, X. (1993). *Chinese Acupuncture and Moxibustion*. Beijing, China: Foreign Languages Press.

Connelly, D. (1979). *Traditional Acupuncture: The Law of the Five Elements*, Columbia, MD: The Center for Traditional Acupuncture.

Henshall, K. (1992). *A Guide to Remembering Japanese Characters*. Rutland, Vermont: Charles E. Tuttle Company.

Jarmey, C. and Mojay, G. (1991). *Shiatsu: The Complete Guide*. Hammersmith, London: Thorsons.

Maciocia, G. (1994). *The Practice of Chinese Medicine: The Treatment of Diseases with Acupuncture and Chinese Herbs*. Edinburgh: Churchill Livingstone.

Masunaga, S. and Ohashi, W. (1977). *Zen Shiatsu: How to Harmonize Yin and Yang for Better Health*. Tokyo: Japan Publications.

Moyers, B. "The Mystery of Chi." Volume 1: *Healing and the Mind*. Video series. Ambrose Video.

Videos

"The Mystery of Chi." From the video series *Healing and the Mind* with Bill Moyers. Volume 1.

WEB SITES

American Organization for Bodywork Therapies of Asia (*www.aobta.org*)

National Certification Commission for Acupuncture and Oriental Medicine (*www.nccaom.org*)

STUDY GUIDE

LEARNING OUTCOMES

Use the learning outcomes at the beginning of the chapter as a guide to your studies. Perform the task given in each outcome, either in writing or verbally into a tape recorder or to a study partner. This may start as an "open book" exercise, and then later from memory.

KEY TERMS/CONCEPTS

To study key words and concepts listed at the beginning of this chapter, choose one or more of the following exercises. Writing or talking about ideas helps you remember them better, and explaining them helps deepen your understanding.

1. Write a one- or two-sentence explanation of each key word and concept.

2. Make study cards by writing the explanation from problem 1 on one side of a 3 × 5 card, and the key word or concept on the other. Shuffle the cards and read one side, trying to recite either the explanation or word on the other side.

3. Repeat problem 2 for history and philosophy terms.

4. Pick out two or three key words or concepts and explain how they are related.

5. With a study partner, take turns explaining key words and concepts verbally.

6. Make up sentences using one or more key words or concepts.

7. Read your sentences to a study partner, who will ask you to clarify your meaning.

STUDY OUTLINE

The following questions test your memory of the main concepts in this chapter. Locate the answers in the text using the page number given for each question.

1. A term used to describe forms of bodywork with roots in Chinese medicine is _____ (ABT). (p. 312)

2. Three Asian countries that have developed forms of ABT are _____, _____, and _____. (p. 312)

3. Several forms of ABT are recognized by _____ (AOBTA®). (p. 312)

4. The scope of practice of ABT includes _____ and _____ of energetic imbalances according to _____ theory. (p. 312)

5. ABT techniques include touching, holding or pressing the body along _____ or on _____. (p. 312)

6. The three branches of Chinese medicine for which there is practitioner certification by NCCAOM are (1) _____, (2) _____, and (3) _____. (p. 312)

7. NCCAOM refers to the _____. (p. 312)

History of ABT

1. Chinese medicine is assumed to have developed from Chinese _____ and thousands of years of _____ evidence. (p. 313)

2. The earliest known text on Chinese medicine is the _____, traditionally ascribed to the legendary _____ in c. 2500 BCE. (p. 313)

3. The earliest reference to Yin and Yang is thought to be in the _____, written in about 700 BCE. (p. 313)

4. Chinese medicine originated in the lands north of the _____ in China over 5000 years ago. (p. 313)

   a. Inhabitants there used _____, _____, and _____ (i.e., bodywork) to treat various ailments. (p. 313)

   b. Over many years, the Chinese people identified _____ pathways and _____ on the body that now form the energetic anatomy of Chinese medicine. (p. 313)

5. Different schools of philosophy including the _____ and the _____ schools combined with practical healing methods to make up Chinese medicine. (p. 313)

6. Chinese medicine eventually spread to _____ and Japan, reaching Japan in about _____ CE. (p. 313)

7. _____ from Asia have brought Chinese medicine to many Western countries. (p. 315)

8. _____ returning from Imperial China brought information about Chinese culture to Europe in the 17th century. (p. 315)

9. A French diplomat named _____ published writings on acupuncture in 1940 that captured the interest of Westerners. (p. 315)

10. _____ taught Japanese shiatsu in the United States between 1953 and 1960. (p. 315)

11. Different teachers introduced a variety of forms of Japanese bodywork to the United States and other Western countries in the year _____. (p. 315)

12. In the West, Chinese medicine is called _____ (TAM) to acknowledge its origins in East Asia. (p. 313)

13. _____ medicine has been integrated into the healing practices of China and Japan in the past 50 years. (p. 315)

Yin and Yang

1. Yin and Yang illustrate the concept of _____ and _____ of all. (p. 316)

2. The Chinese character for Yin depicts _____. (p. 316)

3. Yin (in relation to Yang) is _____, _____, _____ aspect of the universe. Yin is characterized by _____, _____, _____, _____, _____, and _____. (p. 316)

4. The Chinese character for Yang is _____. (p. 316)

5. Yang (in relation to Yin) is the _____, _____, _____ aspect of the universe. Yang is characterized by _____, _____, _____, _____, _____, _____, _____. (p. 316)

6. Five principles of the Yin and Yang relationship are _____, _____, _____, _____, _____. (p. 317)

Concept of Qi

1. In a large sense, everything in the _____ is Qi, sometimes called the _____ Qi. (p. 317)

2. Qi is a continuous form of energy in material form when it _____, and nonmaterial when it _____. (p. 317)

3. In a more narrow sense, Qi or Little Qi, may be translated as life _____ or life _____. (p. 317)

4. Qi extracted from _____ and _____ circulates in the body through a network of channels. (p. 317)

5. If Qi is deficient, one _____ it. If it is excess, one _____ it. If it is stagnant, one _____ it. If it is sinking, one _____ it. If it rebellious, one _____ it. This is the purpose of ABT techniques. (p. 318)

6. The functions of Qi include: _____, _____, _____, _____ and _____. (pp. 318)

Five Elements and Their Orbs of Influence

1. The five elements depict the _____ of life. (p. 318)

2. Match the following elements with the general characteristics below: (pp. 319–320)

   a. Wood

   b. Fire

   c. Earth

   d. Water

   e. Metal

   _____ Yang, Summer, heat and light, sweat, the tongue, propriety, insight

   _____ Transition, late Summer, damp, rooted, sweet, fragrant, integrity

   _____ Yin, Autumn, letting go, pungent taste, mucus, inspired, receptive

   _____ Yang, Spring, sunrise, green, wind, sour taste, benevolence, patience

_____ Yin, Winter, night, hearing, groaning, salty taste, yielding, wisdom

3. Match the elements with their corresponding channels and organs: (Figure 17–1)

    a. Wood

    b. Fire

    c. Earth

    d. Water

    e. Metal

_____ Stomach and Spleen

_____ Lung, Large Intestine

_____ Gall Bladder, Liver

_____ Heart, Small Intestine, Pericardium, Triple Burner

_____ Bladder, Kidney

4. Two important cycles involving the five elements are the _____ or generating cycle, and the _____ or controlling cycle. (p. 320)

Chinese Body Clock

1. The energy channels flow through the body according to a natural rhythmic _____ called the Chinese body clock. (p. 321)

2. Identify the primary energy channel associated with each time of the day listed below: (Table 17–2)

    3:00–5:00 a.m. _____

    5:00–7:00 a.m. _____

    7:00–9:00 a.m. _____

    9:00–11:00 a.m. _____

    11:00 a.m.–1:00 p.m. _____

    1:00–3:00 p.m. _____

    3:00–5:00 p.m. _____

    5:00–7:00 p.m. _____

    7:00–9:00 p.m. _____

    9:00–11:00 p.m. _____

    11:00 p.m.–1:00 a.m. _____

    1:00–3:00 a.m. _____

The Four Pillars of Assessment

1. The four pillars of assessment are _____, _____, _____, _____. (p. 324)

2. The practitioner observes the following about the client: _____, _____, _____, _____, _____. (p. 324)

3. Assessment of the tongue includes looking at _____, _____, _____. (p. 324)

4. Areas of the body are touched to determine _____ or _____. (p. 324)

5. Each hand has _____ that can be assessed. (p. 324)

6. The client may have a smell about them that corresponds to one of the _____. (p. 324)

7. Listening to the _____ of the voice can give clues to imbalances. (p. 324)

8. Questions asked to give further assessment include _____, _____, _____, _____. (p. 324)

9. Using the four pillars of assessment, a _____ is developed. (p. 324)

Acupoints

1. Acupoints are specific spots along an _____ which, when properly located and palpated, can effect the flow of Qi. (p. 325)

2. The effectiveness of acupoints depends on accurate _____. (p. 325)

3. Acupoints may not work as expected if used in a Western _____ fashion. (p. 325)

4. Acupoints contraindicated during pregnancy include _____, _____, _____, and _____. (p. 325)

5. The commonality that binds Asian bodywork therapists is _____, _____, and _____. (p. 331)

FOR GREATER UNDERSTANDING

The following exercises are designed to take you from the realm of theory into the real world. They will help give you a deeper understanding of the subjects covered in this chapter. Action words are underlined to emphasize the variety of activities presented to address different learning styles, and to encourage deeper thinking.

1. Receive an Asian Bodywork Therapy session from a certified practitioner. Notice their methods of assessment. Be aware of any feeling of the movement of energy as the practitioner performs various techniques. Identify acupoints that were stimulated in the session. Discuss your experience with the practitioner and later with a study partner.

2. Observe a trained ABT practitioner give a session. Note how it is different from a Western massage session. Write your observations and/or discuss them with a study partner. (Alternative: Watch a video of an ABT demonstration.)

3. Repeat problem 1 or problem 2 with a different form of ABT. Compare and contrast the two experiences.

4. Interview a certified ABT practitioner. Ask about the form of ABT they practice, including its history, theory, and techniques. Ask about their training, requirements for certification, and types of clients in their practice. Share your findings with a study partner or group.

5. Draw the twelve primary energy channels on a partner using a chart as a guide. Locate the 20 important acupoints. (Alternative: Draw on a diagram of the body.)

6. Take an introductory class to some form of ABT. Notice how TAM theory is applied in this specific form. Discuss your experience with a study partner.

7. Visit the Web site of the American Organization for Bodywork Therapies of Asia (*aobta.org*.) Read about ABT, practitioner certification, and other information. Report your findings to a study partner or group.

8. Visit the Web site of the National Certification Commission for Acupuncture and Oriental Medicine (NCCAOM). Read about the organization and the ABT certification process. Report your findings to a study partner or group.

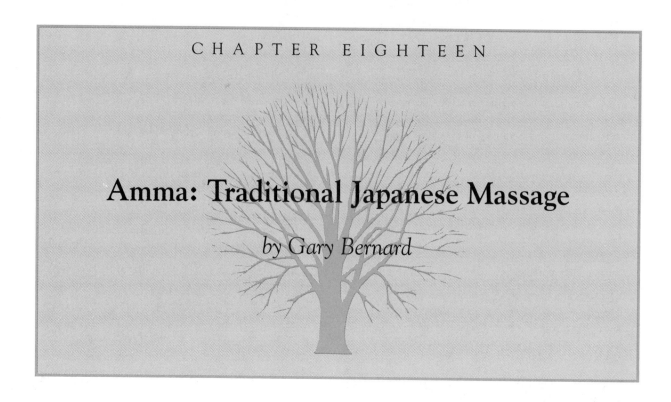

CHAPTER EIGHTEEN

Amma: Traditional Japanese Massage

by Gary Bernard

LEARNING OUTCOMES

After studying this chapter, the student will have information to:

1. Trace the history of amma in Japan and the United States.
2. Screen clients for important information.
3. List important characteristics of the one-hour amma form.
4. Describe the general sequence of techniques for a one-hour amma kata.
5. Use proper body mechanics when giving amma.
6. List the techniques of a model amma routine.
7. Appreciate the usefulness of kata in learning amma.

HISTORICAL PEOPLE AND DEVELOPMENTS

Amma Institute of Traditional
  Japanese Massage
Anmo
Blind ammas
Palmer, David
Kaneko, DoAnn

Edo period
Keller, Helen
Kabuki Hot Springs
Kampo
Meiji Restoration
Yamamoto, Shizuko

Masunaga, Shizuto
Nakamura, Takashi
Namikoshi, Torujiro
Ohashi, Wataru

MEDIALINK

A companion CD-ROM, included free with each new copy of this book, supplements the techniques presented in this chapter. Insert the CD-ROM to watch video clips of massage techniques being demonstrated. This multimedia feature is designed to help you add a new dimension to your learning.

KEY TERMS/CONCEPTS

Acupoint	Kata	Traditional Asian medicine
Amma	Perpendicularity	(TAM)
Amma kata	Screening process	Tsubo
Back straight	Shiatsu	Weight transfer
Body mechanics	Stacking the joints	

Amma, traditional Japanese massage, dates back 4,500 years to the northern regions of China and the beginning of Chinese medicine. In the United States today, amma continues to grow and evolve as a versatile and effective contemporary style of massage.

HISTORY OF AMMA IN JAPAN

The two Chinese characters pronounced **anmo** mean "to calm by rubbing." The Japanese pronounce the same two characters **amma,** which is sometimes spelled *anma*. Amma is the foundation of all forms of Japanese massage including the modern-day forms of shiatsu.

Amma originated in the tradition of Chinese medicine. It was first developed in the northern region of China in the barren lands north of the Yellow River. The inhabitants of this area used acupuncture, moxibustion and anmo, that is, manual methods, to provide cures. Over many years of practice and experience with massage, acupuncture, and moxa, the Chinese people came to identify the points on the body where such therapy produces maximum effects. Eventually these points, called **acupoints,** were documented together with the 14 major meridians or channels of energy that emerged from the patterns created by the acupoints. Today we know this system of meridians and acupressure points as the energetic anatomy of **traditional Asian medicine (TAM)** (Serizawa 1976, 1984).

Anmo was brought to Japan by way of the Korean peninsula at the beginning of the Asuka period in the 6th century CE. It was an integral part of the unified system of Chinese medicine, which the Japanese call **kampo,** "the Chinese way" (Serizawa, 1972, pp. 14–15; Serizawa, 1984). The Japanese assimilated the Chinese medical philosophy into their culture, and amma was born as a therapeutic art form.

Amma was recognized by the official medical authorities in Japan during the Nara period (672–707 CE). By 701 CE, Taiho Law referred to the new massage of Japan with the mention of "amma experts" (Joya 1958).

The literature available in English is very sketchy on the history of amma until the **Edo period** (1603–1857 CE). There are a few references that suggest that the perception of amma as a form of medical intervention changed from time to time. Amma apparently lost its popularity, but experienced a revival in the Edo period (Joya, 1958). Kampo, including amma, was the main medical stream in Japan from the time it was introduced until the end of the Edo period (Serizawa 1972).

Most of the literature agrees that during these 1,000 years, amma developed into a highly specialized style of massage. Amma involves complex techniques, which encompass a myriad of pressing, stroking, stretching, and percussive manipulations with the thumbs, fingers, arms, elbows, and knees to stimulate points along the 14 major meridians of the body.

Amma reached its peak of popularity in the Edo period. During this time, students of medicine were required to study amma to understand and become familiar with the structure and function of the energetic anatomy of the body. Masunaga relates that "their training in this type of manual therapy enabled them to accurately diagnose and administer Chinese herbal medicine as well as locate the tsubos . . . easily for acupuncture treatments" (1977, p. 9).

By the end of the Edo period, two historically significant changes occurred in Japan that dramatically altered both the way amma was taught and the people's perception of kampo and amma. The first event occurred early in the 19th century when the Shogunate authorities decreed that blind persons assume the job of masseur and acupuncturist as a welfare measure (Serizawa, 1984, p. 15). As a result, many schools were created, and high-ranking amma practitioners enjoyed public respect and were honored by the court and government. However, once the schools of amma began training **blind ammas,** amma's status as a healing art gradually began to suffer because it was perceived that "blind people were at a disadvantage in receiving formal study in diagnosis and treatment" (Masunaga, 1977, p. 10). As part of its program to reserve amma as a profession for the blind, the government required that all the ammas, the name given to people who practiced amma, be licensed. The story goes that to avoid these regulations many therapists already in practice changed the name of their type of treatment. Thus, the term **shiatsu** came into use (Masunaga, 1977, p. 9).

The second change occurred during the **Meiji Restoration** (c. 1868 CE) and the modernization of Japan. Western medicine began to influence Japanese medical practices. Serizawa (1976) reports that "Western medical science as known in Germany and Holland began to influence Japanese thought, especially because of its surgical methods and its effectiveness against epidemics" (p. 30). Eventually, kampo was eclipsed by Western medicine, and misconceptions about amma discredited it in Japan.

Consequently, by the beginning of the 1900s kampo and amma had become known as "folk medicine" and amma erroneously associated only with pleasure and comfort. Amma became known as a blind person's profession, and as a result of prejudice, the word *amma* in Japan acquired some stigma as a lowly profession (Serizawa, 1984).

At the outbreak of World War II, over 90 percent of the people practicing amma in Japan were blind. At the end of the war, General MacArthur went into Japan and banned the traditional healing arts of kampo and amma. This left many hundreds of blind ammas out of work with no real prospects for a livelihood. The result was an epidemic of suicides among the amma practitioners. **Helen Keller** was informed of this tragedy and wrote to President Truman, asking him to rescind the order (Ohashi, 1976). He finally did, but the damage had been done. Amma and the traditional healing arts of Japan were being further overshadowed by Western medical science.

Joya writes in her book, *Things Japanese*, "Most amma are still blind people. Formerly they used to blow a small flute as they went about, and the people used to call them in as they heard the sounds. However, except in some rural districts, this amma flute is no longer heard" (1958, p. 61).

Interestingly, many schools that teach massage in Japan today, teach a form of amma. However, most people born after World War II have never heard the word *amma* in reference to massage.

In 1940, **Torujiro Namikoshi** opened the Japan Shiatsu School in Tokyo, which was licensed by the government in 1957. As a result of Namikoshi's marketing skills in the late 1940–1950s, *shiatsu* has become the word most commonly used to refer to massage in Japan. Shiatsu was recognized by the Japanese government as a style of massage separate from amma in 1964. The Director of the Shiatsu Massage School of California in Santa Monica, DoAnn Kaneko, told this author that many of the massage practitioners doing massage in Japan today do both the amma and shiatsu, and call it shiatsu.

AMMA IN THE UNITED STATES

Torujiro Namikoshi, along with his son Toru, introduced shiatsu to the United States in the 1953. Toru Namikoshi spent seven years in the United States introducing shiatsu to students at the Palmer School of Chiropractic in Davenport, Iowa. Torujiro went on to Hawaii to open a massage school. In 1969, Torujiro wrote his first book, *Health and Vitality at Your Fingertips: Shiatsu in English*, and distributed it in the United States, Great Britain, New Zealand, and Australia. This book was later translated into several other languages under the name *Japanese Finger-Pressure Therapy, Shiatsu* (1969) and distributed all over the world. Namikoshi's style of shiatsu was the primary style of Japanese massage taught in the United States until the 1970s.

During the 1970s, a number of other Japanese practitioners brought their styles of shiatsu to the United States, including **DoAnn Kaneko,** who brought a form called Amma Shiatsu; **Shizuto Masunaga,** who developed Zen Shiatsu; **Shizuko Yamamoto,** who developed Barefoot Shiatsu; and **Wataru Ohashi,** who developed Ohashiatsu.

Namikoshi's style of shiatsu involves the simplest of the amma techniques (finger, thumb, and palm pressure), and does not include the traditional meridian system of TAM. Sensitive to the 20th century enthusiasm for Western scientific medicine throughout the world, Namikoshi superimposed his points over Western structural anatomy. Toru Namikoshi details this system with diagrams in *The Complete Book of Shiatsu Therapy* (1981).

Shizuto Masunaga developed an alternative meridian system, which is described in his book *Zen Shiatsu* (1977). His student, Wataru Ohashi, returned to the original traditional Chinese meridian system, which he details in *Do-It-Yourself Shiatsu* (1976). Shizuko Yamamoto does not include a map of their meridian system in her book nor does she include acupressure points in her complete shiatsu treatment. She does, however, suggest a list of acupoints for treating common problems. Mr. Kaneko follows the traditional Chinese meridian system and includes many of the more complicated techniques of amma in his style of shiatsu. As you can see, when someone says, "I do shiatsu," they may be speaking about any one of a number of different forms of this ancient healing art.

Traditional amma was first formally introduced to the United States in 1971, with the opening of **Kabuki Hot Springs** in Japantown, San Francisco, California. Designed as a traditional Japanese spa, Kabuki Hot Springs employed sighted amma practitioners who had been trained in Japan and brought to the United States to work in the new spa. By 1977, the owners of the Hot Springs wanted to develop a local source of qualified practitioners. They asked **Takashi Nakamura,** a practitioner from the Kensai School of Massage, Acupuncture, Moxa, and Cautery in Osaka, Japan, to open a school in San Francisco. Although he taught amma, the school was called the Kabuki Shiatsu School of Massage.

Nakamura developed a highly choreographed one-hour, full-body table sequence using over 25 different hand and arm techniques on over 140 **tsubo,** or acupoints. He taught this sequence in the way that he had been taught in Japan. He demonstrated a small portion of the sequence on each student; they then practiced on one another, and then each student demonstrated his or her ability to repeat that segment on Nakamura. The entire sequence was taught this way, each piece building on the next. By teaching this form appropriate for a spa setting and modeling how the amma forms were taught in Japan, Takashi Nakamura helped to further an understanding of the amma tradition in the United States. Nakamura returned to Japan in 1981, after teaching his student, **David Palmer,** how to teach the amma spa form.

Palmer reopened the school in 1982. Recognizing the significance of the amma tradition and how it differed from the way shiatsu was being taught and practiced in the United States, he renamed the school the **Amma Institute of Traditional Japanese Massage.** In an attempt to make skilled touch more accessible in the United States, Palmer adapted the last part of the one-hour full-body spa sequence and created a 15-minute upper-body form for clients seated in a chair. The 15-minute chair form had made receiving amma appear safe, convenient, and affordable. Massage practitioners can once again bring their service out to the people like the blind ammas of Japan were doing over 80 years ago. In December of 1988, Palmer left the Amma Institute to develop the Skilled Touch Institute of Chair Massage. Each year his trainers introduce the techniques of Japanese massage to hundreds of professional bodyworkers.

OVERVIEW OF A ONE-HOUR AMMA KATA

The one-hour routine or **amma kata** described here was created as a wellness or health maintenance massage. It is given on a table and includes a variety of techniques, including pressing, stroking, stretching, and percussive manipulations. Techniques are performed with the thumbs, fingers, and arms to stimulate over 140 acupressure points along the 14 major energy meridians.

Amma is very rhythmic. The 60-minute form described here is characterized by a four-beat rhythm. The prescribed sequence, called a **kata,** is designed to relax and rejuvenate the body, leaving the receiver feeling refreshed and revitalized.

The intention of this amma form is to facilitate the flow of energy in the body. By improving circulation (i.e., ki and its many manifestations such as blood, lymph, and other body fluids), the amma techniques help the body's own healing mechanisms to operate more effectively. The practitioner's main focus is the comfort of the receiver and the precision of performance of the kata.

A practitioner's first consideration is to determine whether or not the receiver will benefit from amma massage. The second is whether the service that the practitioner is providing is what the recipient is expecting to receive. Clarity of intention helps to ensure the comfort of the amma experience. To learn the receiver's expectations and determine whether or not the amma sequence will offer benefit, each session begins with a screening process.

Screening

During the **screening process,** the practitioner asks five basic questions:

1. Have you ever had massage before?
2. Have you ever had a Japanese massage before?

3. Do you have any recent injuries or illnesses?
4. Are you under a doctor's care or are you taking any medication?
5. Are you pregnant or trying to be pregnant (for women of child-bearing age)?

Amma is contraindicated for pregnancy. Many of the points that we press are used in labor to help stimulate uterine contractions.

If the practitioner is unsure whether or not the recipient would benefit from the massage, they follow one simple rule: When in doubt, don't. The second rule they follow is: Always err on the side of caution.

And finally, before beginning the session the practitioner gives the receiver permission to give feedback regarding the comfort of the massage. The receiver decides how strong the pressure should be, not the practitioner. By following these guidelines, and by always screening, the practitioners ensure that the service they are providing is safe for the recipient and for themselves.

Amma Kata Sequence

To start, the receiver lies face down on a massage table with the arms bent overhead and resting on the table. The hands are by the ears. The practitioner drapes the receiver with a sheet, leaving only the head exposed. All of the techniques are performed through the sheet.

The traditional one-hour kata begins with the practitioner climbing onto the table and straddling the receiver by placing one knee along side of, but not touching, the hip, and the other foot near the receiver's arm pit. See Figure 18–1. This position allows the practitioner to use body leverage to apply pressure to the back.

The practitioner then presses with the palms (*shusho apakuho*) down both sides of the back on the crest of the erector spinae muscles. Start between the scapula and end just superior to the sacrum, pressing in four or five places going down the back.

The practitioner climbs off the table and moves to the shoulders. The sequence then proceeds from the shoulders to the arms all the way out to the fingertips. Once one shoulder and arm have been completed, the practitioner moves to the other shoulder and arm. This symmetry of form continues through the entire massage.

After completing the shoulders and arms, the practitioner massages the neck; from the neck to the back; from the back to the hips and legs all the way to the bottom of the feet. The practitioner completes the first side of the body by returning to the back with bilateral thumb presses and then finishes with a series of percussions. At the end of the final percussion the practitioner asks the client to "turn over, please."

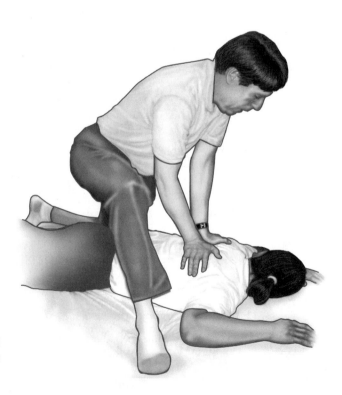

FIGURE 18–1. Amma technique called *shusho apakuho*, applying pressure with the palms.

After draping the receiver with a sheet and wrapping a towel across the ears and eyes, the practitioner begins with the right leg, pressing points along the top, side, and inside of the leg down to the feet and then stretching the leg. After repeating this sequence on the left leg and then stretching the toes bilaterally and shaking the legs, the practitioner moves to the head of the table. Then the practitioner massages the face, the neck, the chest, and the abdomen.

To complete the massage we sit the receiver up and work on the scalp, the neck, and the shoulders, stretch the back and arms, and finish with a closing series of percussions on the upper back and shoulders, which ends with the words "thank you very much." Palmer added "thank you very much" to all the amma sequences that are taught at The Amma Institute. He did this for three reasons: (1) to indicate to the client that the massage is over; (2) to acknowledge that a practitioner–client relationship is a peer relationship and that the practitioner would not be able to do the work they love best without the client, and (3) as a way for the practitioner to practice humility.

Amma Techniques

The most commonly used amma techniques in the one-hour full-body sequence are listed in Table 18–1. Each technique would take pages of description to explain; however, there are four basic concepts pertaining to **body mechanics** that are common to all the techniques that are used to apply pressure.

- Weight transfer
- Perpendicularity
- Stacking the joints
- Keeping the back straight

Weight transfer allows the practitioner to find a comfortable balance, that is, pressure that is comfortable to the receiver. It also ensures that the connection that the practitioner is making comes from the whole body and not from strength. To transfer weight, the practitioner must stand (or kneel) with one foot forward and the other foot (or knee) back. In a standing position the front leg must always be bent with the foot forward enough to be in front of the knee. The back leg is straight. The

Table 18–1   FULL-BODY AMMA SEQUENCE

Shusho Apakuho	Palm pressure
Boshi Apakuho	Thumb pressure
Shusho Junenko	Back and forth movement with palm
Boshi Junenko	Back and forth movement with thumb
Nishi Junenko	Back and forth movement with thumb and index finger
Shishi Junenko	Back and forth movement with four fingers
Haaku Junenko	Back and forth movement by grasping with thumb and finger
Rinjyo Junenko	Circular motion with thumb only
Wansho Junenko	Back and forth movement with forearm
Rotojyo Junenko	Waving motion with the hand
Shusho Keisatsuho	Stroking with the palm
Boshi Keisatsuho	Stroking with the thumb
Shishi Keisatsuho	Stroking with the four fingers
Skukendaho	Percussion with a loose fist
Setsudaho	Percussion with both hands alternating
Gasshadaho	Percussion with both hands joined
Gankidaho	Cupped hands percussion movement
Hakudaho	Cupped hand percussion
Kurumade	Rolling motion from fingertips to back of hand
Tsukide	"Finger dives"
Tsukamide	Finger grasping in quick movements with the wrist
Yanagide	"Willow Tree"
Yokode	Back and forth motion with either side of hand

hips are aligned so that the back is straight. The transfer happens by taking the weight off the front leg and moving it to the heels of the hands, thumbs, or whichever part of the hand or arm is being used to apply pressure.

Perpendicularity is an important part of the precision and efficiency of amma. To make sure that the pressure is sinking straight into an acupressure point, the line from the shoulders to the point of contact (heel of hand or thumb) must be 90 degrees to the plane of the surface of the point on the body. If the line isn't 90 degrees, the client's skin will usually stretch in one direction or another.

Stacking the joints one on top of another is essential to the concept of perpendicularity and weight transfer. For a connection to be made with the whole body, there must be a straight line from the body, either through the shoulder, or through the elbow acting as an extension of the shoulder, to the heel of the hands or the thumbs. For example, imagine the weight moving down from the shoulder into the top third of the fingerprint part of the thumb. The shoulder is stacked over the elbow, which, in turn, is stacked over the wrist and an arched thumb. Stacking the joints in this way allows the pressure to go straight into each point effortlessly.

A **straight back,** that is, an aligned back, is the fourth essential part in all of the amma techniques. If the back is not in alignment, the practitioner often ends up pushing with the upper body instead of the more effortless feeling of transferred weight. The practitioner's weight should be held in the legs, not the back. At first, this may feel uncomfortable; however, some of the biggest muscles in the body are in the legs. They develop quickly and are much more forgiving than the small muscles of the back. If you carry the weight in the back, fatigue sets in more quickly and eventually the pain can become debilitating.

A Simple Exercise To Feel the Significance of These Four Body Mechanic Concepts.   The following is an exercise that puts all of these components together to demonstrate the sensation of transferring weight. Stand facing a wall and put both hands on the wall a shoulder's width apart and at shoulder height. Step back with both feet so that your body is at a 45 degree angle and you're leaning into the wall. Bring your hips forward so that your shoulders, back, and feet are aligned. Notice that all your weight is in your feet and in your hands. Now bring one leg forward and bend it. Make sure your foot is forward enough so that your toes are in front of your knee. The other leg stays back and straight. Keep your hips aligned with your shoulders and your back foot. Your stance should be open with your back leg centered between your hands and the front leg slightly off to the side. Keep your arms straight and relax your shoulders. Your hands are placed with your fingers out to the sides, and the heels of your

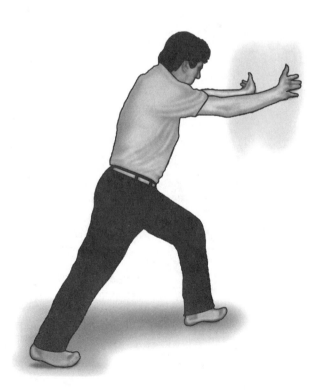

FIGURE 18–2. Wall exercise to practice transfer of weight while applying pressure for techniques like *shusho apakuho*.

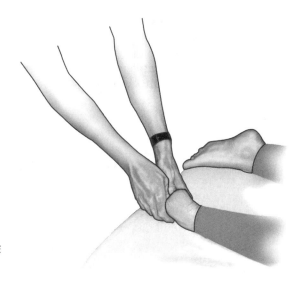

FIGURE 18–3. Amma technique called *boshi apakuho*, applying pressure with the thumbs.

hands are parallel to one another. See Figure 18–2. If you have range of motion limitations in your wrists, adjust your hands so you're comfortable. Sometimes slightly curling your fingers is enough. Now try to hold your weight in your front leg so that your hands are not supporting you at all.

Begin by slowly transferring the weight of your body from your front leg to the heels of your hands. Keep your arms straight and your hips aligned. Your hips don't need to move at all. As you feel the weight transfer to the heels of your hands, you'll notice that weight is also moving to your back foot. The heel of your foot shouldn't be down. The weight is in the ball of your back foot.

To really feel this sensation, actually lift the front foot, keeping the hips quiet and the back straight. Don't bend the arms. As you lift your leg, exhale. Now lower the leg and put weight in the front leg. Remember the front foot should be far enough forward so that the toes are in front of the knee. The hands should not be holding any weight again. The hips should still be in the same place. Do not pull back with the hands. Arms can still be straight out in front. Now, transfer the weight back to the "palms" (really the heel of the hands). The above is an introduction to the first technique of amma—*shusho apakuho* as shown in Figure 18–1.

The amma techniques that are taught in the one-hour full-body spa sequence are listed in Table 18–1. *Apakuho* (thumb pressure) and *wansho junenko* (back and forth motion with the forearms), are shown in Figures 18–3 and 18–4, respectively.

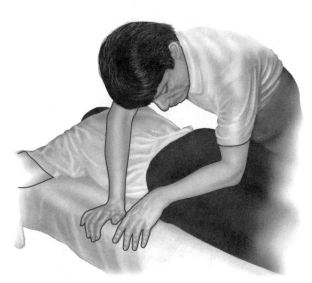

FIGURE 18–4. Amma technique called *wansho junenko*, back and forth motion with the forearms.

USING KATA TO LEARN AMMA

The challenge presented to instructors in the West who are teaching Eastern styles of massage is twofold. First, the instructor needs to understand the philosophical foundation or cosmology that produced the massage form. And second, the instructor needs to be aware of his own culture's cosmology to be able to present the new information in a way that can be easily assimilated by the students.

When Takashi Nakamura began teaching amma in the United States in 1977, he taught a choreographed full-body sequence. The concept of kata is often used to help students understand the significance of the Japanese use of sequence in teaching a physical skill.

There is no exact translation of the word **kata;** however, the basic concept has to do with a form, or sequence, or system of movement that determines precisely how something is accomplished. Katas are studied in all of the Japanese arts; however, in our Western culture the term is most frequently used in the context of the martial arts. Students practice katas, or sequences of movements, over and over again until they become automatic.

Practice is vital to the process involved in learning any physical skill. Teaching students a massage kata allows them to practice skilled touch with the confidence of knowing that the kata is effective in doing what it is designed to do even while the student is still integrating the sequence, the techniques, and the point locations and learning how to touch someone comfortably. The student doesn't have to know Chinese medicine, for example, to give a highly effective amma massage. The kata "knows" Chinese medicine. The student simply has to follow the kata. Palmer (1995) says: "We teach a kata and it is the kata which teaches the student massage" (p. 26).

> The Kata is like a wise elder which has the wisdom of the centuries behind it. The Kata has a long lineage that extends from teacher to teacher and is based on a theoretical foundation and philosophical world view which transcends our individual understanding. If you trust the Kata and develop an honest relationship with it, you will be rewarded with an unlimited stream of insights about the nature of touch, massage, service, relationships, [and] yourself . . . When you practice [a traditional Japanese] massage Kata it eventually becomes something like a beautiful dance or a piece of classical music. Highly structured and choreographed, it is the same each time it is performed and yet, each time, it is also different (Palmer, 1995, pp. 26–27).

SUMMARY

Amma is traditional Japanese massage. It was brought from China, to Korea, and then to Japan during the 6th century CE. Amma reached its peak of popularity in Japan during the Edo period (c. 1600–1857 CE). It eventually became an occupation for the blind in Japan. After World War II, a derivative of amma called shiatsu was developed by Torujiko Namikoshi. Traditional amma was brought from Japan to San Francisco in the 1970s by Takashi Nakamura as a service at the Kabuki Hot Springs. David Palmer took over Nakamura's school in the early 1980s, and developed a form of amma for seated clients.

Amma includes a variety of pressing, stroking, stretching, and percussive techniques applied with the thumbs, fingers, forearms, elbows, and knees. These techniques are combined into sequences of movement that stimulate acupoints along the 14 major meridians or energy channels of the body.

Principles of applying amma techniques safely and effectively are: weight transfer, perpendicularity, stacking the joints, and keeping the back in alignment. A useful method of learning amma is in a sequence or form called a kata. Practicing an amma kata helps students learn point locations, develop technique skills, good body mechanics, confidence, and insights about the nature of touch, massage, service, and themselves.

A look ahead . . .

Several teachers in the modern era have developed their own styles and techniques of ABT, building on the foundation of traditional Japanese amma. Chapter 19 describes one of these adaptations called Zen Shiatsu, developed by Shizuto Masunaga, that was brought to the United States in the 1970s.

REFERENCES

Joya, M. (1958). *Mock Joya's things Japanese*. Tokyo: Tokyo News Service, Ltd.

Masunaga, S. (1977). *Zen shiatsu*. Tokyo: Japan Publications.

Namikoshi, T. (1969). *Japanese finger-pressure, shiatsu*. Tokyo: Japan Publications.

Namikoshi, T. (1981). *The complete book of shiatsu therapy*. Tokyo: Japan Publications.

Ohashi, W. (1976). *Do-it-yourself shiatsu*. New York: E. P. Dutton.

Palmer, D. (1995). What is Kata? *TouchPro massage manual*. San Francisco: Skilled Touch Institute of Chair Massage.

Serizawa, K. (1972). *Massage, the oriental method*. Tokyo: Japan Publications.

Serizawa, K. (1976). *Effective tsubo therapy*. Tokyo: Japan Publications.

Serizawa, K. (1984). *Tsubo: Vital points for oriental therapy*. Tokyo: Japan Publications.

ADDITIONAL REFERENCES

Videos

"Anma: Art of Japanese massage." With Shogo Mochizuki. Boulder, CO: Kotobuki Publications.

S T U D Y   G U I D E

LEARNING OUTCOMES

Use the learning outcomes at the beginning of the chapter as a guide to your studies. Perform the task given in each outcome using the information in the chapter. This may start as an "open book" exercise, and then later from memory.

KEY TERMS/CONCEPTS

To study the key concept and terminology listed at the beginning of this chapter, choose one or more of the following exercises. Writing or talking about ideas helps you remember them better, and explaining them helps deepen your understanding. Some exercises are designed to sharpen your focus on the details of performing the techniques.

1. Write a one-sentence explanation of each of the key words or concepts. Explain them verbally to a study partner.

2. Match important words or concepts that are related and explain their relationship to a study partner.

3. Tell a study partner about the history of amma in Japan and how it came to the United States in the 1970s. What were noteworthy time periods, people, and places? Explain its history as an occupation for the blind.

4. Name and practice the principles of performing amma techniques. Have a study partner observe and give you feedback about your body mechanics.

5. Explain how knowledge of Chinese medicine is used in amma.

6. Explain the concept of kata, and its usefulness in learning amma.

STUDY OUTLINE

The following questions test your memory of the main concepts in this chapter. Locate the answers in the text using the page number given for each question.

History of Amma in Japan

1. Two Chinese characters pronounced anmo mean to _____. (p. 339)

2. The Japanese pronounce the same two characters _____. (p. 339)

3. Amma is the foundation of all forms of Japanese massage, including _____. (p. 339)

4. Amma originated in ancient _____. (p. 339)

5. Amma came to Japan in the _____ century CE from _____. (p. 339)

6. After a period of decline, the practice of amma had a revival during the _____ period in Japan (1603–1857). (p. 339)

7. By this time, amma had developed into a highly specialized style of massage involving complex manual techniques to stimulate points along the _____ of the body. (p. 339)

8. Amma became an occupation for the _____ in Japan by the 1800s. (p. 339)

9. Western medicine began to influence traditional Japanese medical practices during the _____ (c. 1868 CE). (p. 340)

10. By the early 1900s amma was considered a _____ medicine, and associated only with _____ and _____. (p. 340)

11. After World War II amma was banned in Japan, but since it was an occupation for the blind, the ban was rescinded after a plea from _____. (p. 340)

12. Torujiro Namikoshi opened the _____ School in Tokyo in _____, and was instrumental in spreading shiatsu throughout the world. (p. 340)

History of Amma in the United States

1. Torujiro and his son Toru brought shiatsu to the United States in the _____ and taught shiatsu at the Palmer School of _____ in Davenport, Iowa. They also opened a school in _____. (p. 340)

2. A number of other shiatsu practitioners came to the United States from Japan in the _____s. (p. 340)

3. _____ Hot Springs opened in San Francisco in _____ bringing amma, traditional Japanese massage to the United States. (p. 341)

4. _____ opened an amma school in San Francisco in 1977 called the Kabuki Shiatsu School of Massage. (p. 341)

5. _____ reopened the school in 1982, calling it the _____ of Traditional Japanese Massage. (p. 341)

6. Palmer adapted the amma table form to the _____ that he developed, and began the _____ massage movement in the United States. (p. 341)

Overview of One-Hour Amma Kata

1. The one-hour amma kata described here is a _____ or health maintenance massage. (p. 341)

2. It is performed on a table and uses a variety of techniques such as _____, _____, _____, and _____. (p. 341)

3. The amma kata stimulates over 140 _____ along the 14 major _____. Its intention is to stimulate the flow of _____ in the body. (p. 341)

Screening Process

1. Five screening questions: (1) Have you ever _____ before? (2) Have you ever had a _____ massage before? (3) Do you have any recent _____ or _____? (4) Are you under a _____ or taking _____? (5) Are you _____ or trying to become _____? (pp. 341–342)

2. This amma kata is _____ for pregnant women. (p. 342)

Amma Kata Sequence

1. The kata begins with the receiver face _____ on the table covered with a sheet. (p. 342)

2. The kata _____ in prone position is back, shoulder, arms, hands, neck, back, hips, legs, and feet. (p. 342)

3. The kata _____ in supine position begins with the legs, then face, neck, chest, and abdomen. (p. 343)

4. The kata ends in the _____ position with _____ on the back and shoulders. (p. 343)

Amma Techniques

1. Four basic concepts related to body mechanics for the giver are (1) _____ transfer, (2) _____, (3) _____ the joints, and (4) keeping the back _____. (p. 343)

Using Kata to Learn Amma

1. Kata is a form or sequence of movement that determines _____ how something is _____. (p. 346)

2. Students practice kata or movement sequences over and over until they become _____. (p. 346)

3. Palmer says "We teach a kata and it is the kata that _____ the student massage." (p. 346)

FOR GREATER UNDERSTANDING

The following exercises are designed to take you from the realm of theory into practical applications. They will help give you a deeper understanding of the information covered in this chapter. Action words are underlined to emphasize the variety of activities presented to address different learning styles, and to encourage deeper thinking.

1. <u>Receive</u> an amma session from a certified practitioner. <u>Notice</u> the rhythm of the sequence and the techniques used. What did amma feel like? Write up or discuss your findings with a study partner.

2. <u>Observe</u> a certified practitioner perform amma. <u>Notice</u> their body mechanics, and the techniques they use.

<u>Describe</u> what you saw to a study partner. (Alternative: Watch an instructional video or the Asian bodywork section of the CD-ROM video included with this text.)

3. <u>Take an introductory course</u> in amma from a qualified teacher.

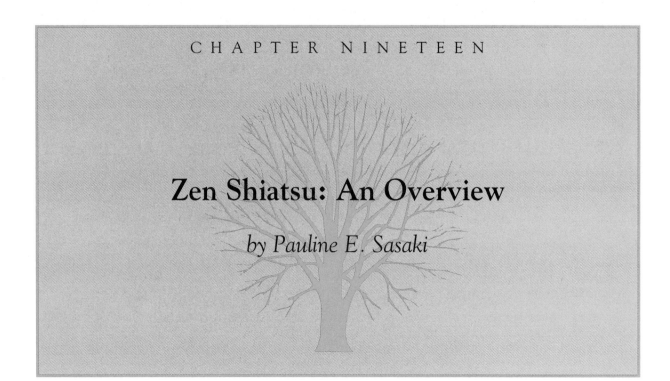

CHAPTER NINETEEN

Zen Shiatsu: An Overview

by Pauline E. Sasaki

LEARNING OUTCOMES

After studying this chapter, the student will have information to:

1. Trace the history of shiatsu.
2. Distinguish three major types of shiatsu.
3. Explain the concepts of energetic structure, ki and meridians.
4. Relate ki and the major meridians to various processes of sustaining life.
5. Relate ki and major meridians to mental and emotional health.
6. Explain the importance of vibrational quality of ki, and the quantity of ki (kyo-jitsu).
7. Describe the procedure of diagnosis in zen shiatsu.
8. Explain the four primary principles of performing shiatsu techniques.

HISTORICAL PEOPLE AND DEVELOPMENTS

Acupressure	Shiatsu massage	Zen shiatsu
Amma (anma)	Masunaga, Shizuto	
Shiatsu	Namikoshi, Torujiro	

KEY TERMS/CONCEPTS

Diagnosis	Jitsu	Ki
Homeostasis	Jitsu meridian	Kyo

MEDIALINK

A companion CD-ROM, included free with each new copy of this book, supplements the techniques presented in this chapter. Insert the CD-ROM to watch video clips of massage techniques being demonstrated. This multimedia feature is designed to help you add a new dimension to your learning.

Kyo meridian	Observation	Transfer of body weight
Life cycle of the meridians	Perpendicular penetration	Tsubos
Meridians	Rhythmic pattern	Vibrational quality

SHIATSU AND ITS HISTORY

Humankind has always recognized that the hand can contribute powerfully to the healing process. No one has to be told that rubbing the eyes or the scalp helps to soothe the pain of a headache, and in Western medicine, the role of the physical therapist has come to be widely accepted. In Japan, however, the use of the hand as a therapeutic tool has a time-honored history and a deep philosophical foundation.

The Japanese art of **shiatsu** (literally, *shi* or finger *atsu* or pressure) is a system for healing and health maintenance that has evolved over the course of thousands of years. Practiced informally since at least 2500 BCE, shiatsu was systematized in the early 1900s and became accepted as a form of therapy widely practiced to this day.

Shiatsu derives both from the ancient healing art of acupuncture and from the traditional form of Japanese massage, **amma** (also **anma**). In Japan, amma was originally considered the equivalent of Chinese acupuncture as the method one studied to treat the human body in illness. It was recognized to have bona fide therapeutic benefits up until the end of the Tokugawa period in the 18th century (Masunaga, 1983, p. 1). Because this was a peaceful period in Japan's history, intellectual inclinations flourished. Simultaneously, however, society became overly enamored of the pleasures and luxuries of life, with the result that amma was reduced to being merely an instrument of psychologic and sexual pleasure. Amma as it was practiced had discarded the historic foundations that had legitimized it as a therapeutic system.

Ultimately, shiatsu developed apart from amma as a therapeutic discipline based once again on its original theory. In the meantime, prior to World War II, amma became a major employer of the blind in Japan. During the American occupation of Japan when General MacArthur was considering outlawing both amma and shiatsu (due to erroneous information that they had sexual connotations), the blind of Japan appealed to Helen Keller in America to intercede on their behalf. Their appeal was successful and shiatsu and amma were permitted to be practiced (Ohashi, 1976, p. 10). Eventually, this approval led to a formal school of shiatsu, the Nippon Shiatsu School, established by **Tokujiro Namikoshi** in the late 1940s. Since then, shiatsu has become a popular medical therapy that is recognized and licensed by the government of Japan.

TYPES OF SHIATSU

Presently, there are three major types of shiatsu being practiced, each of which approaches the goal of balancing energy flow differently: shiatsu massage, acupressure, and zen shiatsu. As explained earlier, **shiatsu massage** is based largely on amma techniques and views the body purely from an anatomic or physiologic perspective. In conjunction with the use of massage techniques and manipulations, hard pressure is applied to the body at certain points to elicit the relief of specific symptoms. The most widely known form of shiatsu massage is the Namikoshi method, developed by Tokujiro Namikoshi (1969), and his son Toru Namikoshi (1981).

Acupressure is similar to shiatsu massage. However, acupressure incorporates the same theory of meridians and *tsubos* used by acupuncture. Acupressure theory and practice is described in detail in books by Katsusuke Serizawa (1976, 1984).

Zen shiatsu recognizes a broader set of meridians and *tsubos* than does acupuncture (Figure 19–1). The level of pressure applied to the *tsubos* and meridians is significantly lighter than that in other types of shiatsu. Also, unlike shiatsu massage and acupressure, zen shiatsu incorporates the diagnostic theory of *kyo-jitsu*. This style of shiatsu was developed by the late **Shizuto Masunaga,** founder and director of the Iokai Shiatsu Center in Japan (Masunaga & Ohashi, 1977). Because this style of shiatsu is unique, its basic concepts will be discussed in detail in this chapter.

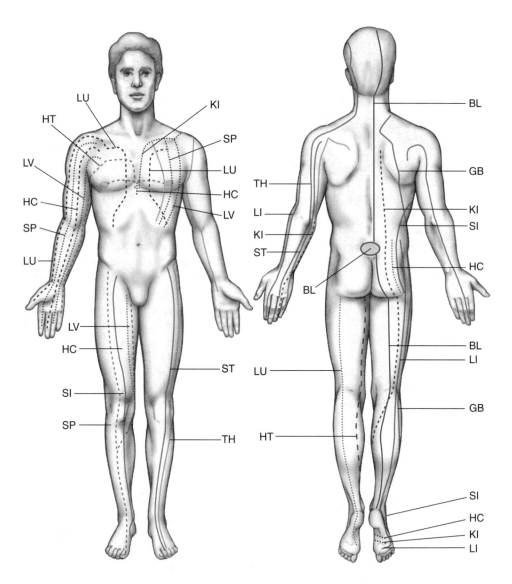

FIGURE 19–1. Meridians used in zen shiatsu.

CONCEPTS OF KI AND MERIDIANS

To understand shiatsu, one must first understand some of the basic concepts shared by acupuncture, shiatsu, and the Eastern healing arts in general. The basic tenets of Eastern medicine can be traced back to China to a time when in the Yellow Emperor's *Classic of Internal Medicine* a system of energy channels called *meridians* was described (Omura, 1982, p. 13). This perception of the body as a system of **meridians** formed at a time when the prevailing religion forbade any type of surgical intrusion into the human body. Denied access to procedures that would reveal the structure and functions of the human body, the Chinese developed a practical metaphor for the anatomy and physiology of the body through observation and intuition. They conceptualized the body as a living, dynamic entity subject to the influences of an underlying network of energy pathways. Thus, meridians represented the energetic, as opposed to the anatomic, structure of the body.

This emphasis on energy rather than structural anatomy is perhaps the fundamental difference between Eastern and Western medicine. When the body is analyzed anatomically, it appears as a collection of separate parts that exist whether the owner of the body is alive or dead. Examined energetically, however, the body appears to function as the result of a dynamic life force or **ki** (also chi or qi) that serves as the common link among all the body's tissues and organs. Ki ties together all bodily structures and functions so that they operate as a single entity. To the Easterner, the organs are not sufficient to sustain life unless the vital force ki is also present to keep the organs functional and properly interrelated. Furthermore, since ki represents the essence of life, this energetic structure ceases to exist once a person dies.

In its role as the life force, ki is always present and active within the body. Moreover, ki affects and even controls a person's entire life structure. To the Eastern mind, the unobstructed, balanced flow of ki along the meridians is both the cause and the effect of good health. Eastern medicine, including the disciplines of acupuncture and shiatsu, is dedicated to maintaining the balanced flow of ki throughout the body and to reestablishing that balance whenever it is thrown askew.

THE STRUCTURE OF MERIDIANS

All bodily processes are associated with various major functions, each of which is in turn associated with one or more **meridians.** Consequently, each meridian has been assigned the name of an organ. (Because the relationship of a meridian to an organ is metaphoric rather than anatomic, many Westerners become confused when they find, for example, that the lung meridian lies along the arm, or that the liver meridian lies along the leg. The name assigned to a meridian refers not to the meridian's external location on the body but to the functional influence of the meridian within the body.) Table 19–1 contains a list of some of the major functions and the meridians with which they are associated.

These general functions illustrate the range of roles ki plays in the human body and how the meridians work symbolically through the physiological systems. The theory of the life cycle of the meridians explains the sequence and the purpose of the various processes for maintaining life.

The **life cycle of the meridians** begins with the lung and large intestine meridians. As a pair, these meridians govern the intake of ki and elimination. The action of inhaling the ki from the outside world and bringing it into the body is represented by the respiratory system. The action of exhaling the extraneous ki is represented by the eliminative system. On a symbolic level, the breath begins life by differentiating between the ki from the outside world and the ki within the human form. An example of this is the birth of a child. A child is not acknowledged as being alive until it takes its first breath. Once the child continues to breathe, its existence as a human being is established.

The ki from the outside world is separated from human ki by the existence of a border, represented by the skin. The skin acts in two ways, i.e., it absorbs ki from the outside, and it excretes waste material from the inside of the body via the pores. If both activities are in balance, the human form remains

Table 19–1   *FUNCTIONS ASSOCIATED WITH MAJOR MERIDIANS*

Function	Meridians
Intake of *ki*	Lung
Process of elimination	Large Intestine
Intake of food	Stomach
Digestion	Spleen
Interpretation of the emotional environment	Heart
Assimilation	Small Intestine
Purification	Bladder
Impetus to move	Kidney
Circulation	Heart Constrictor
Protection	Triple Heater
Storage, distribution	Liver
and detoxification of *ki*	Gallbladder

Modified from S. Masunaga & W. Ohashi. (1977). *Zen Shiatsu*. Tokyo: Japan Publications, pp. 42–47.

an entity. Once this is established, two requirements are necessary for survival: (1) nourishment from an outside source, and (2) emotional stimuli to satisfy the spirit.

Nourishment from Food

The primary external source of nourishment is food. Therefore, the intake of food and its breakdown for human consumption as represented in the process of digestion is an important function that is necessary to replenish expended ki. The stomach and spleen meridians initiate these functions via the actual stomach, esophagus, and duodenum as well as via the digestive enzymes necessary for the breakdown of food.

Nourishment for the Psyche

The second requirement is nourishment of the psyche by giving meaning to all human actions. The heart and small intestine meridians act as the interpreter and assimilator of stimuli that affect the emotions and feelings. A person's interaction with others is dependent on these functions; if a person cannot understand and absorb stimuli from the environment, life has no meaning beyond pure existence, and the reason for relationships and experiences ceases to exist. Of all the meridians, the heart and small intestine are most associated with the spiritual aspect of ki, primarily compassion. They are the connecting links between the physical and heavenly bodies (i.e., our relation to the universe). On a physiologic level, the qualities of the heart are symbolized by the color red in our blood. Therefore, the heart and small intestine meridians are said to influence the quality of the blood.

These three pairs of meridians all deal with extracting ki from the environment. When that function is completed, the ki is then processed internally so it can be utilized. The first step is to filter out the impurities in the ki taken in from the outside world and move it to the meridians that circulate it throughout the body. The bladder and kidney meridians govern the purification and movement process via urination, the autonomic nervous system, and the endocrine gland system.

When the ki is refined, it is sent to the central distributors for circulation and protection. The heart constrictor and triple heater meridians are the central distributors that make ki available to all parts of the body regardless of whether the body is active or inactive. For circulation to occur, a specific temperature must be maintained. The heart constrictor and triple heater meridians carry out these functions via the vascular system, the lymphatic system, and the metabolic processes that regulate body temperature.

When the ki is available for use, the liver and gallbladder meridians control how the ki is distributed to accomplish a specific action. For example, in the action of walking, more ki would be channeled into the moving leg than other parts of the body that are still. However, not all the ki is distributed and used. Much of it is stored for future use so that it does not have to be constantly replenished. The quality of ki is constantly maintained through the process of detoxification. This function of allocating ki for specific actions over a period of time parallels the birth and growth cycle whereby specific actions at different time periods contribute to a pattern of development. This function is represented on the physiologic level in the reproductive system. The liver and gallbladder meridians thus govern the reproductive system. Since life is a process, this cycle is ongoing until life ends.

The meaning of these functions can be interpreted on a variety of different levels including the physical, the emotional, the intellectual, and the spiritual. For example, an imbalance exhibited in the small intestine meridian indicates that the process of assimilation may not be working properly. On the physical plane, this imbalance may indicate faulty absorption of nutrients from the food in the intestines. This imbalance may express itself through physical symptoms such as acne, flatulence, migraine headaches, and intestinal problems. If the remedy addresses the problem of assimilation, the physical symptoms will automatically subside.

On an emotional plane, an assimilation problem might occur if there is an overload of emotional stimuli coming from the environment. Having to process and cope with the reactions to such stimuli disrupts the assimilation mechanism that normally adds meaning to our emotional environment. In cases such as trauma when the person cannot cope with the amount of stimuli derived from the experience, the body halts the assimilation process by going into a state of shock. This imbalance might manifest itself in symptoms such as hypersensitivity, the inability to cope with emotional situations, or the inability to recall traumatic experiences (in cases of shock).

On an intellectual plane, a small intestine meridian imbalance may indicate an inability to fully understand abstract concepts and an inability to follow through on details. Symptoms could include excessive worrying, anxiety, or too much concentration on unimportant details. On a spiritual plane, an assimilation problem may exhibit itself by a person's being overwhelmed with emotion during religious experiences or by a lack of compassion due to an inability to react emotionally.

We can see from this analysis that a variety of symptoms can manifest themselves from one single cause—in this case, poor assimilation. If the imbalance in a particular meridian is rectified, it will have positive repercussions on all of the different planes.

HOMEOSTASIS

Homeostasis is a modern scientific term that happens to describe quite suitably the flow of ki within and among the meridians. The idea behind homeostasis is that dynamic systems (in this case, the human body) naturally seek and maintain a condition of overall balance. Whenever an external force is applied to the system, at least one change must occur in the system in order to establish a new condition of balance.

With regard to the balance of ki, external forces resulting from physical, mental, and spiritual stresses produce internal obstructions that are released at points along the meridians, termed **tsubos.** The character of these obstructions depends not only on the meridian or meridians affected but also on the quality and quantity of the *ki* involved in the imbalance. The study of the quality and quantity of *ki* and how it influences homeostasis in the body involves the concepts of vibration quality and of kyo-jitsu.

Vibrational Quality

Ki can be thought of as a form of vibration that ranges in frequency from low to high. *Ki* with a low **vibrational quality** seems heavy and slow, whereas *ki* with a high vibrational quality seems light and fast. These qualities are additionally influenced by the quantity of ki present, which can be either deficient or excessive. The most common sensations of vibration felt are temperature differences, i.e., high vibration is sensed in heat and low vibration is sensed in the feeling of coldness. However, these are not the only barometers for measuring the quality of vibration. Trained shiatsu practitioners spend years developing sensitivity to the flow of ki within the body and are able to feel subtle vibrational qualities of energy imbalances associated with illness, disease, and pain.

Kyo-Jitsu

The terms **kyo** and **jitsu** refer to the quantity as well as quality of *ki*. The concept of Kyo-Jitsu is explained by Masunaga and Ohashi in the book *Zen Shiatsu* (1977). *Kyo* is defined as an area of deficient and weak *ki*, whereas *jitsu* is defined as an area of excessively strong *ki*. Imbalances generally stem from an absence of *ki* (*kyo*) because this absence retards a meridian's function. When this occurs, the life process is threatened and the remainder of the network becomes distorted as energy is redistributed in order to compensate for the weak area that is malfunctioning. As a consequence of this dynamic redistribution of energy, areas of excess *ki* (*jitsu*) appear and are necessary to sustain the distorted state. This condition persists as long as the malfunctioning area remains weak. Once the weakness is alleviated, the meridian initially affected regains its normal function, the remainder of the body is able to disperse the areas of *jitsu*, and the normal pattern of energy flow becomes re-established.

ROLE OF THE ZEN SHIATSU PRACTITIONER

The zen shiatsu practitioner has three primary goals: (1) diagnosis (to identify the nature and extent of energy imbalances in a patient), (2) treatment (to penetrate meridians in such a way as to alleviate the imbalances that exist), and (3) maintenance (to apply manual pressure in such a way as to sustain and strengthen the existing energy balance).

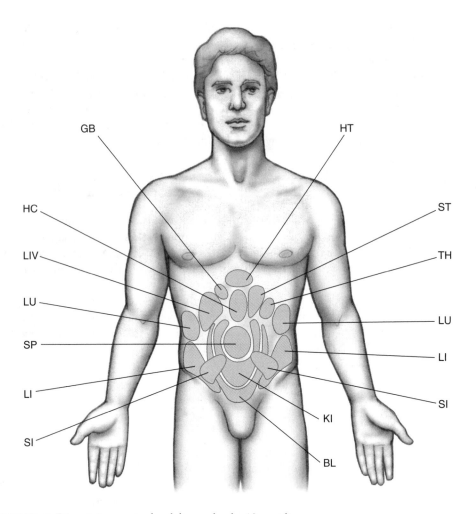

FIGURE 19–2. Diagnostic areas in the abdomen for the 12 meridians.

DIAGNOSIS

The underlying purpose of **diagnosis** in shiatsu is to identify the cause-and-effect relationship between a **kyo meridian** and a **jitsu meridian,** with the goal of altering the cause of the condition so that the effect will take care of itself. (In any cause-and-effect relationship, the effect will persist until the cause is dealt with. For instance, a person lacking adequate food will feel continuously hungry. Once he or she eats, however, the hunger disappears.) Specifically, a jitsu condition (the effect) disperses automatically once the weak kyo condition (the cause) is altered. Because diagnostic areas for each of the 12 meridians are located in the abdomen (Figure 19–2), the primary means of evaluating the state of a person's energy is to palpate the abdominal area. The intent is to use findings of kyo and jitsu areas to identify those meridians in which energy levels and flow are out of balance. (Additional sites on the back can be used for visual diagnosis. When there is an imbalance in a meridian, the area where it pools in the back may appear distorted or out of proportion to the whole. See Figure 19–3.)

Skill in diagnosis is a function of the practitioner's ability to sense kyo and jitsu relationships within the abdomen. Once those relationships have been correctly identified, a talented practitioner can usually draw meaningful conclusions as to how and why the imbalance developed. Typically, a Zen shiatsu session begins with palpation of the patient's abdomen; pressure is then applied to tsubos along the kyo and jitsu meridians; finally, the abdomen is once again palpated. If the practitioner has been effective, the final palpation will indicate that both the kyo and jitsu conditions have been altered and even alleviated entirely.

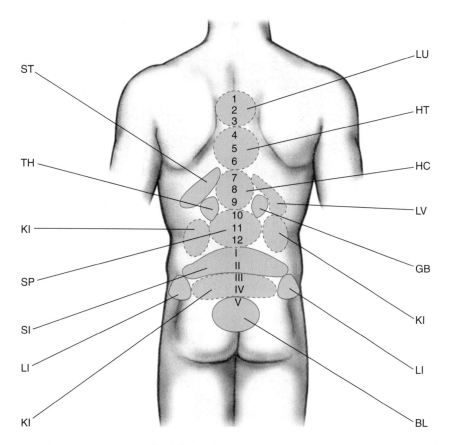

FIGURE 19–3. Diagnostic areas in the back for the 12 meridians.

PERFORMING SHIATSU TECHNIQUES

Four primary principles govern performance of shiatsu techniques:

1. The giver maintains the attitude of an observer.
2. Penetration is perpendicular to the surface of the meridian being treated.
3. Body weight rather than strength is used to allow the hand to penetrate into the meridian that is being worked on.
4. Pressure is applied rhythmically.

The Practitioner as Observer

To tap into the body's natural source of healing energy so that it can remedy an imbalance, the shiatsu practitioner must become attuned to the internal dynamics of the ki structure of the body by the simple device of **observation.** Maintaining a relaxed hand and an attitude devoid of any intention to interfere with the receiver's ki, the practitioner ensures that the focus remains on using the receiver's own energy as the source of healing. The practitioner acts as a catalyst for the healing process.

Perpendicular Penetration

The purpose of shiatsu is to effect changes in the flow of energy in a meridian by manipulating the energy vortices called **tsubos.** In Japanese, the word tsubo means *vase*. The metaphor is of a vessel with a narrow neck. Contacting the flow of ki in a meridian is analogous to pouring water into a vase. Unless water is poured into the vase from directly overhead (i.e., **perpendicular penetration**), much will be lost.

Similarly, in shiatsu, penetration into the tsubo must occur at a 90 degree angle to the tsubo in order to have the optimum impact on the flow of ki within the meridian. At any other angle, the effects will remain on the surface and will not penetrate deeply enough to influence the meridian. Shiatsu techniques that employ perpendicular penetration produce significant changes in the meridian structure that go beyond superficial stimulation.

Body Weight versus Muscle Strength

The type of pressure applied directly affects the nature of the impact a shiatsu session has on the receiver. To apply hard pressure to a meridian, the practitioner would have to tense the upper-body muscles forcefully; to endure such hard pressure, the receiver would have to remain totally passive and would be unable to participate at all in the healing process. Since tension decreases a practitioner's sensitivity, no communication bond between giver and receiver could be established. The practitioner would dominate the process, and the receiver would remain a passive recipient. Techniques that use hard pressure require more upper-body strength than more gentle techniques, and they can produce physical problems in the shoulders and arms of the giver.

In contrast, when penetration of tsubos is achieved through the use of body weight, the practitioner's hand and upper body remain relaxed rather than tense. Pressure is applied by **transferring the body's weight** into the hand. The receiver senses this type of pressure as firm but gentle, with the result that a communication line of energy is established between giver and receiver. This relaxed form of penetration draws the receiver's own energy into the area being touched. The receiver participates by using that energy to rectify the imbalance in the meridian. The communication bond enables the practitioner to detect changes as they take place in the meridian and thereby monitor the receiver's response and progress. Because giver and receiver are providing each other feedback, this type of shiatsu is beneficial to both.

Rhythmic Pattern

The receiver's response to shiatsu is contingent on the quality of the pressure being used on the meridians and tsubos. The intervals at which pressure is felt constitute the **rhythmic pattern** of the technique. The response to rhythm can be seen in a person's response to music. If a piece of music has a slow rhythm, the common reaction to it is one of relaxation or of feeling soothed. A slow rhythm also allows the listener to focus on the composition of the music and how each note is played in relation to the others. If the rhythm is fast, the listener reacts excitedly, responding by moving the body or dancing. Instead of tuning in to the notes being played, the person is carried away with the active response to the beat.

The rhythms of shiatsu technique elicit similar responses. A slow rhythm is produced when perpendicular pressure is held on a *tsubo* for a short length of time (usually the time needed to create a vibrational change in the area being touched). This is the principal technique used when working along the *kyo* meridian because it brings the cause of the imbalance to the attention of the receiver. This results in more permanent changes in the energy pattern. When the pressure is held, it allows the receiver's energy to tune in to the area of weakness and remedy it. At the same time, the slow rhythm relaxes and soothes, making it easier for the receiver to participate in the healing process.

A fast rhythm, on the other hand, causes the *ki* in the *tsubo* being touched to disperse. Fast-moving, perpendicular pressure produces a rapid rhythm that distracts the receiver's attention from the cause of an imbalance. Because of this, sole use of this type of pressure throughout an entire shiatsu session produces very temporary results. This technique is used primarily on the *jitsu* meridian to assist in the redistribution of excess *ki* in an area that is exceptionally obstructed, as in cases of injury.

If these four primary guidelines are adhered to, shiatsu becomes a highly effective method for correcting ki imbalances quickly with the least amount of effort exerted by the giver. When this is accomplished, the healing power of both the giver and receiver is strengthened.

SHIATSU PERSPECTIVE

In Chinese medicine, a therapeutic approach was considered valid if it produced consistently positive results over a long period of time with little or no ill effect. This contrasts with Western medicine, in which the focus is on fast relief of the present symptoms in the shortest period of time, often without regard for the long-range effects. Although Western science still does not recognize the existence of the meridian structure of the body, there is no doubt that the practical application of the basic principles of shiatsu are effective.

Humankind may have changed through the years, but the relationship of the human species to natural law has remained the same. Shiatsu is based on that law, and its tool, the hand, is imbued with the sensitive qualities necessary to evaluate the impact those laws are having on an individual. Just as the ancient system of meridians and tsubos is as effective today as it was thousands of years ago, shiatsu continues to unify body, mind, and spirit and contribute to a life lived to its highest potential through healthful and fulfilling experiences.

SUMMARY

The Japanese art of shiatsu (literally, *shi* or finger *atsu* or pressure) is a method for healing and health maintenance that has evolved over the course of thousands of years. The foundation of shiatsu is ancient Chinese medicine with its system of energy channels called meridians, acupoints called tsubos, and the dynamic life force called "ki" in Japanese. The unobstructed and balanced flow of ki, both the cause and effect of good health, is the aim of shiatsu. Zen shiatsu is a unique form of ABT developed by Shizuto Masunaga.

The meridians, or pathways for ki, are associated with major body functions. These include intake and elimination of ki and of food, emotions, assimilation, purification, circulation, protection, and storage of ki. The theory of the life cycle of the meridians explains the sequence and the purpose of various processes for maintaining life. *Homeostasis* is a modern scientific term that describes the flow of ki within and among the meridians.

The vibrational quality of ki ranges in frequency from low (heavy, slow) to high (light, fast). The quantity of ki can be described as kyo (deficient, weak) or jitsu (excessively strong). The shiatsu practitioner assesses the quality and quantity of ki in the meridians, and by applying shiatsu techniques, balances or restores the flow of ki to a more healthy state. Shiatsu techniques apply finger pressure to tsubos or points on meridians that are imbalanced.

The goals of the shiatsu practitioner are diagnosis of energy imbalances, treatment to alleviate imbalances, and maintenance to sustain balance. Diagnosis of energy imbalances is performed on the abdomen (hara), and on the back for the 12 major meridians. Four principles govern performance of shiatsu techniques: (1) the giver maintains an attitude of observer, (2) penetration or pressure is perpendicular to the surface of the meridian, (3) shifting body weight is used to apply pressure, and (4) pressure is applied rhythmically.

A look ahead . . .

Chapter 20 explores Jin Shin Do®, another form of Asian Bodywork Therapy developed in the 20th century. Jin Shin Do synthesizes ancient practices with modern knowledge of psychology in a transformational process leading to bodymind balance and good health.

REFERENCES

Masunaga, S. (1983). *Keiraku to shiatsu*. Yokosuka: Ido-No-Nihonsha.
Masunaga, S., & Ohashi, W. (1977). *Zen shiatsu*. Tokyo: Japan Publications.
Namikoshi, T. (1969). *Shiatsu*. San Francisco: Japan Publications.
Namikoshi, T. (1981). *The complete book of shiatsu therapy*. Tokyo: Japan Publications.
Ohashi, W. (1976). *Do-it-yourself shiatsu*. New York: Dutton.
Omura, Y. (1982). *Acupuncture medicine*. Tokyo: Japan Publications.
Serizawa, K. (1976). *Tsubo*. Tokyo: Japan Publications.
Serizawa, K. (1984). *Effective tsubo therapy*. Japan Publications.

S T U D Y   G U I D E

LEARNING OUTCOMES

Use the learning outcomes at the beginning of the chapter as a guide to your studies. Perform the task given in each outcome, either in writing or verbally into a tape recorder or to a study partner. This may start as an "open book" exercise, and then later from memory.

KEY TERMS/CONCEPTS

To study key words and concepts listed at the beginning of this chapter, choose one or more of the following exercises. Writing or talking about ideas helps you remember them better, and explaining them helps deepen your understanding.

1. Write a one- or two-sentence explanation of each key word and concept.

2. Make study cards by writing the explanation from problem 1 on one side of a 3 × 5 card, and the key word or concept on the other. Shuffle the cards and read one side, trying to recite either the explanation or word on the other side.

3. Repeat problem 2 using historical people, places, and events.

4. Pick out two or three key words or concepts and explain how they are related.

5. With a study partner, take turns explaining key words and concepts verbally.

STUDY OUTLINE

The following questions test your memory of the main concepts in this chapter. Locate the answers in the text using the page number given for each question.

Shiatsu and Its History

1. Shiatsu means *shi* or _____ + *atsu* or _____. (p. 351)

2. Shiatsu derives from the ancient healing art of acupuncture and from traditional Japanese massage called _____. (p. 351)

3. _____ opened the Nippon Shiatsu School in Tokyo in the 1940s. (p. 351)

4. Since the 1940s, shiatsu has become a popular _____ therapy in Japan, and shiatsu practitioners are _____ by the Japanese government. (p. 351)

Types of Shiatsu

1. There are _____ major types of shiatsu currently being practiced in the United States. (p. 351)

2. _____ uses amma techniques and views the body from an anatomical perspective. An example is the _____ method. (p. 351)

3. _____, is similar to shiatsu massage, but incorporates meridian theory from acupuncture. An example is the work of Katsusuke Serizawa. (p. 351)

4. _____, uses a broader set of acupoints and meridians, and includes kyo-jitsu diagnosis. This style was developed by _____. (p. 351)

Concepts of Ki and Meridians

1. The Chinese developed the concept of _____ pathways or meridians to describe the _____ anatomy of the body. (p. 352)

2. Ki, or dynamic _____, serves as a common link among all body tissues and organs. (p. 352)

3. The unobstructed, balanced flow of ki along the meridians is both the cause and effect of _____. (p. 353)

4. Eastern medicine is dedicated to maintaining the balanced _____ of ki throughout the body, and reestablishing _____ if it is thrown askew. (p. 353)

The Structure of Meridians

1. Each meridian has been assigned a name of an anatomical organ. This is a _____ rather than anatomical description. (p. 353)

2. Each meridian is associated with a major body _____. (p. 353)

3. Meridians used in zen shiatsu are _____ of the traditional meridians. (p. 353)

4. The theory of the life cycle of the meridians explains the _____ and _____ of various processes for maintaining life. (p. 353)

5. The cycle begins with the *lung and large intestine meridians*, which govern the _____ and _____ of ki. (p. 353)

6. The *stomach and spleen meridians* initiate the process of _____ intake and _____ to replenish ki. (p. 354)

7. The *heart and small intestine meridians* act as interpreter and assimilator of stimuli that affect the _____ and _____, and are associated with compassion and the _____ aspect of ki. (p. 354)

8. The *bladder and kidney meridians* govern purification via _____, the _____ nervous system, and the _____ system. (p. 354)

9. The *heart constrictor and triple heater meridians* are the central distributors that make ki available to all parts of the body. They affect _____ and _____ systems, and processes that control body _____. (p. 354)

10. The *liver and gall bladder meridians* control how ki is distributed to accomplish a specific action. They govern the _____ system. (p. 354)

11. The meaning of these functions can be interpreted on _____, _____, _____, and _____ levels. (p. 354)

Homeostasis

1. The idea of homeostasis is that _____ systems like the human body naturally seek and maintain a condition of overall balance. (p. 355)

2. The flow of ki seeks homeostasis by releasing internal _____ at points along meridians, called _____. (p. 355)

3. The _____ and _____ of ki involved in an imbalance affects homeostasis. (p. 355)

4. Vibrational quality of ki ranges in frequency from low (_____, _____) to high (_____, _____). (p. 355)

5. *Kyo* refers to _____ quantity of ki, and *jitsu* refers to _____ quantity of ki. (p. 355)

6. Imbalances generally stem from _____ of ki, which distorts the energy network as it tries to compensate for the weak area. Areas of excess or jitsu appear to _____ the distorted state. (p. 355)

7. Balance is restored as areas of jitsu are _____ and a normal pattern of energy flow is reestablished. (p. 355)

Role of the Zen Shiatsu Practitioner

1. Three goals of the zen shiatsu practitioner are
   (1) _____ of energy imbalance,
   (2) _____ to re-establish balance,
   (3) _____ of existing energy balance.
   (p. 355)

Diagnosis

1. The purpose of diagnosis in zen shiatsu is to identify the cause and effect relationship between a _____ meridian and _____ meridian, i.e., where energy levels and flow are out of balance. (p. 356)

2. The primary means of diagnosing energy imbalance is palpation of the areas of the _____ corresponding to the 12 meridians. (p. 356)

Performing Shiatsu Techniques

1. Four primary principles govern the _____ of shiatsu techniques. (p. 357)

2. The giver maintains the attitude of an _____. (p. 357)

3. Penetration is _____ to the surface of the meridian being treated. (p. 357)

4. Transfer of _____ rather than muscular strength is used to apply pressure. (p. 357)

5. Pressure is applied _____. (p. 357)

Shiatsu Perspective

1. Shiatsu is a therapeutic approach that has provided positive results consistently over a long _____ with little or no _____ effects. (p. 358)

2. Shiatsu continues to unify _____, _____, and _____, and contribute to life lived to its _____ potential. (p. 359)

FOR GREATER UNDERSTANDING

The following exercises are designed to take you from the realm of theory into the real world. They will help give you a deeper understanding of the subjects covered in this chapter. Action words are underlined to emphasize the variety of activities presented to address different learning styles, and to encourage deeper thinking.

1. Receive a Zen Shiatsu session from a certified practitioner. Notice their methods of diagnosis. Be aware of any feeling of the movement of energy as the practitioner performs various techniques. Compare how you felt before and after the session. Discuss your experience with the practitioner and later with a study partner.

2. Observe a trained Zen Shiatsu practitioner give a session. Note how it is different from a Western massage session. Write your observations and/or discuss them with a study partner. [Alternative: Watch a video of a Zen Shiatsu demonstration.]

3. Interview a certified Zen Shiatsu practitioner. Ask about their training, requirements for certification, and types of clients in their practice. Share your findings with a study partner or group. (Can combine with problem 1 after the session.)

4. Take an introductory class in Zen Shiatsu. Notice how TAM theory is applied in this specific form of ABT. Discuss your experience with a study partner.

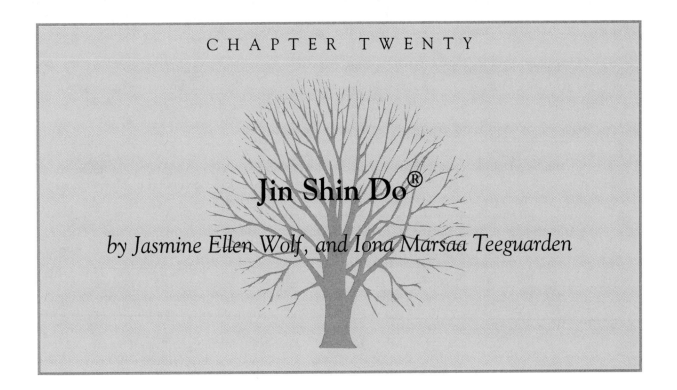

CHAPTER TWENTY

Jin Shin Do®

by Jasmine Ellen Wolf, and Iona Marsaa Teeguarden

LEARNING OUTCOMES

After studying this chapter, the student will have information to:

1. Discuss the development of Jin Shin Do®.
2. Define acupoint, and describe armored acupoints.
3. Describe strange flows and their importance in Jin Shin Do.
4. Discuss the relationship between the 5 elements and the 12 major meridians.
5. Describe assessment of energy flow.
6. Discuss the importance of working in body segments.
7. Describe the use of acupoints in giving Jin Shin Do.
8. List the psychological and physical benefits of Jin Shin Do.

HISTORICAL PEOPLE AND DEVELOPMENTS

Teeguarden, Iona Marsaa   Jin Shin Do Foundation

KEY TERMS/CONCEPTS

Acupoint   Assessment of meridians   Distal point
Armoring   Body segments   Four pairs of strange flows

MEDIALINK

A companion CD-ROM, included free with each new copy of this book, supplements the techniques presented in this chapter. Insert the CD-ROM to watch video clips of massage techniques being demonstrated. This multimedia feature is designed to help you add a new dimension to your learning.

Great central channel (GCC)	Local point	Strange flows
Jin Shin Do	Meridian	Transformational process

INTRODUCTION TO JIN SHIN DO

Jin Shin Do is a method of releasing muscular tension and stress by applying deepening finger pressure to combinations of specific points on the body. These points, called **acupoints,** are highly energized spots along the meridians—pathways of energy associated with body organs.

Jin Shin Do, which may be translated as *the way of the compassionate spirit,* is a modern synthesis of traditional Asian acupressure–acupuncture theory and techniques, breathing exercises, Taoist philosophy, and modern psychology. It integrates Reichian ideas about emotions and armoring with acupressure theories about the relationship between the emotions and energy meridians.

Iona Marsaa Teeguarden researched various acupressure techniques and wrote *Acupressure Way of Health* in 1978. This book describes the basic principles behind her synthesis, which she calls Jin Shin Do. In the ensuing years, she added psychology to this synthesis, as described in *The Joy of Feeling: Bodymind Acupressure™* (1987).

In 1982, Teeguarden founded the **Jin Shin Do Foundation** to train, certify, and network authorized teachers of this method. Jin Shin Do is a registered trademark, and those wishing to learn this form of ABT should seek instruction from an approved instructor. (For a more complete history refer to *The Development of Jin Shin Do® Bodymind Acupressure* by Iona Marsaa Teeguarden at www.jinshindo.org.)

ARMORED ACUPOINTS

Applying simple, direct finger pressure to acupoints helps release tension and reduce physical and emotional stress. In Chinese medicine terms, these **acupoints** are places along the meridians where the life force energy comes close to the surface of the body. In Western terms, they are places of high electrical conductivity or low electrical resistance, compared to the surrounding area.

When a person experiences stress due to environmental, social, emotional, or physical stimuli, tension (and energy) tends to collect at some of these points. If the tension is not released, it acts like a record of the stressful experience or situation. Future incidents may remind the person unconsciously of the original stress or trauma. For instance, a child who is physically or emotionally abused may tighten certain body parts to numb the pain or to suppress tears or shouts in order to avoid further punishment. Stress may be induced years later by the replication of smells, sights, or sounds experienced during these early traumatic events, but the person may not be aware of why she or he is feeling more stressed in these situations. Meanwhile, the points of tension (e.g., in the neck, shoulders, or back) become tighter and tighter and feel increasingly hard to the touch. This chronic tension, called **armoring,** is often located on the acupoints.

Because armored points contain a psychological history, suppressed emotions or old defensive attitudes will sometimes surface to conscious awareness during the release of these points. Jin Shin Do practitioners are trained to empathize with and help people go through such emotional releases as well as to help release physical stress and refer people to psychotherapists and doctors when appropriate. Jin Shin Do is not a medical treatment. It is a **transformational process,** involving consciousness in restoring balance to body, mind, emotions, and spirit.

Jin Shin Do is a gentle way to release muscular tension and armoring. The practitioner starts with light pressure and penetrates deeper when "invited in" by the client. The practitioner stays on the point for a relatively long time and is, therefore, able to work deeply. While one hand is holding a tense place, the other hand holds a series of other points, which helps release the tension and balance the body energy, enabling the release to be more pleasurable and more effective. Even so, it is rarely possible or advisable to release all the tension from an armored area in a single session. People are usually not able to handle too revolutionary a change at once, just as they are not prepared to confront their entire psychologic history too quickly.

Trained practitioners help people pay attention to the sensations and feelings that accompany release or armoring, and to learn and grow from the emotions and imagery that arise. Release is often accompanied by deep relaxation, or occasionally by tingling and trembling, crying or shouting. Sometimes, the process is peaceful and internal, perhaps with the recipient falling asleep during the session. Often the release is followed by a new resolution, on a conscious or unconscious level, and a renewed ability to live joyfully.

STRANGE FLOWS

Ancient Chinese philosophers believed that the body is a microcosm of what is on earth and in the universe. These philosophers observed that when rivers overflow, the excess water forms channels and flows to a river that lacks water. Therefore, these philosophers postulated that when a meridian becomes excessively filled with energy, the excess collects in channels and is redistributed to deficient meridians. These channels are called **strange flows** or *wondrous channels*.

Unlike the flow through the meridians, energy does not flow continuously through the strange flows, but only when the energy is unevenly distributed among the meridians. The strange flows have no acupoints of their own—all their points are on major meridians. An exception is the **great central channel** (GCC) formed by the conception vessel (CV) and the governing vessel (GV) combined.

If the strange flows were free from blockage, the body would maintain harmony and balance through the meridians. However, the strange flows are also subject to armoring and blockages. A Jin Shin Do practitioner can balance the meridians without assessing them by releasing the strange flows.

There are **four pairs of strange flows**—the yin and yang great regulator channels (GRC), the yin and yang great bridge channel (GBC), the belt channel (BC) and penetrating channel (PC), and the conception vessel (CV) and governing vessel (GV). The CV and GV combined are the GCC. Release of the GCC (which is shown in a simplified form in Figures 20–1 and 20–2) is good for people with minor spinal or constitutional disorders (check with their doctor or chiropractor first) and it is used to balance the reproductive system, particularly in women. It is also effective for helping psychic energy flow.

The yin and yang GRCs are used for people who are suffering from shoulder or neck tension or from nervous tension. The yin and yang GBCs are chosen for people with back tension. They also help

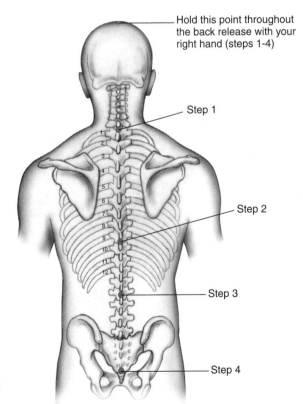

Hold this point throughout the back release with your right hand (steps 1-4)

Step 1

Step 2

Step 3

Step 4

FIGURE 20–1. Location of points for the back release. The back release for the Great Central Channel is performed with the receiver face up. The practitioner sits on the receiver's left side, and places a finger or the palm of the right hand on top of the receiver's head. The right hand remains in place for the entire release. The left hand reaches under the receiver's back, and *gently* presses straight up into each point on the back. *Step 1* is between the seventh cervical and first thoracic vertebrae. *Step 2* is between the ninth and tenth thoracic vertebrae. *Step 3* is between the second and third lumbar vertebrae. *Step 4* is placement of the palm of the left hand against the receiver's coccyx.

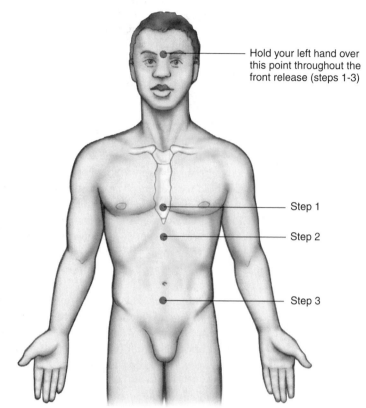

Hold your left hand over this point throughout the front release (steps 1-3)

Step 1

Step 2

Step 3

FIGURE 20–2. The front or conception vessel release. The practitioner should sit on the right. The receiver lies face up. *Step 1.* Place the palm of your left hand over the receiver's "third eye" (just above and between the eyes). Your left hand will stay on the third eye throughout the next three steps. Place either one finger or the palm of your right hand over the midpoint between the receiver's nipples and press. *Step 2.* Place your right palm over the receiver's solar plexus and press. *Step 3.* Place your right palm over the receiver's lower abdomen (hara).

increase a person's energy and are the channels that are traditionally released on athletes. The PC and BC help release the abdominal and low back areas and strengthen the sexual energy and organs. Detailed instructions for releasing all the strange flows can be found in Teeguarden (1978), *The Acupressure Way of Health*, and (1996), *A Complete Guide to Acupressure*.

ASSESSMENT OF MERIDIANS

Although the strange flows can be released without **meridian assessment,** a more accurate meridian balancing requires assessment of the energy flow. Theoretically, if the energy were flowing freely, our bodies would be working perfectly, and we would not experience physical, mental, emotional, or spiritual tension or disease. In Jin Shin Do, releasing tension and enhancing bodymind wellbeing involves the assessment of which meridians and flows are imbalanced, as well as of which parts of the body are most tense or armored.

The emphasis is on energetic imbalance and muscular relaxation, not on symptoms. For example, in the case of the common cold, there may be imbalance of the lung meridian, which would be the most obvious possibility. Nevertheless, assessment of the meridians may indicate that the problem is imbalance of the triple-warmer meridian (which pertains to the maintenance of homeostasis of body temperature and energy production). Or the problem may have begun with a liver meridian imbalance; perhaps the patient is having a problem with toxicity (perhaps toxic anger). Or there may be a kidney meridian imbalance, indicating that the patient's reserve energy is drained (perhaps due to chronic stress). People with imbalanced gallbladder meridians may be so tortured by decision-making that they make themselves sick. Wherever the imbalance starts, if it is not corrected, other meridians may gradually be affected in a domino-like fashion. According to the traditional theory behind Jin Shin Do, the bodymind is one whole, and problems in one part of the system will affect other parts.

It is important to note that we are assessing meridians, *not* organs. A meridian can be out of balance, and yet the person can be physically healthy. For instance, a heart meridian imbalance is much more likely to indicate heartache or difficulty with intimate relationships than physical heart problems. Meridians are symbols, and as such they have many meanings. In Chinese medicine theory, the meridians are associated not only with body organs, but also with specific senses, colors, expressions, emotions, tastes, and activities. An imbalance in a meridian may be reflected as either excess or deficiency in these areas. There are seasons and times of day when the energy is strongest in each meridian. During a meridian's associated "time" or "season" strengths and weaknesses of the meridian are accented.

The 12 "organ meridians" fall within the five categories of metal, earth, fire, water, and wood. These elements are symbols for five energic tendencies, or for five aspects of the bodymind whole.

Some key associations for each meridian are listed in Table 20–1. This is not a definitive list, but these functional relationships will give the reader some idea of the essentially holistic concepts of acupressure theory.

There are several ways to assess the related meridians, including pulse reading and assessing the abdomen (hara) and back. Another method is to observe and ask questions, designing the questions to find out information such as that given in Table 20–1. Let us consider some examples.

Which sense is most important, or works best for the recipient? Which sense is weak? If a recipient has a problem with a sense organ, weakness in the corresponding meridian may be indicated. For example, depending extensively on the sense of sight and not being able to smell very well may indicate both metal and wood imbalance. Similarly, too much or too little of a body liquid could indicate an imbalance. For instance, if a person creates too much mucus or too little there may be an imbalance in the metal element—either the lung or large intestine meridian.

Look at the colors a person wears and the hue of the person's face. For instance, asthmatics are often very white, indicating a lung meridian imbalance. People with metal imbalances may love white or hate it. Listen to the patient. Some people have voices that sing (earth) and others are always shouting

Table 20–1 KEY ASSOCIATIONS OF ELEMENTS AND MERIDIANS

Element	Metal	Earth	Fire	Water	Wood
Yin	Lung	Spleen	Heart & pericardium	Kidney	Liver
Yang	Large intestine	Stomach	Triple warmer & small intestine	Bladder	Gallbladder
Sense	Smell	Taste	Speech	Hearing	Sight
Sense organ	Nose	Mouth, lips	Tongue	Ears	Eyes
Liquid	Mucus	Saliva	Sweat	Urine	Tears
Color	White	Yellow	Red	Blue, black	Green
Expression	Weeping	Singing	Laughing	Groaning	Shouting
Extreme emotion	Grief, anxiety	Worry, reminiscence	Shock, overjoy	Fear	Anger
Balanced emotion	Openness, receptivity	Sympathy, empathy	Joy, compassion	Resolution, trust, motivation	Assertion
Taste	Pungent, spicy	Sweet	Bitter, burned	Salty	Sour
Season	Fall	Indian summer	Summer	Winter	Spring
Related activity	Letting go	Mental activity	Inspiration & intimacy	Willpower & vitality	Planning & decision making
Times	Lung, 3–5 AM	Stomach, 7–9 AM	Heart, 11 AM–1 PM	Bladder, 3–5 PM	Gallbladder 11 PM–1 AM
	Large intestine, 5–7 AM	Spleen, 9–11 AM	Small intestine, 1–3 PM	Kidney, 5–7 PM	Pericardium, 7–9 PM
					Triple warmer 9–11 PM

(wood imbalance). Some people giggle at inappropriate times, for example, when they talk about having been hurt (fire imbalance).

Which emotions cause problems? Some people are so sympathetic that they are swallowed by other people's sorrows, whereas others are unable to feel or express their sympathy. In both cases there is likely to be an earth imbalance.

Times of day when a person feels tired or uncomfortable can help point out imbalances. A person who feels tired at 2 p.m. probably has a small intestine meridian imbalance since the small intestine "time" is from 1 to 3 p.m.

The way people express themselves also reveals imbalances. For example, intellectuals tend to have earth imbalances as do people who scorn the intellect, whereas a fear of intimacy suggests a fire imbalance.

Assessment is nonjudgmental. In the Chinese philosophy frame of mind, nothing is good or bad. In Western society, anger is often considered "bad." Notice that anger is a wood element quality along with spring and green. When it flows smoothly, anger is an honest, spontaneous emotion from the heart, and such anger is often felt toward a loved one or someone considered important. Healthy anger can be a renewal because it can clear away the debris in a relationship. On the other hand, stifled anger festers and becomes toxic, and like explosive anger it suggests a wood imbalance.

Another way to assess meridians in the body is to touch the *associated points* and determine whether they are tense or sore. These points are located on the back along the two bladder meridian lines that are on the edges of the erector spinae. On these lines, the points parallel to the spaces between the vertebrae correspond to specific meridians (Figure 20–3). If the tension is mostly on the me-

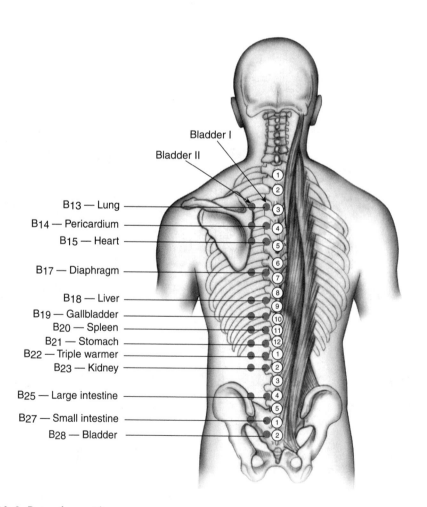

FIGURE 20–3. Points for meridian assessment.

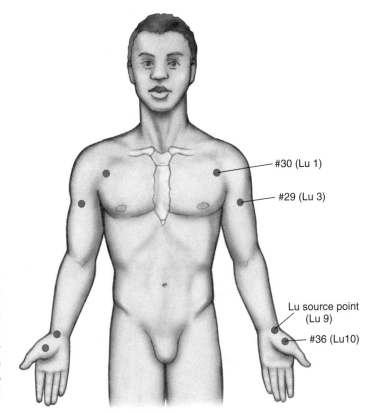

FIGURE 20–4. Lung meridian release. Some release points on the lung meridian. While one hand holds the local point known as #30 in Jin Shin Do numbering (called Lung 1 in acupuncture), the other could hold several distal points along the lung meridian, such as point #36 (Lung 10 in acupuncture) at the base of the thumb.

dial edge of the erector spinae, then the problem is short term or in the early stages of development, and if the tension is on the outer edge of the muscle then the imbalance is chronic. For instance, the points on these lines that are next to the discs between the third and fourth thoracic vertebrae are associated with the lung meridian. If the lung meridian is weak, then the third or fourth thoracic vertebrae may be out of alignment or the area around one or both of the lung-associated points may be tense or lifeless, colorless or excessively colored, hot or cold, or may have some other unusual quality. These points may be sore when touched or may be so armored that they are numb. There may also be muscle spasms in this area.

In Jin Shin Do, the practitioner first chooses a meridian to work with and then chooses a point on that meridian needing to be released. For instance, in working with the lung meridian, a point called #30 is a good choice for a **local point,** that is, a point that is the site of the problem or of excessive tension. This point is held for about two minutes while at least two other points on the lung meridian are pressed, one after the other. These points are called **distal points** because they are distant from the site of the problem, but they facilitate deeper release of the local point. Because of the connection created between the two stimulated points, both points are released more efficiently than they would be if only one point were held at a time. It is necessary to study Jin Shin Do with a trained practitioner in order to know how to effectively release the meridians, but Figure 20–4 provides an example of how you might work with the lung meridian.

BODY SEGMENTS

Jin Shin Do practitioners also work in terms of **body segments.** These are groups of muscles that are functionally related and that work together to make expressive movements and gestures. For example, if you grit your teeth, you can feel the back of your neck tensing. Therefore, these areas are part of the

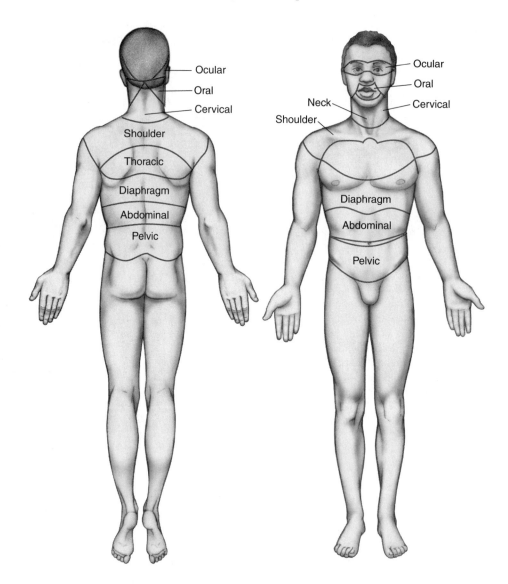

FIGURE 20–5. Major body segments, posterior and anterior.

same segment. For this reason it is impossible to fully release the neck until tension is released from the jaw. The major body segments are shown in Figure 20–5.

Determining which segments are tense also helps the practitioner understand a patient's emotional conflicts. The chest, for instance, reveals how we do or do not let our feelings flow. People with inflated chests are likely to have a macho facade and to act stronger than they really are. One way to correlate the segments and emotions is to think of clichés associated with the tight segments, such as "carrying the weight of the world on my shoulders," or "I can't stomach the situation." Table 20–2 provides examples of emotional correlations with the major body segments.

Usually, all the segments need some release. In Jin Shin Do, the usual procedure is to release the segments from the top down, first freeing the areas related to self-expression. Then, when energy is released in the lower segments, it does not get stuck when it flows up the back along the strange flows. When the upper segments are free, the person is more able to release stagnated energy through vocal expression. All Jin Shin Do sessions end with a neck release to be sure that this often tense area is relaxed—and because the neck release is very pleasurable (Figure 20–6).

Table 20–2 EMOTIONAL ASSOCIATIONS WITH THE BODY SEGMENTS

Body Segment	Emotional Association
Ocular and oral	Expression of feelings
	Rational thinking
Neck	Division between rational and feeling parts of the body
	Choking down feelings
	Difficulty in expression
Shoulder	Responsibility
	Judgment (including self-judgment)
Chest	Restricting the flow of our emotions
	Restricting breathing is the way to restrict feelings
	In the heart segment we experience appreciation and love as well as the loss of love (heartache or heartbreak)
Diaphragm and abdominal	Emotional and intrapersonal power
	Fear of losing oneself to one's feelings
	In this society we are told to hold our stomachs in, an area related to our personal power and gut feelings. In the Orient, by contrast, the ideal is a relaxed belly
Pelvic	This is the segment we cannot talk about in social settings—sex and elimination
	Fear of our primary survival needs or of losing control to our primal self

More information on the segments is found in Iona Marsaa Teeguarden (1987) *The joy of feeling: Bodymind acupressure™*, and (1996) *A complete guide to acupressure*.

HOW TO GIVE JIN SHIN DO SESSIONS

It is very simple to learn to use Jin Shin Do at a basic level for self-help and to help family and friends. After studying the 40-hour basic course, students are able to give many types of full sessions by following various release examples, or by creating their own combination of points. The only motion in a Jin Shin Do session is pressing points and holding them. The point most requiring release is called the local point. The local point is held continuously while at least two distal points are held, one after the other. The distal points are chosen by their relationship to the local point. Usually, the two points are in the same segment, on the same meridian, or on the same strange flow.

A pressure point is held by pressing a finger against the point firmly, but not so deeply that the recipient cannot relax. As the point releases, the practitioner's finger will automatically sink

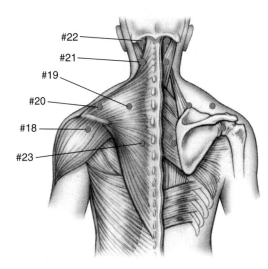

FIGURE 20–6. Neck and shoulder release. The recipient lies on his or her back; the operator sits at the head. Place hands under the shoulders and use one finger of each hand to hold both 23s until they release. Then hold both 18s until they release. Then with the fingers over the shoulders, press the thumbs into the 19s until they release, followed by thumb pressure to the 20s until they release. Next, press the 21s with the fingers. The operator finishes by pulling the occipital ridge toward him or her, pressing the 22s until they release. Adapted from JSD Neck Release (Teeguarden, 1978).

deeper into the point. The points are held for an average of one to two minutes or until the following occurs:

1. The practitioner feels the muscle relax to a significant degree.
2. The practitioner feels a pulsation or an increase in pulsation. (It might take practice to be able to feel this.)
3. The recipient feels a decrease (or sometimes, first, an increase) in sensitivity.

BENEFITS OF JIN SHIN DO

Psychological Benefits

Much disease is associated with destructive thought patterns often created in early childhood as an adaptive mechanism. An example of this kind of destructive thought pattern follows.

Now a woman in her 30s, Andrea was taught by her father not to be an "overemotional wimp." When Andrea first came to the author for treatment, she had severe asthma and had taken medication nightly for the past 12 years. The medication was no longer of value. Andrea told the author that she never cried and that she held her anger inside until she exploded uncontrollably. When she was angry she would grit her teeth, sometimes to the point of breaking them. Andrea had a very white complexion and assessment indicated that the energy in her lung meridian was excessive. The author used the lung meridian release in the *Jin Shin Do Handbook* (1981, p. 8), which includes #30 (Lung 1), several other lung meridian points, and other points on the chest segment.

During the sessions, Andrea explained that her asthma had been very severe for the past month. Asked if anything significant had happened in her life a month ago, Andrea explained that her aunt had died, but true to her training, she had not cried. When the author explained that Andrea might be choking on her own emotions, Andrea agreed to let herself cry rather than suffocate herself. By the end of the session, her complexion was red. She did not need to use her medication once for as long as the author kept in contact with her, which was nine months. Although hiding her emotions was destructive, this behavior was originally adaptive, for it had helped Andrea to win her father's love.

One purpose of Jin Shin Do is to help people become aware of the bodymind connection. Very often, people believe their body is "doing it to them." Our bodies are not separate entities that are giving us pain. When we learn to look for the cause of our pain within ourselves, we can accept it and then be ready to use our minds to transform our health. It is important to learn from our tensions rather than judge them. The Chinese word for crisis is composed of two characters—"danger" and "opportunity." It is the practitioner's job to help the client become aware of the opportunity for growth that is contained in tensions, pains, or other health crises. Patients can use this knowledge as they wish. Some people need their diseases.

Jin Shin Do practitioners are not magical healers. They are more like midwives to a client's self-healing. They assist the self-healing process by holding acupoints and by making suggestions to facilitate release. People can only heal themselves. (As noted earlier, they occasionally need the help of doctors, physical therapists, or psychotherapists to do so.)

In Jin Shin Do practice, health is seen as a balance of the vital energies and of the bodymind–spirit. Health is not an achievement to be maintained, but a continual process that includes growth and knowledge of ourselves and the world.

Physical Benefits

Because both the length and depth of pressure are paced to the receiver's needs, Jin Shin Do helps provide gentle and deep release of tensions, as well as reduction of stress. As Jin Shin Do involves no movement, it is excellent for people who cannot be moved or who must be worked in a specific position. Although only a small area is touched, muscles and meridians are affected all over the body.

Jin Shin Do is, therefore, effective in conditions that cannot be touched. For example, a practitioner could not work directly on an injured disc, but could help the surrounding muscles to relax. In such cases, the practitioner must always work with the permission of a chiropractor or a doctor. Jin Shin Do is excellent to use just before a chiropractic adjustment because the adjustment is likely to be easier and to last.

Project PRES (Physical Response Education System) conducted research in California on effects of weekly Jin Shin Do sessions on handicapped children. More recently, Steve Schumacher in Kentucky has conducted similar studies as described in Chapter 20 of *A Complete Guide to Acupressure* (Teeguarden, 1996). The research has demonstrated many benefits to these children, including improvement in learning and decrease in allergies, seizures, bedwetting, constipation, night coughing, lung congestion, ear infections, runny noses, nosebleeds, skin conditions, and weight problems. The researchers reported that children were less hyperactive, less angry, and happier. One child who had never talked began to talk in three-word sentences. Another child made a gain of almost two grade levels in language development. This study suggests that the use of Jin Shin Do with normal children might be of great benefit (Teeguarden, 1985, p. 22).

SUMMARY

Jin Shin Do® is a form of acupressure that improves energy flow and harmonizes mind, body, and spirit. It integrates Reichian ideas about emotions and armoring with acupressure theories about the relationship between the emotions and the energy meridians of Chinese medicine. It is a gentle way to release tension in groups of muscles or body segments.

The basic technique of Jin Shin Do is to hold two acupoints for one or two minutes using finger pressure. While one finger presses into the point of tension (i.e., local point), the other holds a series of other points (i.e., distal points) in systematic order. As the points release and muscles relax, the fingers will sink deeper into the tissues, the practitioner may feel pulsation, and the recipient feels a decrease in sensitivity.

Psychological benefits of Jin Shin Do include increased bodymind awareness, and stress reduction. A physical benefit is release of muscular tension. Research has demonstrated benefits to children with a number of different medical conditions. Jin Shin Do practitioners are not magical healers, but are more like midwives to the client's self-healing process.

A look ahead . . .

Parts I–IV of this text described the theory and practice of Western massage and Asian Bodywork Therapy in detail. Part V will explore the applications of massage and bodywork for special populations such as athletes, mothers, infants, older adults, the terminally ill, and for the workplace. Chapter 21 looks at how massage is used to help athletes in their training, and to enhance performance.

REFERENCES

Teeguarden, I. M. (1978). *Acupressure way of health: Jin Shin Do*. New York/Tokyo: Japan Publications (distributed by Putnam).

Teeguarden, I. M. (1985). Acupressure in the classroom. *East West Journal, 15* (August), 22.

Teeguarden, I. M. (1981). *Jin Shin Do handbook*, 2nd ed. Felton, CA: Jin Shin Do Foundation.

Teeguarden, I. M. (1987). *Joy of feeling: Bodymind acupressure™*. New York/Tokyo: Japan Publications (distributed by Putnam). Harper & Row.

Teeguarden, I. M. (1996). *A complete guide to acupressure*. New York/Tokyo: Japan Publications (distributed by Putnam).

ADDITIONAL RESOURCES

WEB SITE

(www.jinshindo.org) Jin Shin Do® Foundation

STUDY GUIDE

LEARNING OUTCOMES

Use the learning outcomes at the beginning of the chapter as a guide to your studies. Perform the task given in each outcome, either in writing or verbally into a tape recorder or to a study partner. This may start as an "open book" exercise, and then later from memory.

KEY TERMS/CONCEPTS

To study key words and concepts listed at the beginning of this chapter, choose one or more of the following exercises. Writing or talking about ideas helps you remember them better, and explaining them helps deepen your understanding.

1. Write a one- or two-sentence explanation of each key word and concept.

2. Make study cards by writing the explanation from problem 1 on one side of a 3 × 5 card, and the key word or concept on the other. Shuffle the cards and read one side, trying to recite either the explanation or word on the other side.

3. Repeat problem 2 using historical people, places, and events.

4. Pick out two or three key words or concepts and explain how they are related.

5. With a study partner, take turns explaining key words and concepts verbally.

STUDY OUTLINE

The following questions test your memory of the main concepts in this chapter. Locate the answers in the text using the page number given for each question.

1. Jin Shin Do is a method of releasing muscular tension and stress by applying _____ to combinations of specific points on the body. (p. 364)

2. These points, called _____, are highly energized spots along the meridians or pathways of _____ associated with body organs. (p. 364)

3. Jin Shin Do means *way of the* _____. (p. 364)

4. Jin Shin Do is a synthesis of _____ theory and techniques, breathing exercises, _____ philosophy, and modern _____. (p. 364)

5. Jin Shin Do was developed by _____ in the 1970s. (p. 364)

6. The Jin Shin Do Foundation was established in 1982 to train, certify, and network _____ of this method. (p. 364)

low _____ resistance, compared to the surrounding area. (p. 364)

3. _____ tends to collect at acupoints when a person experiences environmental, social, emotional, or physical stress. Over time, the _____ may become chronic. (p. 364)

4. Chronic tension called _____, often collects at acupoints. (p. 364)

5. Sometimes suppressed _____ or old _____ patterns emerge when armored acupoints are released. (p. 364)

6. Jin Shin Do is a _____ process, involving consciousness in restoring _____ to body, mind, emotions, and spirit. (p.364)

7. Jin Shin Do is a _____ way to release muscular tension and armoring. (p. 364)

Armored Acupoints

1. In Chinese medicine, acupoints are places along the energy meridians where the _____ comes close to the surface of the body. (p. 364)

2. In Western science, acupoints may be described as places of high _____ conductivity or

Strange Flows

1. Strange flows are channels that collect _____ energy from meridians. (p. 365)

2. Strange flows do not have _____ of their own. _____ on major meridians affect strange flows. (p. 365)

3. There are _____ pairs of strange flows. (p. 365)

4. Each pair of channels is associated with certain types of _____. (p. 365)

5. GCC with minor _____ or _____ disorders, _____, and _____ energy flow. (p. 365)

6. GRCs with _____, _____ or _____ tension. (p. 365)

7. GBCs with _____ tension, and for increased _____. (pp. 365–366)

8. PC and BC with _____ and _____ back areas, and to strengthen _____ energy and organs. (p. 366)

Assessment of Meridians

1. The emphasis in Jin Shin Do is on energetic _____ and muscular relaxation, not _____. (p. 366)

2. Wherever an _____ starts, if not corrected, it can affect other meridians and eventually the body as a _____. (p. 366)

3. The 12 traditional organ meridians are associated with the 5 _____, 5 energetic _____, and 5 aspects of the body as a _____. (p. 367)

4. Meridian assessment may be accomplished by _____ reading, _____ and back assessment, _____, and asking _____. (p. 367)

5. Assessment may include touching associated points to determine whether they are _____ or _____, _____, or near muscle _____. (p. 368)

6. Assessment is non-_____. (p. 368)

7. A _____ point is a point at the site of a problem or of excessive tension. (p. 369)

8. _____ points are distant from the site of a problem, but facilitate deeper release of the local point. (p. 369)

Body Segments

1. Jin Shin Do practitioners work with body segments, i.e., groups of _____ that are functionally related and work together to make _____ movements and _____. (p. 369)

How to Give Jin Shin Do Sessions

1. The only motion in a Jin Shin Do session is _____ points and _____ them. (p. 371)

2. The local point is the point requiring _____. (p. 371)

3. The local point is held _____ while at least two distal points are held, one _____. (p. 371)

4. An acupoint is held by pressing a finger against the point _____, but not so deeply that the receiver cannot _____. (p. 371)

5. As the point releases, the practitioner's finger will _____ deeper into the point. (pp. 311–372)

6. Points are held for _____ or _____ minutes, or until you feel the muscle _____ to a significant degree, you feel a _____, or the receiver feels a decrease in _____. (p. 372)

Benefits of Jin Shin Do

1. Jin Shin Do can help people become aware of the _____ connection, and release _____ emotions. (p. 372)

2. Jin Shin Do can help clients become aware of the opportunity for growth contained in their _____, _____, or _____ crises. (p. 372)

3. Jin Shin Do can provide gentle yet deep release of _____ and _____. (p. 372)

4. Jin Shin Do is good for people who cannot be _____ or who must maintain a certain _____. (p. 372)

5. Jin Shin Do is effective for conditions that cannot be _____ directly. (p. 372)

6. Jin Shin Do is proven effective for a variety of _____ in children. (p. 373)

FOR GREATER UNDERSTANDING

The following exercises are practical applications of the guidelines presented in this chapter. Action words are underlined to emphasize the variety of activities presented, and to encourage advanced skill development. These exercises can be done with a study partner or group, or in class.

1. <u>Receive</u> a Jin Shin Do session from a trained practitioner. <u>Notice</u> how techniques are performed, and how you feel before and after the session. <u>Discuss</u> your experience with the practitioner and later with a study partner.

2. <u>Observe</u> a trained Jin Shin Do practitioner give a session. <u>Note</u> how it is different from Western massage, and other forms of Asian bodywork you may have received. <u>Write</u> your observations and/or discuss them with a study partner. [Alternative: Watch a video of a Jin Shin Do demonstration.]

3. <u>Practice</u> the Jin Shin Do back release, front release, and/or neck and shoulder release described in the chapter. <u>Note</u> any releasing or energy flow that you feel. <u>Discuss</u> the session with your practice partner.

4. <u>Practice</u> releasing the points on the lung meridian as described in the chapter. <u>Note</u> any releasing or energy flow that you feel. <u>Discuss</u> the session with your practice partner.

5. <u>Take</u> an introductory Jin Shin Do® course from a certified instructor.

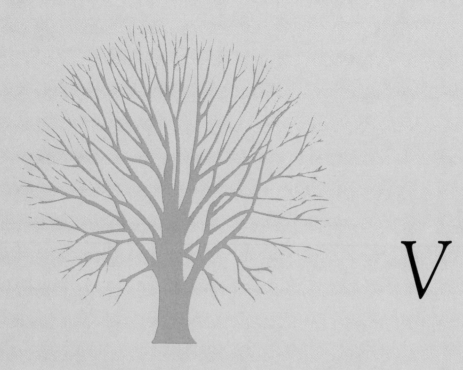

V

Applications of Massage

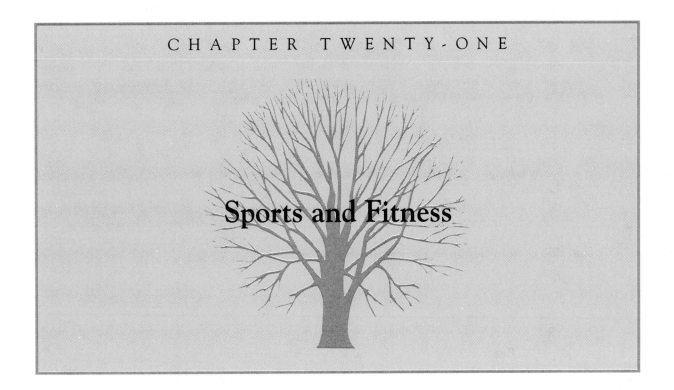

CHAPTER TWENTY-ONE

Sports and Fitness

LEARNING OUTCOMES

After studying this chapter, the student will have information to:

1. Define sports massage.
2. Explain five applications of sports massage.
3. Plan a sports massage session for recovery.
4. Describe remedial applications of sports massage.
5. Explain how massage is used for rehabilitation.
6. Plan a maintenance sports massage session.
7. Plan massage sessions to meet the needs of athletes at sports events.

KEY TERMS/CONCEPTS

Event	Post-event	Remedial massage
Five major applications	Pre-event	Sports massage
Inter-event	Recovery	
Maintenance	Rehabilitation	

MEDIALINK

A companion CD-ROM, included free with each new copy of this book, supplements the techniques presented in this chapter. Insert the CD-ROM to watch video clips of massage techniques being demonstrated. This multimedia feature is designed to help you add a new dimension to your learning.

Massage has been used since ancient times on the training of athletes. This tradition from ancient Greece and Rome is carried on today in a specialization called sports massage. Chapter 2 contains a brief historical survey of sports massage in ancient and modern times.

DEFINITION OF SPORTS MASSAGE

Sports massage is defined as "the science and art of applying massage and related techniques to ensure the health and well-being of the athlete and to enhance athletic performance" (Benjamin & Lamp, 1996). Most of the principles of sports massage are applicable to anyone engaged in physical fitness activities. Many fitness participants train just as hard as athletes and have similar needs, even though they may not enter competitions. Massage helps care for the wear and tear and minor injuries sustained in the performance of any strenuous physical activity.

FIVE APPLICATIONS

There are **five major applications** of massage for athletes as described by Benjamin and Lamp (1996).

1. **Recovery.** To enhance physical and mental recovery from strenuous physical activity
2. **Remedial.** To improve a debilitating condition
3. **Rehabilitation.** To facilitate healing after a disabling injury
4. **Maintenance.** To enhance recovery from strenuous exertion, to treat debilitating conditions, and to help the athlete maintain optimal health
5. **Event.** To help the athlete prepare for and recover from a specific competitive event

TECHNIQUES AND KNOWLEDGE

Sports massage as practiced in the United States today is based in traditional Western massage. Some techniques are used more than others, depending on the situation and the desired results. For example, compression is used to increase circulation in pre-event and post-event situations when athletes are clothed (see Fig. 21–1), while effleurage (sliding) and petrissage (kneading) are more often per-

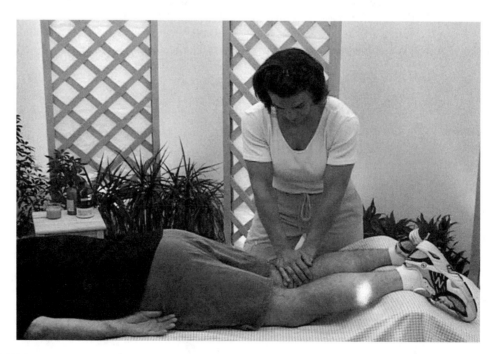

FIGURE 21–1. Compression used to increase circulation in pre-event and post-event situations when athletes are clothed.

formed in maintenance and recovery sessions where athletes are unclothed and draped, and oil is used.

Because of the recurring stress, overload, and trauma to the body, athletes often need specific remedial work in their maintenance sessions. Myofascial massage techniques are useful for freeing fascia and restoring optimal mobility, as described in Chapter 12. Neuromuscular therapy zeros in on locating and deactivating trigger points that cause pain and limit performance, as described in Chapter 13. Lymphatic drainage massage reduces swelling around joints and enhances tissue repair, as explained in Chapter 14.

Techniques are applied very specifically to certain muscles and tendons; therefore, sports massage specialists should have well developed palpation skills and knowledge of musculo-skeletal anatomy. Understanding of the biomechanics of specific sports and fitness activities is useful in planning sessions and locating areas of stress. Practitioners working with athletes and fitness participants should be well versed in their special needs and be able to adapt their massage sessions accordingly.

RECOVERY

Recovery from strenuous exertion is a major application of sports massage. Recovery massage addresses the tight, stiff, and sore muscles that often accompany exercise, and helps the body in healing minor tissue damage. Recovery is a major component of maintenance sports massage. For recovery, the practitioner spends more time on body areas most stressed during an athlete's performance in a specific sport or in a fitness participant's exercise routine.

Recovery massage generally includes techniques to improve circulation, promote both muscular and general relaxation, and enhance flexibility. Effleurage and petissage are used to improve circulation and, thereby, bring nutrients to an area, flush out metabolic waste products, and enhance tissue repair. When the recipient is clothed, compression is the technique of choice to improve circulation.

Joint movements and stretching help muscles relax and lengthen. Jostling and rocking are good techniques to encourage "letting go" of tension held unconsciously in muscles. Broadening techniques help separate muscle fibers, which may be adhering due to the stress endured during exercise. See Figures 21–2 and 21–3 for illustrations of joint movement and broadening techniques used in recovery sports massage given after an event.

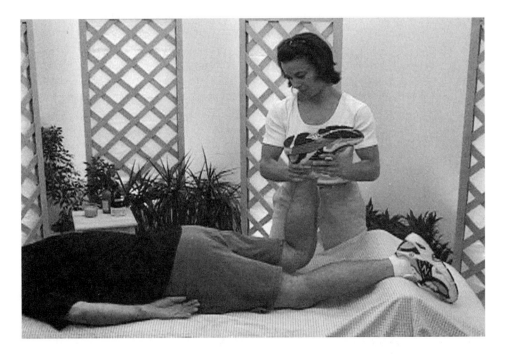

FIGURE 21–2. Joint movements of the lower leg for recovery after strenuous exercise.

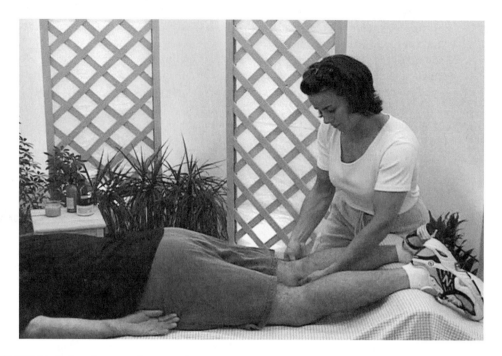

FIGURE 21–3. Broadening technique to hamstring muscles to facilitate recovery after strenuous exercise.

An important component of **recovery** is general relaxation. Stress interferes with the body's capacity to heal itself, and relaxation promotes the healing process. The relaxation response may be evoked with long flowing effleurage techniques or light rhythmic compressions. The environment should be as relaxing as possible with low light and little distracting noise. A hot shower, whirlpool, sauna, or steam room before the recovery massage will enhance its effects.

REMEDIAL MASSAGE AND REHABILITATION

Remedial and **rehabilitation** applications of massage with athletes are the same as with other populations. The most common situations involve muscle tension and inflexibility, muscle soreness, trigger points, edema, tendinitis, tenosynovitis, strains, sprains, and general stress. Deep friction massage is especially useful in the development of healthy mobile scar tissue and freeing adhesions in tissues after trauma. Massage techniques used to address these situations (e.g., myofascial massage, neuromuscular therapy, and lymphatic drainage massage) are described elsewhere in the text.

MAINTENANCE

Maintenance is a term used to describe an all-purpose massage session received regularly that addresses the unique needs of the athlete. In maintenance sessions, extra attention is given to areas commonly stressed in the recipient's sport or fitness activity. The goal of the session is to keep athletes in optimal condition as they are training. Maintenance sessions last from 60 to 90 minutes. Their foundation is massage designed for recovery and also includes remedial massage for problem conditions as needed.

EVENTS

Applications of massage at athletic events include **pre-event, inter-** or **intra-event,** and **post-event.** These applications help the athlete prepare for and recover from the effects of the all-out effort of competition. Special areas are often set aside at organized competitions for athletes to receive sports massage; for example, tents are often used to shelter sports massage at outdoor events.

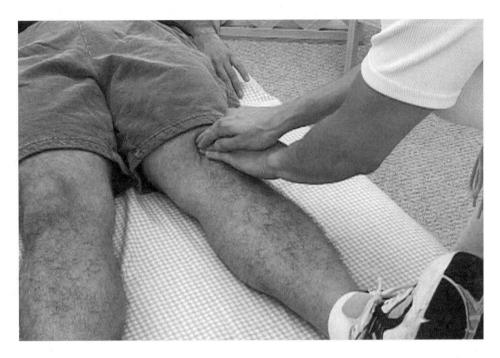

FIGURE 21–4. Friction around knee in pre-event sports massage.

Pre-event massage is very different from the other applications of sports massage described thus far. The purpose of pre-event massage is to help the athlete prepare physically and mentally for the upcoming event. It may be part of the athlete's warm-up routine.

Pre-event massage should be 15 to 20 minutes in duration, have an upbeat tempo, avoid causing discomfort, concentrate on the major muscle groups to be used in the upcoming performance, and adjust for psychological readiness. If the athlete is anxious, more soothing techniques may be used, but most athletes benefit from a stimulating session. Athletes are usually clothed, and techniques used include compression, direct pressure on stress points, friction, lifting and broadening, percussion, jostling, joint mobilizations, and stretching (Benjamin & Lamp, 1996). Figures 21–4, 21–5 and 21–6

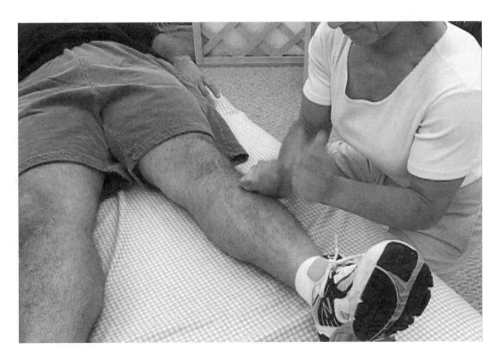

FIGURE 21–5. Percussion on the lower leg in pre-event sports massage.

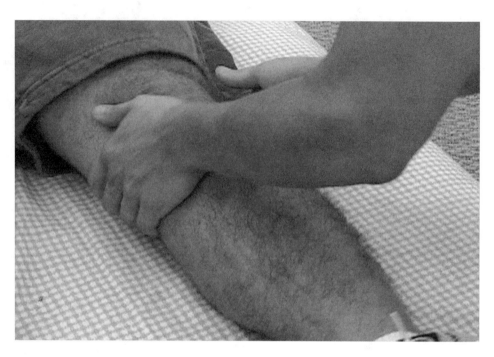

FIGURE 21–6. Jostling of the leg in pre-event sports massage.

illustrate pre-event techniques for the legs including friction around the knee, percussion on the lower leg, and jostling.

Inter-event massage is performed on athletes between events at competitions such as track and swim meets. It is short (10–15 minutes), avoids discomfort, and focuses on recovery of the muscles used most in the preceding event. It must give attention to psychological recovery and also readiness for the upcoming performance. Techniques used are a combination of those used for pre-event and for post-event situations.

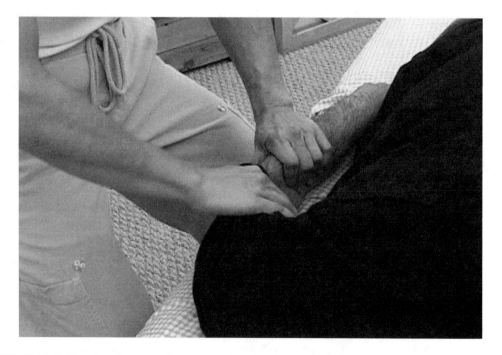

FIGURE 21–7. Kneading the arm without using oil in post-event sports massage.

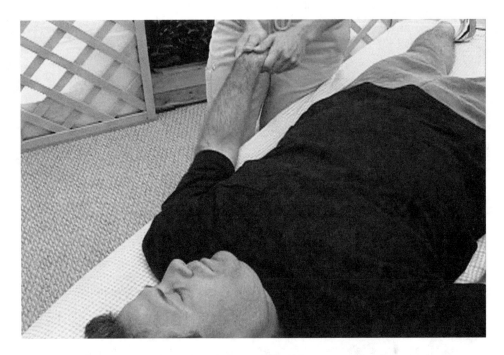

FIGURE 21–8. Joint movement (shaking) of the arm and shoulder in post-event sports massage.

The primary goal of **post-event** massage is physical and psychological recovery of the athlete. If the session takes place close to the time of the event, the practitioner may also identify and assess injuries received during the competition. These may be treated, given first aid, and/or referred to other health care practitioners.

Post-event massage should be short (10–15 minutes) if close to event time, or may be longer (30–90 minutes) if 1 hour or more after an event. The athlete should be cooled down, have taken adequate fluids, and be breathing normally before getting massage. Pressure used is generally lighter, pace is moderate to slow, and special attention is given to muscles used in the event. Techniques known to increase circulation and promote muscular and general relaxation are emphasized. These include compression, sliding strokes, kneading, jostling, positional release, joint movements, and stretching. Figures 21–7 and 21–8 show kneading the arm without using oil, and shaking the arm, techniques that are used in post-event sports massage.

SUMMARY

Sports massage is the science and art of applying massage and related techniques to promote the health and wellbeing of athletes, fitness participants, and others engaged in strenuous physical activity. It is also used to enhance athletic performance. Sports massage practitioners should be well versed in musculo-skeletal anatomy and the biomechanics of sports activities.

Sports massage as practiced in North America is based on traditional Western massage and related therapies. In addition, neuromuscular (trigger point) therapy, myofascial massage, lymphatic massage, and deep transverse friction are used to address the physical stresses of athletes. The compression technique is used frequently when working at athletic events where athletes are clothed and no oil is applied.

The five major applications of sports massage are recovery, remedial, rehabilitation, maintenance, and event. The intent of recovery sports massage is to promote general relaxation and healing from stresses and strains of training and competition. Remedial sports massage addresses problem conditions before they worsen into acute conditions. Rehabilitation applications address repetitive strain and other injuries, and recovery from surgery. Maintenance sessions focus on recovery and remedial applications. Sports massage at events helps athletes prepare for, and recover from the rigors of competition.

A look ahead . . .

Other populations benefit from massage tailored to their special needs. Chapter 22 describes massage to relieve the stresses and strains of pregnancy, and for the growth and development of infants.

REFERENCES

Benjamin, P. J., & Lamp S. P. (1996). *Understanding sports massage*. Champaign, IL: Human Kinetics.

ADDITIONAL REFERENCES

Videos

"Massage for sports health care: For enhanced athletic performance and recovery." (1998) Champaign, IL: Human Kinetics. (*www.humankinetics.com*)

"Sports massage." Nelson, British Columbia, Canada: Sutherland Massage Productions. (*www.sutherlandmassage productions.com*)

S T U D Y   G U I D E

LEARNING OUTCOMES

Use the learning outcomes at the beginning of the chapter as a guide to your studies. Perform the task given in each outcome, either in writing or verbally into a tape recorder or to a study partner. This may start as an "open book" exercise, and then later from memory.

KEY TERMS/CONCEPTS

To study key words and concepts listed at the beginning of this chapter, choose one or more of the following exercises. Writing or talking about ideas helps you remember them better, and explaining helps deepen your understanding.

1. Write a one- or two-sentence explanation of each key word and concept.

2. Make study cards by writing the explanation from problem 1 on one side of a 3 × 5 card, and the key word or concept on the other. Shuffle the cards and read one side, trying to recite either the explanation or word on the other side.

3. With a study partner, take turns explaining key words and concepts verbally.

4. Make up sentences using one or more key words or concepts.

5. Choose a sports figure and make up a story about how he or she might benefit from the five major applications of sports massage. Go through a typical year and explain how sports massage might be applied during different phases of training and the competitive season. Be specific about how the sport is played, training, forms of competition, and the timing of the seasons and off-season (track and field competitive summer season, or football in the fall).

STUDY OUTLINE

The following questions test your memory of the main concepts in this chapter. Locate the answers in the text using the page number given for each question.

1. Sports massage is the science and art of applying massage and related techniques to promote the _____ and _____ of athletes and fitness participants. (p. 380)

2. Sports massage is also used to enhance athletic _____. (p. 380)

3. Five applications of sports massage are for _____, _____, _____, _____, and _____. (p. 380)

Techniques and Knowledge

1. Sports massage as practiced in the United States today is based on _____ massage techniques. (p. 380)

2. _____ and _____ are techniques used in recovery and maintenance sports massage for increasing general circulation, and for muscular and general relaxation. (p. 380)

3. _____ techniques are used in pre-event massage for stimulation. (p. 380)

4. _____ is a technique used at events for massage of clothed athletes. (p. 380)

5. In addition to traditional Western massage, remedial sports massage often includes _____, _____, and _____ massage. (p. 381)

6. Deep friction techniques are used in _____ of musculo-tendinous injuries. (p. 381)

7. Sports massage specialists need well developed _____ skills and knowledge of _____ anatomy. (p. 381)

8. Understanding the _____ of specific sports and fitness activities is useful in planning sports massage sessions. (p. 381)

Recovery

1. Recovery sports massage addresses the _____, _____, and _____ muscles that often accompany physical exertion, and helps in minor _____ repair. (p. 381)

2. The intent of recovery sports massage is to increase _____, promote muscular and general _____, and enhance _____. (p. 381)

3. Typical recovery massage techniques include _____, _____, _____, joint movements and _____. (p. 381)

4. General relaxation is an important aspect of recovery massage that enhances the _____ process. (p. 382)

5. Hydrotherapy such as a hot _____, _____, _____, or _____ before recovery massage will enhance its effects. (p. 382)

Remedial Massage and Rehabilitation

1. The most common remedial situations for athletes include muscle tension and _____, lack of _____, _____ points, _____, _____-itis, _____, _____, and general _____. (p. 382)

2. _____ massage techniques are especially helpful in rehabilitation for the development of healthy _____ tissue and freeing _____. (p. 382)

Maintenance

1. Maintenance is a term used to describe an _____ massage session received _____ that addresses the unique needs of the athlete. (p. 382)

2. Extra _____ is usually given to areas of the body commonly stressed in the athlete's _____ activity. (p. 382)

3. The goal of maintenance sports massage is to keep athletes in _____ condition while they are _____. (p. 382)

4. The basis of maintenance sports massage is _____ plus _____ massage for problem conditions. (p. 382)

Events

Pre-Event

1. The purpose of pre-event massage is to help the athlete prepare _____ and _____ for an upcoming event or competition. (p. 383)

2. Pre-event massage is performed without _____, with the athlete clothed, and should be _____ minutes in duration, have an _____ tempo, avoid causing _____, concentrate on _____ to be used in the upcoming event, and adjust for psychological _____. (p. 383)

3. Techniques commonly used in pre-event sports massage are _____ for increased circulation, direct pressure on stress _____, _____ friction, lifting and _____, _____ for stimulation, and joint movements like _____ and _____. (p. 383)

Inter-Event

1. Inter-event sports massage is performed on athletes between events at competitions such as _____. (p. 384)

2. Inter-event massage is performed without oil with the athlete clothed, and should be short (_____ minutes), avoid _____, focus on _____ of muscles used recently, and take into consideration _____ for the upcoming event. (p. 384)

3. Techniques used in inter-event massage are a combination of those used in _____ and _____ sports massage. (p. 384)

Post-Event

1. The primary goal of post-event massage is _____ and _____ recovery. (p. 385)

2. If given right after an event, the practitioner may also help to identify _____, and offer _____. (p. 385)

3. Post-event massage is performed without oil with the athlete clothed, should be short (_____ minutes) if close to event time, or may be longer (_____ minutes) if an hour or more after an event. (p. 385)

4. The athlete should be _____ down, have taken adequate _____, and be breathing _____ before receiving post-event massage. (p. 385)

5. Post-event massage is generally _____ and _____ than pre-event massage, with primary focus on muscles just used. (p. 385)

6. In post-event massage, techniques known to increase _____, and promote muscular and general _____, are emphasized. (p. 385)

FOR GREATER UNDERSTANDING

The following exercises are designed to take you from the realm of theory into the real world. They will help give you a deeper understanding of the subjects covered in this chapter. Action words are underlined to emphasize the variety of activities presented to address different learning styles, and to encourage deeper thinking.

1. Interview an athlete who receives massage regularly. Ask about what he or she feels are the main benefits of receiving massage as an athlete, and what knowledge and skills they expect from a massage therapist to meet their needs. Try to get specific examples from their personal experience. Report findings to a study partner or group, and compare different athletes' responses.

2. Role play pre- and post-event massage with a study partner. Variables for the scenario might include the athlete's sport, their physical problems, their psychological state, and level (e.g., beginner, recreational, or elite athlete). Post-event situation might include injuries or cramps. Write the scenario first, and then begin the role-play with the massage practitioner having to respond and adapt as they go along. Afterward, discuss the role-play with a study group.

3. After practicing pre- and post-event skills in class, join a sports massage team at a sports event. Notice athletes' expectations about sports massage. Did anything unexpected happen? Any injured athletes? How did you or others handle the situation? Discuss with a study partner or group. (Alternative: Observe sports massage at an event or competition.)

4. Observe treatment of athletes at a sports medicine rehabilitation center. Note the roles of physical therapists, athletic trainers, and massage therapists in the setting. How are the roles different? Similar? How did different therapists use massage? What adjunct therapies were offered? Discuss your visit with a study partner or group.

5. Take an introductory sports massage workshop. Notice similarities and differences in sports massage and traditional Western massage. What additional knowledge was presented beyond standard Western massage? Discuss with a study partner or group. (Alternative: Watch a video about sports massage.)

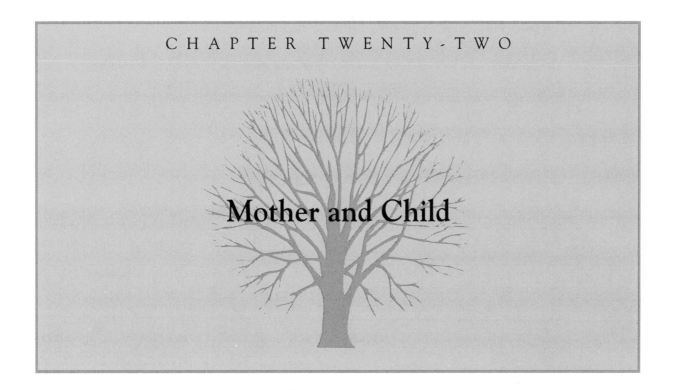

CHAPTER TWENTY-TWO

Mother and Child

LEARNING OUTCOMES

After studying this chapter, the student will have information to:

1. Plan a massage session to meet the special needs of pregnant women.
2. Take into consideration the physical and emotional changes women experience during pregnancy.
3. Identify contraindications and cautions for giving massage to pregnant women.
4. Provide an optimal environment for giving massage to pregnant women.
5. Position pregnant women comfortably on the massage table.
6. Include important elements and techniques in pregnancy massage.
7. Explain how massage can help ease labor, delivery, and recovery.
8. Discuss the benefits of massage for nursing mothers and women with small children.
9. Plan a massage session to meet the special needs of infants.
10. Perform massage for the optimal growth and development of infants.

KEY TERMS/CONCEPTS

Breast massage
Gall bladder channel
Infant massage

Kinesthetic stimulation
LI4 and Sp6
Pregnancy posture

Reclining position
Side-lying position
Tactile stimulation

MEDIALINK

A companion CD-ROM, included free with each new copy of this book, supplements the techniques presented in this chapter. Insert the CD-ROM to watch video clips of massage techniques being demonstrated. This multimedia feature is designed to help you add a new dimension to your learning.

Massage can relieve some of the physical and emotional stresses women experience during pregnancy. For example, massage addresses the strain put on the spine and lower extremities by the extra weight gained while carrying a child. Women confined to bed during pregnancy can benefit from the improved circulation, joint movements, and social contact during massage. Women are especially grateful for the anxiety reducing and relaxing benefits of massage during pregnancy.

BENEFITS OF PREGNANCY MASSAGE

Pregnancy is a special time in which a woman's body undergoes significant changes as it nurtures, carries, and prepares to deliver the growing baby. These changes include hormonal, structural, and postural deviations from the nonpregnant state. Some of the changes cause discomfort and distress that can be relieved with massage.

Many women experience mood swings and greater emotional reactions as hormone activity increases. Insomnia may be a problem for some.

Structural changes include enlarged breasts and additional weight anteriorly as the fetus grows. This shifting weight distribution causes postural distortion that puts pressure on the lower back, and results in neck strain. A typical **pregnancy posture** may be described as head forward, chest back, belly out, and hips tilted forward, locked knees, and feet turned out. Figure 22–1 shows the typical posture of a pregnant woman and major areas of stress. Pressure from the additional weight being carried and decreased physical activity as the pregnancy progresses may cause swelling of the hands, legs, and feet.

During pregnancy, there is a softening of the connective tissue of the body, including cartilage and ligaments. This facilitates normal delivery of the baby. It may also cause instability and pain in the joints.

The intent of pregnancy massage includes helping the mother relax and release emotional stress, and addressing the strain felt in the lower back, neck, legs, and feet. Massage may also help reduce edema in upper and lower extremities. Research shows massage to have potential for reducing obstetric and postnatal complications including lower prematurity rates (Field, T. et al 1999).

CONTRAINDICATIONS AND CAUTIONS

Because each woman is unique, and many complications are possible during pregnancy, it is best to get permission from the primary health care provider before giving massage. Massage may be contraindicated totally in a few cases, or there may be cautions or restrictions to take into consideration. It is important for practitioners working with pregnant women to understand what is happening in a woman's body during that time in order to give massage safely.

Abdominal massage is contraindicated during pregnancy. A few nerve strokes, passive touch, and some forms of energy work may be performed safely. It is best to use extreme caution in the area of the belly.

Elaine Stillerman, in her book *Mother-Massage* (1992), lists the following general contraindications for massage of pregnant women: morning sickness, nausea, or vomiting; any vaginal bleeding or discharge; fever; a decrease in fetal movement over a 24-hour period; diarrhea; pain in the abdomen or anywhere else in your body; excessive swelling in arms or legs; immediately after eating (wait two hours); over a bruise or skin irritation (local contraindication).

According to Chinese medicine, strong pressure should be avoided on the **gall bladder channel** at the top of the shoulders, and points **LI4** and **Sp6**. If there is worry about miscarriage in the early months of pregnancy, also avoid pressure on the Yin Channels on the inside of the lower legs (Lundberg 1992, p. 176).

SETTING THE ENVIRONMENT

There are some things about the general environment and your equipment to keep in mind when preparing to give massage to pregnant women. They are often warm, and so the room should generally be kept 5–10 degrees cooler than usual for massage. Good air flow and fresh air are desirable. The

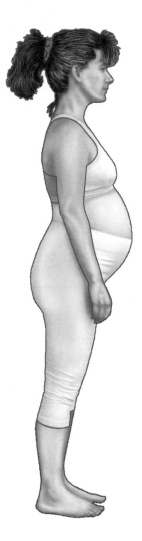

FIGURE 22–1. Typical posture of a pregnant woman—head forward, chest back, belly out and hips tilted forward, locked knees.

massage space should be near a bathroom if possible, because pregnant women feel the need to urinate frequently. The atmosphere should be relaxing, including any music played.

Your table height should be lower than usual, especially when the woman is further along in the pregnancy. As she gets larger, and especially in the side-lying position, you will be better able to use good body mechanics with a lower table. Have several bolsters or pillows to use as props for comfortable positioning of the pregnant recipient. A glass of water should be in reach for the recipient, and tissues handy.

A stepping stool may be useful for the woman to use to get up onto the table. You may also want to be present to assist the recipient and help her get into a comfortable position. This is especially true in the later stages of pregnancy.

POSITIONING OPTIONS

It is important for the recipient to be in a safe and comfortable position while receiving massage. The prone, supine, reclining, and side-lying positions each have their place in giving massage to pregnant women.

In the first few months, women may be comfortably prone or supine as usual for massage. Once the fetus has grown and the mother's belly starts to get larger, other positions may be more comfortable. Later in the pregnancy, the mother may not be able to lie supine without the fetus putting pressure on the descending aorta, impeding the flow of blood to the placenta and causing shortness of breath. Lying flat on the back may also put pressure on the inferior vena cava, resulting in feelings of lightheadedness, nausea, and backache. Lying prone may be difficult, although with proper bolstering, it may be quite comfortable.

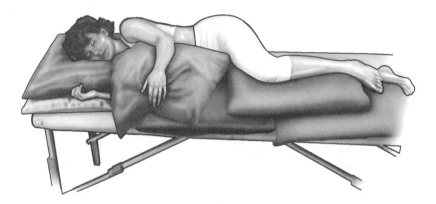

FIGURE 22–2. Props for side-lying position for pregnant woman; pillows under and around the belly, under the head, and under the top arm and leg.

Reclining, or half-sitting, may be a good alternative to lying supine. Bolsters may be used to prop the recipient into a half-sitting position. Some stationary massage tables have an adjustment to convert the flat tabletop into one with a back support.

Side-lying is perhaps the most common position for pregnant women receiving massage. Some doctors caution against pregnant women lying on the left side while sleeping. This may not be a problem for the short duration of massage, but it doesn't hurt to check with the woman's physician for his advice on positioning, especially if there is any complicating health factor.

A general rule of thumb for positioning and propping pregnant women is to fill in any spaces you find with bolsters, pillows, or rolled-up towels. In the supine and reclining positions, a bolster under the knees is useful to take pressure off of the lower back. In the prone position, props may be placed under the shoulders, under the ankles, and as needed around the belly. In the side-lying position, pillows are placed around the belly for support, under the top arm, and under the top leg or between the legs. A pillow may also be needed under the head. Figure 22–2 illustrates the props for the side-lying position, and Figure 22-3 shows draping in side-lying while massaging the legs.

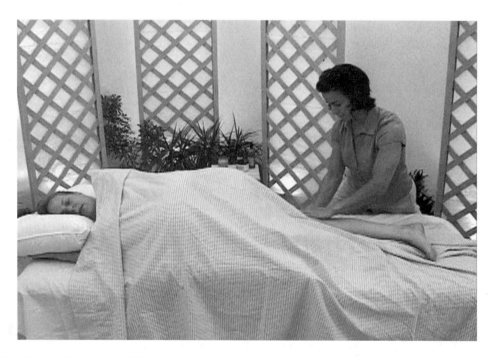

FIGURE 22–3. Draping in side-lying position for massage of legs.

PREGNANCY MASSAGE SESSION

The massage should generally be gentle and relaxing. Traditional Western massage and its variations, various forms of acupressure and other energy work, reflexology, and other forms of massage and body-work may be used to address the wellness of pregnant women.

While there are no special techniques for massage during pregnancy, there are some places on the body that need special attention, for example, neck, chest, lower back, hips, legs, and feet. Suggestions for massaging specific areas are described below.

Because of the forward head posture, the neck and upper back may feel strained. This may also re-sult in tension headache. The neck is most easily accessed in the supine or side-lying positions. Ef-fleurage, deep friction, and compression are effective in reducing tension in the muscles of the neck and upper back. There may be trigger points to be relieved. Direct pressure to certain acupressure points can also reduce neck tension. Figures 22–4 and 22–5 show massage around the scapula and to the neck with pregnant client in side-lying position.

The chest may become sunken or depressed as the pregnancy progresses. The enlarged uterus also takes up a lot of room in the abdomen, making it hard for pregnant women to breathe. Therefore, mas-sage that frees up the rib cage and diaphragm can be important. Massage of the skeletal muscles involved in respiration can relieve tension and promote easier breathing.

An exaggerated lordosis that puts pressure on the lower back often results from pregnancy. This can be addressed effectively in the side-lying position, which itself relieves pressure in the lower back. A simple technique to help relieve tension in muscles of the back is a firm effleurage with the palm of the hand from the upper back to the sacrum. When over the sacrum, apply a little more pressure to help reduce the lordotic curve. Repeat several times.

Childbearing puts strain on the entire lower body. The muscles of the hips and legs have to work harder to carry the added weight accumulated during pregnancy. The lower extremities are massaged as usual, ending with distal to proximal effleurage to help accumulated fluid move out of the area. Deep work on inner thighs should be avoided in advanced stages of pregnancy.

When massaging the feet, you may want to apply some reflexology. Areas to stimulate include along the medial border, which corresponds to the hips and spine, and on the inside of the foot below the ankle bone, which corresponds to the uterus. It is now considered a myth that reflexology can cause miscarriage. Kunz and Kunz believe that reflexology is safe for pregnant women and that it has never

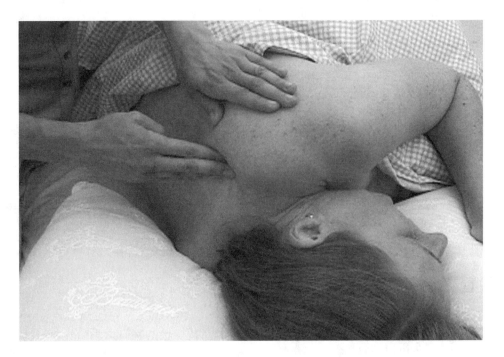

FIGURE 22–4. Friction around the scapula with pregnant client in side-lying position.

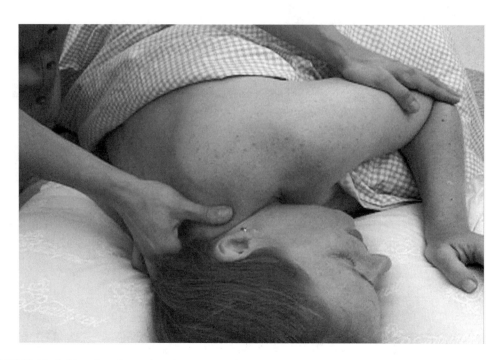

FIGURE 22–5. Kneading the neck with pregnant client in side-lying position.

been shown to have caused the body to do something it didn't want to do. It merely helps the body seek its own equilibrium (1980).

LABOR, DELIVERY, AND RECOVERY

Midwives, childbirth assistants, and others in the delivery room may use massage during labor and delivery, as desired by the mother. This may be as simple as gentle stroking to reduce anxiety. Massage has been shown to reduce anxiety and labor pain, and for some women to decrease the length of labor and need for medication (Field, T. et al. 1997).

There are also certain acupressure points that may be pressed to relieve labor pain. These include the Shoulder Well (GB21) on the trapezius; Sacral Points (GB 27–34); Hoku or Joining the Valley (LI4) in the web of the thumb; Bigger Stream (K3) near the Achilles tendon; and Reaching Inside (B67) on the little toe (Gach, 1990).

Massage may be used during recovery from labor and delivery. Traditional Western techniques help relax stressed and sore muscles and soothe nerves. Acupressure points to press for postpartum recovery include Sea of Energy (CV6) just below the navel; Inner Gate (P6) inside of the forearm just above the wrist; Sea of Vitality (B23 and B47) across the back at waist level; Womb and Vitals (B48) lateral to the sacrum; Three Mile Point (St36) just below the kneecap lateral to the shin bone; and Bigger Rushing (Lv3) on top of the foot between the big toe and the second toe (Gach, 1990).

After an appropriate amount of healing has taken place, women who have delivered their babies by C-section may benefit from abdominal massage and massage around and on the scar itself. Deep transverse friction can help prevent adhesions and promote mobile scar tissue as in any wound healing situation.

WOMEN WITH INFANTS AND TODDLERS

Women with infants and toddlers have a new set of stresses from the demands of motherhood. Massage affords an opportunity to take time out and relax. It may also address the stress on the upper back, neck, and arms from picking up, holding, and nursing the growing babies. Nursing mothers may find **breast massage** useful for relieving the discomforts of nursing. (Refer to *Breast Massage* by Debra Curties, 1999.)

INFANT MASSAGE

Benefits

Massage given by parents and other caregivers is an excellent way to provide the **tactile and kinesthetic stimulation** essential for the healthy growth and development of infants. A significant body of evidence confirms that massage not only contributes to the healthy development of normal infants, but is also effective in promoting recovery of preterm, cocaine-exposed, HIV-exposed, and other high-risk infants (Field 2000; Dieter, Emory 2002).

Massage has other benefits for infants, including releasing tension and learning to relax, bonding with parents, aiding digestion and elimination, improving sleep, easing growing pains, and helping calm colicky babies. In addition, touching and handling her baby promotes milk production in the mother by stimulating the secretion of prolactin. Massage can also provide fathers with an opportunity to touch and interact with their babies in a way that is satisfying and also builds confidence in handling the child (Schneider, 1982).

Infant Massage Techniques

Infant massage is a simple, gentle, yet firm application of stroking, pressing, squeezing, and movement of the limbs. Examples of infant massage techniques include soft circular motions with fingertips all over the baby's head; gentle but firm squeezing and twisting the soft tissues of the legs; strokes with the thumbs on the bottom of the feet; circular massage of the abdomen; broad strokes on the chest; milking the arms; and small circles all around the back with the fingertips.

It is important that the massage giver be relaxed and comfortable throughout the session. Givers may sit on the floor with legs extended and back straight, perhaps supported against a wall or piece of furniture. The infant is placed supine on or between the giver's legs, or prone across the legs. Figures 22–6 to 22–14 illustrate positioning and important infant massage techniques using a doll.

Figure 22–14 shows the squeeze and twist technique used on the legs and arms. Grasp the limb like holding a baseball bat, then gently squeeze and twist the hands in opposite directions. Continue the motion while traveling up the leg from buttocks to feet. This gentle twist primarily causes movement in the superficial tissues, and should not be confused with deep effleurage on adults that is always performed distal to proximal.

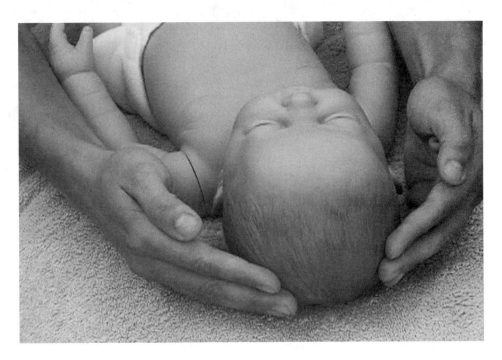

FIGURE 22–6. Gentle circles over the infant's head.

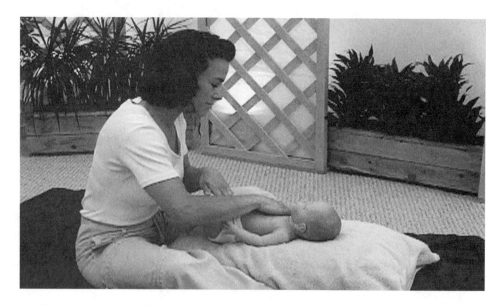

FIGURE 22–7. Applying oil to the chest with effleurage applied diagonally from rib cage to shoulder.

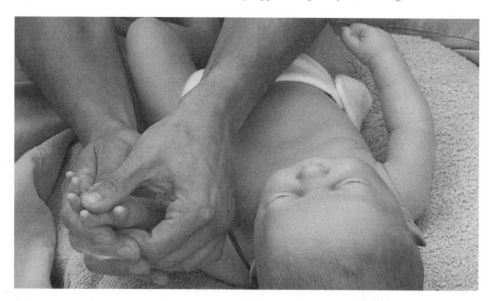

FIGURE 22–8. Thumb strokes to the infant's palms and fingers.

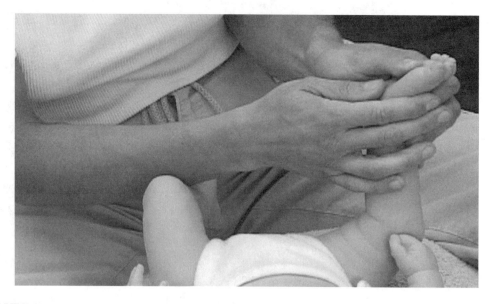

FIGURE 22–9. Thumb strokes to the bottoms of the feet.

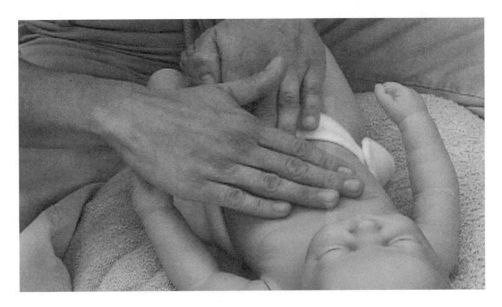

FIGURE 22–10. Circular effleurage clockwise over the abdomen.

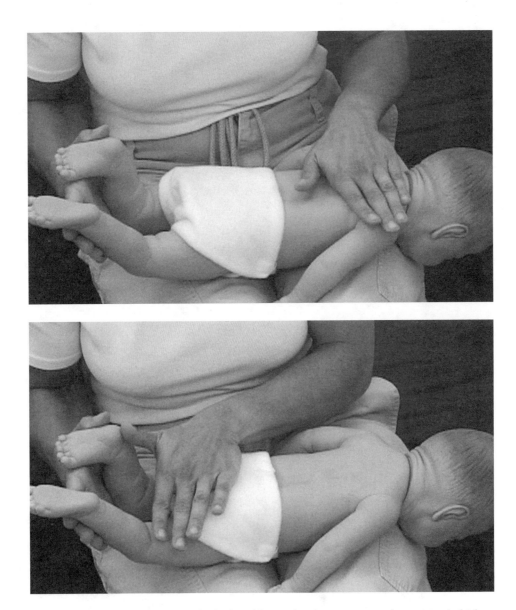

FIGURE 22–11 A–C. Long stroke over the back and legs with infant prone over the caregiver's thighs.

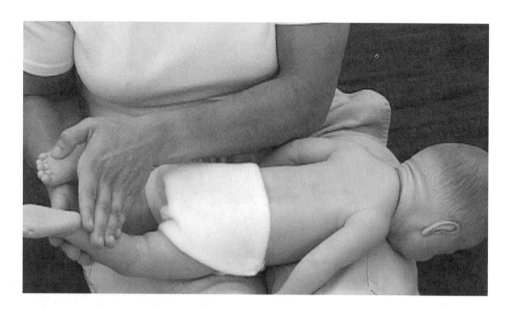

FIGURE 22–11. *(Continued)*

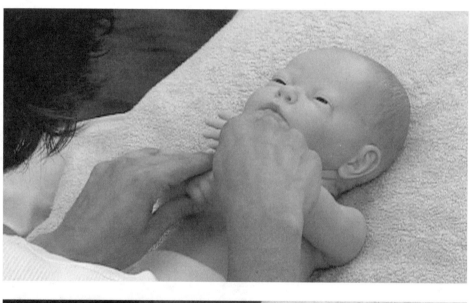

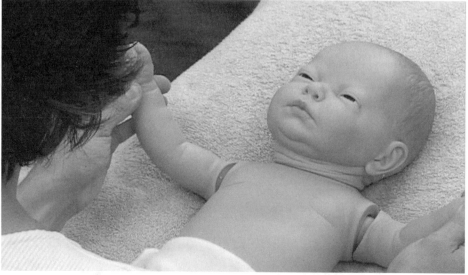

FIGURE 22–12 A, B. Arm movement across chest (hug) and then out to the side.

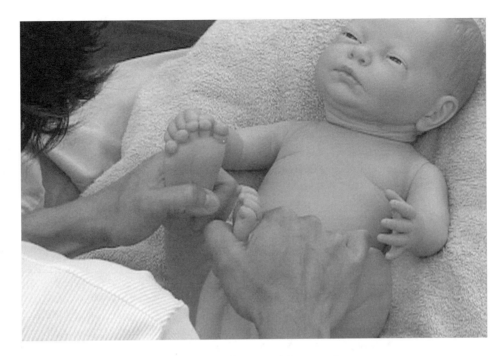

FIGURE 22–13. Leg movement with knees to abdomen and then straightening.

Caregivers should maintain eye contact and talk or sing to the child throughout the massage. It can be a time of connecting and playful interaction that helps in the infant's emotional and social development, as well as the physical.

Massage practitioners may include training in infant massage in their services to pregnant clients before or after delivery. Dolls may be used to introduce massage techniques before the baby is delivered.

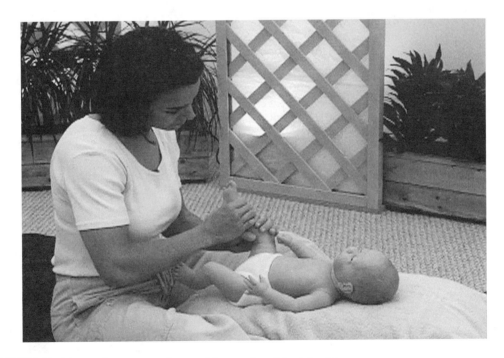

FIGURE 22–14. Gentle squeeze and twist of the muscles of the infant's leg.

SUMMARY

Massage helps relieve some of the stresses women experience during pregnancy, including strain on the spine and lower extremities. It can also be a time of relaxation and emotional relief. Massage is safe in most cases of pregnancy, but it is best to check with the mother's physician for any special cautions or directions. Abdominal massage is contraindicated, and massage should be avoided if the mother is experiencing nausea, vomiting, diarrhea, or any unusual pain, swelling, or bleeding.

In the first few weeks of pregnancy, women may lie supine or prone. As the belly gets larger, switch to the reclining or side-lying position. Use pillows and other props to support the body comfortably. The room temperature may be kept a little cooler than usual for massage. Air should be fresh and flowing, and music relaxing. A bathroom should be accessible. A stepping stool may be useful for the recipient to get onto the table.

Techniques should be gentle and relaxing. Western massage, acupressure, and reflexology have been found effective to address pregnant women's needs. Focus of the sessions is on neck, lower back, legs, and feet, and general relaxation. Massage may be performed during delivery to help reduce anxiety and ease labor pain.

Massage received during the weeks after delivery helps recondition areas stressed during the birth process. Women who have cesarean sections may also benefit from massage during recovery and from techniques that help form healthy scar tissue. Women with infants and children may benefit from taking time for themselves and receiving relaxing massage as part of their regular self-care.

Massage given to infants by parents and other caregivers is an excellent way to provide the tactile and kinesthetic stimulation essential for their healthy growth and development. Massage also helps infants to release tension and learn to relax, and bond with caregivers. It aids digestion and elimination, improves sleep, eases growing pains, and calms colicky babies. Massage techniques for infants include gentle stroking, pressing, squeezing, and movement of the limbs.

A look ahead . . .

Massage is also beneficial for those further along in the life cycle. Chapter 23 addresses the special needs of adults in midlife and beyond, and the applications of massage for maintaining lifelong health and vigor.

REFERENCES

Curties, D. (1999). *Breast massage.* Moncton, New Brunswick, Canada: Curties-Overzet Publications.

Dieter, J. N. I., & E. K. Emory (2002). "Supplemental tactile and kinesthetic stimulation for preterm infants." Chapter 7 in *Massage therapy: The evidence for practice.* Rich, G. J., Editor. New York: Mosby.

Field, T. (2000). "Enhancing growth." Chapter 1 in *Touch Therapy.* New York: Churchhill Livingston.

Field, T., Hernandez-Reif, M., Hart, S., & Teakston, H. (1999). "Pregnant women benefit from massage therapy." *Journal of Psychosomatic Obstetrics and Gynecology, 19.*

Field, T., Hernandez-Reif, M., Taylor, S., Quintino, O., & Burman, I. (1997). "Labor pain is reduced by massage therapy." *Journal of Psychosomatic Obstetrics and Gynecology, 18,* pp. 286–291.

Gach, M. R. (1990). *Acupressure's potent points: A guide to self-care for common ailments.* New York: Bantam Books.

Kunz, K., & Kunz, B. (1991). *The complete guide to foot reflexology.* Englewood Cliffs, NJ: Prentice-Hall.

Lundberg, P. (1992). *The book of shiatsu.* New York: Simon & Schuster.

Schneider, Vimala (1982). *Infant massage: A handbook for loving parents.* New York: Bantam Books.

Stillerman, E. (1992). *Mother-massage: A handbook for relieving the discomforts of pregnancy.* New York: Delta/Delcorte.

ADDITIONAL RESOURCES

Books

Osborne-Sheets, C. (1998) *Pre- and perinatal massage therapy: A comprehensive practitioner's guide to pregnancy, labor, postpartum.* San Diego, CA: Body Therapy Associates.

WEB SITES

> *www.bodytherapyassociates.com* (Pre- and Perinatal Massage Therapy)
> *www.lovingtouch.com* (International Loving Touch Foundation)
> *www.iaimi.com* (International Association of Infant Massage Instructors)

Videos

> "Gentle touch infant massage." (2003) Goldhil Home Media.
> "Infant massage: A gift of love." (1999) With Cheryl Brenman. Sedona, AZ: Brenman Productions.
> "Infant massage: The power of touch." (1995). View Video.
> "Living Arts massage practice for infants." Gaiam/Living Arts. (*www.gaiam.com*)
> "Living Arts massage practice for pregnancy." (2000) With Michelle Kluck. Gaiam/Living Arts. (*www.gaiam.com*)

S T U D Y   G U I D E

LEARNING OUTCOMES

Use the learning outcomes at the beginning of the chapter as a guide to your studies. Perform the task given in each outcome, either in writing or verbally into a tape recorder or to a study partner. This may start as an "open book" exercise, and then later from memory.

KEY TERMS/CONCEPTS

To study key words and concepts listed at the beginning of this chapter, choose one or more of the following exercises. Writing or talking about ideas helps you remember them better, and explaining them helps deepen your understanding.

1. Write a one- or two-sentence explanation of each key word and concept.

2. With a study partner, take turns explaining key words and concepts verbally.

3. Make up sentences using one or more key words or concepts.

STUDY OUTLINE

The following questions test your memory of the main concepts in this chapter. Locate the answers in the text using the page number given for each question.

Benefits of Pregnancy Massage

1. Deviations from the nonpregnant state that cause discomforts that can be relieved by massage include _____, _____, and _____ deviations. (p. 390)

2. Typical pregnancy posture may be described as head _____, chest _____, belly _____, hips tilted _____, _____ knees, and feet turned _____. (p. 390)

3. Massage can help relieve strain on the _____ and _____ caused by pregnancy posture. (p. 390)

4. Pressure from the additional weight carried during pregnancy often causes _____ of the hands, legs, and feet. (p. 390)

5. Softening of _____ tissue during pregnancy causes joint instability and pain. (p. 390)

Contraindications and Cautions

1. Massage is _____ in most cases of pregnancy, but it is best to check with the mother's physician for any special _____ or _____. (p. 390)

2. Massage of the abdomen is _____ for pregnant women. (p. 390)

3. Massage should be avoided if the mother is experiencing _____, _____, _____, or any unusual _____, _____ or _____. (p. 390)

4. Chinese medicine dictates that heavy pressure over the _____ channel, and (choose one: yin or yang) meridians on inside of the lower legs, and _____ to LI4 and Sp6 should be avoided on pregnant women. (p. 390)

Positioning and Environment

1. The room temperature is kept a little _____ than usual for pregnancy massage. (p. 390)

2. Air should be _____ and _____. (p. 390)

3. Atmosphere and music should be _____. (p. 391)

4. A _____ should be accessible since pregnant women have to urinate frequently. (p. 391)

5. The massage table may be adjusted (choose one: higher or lower) than usual. (p. 391)

6. A _____ may be useful for the recipient to get onto the table. (p. 391)

7. In the first few weeks of pregnancy, women may lie _____ or _____. (p. 391)

8. As the belly gets larger, switch to the _____ or _____ positions. (p. 391)

9. Some doctors caution against pregnant women lying on their (choose one: right or left) side. (p. 392)

10. In side-lying position, pillows are placed under the client's _____, _____, and _____. (p. 392)

11. Use _____ to support the body comfortably. (p. 392)

Pregnancy Massage Session

1. The characteristics of pregnancy massage can be described as _____ and _____. (p. 393)

2. Traditional Western massage, _____, and _____ are types of bodywork found to address pregnant women's needs. (p. 393)

3. Focus of the pregnancy massage sessions is on these parts of the body: _____, _____, _____, and _____. (p. 393)

4. A goal of pregnancy massage is general _____. (p. 393)

5. Massage may be performed during _____ to help reduce anxiety and ease labor pain. (p. 394)

Massage After Delivery

1. Massage may be received during the weeks after birth to help _____ areas stressed during delivery. (p. 394)

2. Women who receive _____ may also benefit from massage during recovery and from techniques that help form healthy _____ tissue. (p. 394)

3. Women with infants and small children may benefit from taking time for _____ and receiving _____ massage as part of their regular self-care. (p. 394)

4. Breast massage has been found useful for relieving the discomforts of mothers _____ their infants. (p. 394)

Infant Massage

1. Massage given to newborns by parents, grandparents, and other caregivers is an excellent way to provide the _____ and _____ stimulation essential for healthy growth and development of infants. (p. 395)

2. Research has shown infant massage to be beneficial not only for healthy babies, but also for promoting recovery of _____, _____, _____, and other high risk infants. (p. 395)

3. Other benefits for infants include releasing _____, learning to _____, _____ with parents, aiding _____ and elimination, improving _____, easing _____ pains, and helping calm _____ babies. (p. 395)

4. Infant massage techniques include gentle _____, _____, _____, and _____. (p. 395)

5. Caregivers should maintain _____ contact during massage when the infant is supine. (p. 399)

FOR GREATER UNDERSTANDING

The following exercises are designed to take you from the realm of theory into the real world. They will help give you a deeper understanding of the subjects covered in this chapter. Action words are underlined to emphasize the variety of activities presented to address different learning styles, and to encourage deeper thinking.

1. <u>Interview</u> a pregnant woman, and <u>ask</u> what changes she has noticed in her body and emotions as her pregnancy progresses. <u>Observe</u> her posture, how she moves, and other physical challenges. <u>Write</u> a report of your findings, and in it, discuss how massage might meet the needs of this particular woman.

2. <u>Analyze</u> a massage practice space in a private office, health club, or spa to determine how conducive it is for pregnancy massage. <u>Draw</u> the space and note its proximity to a bathroom. <u>Evaluate</u> other aspects of the environment and the equipment available for pregnancy massage. <u>Write</u> a report and share with a study partner or group.

3. <u>Observe</u> massage of a pregnant woman in the side-lying or reclining position. How did the massage practitioner position the woman? How was draping handled? What areas did the practitioner concentrate on? What specific techniques were used? <u>Write a report</u> of your observations and share it with a study partner

or group. (Alternative: Watch a video of massage given to a pregnant woman.)

4. <u>Observe</u> infant massage given by a caregiver trained by a certified practitioner. <u>Write a report</u> describing how techniques were applied, how they were adapted for the individual infant, and the reaction of the infant and the caregiver. <u>Interview</u> the caregiver regarding the benefits they have observed from infant massage.

5. <u>Take a training</u> in infant massage, and practice techniques on a doll. How are they similar and different from massage of an adult?

6. <u>Visit the Web sites</u> mentioned in Additional Resources. What organizations exist for infant massage? What are their missions? What resources do they have available? What training and certifications? Report your findings to a study partner or group.

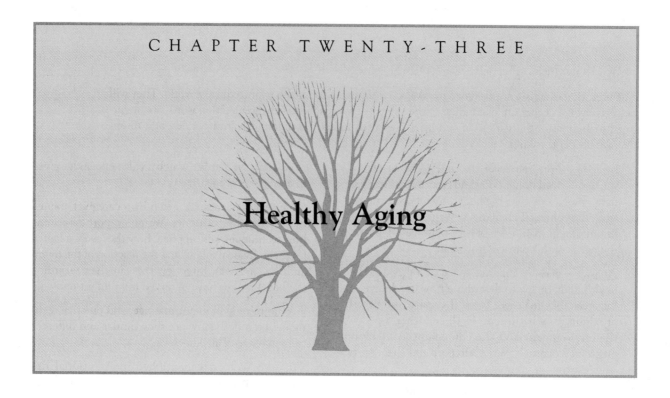

CHAPTER TWENTY-THREE

Healthy Aging

LEARNING OUTCOMES

After studying this chapter, the student will have information to:

1. Describe the effects of aging.
2. Explain the benefits of massage for healthy aging.
3. Identify the benefits of massage for elders.
4. Distinguish between physiological and chronological age.
5. Distinguish among robust, age-appropriate, and frail elders.
6. Plan a massage session to meet the special needs of elders.
7. Observe appropriate cautions in working with elders.

KEY TERMS/CONCEPTS

Age-appropriate	Frail elderly	Physiological age
Chronological age	Life-long wellness	Robust elderly
Elders	Physical effects of aging	

MEDIALINK

A companion CD-ROM, included free with each new copy of this book, supplements the techniques presented in this chapter. Insert the CD-ROM to watch video clips of massage techniques being demonstrated. This multimedia feature is designed to help you add a new dimension to your learning.

Massage can be an important component of **life-long wellness.** It promotes general physical and emotional wellbeing, addresses conditions commonly associated with aging, and enhances the quality of life. Massage can help slow the aging process and maintain youthful characteristics longer.

Massage works best if received regularly and over a period of years. As we grow older, our state of wellbeing is a reflection of a lifetime of both good and poor health practices. Along with good eating and exercise habits, regular massage can help prevent or retard some of the decreases in condition and function associated with age. Massage can help improve an already deteriorated condition, but works best as a measure of prevention.

EFFECTS OF AGING AND BENEFITS OF MASSAGE

The **physical effects of aging** are perhaps the most visible, and begin noticeably for most around age 30. These include decrease in general mobility and muscular strength, slower nerve conduction, less efficient circulation, less tissue elasticity, thinner and drier skin, loss of bone mass, decreased function of the senses, and a less efficient immune system. This is experienced as general aches and pains, slower movement, and less stamina. Research has found that many of these "biomarkers" can be slowed considerably with a healthy lifestyle, including good nutrition and exercise (Evans & Rosenberg, 1991).

Massage addresses many of the effects of aging directly. For example, it promotes well nourished skin by increasing superficial circulation, and moisturizes skin through the use of oils and lotions. Massage improves general blood circulation, especially in the extremities. Immune system function is strengthened with improved lymph flow and general relaxation.

It has been found that chronic stress and inactivity accelerate the aging process (Evans & Rosenberg, 1991). Massage helps reduce the physical and mental effects of stress and anxiety. It is known to trigger the relaxation response, relieve muscular tension, reduce anxiety, improve sleep, and increase feelings of wellbeing. Older adults find massage useful for reducing the muscular tension, aches and stiffness that can accompany exercise programs. By keeping muscles more pliable and increasing flexibility, massage reduces the potential for injury during workouts. Chapters 3 and 4 review the research on the effects of massage discussed in this section.

BENEFITS FOR ELDERS

Massage has special benefits for **elders,** that is, people 65 years and older. Along with exercise, it helps elders keep the flexibility and strength needed to do simple things like get up out of a chair, dress and undress, climb stairs, and get in and out of a bathtub. Therefore, it contributes to maintaining independence.

Another physical benefit is improved digestion and elimination. Abdominal massage improves large intestine function, and helps alleviate constipation. See Figure 23–1.

Massage helps ease the pain of loss, frustration, and fear about the future. Elders are often confronted with loss of work, home, spouse, family, friends, independence, and financial security. The caring touch and relaxing benefits of massage help ease these emotional pains. Relaxing massage of the face is shown Figure 23–2.

Massage also provides an avenue for social interaction, especially for elders in nursing homes or homebound. The personal interaction with the practitioner helps reduce feelings of social isolation, and the inherent touch of massage provides a special connection to others.

In her book *Compassionate Touch*, Dawn Nelson lists some of the common conditions that the elderly experience and that massage can help alleviate. These include insomnia, loss of appetite, constipation, immobility, poor circulation, decreased immune system functioning, skin problems such as loss of elasticity and dryness, bedsores, physical discomfort and pain, chronic stress, chronic depression, feeling alone and useless (1994).

Some of the research about elders and massage in clinical settings is reviewed in Chapter 4 of this text. Studies have shown massage to be beneficial to those hospitalized for a number of conditions, including heart disease, cancer, and psychiatric problems. The benefits of back massage to institutionalized elderly included relaxation, improved communication, and reducing the common dehumanizing

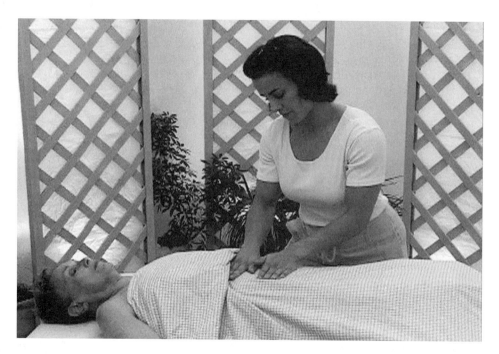

FIGURE 23–1. Abdominal massage aids elimination and relieves constipation.

effects of institutional care (Frazer & Kerr, 1993). These results were confirmed by another study of slow-stroke back rub for the elderly by nurses (Fakouri & Jones, 1987).

There is promising research on massage for the agitated elderly in institutions and for those with Alzheimer's disease and dementia. Several studies have found reduction in certain agitated behaviors with regular 10-minute massage. Massage performed in the studies can be characterized as using light pressure, even rhythm, and slow strokes (Remington 2002).

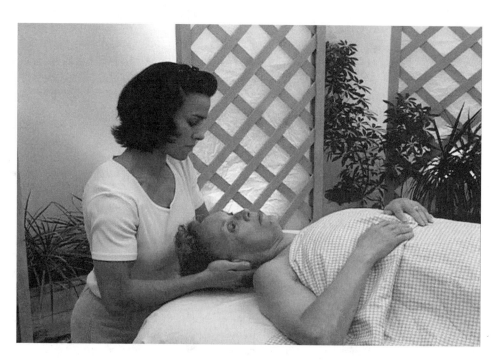

FIGURE 23–2. Massage of the face during general relaxation massage.

WORKING WITH THE ELDERLY

Elders are perhaps the most distinctive population to work with. Individuals in this age group are more different from each other than those in other age groups. By the time people have reached 65+ years of age, they exhibit the accumulated effects of a lifetime of good and poor health habits, diseases and injuries, and life experiences. They are more likely to have chronic health problems and to be on medications. Care should be taken in learning about each individual and in planning their massage sessions.

It is useful to think about older adults in terms of **physiological age,** rather than **chronological age.** People age at different rates depending on their genetic makeup, life-long health habits, and unusual life events such as car accidents, work accidents, and sports injuries. Diseases experienced earlier in life may have an effect later, such as the incidences of post-polio syndrome affecting people 40–50 years after the acute phase.

Elders may be thought of as falling into one of three categories: robust, age appropriate, and frail. **Robust elders** show few outward signs of impaired health, look younger than their chronologic age, are mentally sharp and physically active. People who show some of the typical signs of aging are considered **age appropriate. Frail elders** look and feel fragile to touch (Meisler, 1990).

Robust elders can generally be treated like the typical middle-aged recipient of massage. Information obtained on a health questionnaire can help you identify any areas of caution that are not obvious.

Age-appropriate elders will have some problems associated with aging. Information from a health questionnaire is useful to identify contraindications and areas of caution. Use pillows and bolsters to ensure maximum comfort and the least stress on joints. Limit the prone position to 15–20 minutes. After the session, help the recipient sit up, or at least stay until he or she is sitting up. Leave the room only when you are sure that the recipient is not lightheaded and can get off the table safely.

Frail elders need special care. Check with their physicians before massaging the very frail. Frail elders will probably need assistance getting onto and off of the table. You might find it necessary to massage them in a regular chair or on their beds. Limit the session to 15–20 minutes until you know that they can handle longer sessions. Watch them carefully in the prone position on the table to be sure that they can lie there comfortably. Be extra gentle in lifting frail elders, avoiding pulling on their arms to help them up. Cradle their bodies to help them change position (Meisler, 1990).

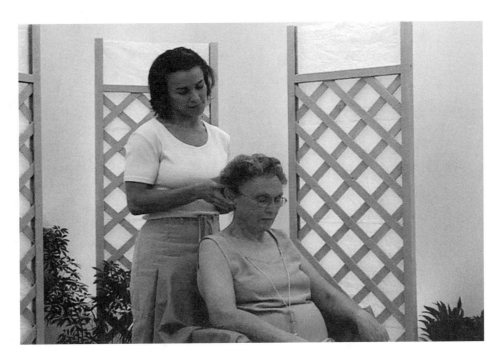

FIGURE 23–3. Massage of the head to a seated elder client.

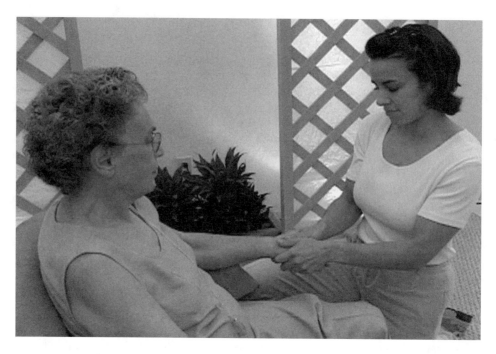

FIGURE 23–4. Massage of the hands of a seated elder client.

MASSAGE FOR ELDERS IN CHAIRS

Massage with the elderly client in a chair can be very pleasant and effective. Remember to use good body mechanics when giving massage to a seated client, keeping your neck and back in alignment. Massage of the head, hands and feet of a seated elder is shown in Figures 23–3, 23–4 and 23–5.

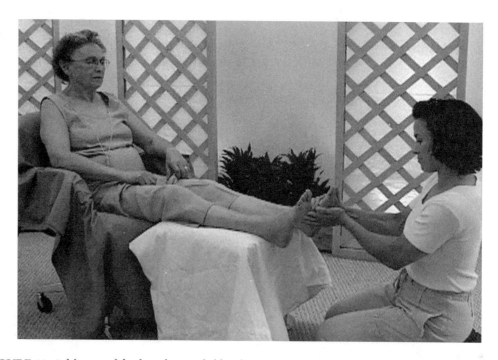

FIGURE 23–5. Massage of the feet of a seated elder client.

MASSAGE SESSION FOR HEALTHY AGING

There are no special massage "techniques" that slow the aging process. However, there are certain points to keep in mind in working with adults, and especially with the elderly.

Do include the following in a massage session for healthy aging:

- Techniques to improve circulation in the extremities. Effleurage moving distal to proximal enhances venous return, and relaxing the muscles with kneading and jostling improves local circulation.
- Kneading, compression, and other petrissage movements that help keep muscle and connective tissue pliable and elastic.
- Joint movements and stretches of the lower extremities for improved mobility and flexibility. Spend time on the feet to relieve soreness, improve circulation, and mobilize joints. Mobilizing the legs and feet can help increase kinesthetic awareness, and thereby improve movements such as walking and climbing stairs.
- Movements and stretches for the shoulders to help maintain some important daily living functions such as getting dressed and undressed and reaching for things overhead. The hands may benefit from special attention to help them to stay mobile and sensitive.
- Passive motion and stretches for the cervical muscles to help maintain normal range of motion in the head and neck. With declining peripheral vision, the ability to turn the head to see things in the environment is important. This is essential for the safety of elders who drive motor vehicles.
- Techniques that focus on lengthening the front of the body, especially abdominal and pectoral muscles, to help maintain an erect posture. Exercises are also needed to keep postural muscles strong and to avoid a bent-over or collapsed condition later in life.
- Abdominal massage for the viscera, which may be important for sedentary elders to improve digestion and elimination. Use gentle but firm pressure, always going clockwise during circular movements.

CAUTIONS

Some problem conditions are more common in older adults and warrant special awareness. Massage is rarely contraindicated totally, but certain cautions apply with the conditions mentioned below. It is important to take a thorough health history to identify the conditions that are contraindicated or for which cautions are important. Always consult the recipient's physician when in doubt about a condition or disease mentioned by a recipient of massage.

- Massage may be contraindicated with certain medications. If you work regularly with older adults and elders, it would be wise to have a reference book that explains the effects and possible side effects of common medications. (Refer to *Massage Therapy & Medications* by Randal S. Persad, 2001.) Check with the recipient's physician if in doubt about the advisability of his or her receiving massage while taking a certain medication.
- Elders usually have thin and delicate skin and bruise more easily than younger people. Pressure used in massage should be gentle to moderate depending on the recipient's general condition.
- Watch for varicose veins in the legs, and do not perform deep effleurage or strong kneading over them. Light effleurage and jostling movements are better for circulation in this case. Elevating the legs slightly when the recipient is supine will help venous return during the massage.
- Older adults and elders may have diagnosed or undiagnosed atherosclerosis, or hardening of the arteries. This is especially dangerous in the cerebral arteries, which pass through the neck. Avoid deep work in the lateral neck area. Avoid movements that put the neck in hyperextension or increase the cervical curve, since this position may further occlude blood vessels to the head and cause fainting.
- Use great care in performing joint movements and stretches involving the hip joint for those who have had hip replacements. Avoid movements involving abduction and circumduction.

Consult the recipient's health care provider for instructions. Extreme care should be taken in the case of any joint replacement because of the potential instability of the joint.

- In the case of cancer patients, always check with the physician before performing massage. Some types of cancer may spread with massage, while some will not be affected. It may be possible to perform massage away from the site of the cancer and do no harm. Observe appropriate cautions with those receiving chemotherapy or radiation cancer treatments.
- Older adults and elders tend to have problems in their joints, including osteo- and rheumatoid arthritis. Massage of the area should be avoided if the joint is inflamed. When there is no inflammation, massage of the surrounding muscles is indicated to help relieve stress on the joint. Holding and warming arthritic and sore joints can be soothing.
- Because massage is commonly done directly on the skin, practitioners may detect skin cancers of which recipients of massage are unaware. Basal and squamous cell carcinoma and malignant melanoma usually appear on sun-exposed areas of the body, including the face, arms, and chest. Malignant melanoma may develop at the site of a mole. Report any lesion or suspicious-looking skin condition to the recipient, or to the caregiver in the case of frail elders, and suggest that it be checked by a physician or dermatologist. Do not massage directly over the site.

SUMMARY

Regular massage can help retard some of the decreases in function and condition that are a part of the normal aging process. Massage promotes well nourished skin, improves general blood circulation and lymph flow, helps keep fascia and muscles more pliable, improves joint flexibility, and strengthens immune system function. It helps reduce physical and mental effects of stress that accelerate the aging process.

Massage is especially beneficial for elders of 65 years old or more. It helps them maintain mobility and independence longer, and eases the emotional pain of loss and frustration often experienced in later years. It alleviates some common problems such as insomnia, constipation, and depression. Massage offers regular caring touch, relaxation, and social interaction to homebound elders and those in institutions.

It is useful to think of older adults in terms of physiological, rather than chronological, age. Elders may be robust, age appropriate, or frail. Contraindications and conditions that warrant caution include certain medications, thinning skin, skin growths, circulatory problems, joint disease, and joint replacements.

There are no massage techniques that slow the aging process. However, massage sessions may be planned to meet the needs of aging adults: for example, to maintain healthy tissues, mobility, good posture, independence, and functions such as digestion and elimination. Massage can be an important part of a life-long personal wellness program, and an aid to caring for elders in institutions.

A look ahead . . .

Massage has special benefits for those at the end of their lives due to old age or illness. Chapter 24 will give information and guidelines for providing massage to this very unique population.

REFERENCES

Evans, W., & Rosenberg, E. H. (1991). *Biomarkers*. New York: Simon & Schuster.

Fakouri, C., & Jones, P. (1987). Relaxation ℞: Slow stroke back rub. *Journal of Gerontological Nursing, 13*(2), pp. 32–35.

Frazer, J., & Kerr, J. R. (1993). Psychophysiological effects of back massage on elderly institutionalized patients. *Journal of Advanced Nursing, 18*, pp. 238–245.

Miesler, D. W. (1990). *Geriatric massage techniques: Topics for bodyworkers no. 2*. Guerneville, CA: Day-Break Productions.

Nelson, D. (1994). *Compassionate touch: Hands-on caregiving for the elderly, the ill, and the dying*. Barrytown, NY: Station Hill Press.

Persad, R. (2001). *Massage therapy & medications: General treatment principles*. Toronto: Curties-Overzet Publications.

Remington, R. (2002). "Hand massage in the agitated elderly." Chapter 8 in *Massage therapy: The evidence for practice* by G.J. Rich, editor. New York: Mosby.

ADDITIONAL RESOURCES

Books

Nelson, Dawn (2001). *From the heart through the hands: The power of touch in caregiving*. Forres, Scotland: Findhorn Press.

Video Tapes

"ABC's of Geriatric Massage." Day-Break Massage Institute (*www.daybreak-massage.com*).

WEBSITES

Aging Research Centre (ARC) (*www.arclab.org*)
American Society on Aging (*www.asaging.org*)
Day-Break Geriatric Massage Institute (*www.daybreak-massage.com*)
National Council on Aging (NCOA) (*www.ncoa.org*)
National Institute on Aging at the National Institutes of Health (*www.nia.nih.gov*)
U.S. Administration on Aging (AoA) (*www.aoa.gov*)

S T U D Y   G U I D E

LEARNING OUTCOMES

Use the learning outcomes at the beginning of the chapter as a guide to your studies. Perform the task given in each outcome, either in writing or verbally into a tape recorder or to a study partner. This may start as an "open book" exercise, and then later from memory.

KEY TERMS/CONCEPTS

To study key words and concepts listed at the beginning of this chapter, choose one or more of the following exercises. Writing or talking about ideas helps you remember them better, and explaining them helps deepen your understanding.

1. Write a one- or two-sentence explanation of each key word and concept.

2. Make study cards by writing the explanation from problem 1 on one side of a 3 × 5 card, and the key word or concept on the other. Shuffle the cards and read one side, trying to recite either the explanation or word on the other side.

3. With a study partner, take turns explaining key words and concepts verbally.

STUDY OUTLINE

The following questions test your memory of the main concepts in this chapter. Locate the answers in the text using the page number given for each question.

1. Massage can be an important part of life-long _____, and an aid to caring for elders in _____ settings. (p. 405)

Effects of Aging and Benefits of Aging

1. The physical effects of aging begin around age _____ and include decrease in general mobility, slower _____ conduction, less _____ circulation, less _____ elasticity, _____ and _____ skin, loss of bone _____, decreased sensory function, and a less _____ immune system. (p. 405)

2. Regular massage can help retard some of the decreases in function and condition that are part of the normal aging process. For example, massage promotes _____ skin, improves general blood _____ and lymph _____, helps keep fascia and muscles more _____, improves joint _____, and _____ immune system function. (p. 405)

3. Massage also reduces the physical and mental effects of _____ that may accelerate the _____ process. (p. 405)

Benefits for Elders

1. Massage is especially beneficial for elders of _____ years or older. (p. 405)

2. Massage helps elders maintain mobility and _____ longer, and helps ease the emotional pain of loss and _____ experienced in later years. (p. 405)

3. Massage may alleviate some common physical problems of the elderly such as _____, _____, _____, physical discomfort, and _____. (p. 405)

4. Massage may also alleviate some common emotional problems such as _____, _____, _____, feeling alone, and _____. (p. 405)

5. Massage offers regular caring _____, _____, and _____ interaction to homebound elders and those in _____. (p. 405)

6. Benefits of massage for elders in hospitals include relaxation, improved _____, and reducing the _____ effects of institutional care. (pp. 405–406)

7. Massage has been found to reduce negative behavior in some _____ elderly in nursing homes. (p. 406)

Working with the Elderly

1. It is useful to think of older adults in terms of _____ age rather than _____ age. (p. 407)

2. _____ elders show few outward signs of impaired health. (p. 407)

3. _____ elders show typical signs of aging. (p. 407)

4. _____ elders look and feel fragile to touch. (p. 407)

5. After the massage, leave the room only when you are sure that the recipient is not _____ and can get off of the table _____. (p. 407)

6. Be gentle in lifting _____ elders. _____ their bodies to help them change position. (p. 407)

Massage for Elders

1. Limit the prone position of elders to _____ minutes. (p. 407)

2. Use bolsters to relieve stress on _____. (p. 407)

3. There are no special massage techniques that _____ the aging process. (p. 409)

4. Elements to include in massage sessions for older people. (p. 409)

   a. _____ enhancing massage, e.g., effleurage.

   b. Petrissage for _____ and _____ connective tissue.

   c. Joint movements to improve _____ and _____.

   d. Joint movements in upper extremities to improve _____ functions.

   e. Passive movement of cervical muscles to improve _____ rotation.

f. Techniques to improve upright _____.

g. _____ massage for improved digestion and elimination.

Cautions

1. Common conditions of the elderly that may be contraindications, or for which special cautions apply, include use of prescribed _____, thinning _____, _____ growths, cancer, circulatory problems such as _____ veins and _____, and joint disease such as _____. (p. 409)

2. Observe limitations around _____ replacements. (p. 409)

3. Avoid _____ and _____ with hip replacements. (p. 409)

4. Avoid massage of the _____ neck. (p. 409)

5. Pressure used to apply techniques should be light to moderate to avoid _____. (p. 409)

6. Tell the client of any skin growths that you suspect may be _____. (p. 409)

FOR GREATER UNDERSTANDING

The following exercises are designed to take you from the realm of theory into the real world. They will help give you a deeper understanding of the subjects covered in this chapter. Action words are underlined to emphasize the variety of activities presented to address different learning styles, and to encourage deeper thinking.

1. Observe people of a variety of ages in a public place like a park or shopping mall. Note differences in the way they move, their posture, and other visible characteristics. Compare and contrast children, young adults, older adults, and the elderly. Summarize your findings in writing and report to a study partner or group.

2. Observe a number of different elderly people. Categorize them as robust, age appropriate, or frail. Explain the basis for your decisions. Summarize your findings in writing and report to a study partner or group.

3. Visit a nursing home or extended care facility for the elderly. Observe the patients' mobility, activity, and limitations. Describe your observations and how massage could add to their health and wellbeing. Report to a study partner or group.

4. Interview an older adult (50–65 years old) and ask them what changes they have noticed in themselves as they age. Describe what specific effects of massage may apply directly to improving their lives. Plan a massage session including approaches to address their unique needs.

5. Give a massage to an older adult or elder. How does it differ from massage of a younger person? Note contraindications and cautions, medications, skin condition, quality of tissues, flexibility, past injuries, and other factors related to age. Report your experience.

6. Volunteer to give seated massage (head, shoulders, hands or feet) to the elderly in a senior center, nursing home, or other facility. How did you modify the massage for each person? What was their reaction to you and the massage? What benefit do you think they got from the experience? What benefit did you get from the experience? Report your experience.

7. Visit the Web sites of organizations for the elderly listed as additional resources at the end of the chapter. What are their missions, and in what way do they benefit older people? Do they have anything of value to offer massage therapists? Report your findings.

8. Take a training specifically for massage of the elderly. How is massage modified to address the needs of this special population?

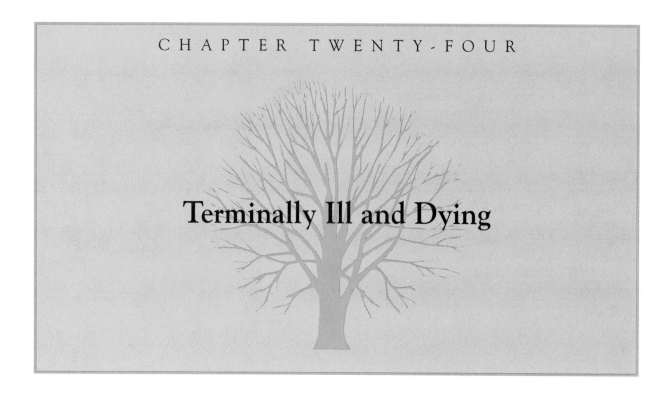

CHAPTER TWENTY-FOUR

Terminally Ill and Dying

LEARNING OUTCOMES

After studying this chapter, the student will have information to:

1. Explain the value of massage for the terminally ill from a wellness perspective.
2. Describe different approaches to massage for the dying.
3. Seek knowledge and skills needed to work with seriously ill and dying people.
4. Plan a massage session for someone seriously ill or dying.
5. Practice self-care while working with the terminally ill and dying.

KEY TERMS/CONCEPTS

Comforting touch
Conscious self-care
Emotional distress

Hospice
Nonverbal communication
Nurturing touch

Palliative care
Touch deprivation

MEDIALINK

A companion CD-ROM, included free with each new copy of this book, supplements the techniques presented in this chapter. Insert the CD-ROM to watch video clips of massage techniques being demonstrated. This multimedia feature is designed to help you add a new dimension to your learning.

Massage is used to bring caring and **comforting touch** to the terminally ill and dying. It is a valuable complementary therapy in hospitals, hospice, and home care. Simple massage techniques may be used by health practitioners, and taught to nonprofessional caregivers, to aid those seriously ill or approaching the end of their lives.

CARING TOUCH OF MASSAGE

From the wellness perspective, even those with terminal illnesses or nearing death continue to strive for optimal wellbeing in their unique life circumstances. Although massage will not cure or save someone from imminent death, it can help improve physical function and ease some of the pain and anxiety felt. As Dawn Nelson points out in her book *Compassionate Touch*, "attentive **nurturing touch** can be a significant therapeutic factor in treating despondency in the aging and/or the ill because of its multiple psycho-social, mental, emotional, and physical benefits" (1994, p. 12). Nurturing touch provides food for the soul as well as for the body and mind.

General relaxation, improved circulation of blood and lymph, reduced muscular tension, and skin stimulation are effects of massage with benefits for everyone. These effects are relevant to the special needs of those who have been physically inactive or bedridden for a long period of time. Massage helps alleviate problems with insomnia, digestion, constipation, difficulty in breathing, and skin degeneration. It can help prevent bedsores.

The terminally ill and dying experience **emotional distress** for a number of reasons. They may feel isolation, grief from the loss of freedom and friends, fear of abandonment, fear of the disease or aging, or fear of dying. Depression is common among the seriously ill and elderly, and may be caused or deepened by **touch deprivation**. Touch is essential nourishment for optimal wellbeing at all stages of life.

Gentle relaxation massage is known to reduce anxiety, provide a sense of connection, and generate feelings of general wellbeing. Massage may also facilitate a release of pent-up feelings, frustrations, sadness, and emotional energy. Pain that is aggravated by stress may be lessened with relaxing massage.

HOSPICE AND PALLIATIVE CARE

Hospice and **palliative care** programs are provided in freestanding facilities, hospitals, nursing homes, and other long-term care facilities. They provide compassionate care at the end of life, and typically involve a team-oriented approach to medical care, pain management, and emotional and spiritual support tailored to the needs of the dying. Hospice services include nursing care, personal care, social services, physician visits, counseling, and domestic services. The goal is to provide high quality palliative care. (Refer to National Hospice Foundation at www.hospiceinfo.org; and Center to Advance Palliative Care at www.capc.org.)

Massage therapy is one of the services increasingly available in hospice settings. The value of massage as a palliative care method has been studied and validated in integrative medical settings (Ellis et al., 1995; Howdyshell, 1998; Ruebottom, 1989).

MASSAGE FOR THE DYING

Near the end of life, massage can provide comforting touch, and communicate caring and love in a **nonverbal** way. The quality of touch for the dying should be gentle, and the techniques simple, such as stroking and holding.

In his book *Touching is Healing* (1982), Jules Older describes a program in New Zealand for the seriously ill and dying called the TLP Programme. TLP stands for Tender Loving Physiotherapy. The function of TLP is short-term rehabilitation and clearing the chest, and if appropriate, easing the transition from life to death. When death is near, smooth, soothing touch is used as a form of comfort and a means of communication. Some technical skills are needed to avoid causing pain or damaging delicate tissues.

Cathleen Farnslow, RN, describes how she uses Therapeutic Touch with the dying in *The Many Facets of Touch* (1984):

> When treating people near the end of the life continuum, I am drawn to place my hands on or near the heart, since this is the area of relationship and fear and requires life energy so that the dying can make

amends and say good-bye, I'm sorry, or I love you before death occurs. As I hold my hands on or near the heart I am consciously sending thoughts of peace, love, and wholeness, which makes energy available for patients to finish their business with those who remain here and decreases pre-death anxiety. The elders feel deep warmth penetrating the heart area and report a sense of peace and deep calm (p. 187).

In hospice and home-care situations, family members and other caregivers can be taught simple ways of giving massage to the dying person. This has benefits for both parties, since it offers caregivers something active to do with their loved one and provides a means of connection even for those who may not be able to speak.

KNOWLEDGE AND SKILLS

A medical profile of the recipient is essential in working with the seriously ill and dying to protect both them and you. As with any other massage, identify contraindications and areas of caution before proceeding with a session. It may also be useful to understand the symptoms expected as a specific disease or condition progresses.

Specific techniques are less important than other essential skills when working with the terminally ill and dying. Dawn Nelson points out that:

If you develop the ability to "see" an individual rather than just looking at a body, and if you reach out to that individual with a caring and open heart, your touch is likely to be far more effective than that of a highly trained professional who may be simply going through the mechanics of manipulating a physical body. Out of your real and pure contact with the individual, you will intuitively know what to do and how to proceed (1994, p. 43).

Intuition and sensitivity to others are important qualities for giving massage to the terminally ill and dying. Other characteristics and abilities recommended by Nelson (1994) include being touch oriented, able to adapt, open-hearted, able to focus energy, willing to face death, and able to focus on the individual. The skills she identifies as important include sensitive massage, active holding, listening and feedback, visualization and guided fantasy, guided meditation, shared breathing, and communicating with the dying. While some of these skills seem outside of the normal scope of a massage practitioner, they are useful in working with this special population.

In planning massage sessions for the terminally ill or dying, there are no specific procedures to follow or ironclad rules to memorize. Each individual will be different in how he or she experiences dying and in how massage might be of benefit. However, there are some general guidelines to keep in mind.

In general, massage sessions with the dying should be softer, gentler, and shorter. A person may only be able to benefit from 10–20 minutes of contact. Techniques may vary from simple hand holding to full-body massage. Massage may be given with the receiver lying on a standard massage table, sitting in a chair or wheel chair, or lying in bed. Patients may be in hospital beds with tubes or IVs in their bodies. Massage practitioners in these situations need to be versatile and able to adapt to the circumstances. Listening and feedback skills are important since communication may be a great need for someone facing death. The key is to be caring, supportive, and accepting.

Hand and arm massage is a useful approach for getting to know a new patient or client and for nursing home and hospice volunteers to give. The hands are easily accessible, relatively safe to massage, benefit from the application of lotion, and are a familiar place of contact with other people. Having the hands touched is comforting in itself and affords the opportunity for eye contact while talking.

SELF-CARE

Working with the terminally ill and dying can be physically and emotionally challenging. It is important to practice **conscious self-care** to help maintain your own wellbeing.

The actual massage techniques used with the seriously ill or elderly tend to be simple and light and easy on the practitioner's hands. However, maintaining good body mechanics may be difficult when working with people in chairs or in bed. The general principles of good mechanics apply here also, and you need to find ways to keep your back straight and spine and neck in good alignment.

If the recipient has a communicable disease, proper precautions and hygiene should be observed. Although potentially awkward, either latex or another type of glove should be worn if necessary for protection.

Maintaining emotional wellbeing involves a variety of factors. It helps to have confronted your own issues and fears around illness and death to a point of acceptance. Conscious awareness of how you feel when you are with someone seriously ill or nearing death can help you work through those feelings later with a friend, co-worker, or supervisor.

Eventual loss is expected in working with the dying. It is natural to develop caring relationships with your patients or clients. When one of them dies, be sensitive to your own process of grieving and letting go. Ongoing professional supervision or peer counseling may be of benefit when working with this special population.

SUMMARY

Massage brings comfort and caring touch to the terminally ill and dying. Simple massage techniques can be used by health practitioners, and taught to nonprofessional caregivers, to help improve the wellbeing of those approaching the end of life. Gentle, soothing stroking and holding are the main techniques used to relieve anxiety and produce a sense of calm. Massage has benefits related to improved circulation, healthy skin, and general relaxation. Touching itself communicates caring nonverbally, and helps those suffering from depression and touch deprivation.

Hospice and palliative care programs provide compassionate care at the end of life, and typically involve a team-oriented approach. The value of massage as a palliative care method has been studied and validated in integrative medical settings.

Massage sessions with the dying are softer, gentler, and shorter than with most other populations. Practitioners use intuition and sensitivity in determining how to approach each person. Knowledge of the recipient's medical profile helps practitioners plan effective massage sessions, and provide a safe environment for both giver and receiver. Physical and emotional self-care practices help practitioners maintain their own wellbeing while working under unique circumstances, and in facing loss encountered when working with the terminally ill and dying.

A look ahead . . .

The invention of the modern massage chair has brought massage into public places like trade shows, conferences, airports, shopping malls, and street fairs. Chapter 25 takes a look at the popularity of seated massage in an environment where millions of people spend a good portion of their waking hours—at their jobs.

REFERENCES

Ellis, V., Hill, & Campbell, H. (1995) Strengthening the family unity through the healing power of massage. *Journal of Hospice & Palliative Care*, V.12, pp. 19–20.

Fanslow, C. (1984). Touch and the elderly. In *The many facets of touch*, edited by C. C. Brown. Skillman, NJ: Johnson & Johnson Baby Products Company.

Howdyshell, C. (1998). Complementary therapy: Aromatherapy with massage for geriatric and hospice care for a holistic approach. *Hospice Journal*, V.13, pp. 69–75.

Nelson, D. (1994). *Compassionate touch: Hands-on caregiving for the elderly, the ill and the dying.* New York: Station Hill Press.

Older, J. (1982). *Touching is healing.* New York: Stein & Day.

Ruebottom, A., Lee, C., & Dryden, P. J. (1989). Massage for terminally ill AIDS patients. *International Conference on AIDS*, June.

ADDITIONAL RESOURCES

Books

Nelson, Dawn (2001). *From the heart through the hands: The power of touch in caregiving.* Forres, Scotland: Findhorn Press.

Videos

"Cancer massage video." Canada Institute of Palliative Massage. Nelson, British Columbia, Canada: Sutherland Massage Productions. (*www.sutherlandmassageproductions.com*)

"AIDS massage video." Canada Institute of Palliative Massage. Nelson, British Columbia, Canada: Sutherland Massage Productions. (*www.sutherlandmassageproductions.com*)

WEB SITES

Center to Advance Palliative Care (*www.capc.org*)

National Hospice and Palliative Care Organization (*www.nhpco.org*)

National Hospice Foundation (*www.hospiceinfo.org*)

S T U D Y   G U I D E

LEARNING OUTCOMES

Use the learning outcomes at the beginning of the chapter as a guide to your studies. Perform the task given in each outcome, either in writing or verbally into a tape recorder or to a study partner. This may start as an "open book" exercise, and then later from memory.

KEY TERMS/CONCEPTS

To study key words and concepts listed at the beginning of this chapter, choose one or more of the following exercises. Writing or talking about ideas helps you remember them better, and explaining them helps deepen your understanding.

1. Write a one- or two-sentence explanation of each key word and concept.

2. Pick out two or three key words or concepts and explain how they are related.

3. With a study partner, take turns explaining key words and concepts verbally.

4. Make up sentences using one or more key words or concepts.

STUDY OUTLINE

The following questions test your memory of the main concepts in this chapter. Locate the answers in the text using the page number given for each question.

1. Massage may be used to bring caring and comforting touch to the terminally ill and dying in _____, _____, and _____ care. (p. 415)

2. Simple massage techniques may be used by health practitioners and taught to _____ caregivers to help improve the physical and _____ wellbeing of those approaching the end of life. (p. 415)

Caring Touch of Massage

1. From the _____ perspective, even those with terminal illness or nearing death continue to strive for optimal _____ in their life circumstances. (p. 415)

2. Although massage will not _____ or save someone from imminent _____, it can help improve physical function and ease some of the pain and _____ felt. (p. 415)

3. Massage can address some of the special problems of those who have been physically _____ or _____ for a long period of time. (p. 415)

4. These people often suffer from poor _____, _____, _____ and _____, difficulty _____, and skin _____. (p. 415)

5. Massage can help prevent bed _____. (p. 415)

6. Relaxing massage can help alleviate emotional distress from feelings of _____, _____, _____, _____, _____, and touch _____. (p. 415)

7. Massage can provide a sense of _____, and generate feelings of general _____. (p. 415)

Hospice and Palliative Care

1. Hospice and palliative care programs provide _____ care at the end of life, and typically involve a _____- oriented approach. (p. 415)

2. Hospice services include _____ care, _____ care, _____ services, _____ visits, _____, and _____ services. (p. 415)

3. The value of massage as a palliative care method has been studied and _____ in _____ medical settings. (p. 415)

Massage for the Dying

1. Massage can communicate caring and love in a _____ way. (p. 415)

2. TLP (Tender Loving _____) is a program in New Zealand for the dying that provides short-term _____ to ease the transition from life to death. (p. 415)

3. Therapeutic Touch has been used to help the dying experience a feeling of _____ and deep _____. (pp. 415–416)

4. Massage offered by caregivers in hospice settings provides a means of _____, even for patients unable to speak. (p. 416)

Knowledge and Skills

1. A medical profile of the terminally ill person is essential for _____ a massage session, and _____ both the recipient and the practitioner. (p. 416)

2. Specific technique is less important when working with the terminally ill than qualities such as _____ and _____. (p. 416)

3. Other useful skills include active _____, listening and _____, _____, guided _____, shared _____. (p. 416)

4. In general, massage sessions with the dying are _____, _____, and _____. (p. 416)

5. Massage sessions with the dying last about _____ minutes. (p. 416)

6. The recipient may be lying on a massage table, sitting in a regular chair or _____ chair, or lying in a _____ or _____ bed. (p. 416)

7. The key to massage for the dying is to be _____, _____, and _____. (p. 416)

Self-Care

1. Working with the terminally ill and dying calls for a strategy of _____ self-care on the part of the massage practitioner. (p. 416)

2. Practitioners should maintain good _____ while working with recipients in chairs and lying in bed. (p. 416)

3. Proper _____ should be observed when recipients have communicable diseases. (p. 417)

4. Maintaining _____ wellness when working with the dying may involve confronting your own issues about illness and dying, and discussing those feelings with a _____, _____ or _____. (p. 417)

5. Eventual _____ of your client is to be expected and ongoing professional supervision may be helpful in your own process of _____ and _____. (p. 417)

FOR GREATER UNDERSTANDING

The following exercises are designed to take you from the realm of theory into the real world. They will help give you a deeper understanding of the subjects covered in this chapter. Action words are underlined to emphasize the variety of activities presented to address different learning styles, and to encourage deeper thinking.

1. <u>Interview</u> a health professional who is working or who has worked with the terminally ill or dying. Ask them about the type of setting, and their personal challenges working in that environment. What were their patients' greatest needs? Inquire about the role of massage, if any, where they worked, and the potential benefits of massage for this special population. Discuss your findings with a study partner or group.

2. <u>Repeat Problem 1</u> with a massage therapist who is working or who has worked with the terminally ill or dying.

3. <u>Visit</u> a hospice or palliative care facility. What is the approach to providing care at the end of life? What types of services do they offer, and what types of health professionals do they employ? <u>Report</u> your findings to a study partner, and <u>compare</u> with others who also completed the assignment.

4. <u>Visit the Web sites</u> given as additional resources at the end of the chapter, and any others you find related to hospice and palliative care programs. What is the mission of the organization? Services offered? Any mention of massage? <u>Report</u> your findings to a study partner or group.

5. <u>Volunteer</u> to give massage at a hospice or in a palliative care program. <u>Take training</u> offered to orient you to the setting. <u>Keep a journal</u> of your experience.

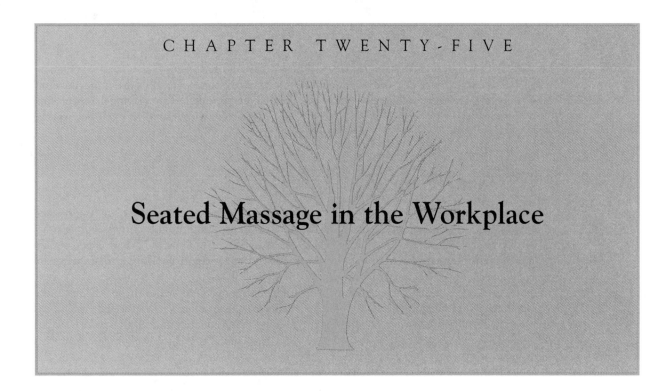

CHAPTER TWENTY-FIVE

Seated Massage in the Workplace

LEARNING OUTCOMES

After studying this chapter, the student will have the information to:

1. Trace the history of workplace massage.
2. Explain the benefits of massage in workplace wellness programs.
3. Choose and adapt techniques for seated massage.
4. Explain the popularity of workplace massage.

KEY TERMS/CONCEPTS

Ergonomics	Repetitive strain injuries (RSI)	Workplace wellness programs
Massage chair	Seated massage	
On-site massage	Worker productivity	

MEDIALINK

A companion CD-ROM, included free with each new copy of this book, supplements the techniques presented in this chapter. Insert the CD-ROM to watch video clips of massage techniques being demonstrated. This multimedia feature is designed to help you add a new dimension to your learning.

Massage is increasingly popular in **workplace wellness programs.** These employer-sponsored programs make services and activities available to employees to improve their overall health and wellbeing. Many businesses recognize the benefits of massage for their employees and are making massage available at the work site itself. Seated massage, in particular, is popular with businesses exploring ways to reduce stress on the job and to minimize job-related injuries.

HISTORY OF WORKPLACE MASSAGE

In the late 19th and early 20th centuries, massage was available at businesses such as large factories and retail stores as part of employee benefits. Industrial recreation programs provided fitness and sport activities that likely included massage. Large businesses often had on-site medical departments, including physiotherapy. Some large companies provided massage for their executives. These in-house programs largely disappeared by the mid-20th century.

In the 1980s, businesses began to rediscover the importance of employee health, and to implement programs to encourage healthy life habits. These include programs such as exercise, weight loss, smoking cessation, and stress reduction. Healthy employees are more productive and lose less work time due to illness or injury. Workplace wellness programs have been found to reduce workers' compensation claims and absenteeism.

The invention of a specially designed chair that allows people to receive massage in a seated position has had a dramatic impact on the availability of massage in offices and other work settings. The first modern **massage chair** was designed in the 1980s by David Palmer of San Francisco, CA, and promoted as the foundation for on-site massage. **On-site massage** means that the massage practitioner goes to where the potential clients are (e.g., at work, in stores, at airports, on the street), making massage more accessible. One of the first large corporations to provide on-site massage for their employees in 1985 was Apple Computer Corporation (Palmer, 1995).

The idea of the massage chair was to make receiving massage more readily available to the general public. It can be transported easily, takes up less room than a massage table, and allows recipients to receive massage sitting up and with their clothes on. Massage techniques that do not need oil, such as compression, direct pressure and kneading, are generally used for seated massage.

BENEFITS OF MASSAGE IN THE WORKPLACE

Many of the tasks performed by workers in the past are now done by sophisticated machines run by computers. However, many workers still sit at workstations for long periods of time performing repetitive tasks such as using computer keyboards, and sorting or assembly. Tradesmen, craftsmen, artists and musicians repeat certain movements over and over, stressing their bodies. Repetitive tasks can cause aching, tenderness, swelling, tingling and numbness, weakness, loss of flexibility, or spasms in the muscles affected.

Repetitive strain injuries (RSI) are common in a number of occupations. RSIs include tendinitis (inflammation of tendons), bursitis (inflammation of fluid sacs around a joint), ganglion cysts (a mass formed over a tendon), and nerve impingement.

Attention to **ergonomics** (i.e., good posture and body mechanics) in the work environment has alleviated some potentially damaging conditions. For example, computer keyboards and monitors are placed in the proper spacial relationship to the user to reduce strain, adjustable chairs that support good sitting posture are used, and phone headsets help prevent neck strain. While these practices can lessen the negative impact on employees, they do not eliminate problems altogether.

The stress level of employees is also a major wellness factor. The dizzying pace of modern times, at work and in everyday life adds to the stress of employees. A high level of chronic stress is known to have a negative effect on health. Tension headaches are common at work.

Massage can help address many of the potentially harmful conditions mentioned above, and it has also been found to increase mental clarity and alertness (Field 1993; *Massage* 1996). This can only enhance **worker productivity.** Practitioners can adapt massage sessions to address the needs of workers, and the use of massage chairs makes offering this service in the workplace convenient.

A recent study on work-site acupressure massage (WSAM) found that the group receiving the specific massage protocol enjoyed significant health benefits. The massage was a 20-minute session received twice weekly for a period of eight weeks. The recipients were fully clothed. Techniques included Western massage, acupressure and reflexology. Results showed that people receiving massage had a significant decrease in anxiety, increase in emotional control, decrease in perceived sleep disturbances, decreased blood pressure, improved cognition, and a decrease in perception of muscle tightness (Hodge et al. 2002).

A summary of the benefits of workplace massage, especially seated massage, are listed below. The list was adapted from the information brochure, *On-Site Therapeutic Massage: Investment for a Healthy Business* (Benjamin, 1994):

- Reduces the physical and mental effects of stress; thus helps prevent burnout and stress-related diseases
- Reduces the adverse effects of sitting for long periods of time in the same position, such as at a desk or other workstation
- Relieves physical problems associated with repetitive tasks such as computer keyboard use, sorting, filing, and assembly-line tasks
- Improves alertness and ability to focus, an antidote for work slumps
- Helps relieve common problem conditions such as tension headaches and stiff and sore muscles
- Improves immune system functioning for better general health and resistance to colds and other illnesses
- Employees feel revitalized and ready to return to work.

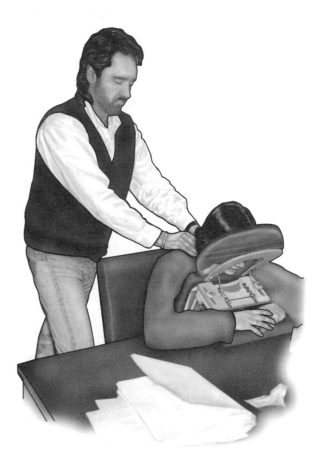

FIGURE 25–1. Portable table-top equipment that provides support for recipients receiving massage at their workstations.

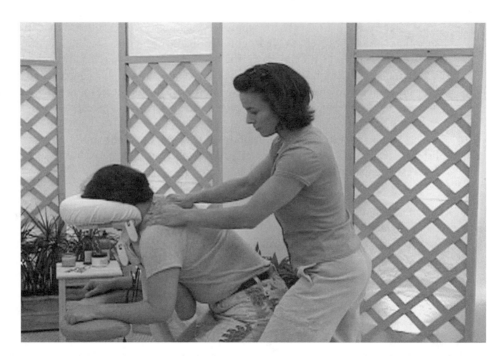

FIGURE 25–2. Kneading the shoulders during seated massage.

SEATED MASSAGE FOR OFFICE WORKERS

Seated massage is massage given to a recipient in a seated position. It may be given at a workstation, in an empty office or cubicle, or in any small space such as the corner of a conference or workroom. Seated massage sessions for office workers typically last from 15 to 20 minutes. Recipients may be seated at their workstations or may be in portable massage chairs. Figure 25–1 shows a tabletop unit that offers recipients support when receiving massage at desks.

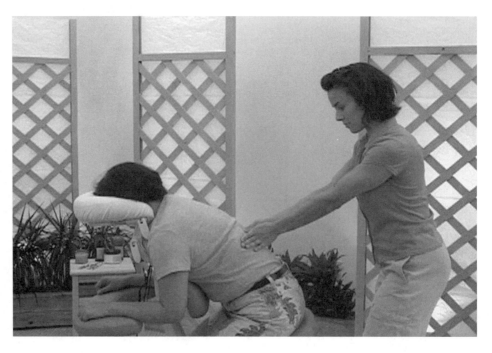

FIGURE 25–3. Direct pressure to muscles along the spine during seated massage.

The recipient is clothed, but removes his or her jacket, tie, large jewelry, or other things that might interfere with the massage. Practitioners should ask permission to work on the face if the recipient is wearing makeup, or on the scalp if massage would disturb the hair.

Seated massage sessions focus on the upper body. Areas of concern are the neck and shoulders, head and scalp, upper back, and forearms, wrists, and hands. Techniques that are effective without the use of oil are used; for example, forms of petrissage (i.e., kneading and compression), friction, tapotement, light stroking, and joint movements. Forms of energy balancing such as polarity therapy may be incorporated into a session. Shiatsu and other forms of Asian bodywork are particularly adaptable for seated massage, since they are given without lubricant and include techniques such as direct pressure, compressions, and percussion.

Seated massage includes kneading the shoulders (Figure 25–2), and direct pressure to points on either side of the spine (Figure 25–3). The upper extremities can be accessed with the arms hanging down or relaxing on the arm rest. Hand and wrist massage using the arm rest is shown in Figure 25–4.

Neck massage can be performed with the client positioned in the face cradle (Figure 25–5). Friction to the small muscles of the head and scalp is shown in Figure 25–6. A combination of kneading the neck and shoulders, pressure points along the trapezius and cervical muscles, and friction to the head and scalp can help relieve tension headache.

Light tapotement to the head as shown in Figure 25–7 is stimulating and increases alertness before getting back to work. (Refer to TouchPro Institute—www.touchpro.org —for information on chair massage training.)

POPULARITY OF WORKPLACE MASSAGE

Massage is popular with employers and employees for a number of reasons. It has immediate positive effects, since recipients usually feel better right away. It may alleviate some of the physical aches and pains developed from sitting long hours doing deskwork. In contrast to other wellness practices,

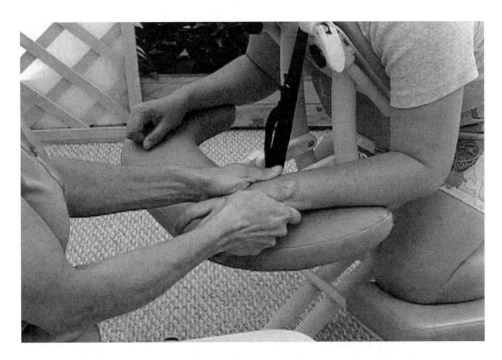

FIGURE 25–4. Hand and wrist massage with arms relaxing on the arm rest during seated massage.

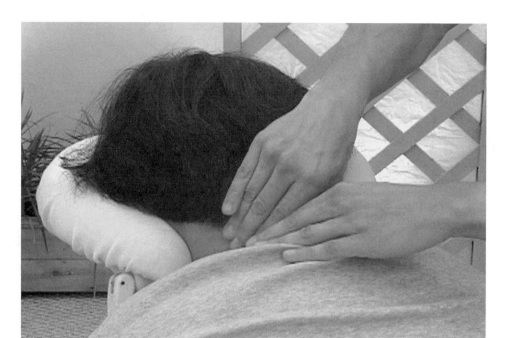

FIGURE 25–5. Neck massage with client positioned in the face cradle during seated massage.

massage requires no practice or effort on the part of the recipient. It complements other health practices such as exercise and stress-reduction programs.

Massage programs help increase good feelings about the workplace and loyalty to businesses that show caring for their employees' wellbeing. They boost productivity, and may be taken advantage of by most workers (Benjamin, 1994).

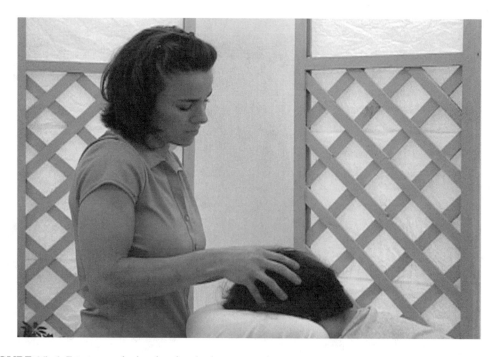

FIGURE 25–6. Friction to the head and scalp during seated massage.

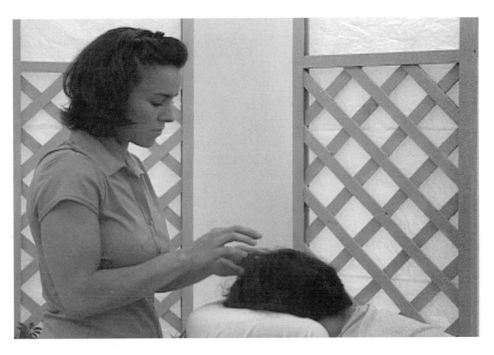

FIGURE 25–7. Light tapotement to the head to conclude seated massage session.

SUMMARY

Massage is an increasingly popular part of workplace wellness programs. Employers recognize the benefits of massage for helping workers stay healthy and productive. Massage can relieve muscular tension caused by prolonged sitting at workstations, and by repetitive tasks. It helps reduce the stresses of the work environment. Studies show that massage can increase mental clarity and alertness. It leaves workers feeling revitalized and ready to return to work.

The invention of a special massage chair in the 1980s has made massage more accessible to the workplace. With the special chair, massage can be given in small spaces to workers who are fully clothed.

In seated massage for the workplace, recipients are asked to take off their jackets, ties, jewelry, and other things that may interfere with the massage. Massage techniques that do not require oil are used, e.g., compression and kneading (petrissage), friction, tapotement, and other forms of bodywork such as amma, shiatsu, and polarity therapy. Areas massaged usually include neck and shoulders, head and scalp, upper back, forearms, wrists and hands.

Effective seated massage techniques include kneading the shoulders, direct pressure on either side of the spine, and arm and hand massage. Tension headaches are relieved by kneading the neck and shoulders, pressure to points along the trapezius and cervical muscles, and friction to the head and scalp. Light tapotement on the head is stimulating and increases alertness before getting back to work.

Seated massage is popular with both employers and employees since it has immediate positive effects, complements other heath practices, increases good feelings about the workplace, and improves worker productivity.

REFERENCES

No author (1996). Massage helps lower stress of working, taking final exams. In *Massage, 62* (July/August), p. 148.

Benjamin, P. J. (1994). *On-site therapeutic massage: Investment for a healthy business.* Information brochure. Rockford, IL: Hemingway Publications.

Field, T. M., Fox, N., Pickens, J., Ironsong, G., & Scafidi, F. (1993). Job stress survey. Unpublished manuscript, Touch Research Institute, University of Miami School of Medicine. Reported in *Touchpoints: Touch Research Abstracts, 1*(1).

Hodge, M., Robinson, C., Boehmer, J., & Klein, S. (2002). "Employee outcomes following work-site acupressure and massage." Chapter 9 in *Massage therapy: The evidence for practice*. New York: Mosby.

Palmer, D. (1995). The death of on-site massage? *Massage Therapy Journal, 34*(3), pp. 119–120.

WEBSITE

TouchPro Institute (*www.touchpro.org*)

ADDITIONAL RESOURCES

Videos

"Chair Massage with Connie Scholl." Riverside, CT: At Peace Media. (*www.atpeacemedia.com*)

"Japanese Chair Massage Video." (2002) By Shogo Mochizuki. Boulder, CO: Kotobuki Publications.

S T U D Y   G U I D E

LEARNING OUTCOMES

Use the learning outcomes at the beginning of the chapter as a guide to your studies. Perform the task given in each outcome, either in writing or verbally into a tape recorder or to a study partner. This may start as an "open book" exercise, and then later from memory.

KEY TERMS/CONCEPTS

To study key words and concepts listed at the beginning of this chapter, choose one or more of the following exercises. Writing or talking about ideas helps you remember them better, and explaining them helps deepen your understanding.

1. Write a one- or two-sentence explanation of each key word and concept.

2. Pick out two or three key words or concepts and explain how they are related.

3. With a study partner, take turns explaining key words and concepts verbally.

4. Make up sentences using one or more key words or concepts.

STUDY OUTLINE

The following questions test your memory of the main concepts in this chapter. Locate the answers in the text using the page number given for each question.

1. Massage is an increasingly popular workplace _____ offering. (p. 422)

2. Seated massage is popular with businesses exploring ways to reduce _____ on the job, and to minimize job-related _____. (p. 422)

History of Workplace Massage

1. In the late 19th and early 20th centuries, massage and physiotherapy were offered by many businesses as part of their employee _____. These in-house wellness programs largely _____ by mid-20th century. (p. 422)

2. Workplace wellness programs were revived in _____ as an offshoot of the larger _____ movement. (p. 422)

3. The invention of the _____ in the 1980s by David Palmer made massage at the workplace more convenient. (p. 422)

4. The term _____ massage was coined to describe offering massage in massage chairs in public places like parks, stores, and the workplace. (p. 422)

5. Massage chairs can be easily _____, use less _____ than a massage table, and allow people to receive massage in a seated position with their _____ on. (p. 422)

Benefits of Massage in the Workplace

1. Massage in the workplace may help minimize _____ injuries (RSI), and reduces _____ among employees. (p. 422)

2. Massage has been found to increase _____ clarity and _____ that can only enhance worker productivity. (p. 422)

3. Massage can help reduce the adverse effects of _____ for long periods of time. (p. 423)

4. Massage can address problems such as _____ headaches and _____ and _____ muscles. (p. 423)

5. Massage improves _____ function for more healthy employees. (p. 423)

6. Massage leaves employees feeling _____ and ready for _____. (p. 423)

Seated Massage for Office Workers

1. Seated massage in the workplace typically lasts _____ minutes. (p. 424)

2. Sessions mainly focus on the _____ body. (p. 425)

3. Techniques that work well without _____ are emphasized. (p. 425)

4. Seated massage techniques include _____, _____, _____, _____, light _____, and _____ movements. (p. 425)

5. Shiatsu and other forms of _____ bodywork are particularly adaptable for seated massage. (p. 425)

6. A technique combination to alleviate tension headache includes _____ of the neck and shoulders, _____ on either side of the spine, and _____ of the head and scalp. (p. 425)

Popularity of Workplace Massage

1. Workplace massage is popular because it has immediate _____ effects, addresses aches and pains related to _____, requires no _____ on the part of the recipient, and complements other health practices like _____ reduction. (p. 425)

2. Workplace massage promotes loyalty, and boosts _____. (p. 426)

FOR GREATER UNDERSTANDING

The following exercises are designed to take you from the realm of theory into the real world. They will help give you a deeper understanding of the subjects covered in this chapter. Action words are underlined to emphasize the variety of activities presented to address different learning styles, and to encourage deeper thinking.

1. Interview a massage practitioner who specializes in seated massage. Ask them about the goals of their sessions, the approach and techniques used, and what type of clients they have. How do they market their practices? Report your findings to a study partner or group.

2. Receive a seated massage offered in a public place like a shopping mall, airport, or street fair. How did the practitioner prepare you for the session? Adjust the chair? What techniques were used? How long did it last? How did you feel afterwards? Report your experience to a study partner or group.

3. Interview someone who receives massage at their workplace. Ask them to describe the seated massage sessions. What benefits do they experience personally? Report your findings to a study partner or group.

4. Observe workplace seated massage sessions. Notice the physical space and environment for massage. Watch how the practitioner greets and prepares the recipient for seated massage. Observe the body mechanics and techniques used. Observe how the recipients respond during and after the session. Report your observations to a study partner or group.

5. Take a training in seated massage. Note the differences in body mechanics and techniques used compared to regular table massage.

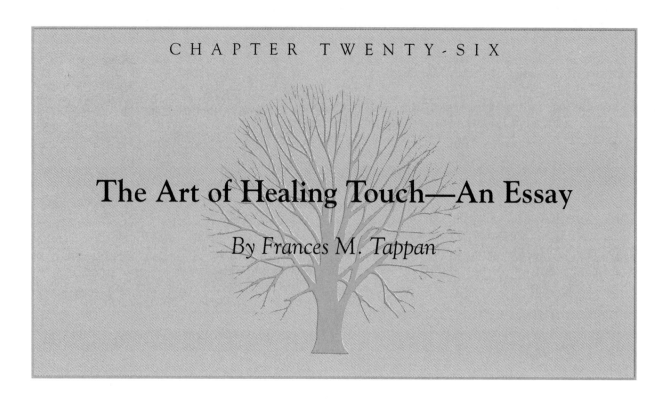

CHAPTER TWENTY-SIX

The Art of Healing Touch—An Essay

By Frances M. Tappan

The following essay written by Frances M. Tappan in the 1980s summarizes her philosophy of the power of touch, and of massage as a healing art. She offers her insights into the human experience of health and disease, and the importance of relationships with patients and clients.

The art of healing touch is a two-way street. A massage that includes the client or patient as a partner will be remarkably more effective than one given as a mere technique of body manipulation. The practitioner who devotes total attention by communicating concern, empathy, and a sincere desire to promote the healing process will spur the receiver of massage to participate more fully in the effort toward regaining health.

The objective of both the practitioner and the recipient is to replace the recipient's dependency with a collaborative effort. To establish this relationship, the client or patient must participate in discussions that include an exchange of ideas, rather than simply receive instructions given by the practitioner. Such an approach will strengthen positive attitudes and minimize feelings of despair.

A pleasant atmosphere, the exchange of laughter, a sense of strength or determination, and feelings of love will strongly encourage the human body toward its own constant search for homeostasis. The body itself will then produce more complicated and comprehensive chemotherapy than is available at any medical center in the world—be it via Eastern or Western medical approaches.

While giving massage, one can encourage the receiver to understand the potential source of healing in his or her own consciousness. The recipient can be encouraged not to be helpless, passive, depressed, or desperate, but rather capable and active in his or her own treatments. According to Bernie Siegel, "The body heals, not the therapy . . . the body can utilize any form of energy for healing . . . even plain water—as long as the patient believes in it" (1986a, p. 129). Everyone wants to love and be loved. Skillful encouragement can stimulate the human body's defense and healing mechanisms.

Current research done with plants, animals, and human beings is proving that positive effects are possible through the "laying-on of hands." In an experiment conducted in 1964, Bernard Grad used barley seeds that had been soaked in saline to simulate a "sick" condition. Oskar Estebany worked with Grad as a "healer" and held flasks of water as he would were he doing laying-on of hands. An identical saline flask of barley seeds was not treated by the laying-on of hands. The seeds held by Estebany sprouted more quickly, grew taller, and contained more chlorophyll (Grad et al. 1964).

In the book *The Secret Life of Plants* (1973), Peter Tompkins and Christopher Bird recorded how Cleve Backster proved without doubt that plants respond if touched with affection. By using lie detector equipment he confirmed Grad's studies that plants respond to loving care and soft music in a positive way. Conversely, they respond negatively to hard rock music and feelings of hate.

Backster conceived a threat that he would burn an actual leaf of a dracaena plant to which his lie machine galvanometer was attached. The instant he got the picture of a flame in his mind, and before he could move for a match, there was a dramatic change in the tracing pattern on the graph in the form of a prolonged upward sweep of the recording pen. Backster had not moved either toward the plant or toward the recording machine. Could the plant have been reading his mind?

There is a lamp on the market, the base of which holds potted plants. When a leaf is touched, a light bulb will go on. A three-way light bulb will cycle through low, medium, and high to off, each time a leaf is touched. During demonstrations, the light refused to go on, although the pot had been recently watered. After several people had tried to transfer enough energy to light the bulb and had failed, the demonstrator suggested that the plant must be thirsty and requested a glass of water that was handed to her in a paper cup. Before the plant had even been touched (in fact, the cup of water was at least four inches from the plant), the lamp light turned on. The demonstrator pulled her hand back and the light went off, again before being touched at all. This plant was considered further proof of Backster's theory that plants respond to human thought or mental intent.

In Eastern cultures the transference of attitudes between the healer and the subject is believed to occur via a state of matter for which Western culture has neither a word nor a concept. It is called *prana* in Sanskrit. The nearest translation in English is vitality or vigor. The Chinese call it *chi*, which translates as energy. Regardless of what it is called, however, this phenomenon refers to the balanced functioning of the human body and the vital life force of energy, which keeps people in good physiologic and psychologic health. Think of the world as having a "collective consciousness" and join the "self" to that strength. Lessen thoughts of yourself as "only one."

Advocates of this concept believe that positive energy can be transferred from the healer to the patient through touch (via any medical approach—pulse reading, acupuncture, or more modern medical methods) to return the patient to normal health. They also believe that it is absolutely necessary for the patient to have faith in the healer and to possess a strong will to get well. In an article called *Love Medicine* (1986b), Siegel tells of a woman in the hospital who visualized her X-ray therapy as a "golden beam of sunshine entering her body." He also believes that people set up defenses against sharing their innermost feelings with anyone. If they feel their ability to love shriveling up, they create a vicious cycle that leads to further despair. Anger can really be a cry for help.

Massage and other therapies that are performed with the practitioner's hands are some of the best ways to transfer the strong healing energy from the giver to the receiver. In a controlled study, Kreiger (1976) proved that Therapeutic Touch, or the laying-on of hands, is a uniquely effective human act of healing. Her results showed significant measurable changes in hemoglobin values of patients after receiving Therapeutic Touch. By touching with the intent to help or heal, the patient would feel that heat within the area beneath the hand. Recipients reported feeling profoundly relaxed and having a sense of wellbeing.

In *Anatomy of an Illness as Perceived by the Patient* (1979), Norman Cousins records how he became, with his doctor, William Hitzig, a participant in the accomplishment of his own recovery. Together they proved that a cheerful atmosphere and an open-minded exchange of ideas related to recovery actually reduced the high sedimentation rate causing his illness. He achieved an almost complete recovery and returned to functional health.

Such attitudes do not develop without concentrated effort on the part of the healer and the one desiring to be healed. All patients are individuals with problems, physical problems that create mental attitudes that may vary all the way from complete rejection of treatment to complete cooperation. Before treating a patient, explain what the treatment will accomplish. Always try to find out what the patient is thinking and feeling by listening more than talking. Work with the patient. Inspire the patient's confidence with a positive attitude that implies that your knowledge and skill are available. This also means that the healer cannot afford to display any personal, negative feelings regardless of anger or rudeness on the part of the patient. A healer's firm, controlled strength of character can guide the patient toward acceptance and belief that the treatment is beneficial.

Sick people become dependent on others in many cases. The health practitioner should strive to replace patient dependency with self-sufficiency; identify important life goals; and eliminate the patient's feelings of despair and loneliness. This can be done by exchanging ideas and sharing knowledge.

Fear can be depressing, if not deadly, so everything possible should be done to strengthen positive attitudes. The atmosphere should always be pleasant. Direct sunlight from windows with a pleasant view is helpful. Tropical fish tanks and tranquil music help the surroundings to be peaceful and interesting. Harmonious relationships should be encouraged.

Illness often follows a crisis that creates a sense of hopelessness and despair. Some theories suggest that each person is ultimately responsible for both illness and the recovery. People from all aspects of health care can help each body in their own special way, but no body is going to heal unless the body itself decides to heal.

The therapist can be most effective by taking careful note of the whole patient at the first moment of contact. Body language can speak louder than words. You can determine how a person feels by the look in her eyes, the way he holds his head, the slump of her shoulders, his tone of voice, or even by noting whether he or she seems to feel happy or depressed.

Above all, the therapist needs to convince the patient that the treatment being given is going to bring relief from pain and recovery from depression. Each patient needs loving support, understanding, a purpose for living, and some sense of satisfaction related to the efforts put forth on his or her behalf.

If massage is to be "healing," both the giver and the receiver will be comfortable with the idea that shared energy and unconditional love provide strong motivation toward healing. Look for the love and light in people. This exchange of healing energy comes in many forms other than massage. It can occur through group concerns with people who share similar problems. People can interact negatively or positively. Never forget, "four hugs a day keep the blues away." People can accept or reject, even subconsciously, the positive energy being extended in their surrounding external environment.

Health practitioners who use touch in their work are in a particularly advantageous position to transfer healing energy by the way in which art, skill, and knowledge are shown during treatment. Each person being treated should be understood by the practitioner as much as possible, relative to the importance of feeling relaxed and at peace, to encourage the caring, loving energy of healing.

There was the case of a dying cancer patient who said to her therapist, "I wish someone would talk to me more about dying! My doctor always changes the subject and my own family refuses to talk about it." The therapist giving massage answered, "You can say anything you want to me." For the remainder of the session they discussed death and the patient's basic beliefs in positive terms.

One person can be terrified under stressful situations, and die of a heart attack. Another person can face the same situation with no terror at all. Those people who are often terrified or angry about situations that occur are less likely to respond to the extension of healing energy.

If you ask seriously ill patients if they would like to live, may of them will say, "No." Nevertheless, ask the same seriously ill people if they would like to live and feel physically well and active, and most of them will say, "Yes!" Do not make the mistake of assuming that all seriously ill people really want to die. An understanding of death at any age is a must for all practitioners, because so many dying people truly need the loving touch of massage.

The human body and mind are *one*. All health practitioners should be aware of their own individual status and know whether they are balanced enough to enhance the healing energy they hope to deliver. They should know how to "center" their own energy toward the wellbeing of their patients.

In class or group sessions, "energy breaks" may be used to keep the positive energy flowing. One technique is to interrupt the presentation and interject without introduction, "Reach out and touch someone." Responses in the group will vary from those who refuse to touch or to be touched, to those who are not satisfied merely to touch but go beyond, even to a hug. It may take several such breaks in a large group before each member trusts the others enough to transfer any healing energy. These breaks can "sneak in" when people learn to trust, and they may be varied as follows:

- Reach out and touch someone.
- Now reach out, touch someone with a warm, caring touch.
- Find a sensitive, painful spot and touch it gently, projecting healing thoughts, and with warmth.
- Massage the tension away from a painful area.

After asking them to "reach out and touch someone," ask each person to make a fist. Tell the person immediately nearby to open the fist. Reaction will range from those who voluntarily open their own fists to those who strongly resist having anyone try to force their fists open. What does this tell us? People are all different, depending on their internal environment and in how they respond to external stimulation.

The author has witnessed a wide range of reactions. Actually, if one is attempting to get a group of strangers into a peaceful state of mind, it is the responsibility of the leader to use instinct, observation, conversation, and careful notation of the peoples' acceptance or resistance to the idea. From that information the leader may attempt to establish a positive relationship for maximum healing results.

Those in the healing professions should realize that what they see and feel about "what's going on" is not necessarily so. All of us "perform" constantly. For example, when asked, "How do you feel today?" the typical answer is "Fine!" Actually, that person may have a splitting headache or the flu, but is not willing to discuss it at the present time or with that particular person.

The health practitioner needs to find out how a patient really feels most of the time. Loving, caring people do not always find support in their daily family or working routine. People may feel negative, or they may think, "Just do the job! Get it done!" If so, the practitioner will find it difficult to evoke relaxation in that person.

Many a busy executive enjoys a "quick fix" massage. This could help reduce stress; it might even relax an exhausted person right into a peaceful snooze. A good practitioner will realize whether a "quick fix" is enough and advise accordingly.

Many organizations are now hiring massage practitioners to provide "quick fix massage" twice a week at the workplace. This procedure is too new to evaluate its permanent value toward enhanced well-being and productivity. If it contributes to employees' feeling content with and good about themselves and their work benefits, it may revolutionize the profession of massage.

All levels of the desire or need to be touched exist in a normal population. Some folks are just born to love, to be touched, hugged, held, and appreciated. If they get this in living surroundings, they are peaceful people. Others are born, or learn, to reject close contacts. They prefer a more reserved approach to touch. If a massage practitioner who understands these differences can help such people to be less inward oriented and become more outgoing, then massage as a "stress buster" may have positive, even healing, effects.

Anyone could die from a heart attack when not even under stress. However, if one truly has (not pretends to have) a peaceful inner life, chances are better for a strong immune system, and much greater health and healing is possible. Belief systems are powerful enough to cure or kill, often with dramatic effects.

Those people who stop and ask, "Would I choose to live with myself as I am right now?" and answer "Yes" usually have a super immune system that works to keep the body in balance, and these people are the easiest to relax with massage techniques. One should ask of oneself, "If I had only a year to live, what would I do?" A peaceful soul would reply, "Maximize good living without compulsive goals or impossible dreams. Adjust as peacefully as possible to all of life's ups and downs."

If these are not the answers, people could try to change their basic living style toward that goal. Not everyone can do this, and some who do may find it takes more energy than expected. Then the work of the giving of unconditional love to others becomes more readily received. This is the challenge of change. It is said that nothing is sure but death and taxes. Yet there is one more thing we can be sure of, and that is change. Change can be hard to deal with. A person may want to change his or her inner being. That is not, however, as easy as deciding to do so. Everyone looks at his or her own environment and reacts to it depending on his or her DNA (inherited genes). From birth—or even while in fetal development—change that shapes and forms character begins to occur. There are those who feel that one cannot change life patterns. Asking the question "What is your purpose in life?" could start one on the road to positive thinking. An evaluation of one's total belief system could be the beginning of change, and striving to be at peace with yourself could improve one's immune system. Massage practitioners must ask themselves all these questions before they will be able to transfer healing energy to others.

It is, therefore, not how a person perceives the immediate environment, but what this means to the inner environment that strengthens or weakens the immune system. Some people may react to others' actions with anger, then hide that emotion and smile outwardly. Another one may yell and scream over a similar action. In the long run, the inner selves who cannot cope are the ones who deplete the strength of their immune system and eventually kill themselves, because no other course of action seems available. In short, it is not the environment outside the self that is deadly. Rather, it is the way the inner self feels in relation to the outside environment that can be damaging.

Someone once said that people can be divided into three groups: Those who make things happen, those who watch things happen, and those who wonder what happened! It is the practitioner's responsibility to encourage the patient to do all in his or her power to "make things happen."

SUMMARY

The art of healing touch through massage is a two-way street that includes the patient and the therapist as partners. The source of healing is in the patient's own being, which is enhanced by the intention, positive energy, and laying-on of hands of the massage practitioner. A healing environment includes external factors such as lighting and sound, as well as the support, understanding, and unconditional love of the therapist.

Stress and anxiety are the source of many of today's ills. The massage practitioner needs to listen to their patients and clients to understand the whole person and the source of their distress. Massage helps to create inner peace, which strengthens the immune system and leads to greater health and healing. It is ultimately the patient's responsibility to change their lives in ways that promote good health. It is the practitioner's responsibility to encourage the patient to do all in his or her power to ensure their own wellbeing.

REFERENCES

Cousins, N. (1979). *Anatomy of an illness as perceived by the patient: Reflections on healing and regeneration.* New York: Norton.

Grad, B. et al. (1964). A telekinetic effort on plant growth, part 2. Experiments involving treatment with saline in stoppered bottles. *International Journal of Parapsychology,* 6, p. 473.

Krieger, D. (1976). Nursing research for a new age. *Nursing Times,* 72 (April), p. 1.

Siegel, B. S. (1986a). *Love, medicine & miracles.* New York: Harper & Row.

Siegel, B. S. (1986b). Love medicine. *New Age Journal,* 50 (April), p. 512.

Tompkins, P., & Bird, C. (1973). *The secret life of plants.* New York: Avon.

STUDY GUIDE

This essay by Frances M. Tappan outlines her views on the art of healing touch through massage. Read the essay again highlighting specific sentences that seem to summarize important points she is trying to make. Make a list of these key sentences and discuss her overall philosophy with a study partner or group.

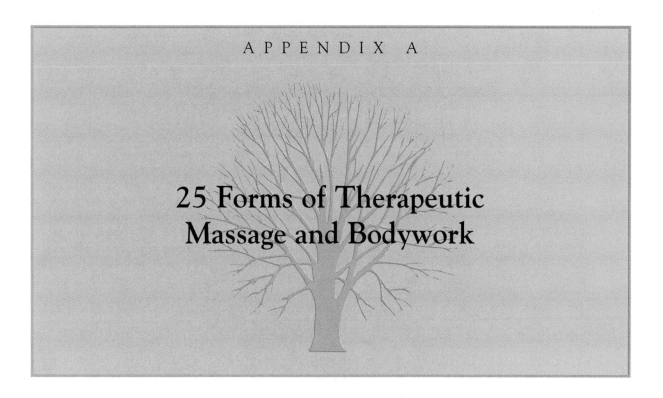

APPENDIX A

25 Forms of Therapeutic Massage and Bodywork

The therapeutic massage and bodywork forms described below are some of the major systems practiced today. Descriptions include a summary of their origins and history, techniques and applications, the theory on which they are based, and some resources for further information. Noncommercial Web sites are listed when available, and books for forms that do not have relevant Web sites (e.g., Ayurvedic massage) are also cited. Readers are encouraged to check the Internet for Web sites appearing after publication of this text.

Many of the forms of massage and bodywork listed are root systems from which other forms or spin-offs have been derived. Because the field of massage therapy is an emerging profession with a large entrepreneurial component, there are several trademarked forms, e.g., Rolfing®. Spin-offs of originals may also be trademarked, or there may be generic spin-offs without trademarks.

For further explanations of these and other forms of massage and bodywork see *Discovering the Body's Wisdom* by Mirka Knaster (New York: Bantam Books, 1996).

1. Alexander Technique

   Origin: Alexander Technique was developed by an Australian named Frederick Matthias Alexander (1869–1955), who practiced in London in the early 1900s. Alexander, a Shakespearean actor, cured himself of loss of voice through correction of faulty posture in the head and neck. He later worked with other actors and public speakers using the same method to improve their vocal abilities.

   Technique: Alexander Technique is a form of contemporary bodywork in which a teacher guides the student through various movements like sitting, walking, and bending. The emphasis is on achieving balance in the head-neck relationship, called Primary Control. Poor habitual patterns are replaced by light, easy, simple, and integrated movement.

   Theory: Proper body alignment and movement patterns are achieved by heightened kinesthetic awareness, and conscious movement.

   Web Sites: Alexander Technique (www.alexandertechnique.com)
   Alexander Technique International (www.ati-net.com)
   American Society for the Alexander Technique (www.alexandertech.org)

2. Aromatherapy Massage

   Origin: The use of natural plant essences for health and therapeutic effects is ancient. The modern term "aromatherapie" was coined by a French chemist named Rene Maurice Gattefosse (1881–1950) as he studied the use of fragrant oils for their healing properties in the 1920–1930s. Later, Madame Marguerite Maury (1895–1968) started prescribing essential oils for her patients, and is credited with the modern use of essential oils for massage. She wrote an important aromatherapy guide in French in 1961 that was translated into English in 1964.

Technique: Aromatherapy massage involves the use of essential oils in massage oil blends for their therapeutic effects. Techniques of Western massage, Ayurvedic massage, and other systems of soft tissue manipulation may be used in the application of aromatherapy massage oils.

Theory: Essential oils are highly concentrated aromatic extracts that are cold-pressed or steam distilled from plants such as grasses, leaves, flowers, fruit peels, wood, and roots. Each essential oil has a specific therapeutic effect such as relaxing, boosting immune system, relieving congestion, or soothing muscular aches and pains. Common massage blends contain essential oils such as peppermint, lavender, citrus, tea tree, and rosemary.

Web Site: National Association for Holistic Aromatherapy (www.naha.org)

3. Ayurvedic Massage

Origin: Ayurvedic massage is one of the healing practices of ancient India. Vedic scriptures of India dating back to 3000 BCE describe healing practices including massage with oil.

Technique: Ayurvedic massage techniques include rubbing, kneading, squeezing, tapping, and pulling or shaking the body. Emphasis is given to massage of the head and feet. Sessions are invigorating and the recipient changes position several times. Pressure is applied to *marmas*, or pressure points on the body.

Theory: Ayurvedic massage is based in traditional Ayurvedic medicine of India. Massage is thought to remove obstructions to the flow of *vayu* (wind) through *siras* or wind-carrying vessels to reduce pain, relieve tension, and encourage more natural breathing patterns. Massage oils are chosen according to body type, the atmosphere and the season.

Reference: *Ayurvedic Massage: Traditional Indian Techniques for Balancing Body and Mind* by Harish Johari (Rochester, VT: Healing Arts Press, 1996).

4. Clinical Massage Therapy

See Medical Massage

5. Craniosacral Therapy (CST)

Origin: Craniosacral therapy stems from the work of an osteopath named Dr. William Garner Sutherland (1873–1954) in the early 1900s. Dr. Sutherland developed the basic theory of CST, including cranial suture movement, rhythmic motion of cerebrospinal fluid (i.e., Breath of Life), and the relationship between craniosacral rhythm and health. John E. Upledger, D.O., has continued development of this work, and added the concept of SomatoEmotional Release (SER) of negative emotions stored in traumatized tissues. The Upledger Foundation was established in 1987 to study CST.

Technique: Craniosacral therapy is a form of contemporary bodywork that uses gentle compression to realign the skull bones and stretch related membranes to balance the craniosacral rhythm (CSR), and improve function of the nervous system.

Theory: CST is based in Western anatomy and physiology, and osteopathic science. The craniosacral system (i.e., cranium, spine, and sacrum) is connected by a fascial membrane called the dura mater that houses the brain and central nervous system. Cerebralspinal fluid is pumped throughout the system, creating a pulse or craniosacral rhythm (CSR). CST techniques aim to balance the CSR so that cerebralspinal fluid flows freely through the system. Once this is achieved, the body's own healing mechanism can function properly.

Web Sites: The Upledger Institute (www.upledger.com)

Craniosacral Therapy Association of North America (www.craniosacraltherapy.org)

6. Esalen Massage

Origin: Esalen massage was developed at the Esalen Institute in Big Sur, California in the 1970s. Its development grew out of the Human Potential Movement and counterculture of the 1960s. Esalen massage was popularized in the classic *The Massage Book* by George Downing, published in 1972.

Technique: Esalen massage is a form of Western massage loosely based in Swedish massage. It emphasizes the sensual qualities of massage, and is associated with scented oils, incense, and New Age music. It initially was performed without draping, but accepted draping standards are now observed in most settings.

Theory: Esalen massage is applied to help the recipient get in touch with their senses, and their inner self, and is considered a meditative and personal growth experience. General health benefits of Swedish massage apply to Esalen massage.

Reference: *The Massage Book* by George Downing (New York: Random House Trade Paperbacks, 1998) (1st edition, 1972).

Web Site: Esalen Institute (www.esalen.org)

7. Feldenkrais Method®

Origin: The Feldenkrais Method was developed by Moshe Feldenkrais (1904–1984), who was an engineer, physicist, judo master, and mathematician. In efforts to heal himself of a knee injury, Feldenkrais developed a system of movement re-education. The Feldenkrais Method came to light during the human potential movement of the 1970–1980s.

Technique: Feldenkrais Method is a form of contemporary bodywork consisting of Functional Integration, i.e., hands-on table work in which the practitioner uses her hands to communicate new sensory movement patterns to the recipient through passive movements. In Awareness Through Movement, a teacher leads a group through structured movement experiences performed on the floor.

Theory: Feldenkrais Method is based in Western anatomy and physiology. Integrated movement patterns are established by re-educating the sensory-motor nervous system through repeated movements.

Web Sites: Feldenkrais Guild® of North America (www.feldenkrais. com) International Feldenkrais Federation (www.feldenkrais-method.org)

8. Infant Massage

Origin: Massage has been given to infants from time immemorial by their mothers, grandmothers and other caregivers. Instances of infant massage are found among native tribes in Africa, South Sea Islands, and North America, in ancient and modern India, and folk cultures of Europe. Recent interest in infant massage was revived by Vimala Schneider in the 1980s, and by the research of Dr. Tiffany Fields at the University of Miami in the 1990s.

Technique: Infant massage is a specialty within Western massage and consists of simple techniques like stroking, kneading, twisting, and pressing performed with gentle pressure. Some passive joint movements are incorporated. Eye contact and communication with the infant are emphasized.

Theory: Infant massage is based in Western anatomy, physiology, and theories of child development. It aims to help the infant relax, improve circulation and other body functions, improve immune function, and promote neurological development. Research confirms the necessity of touch and movement for healthy human development, and the benefits of massage for premature infants.

Reference: *Infant Massage: A Handbook for Loving Parents* by Vimala Schneider McClure, revised edition (New York: Bantam Doubleday Dell, 2000).

Web Sites: International Institute of Infant Massage (www.infantmassageinstitute.com) Loving Touch Foundation (www.lovingtouch.com) infant massage Touch Research Institute (www.miami.edu/touch-research)

9. Lomi-Lomi

Origin: Lomi-lomi is a traditional massage of the natives of the Hawaiian Islands practiced from time immemorial. Different styles of lomi-lomi were developed within families. Typically a tutu, i.e., grandmother, or other respected family member was the keeper of the tradition. Its modern form was popularized by Aunty Margaret Machado of Kona, Hawaii in the 1970–1980s.

Technique: Lomi-lomi is a form of traditional native massage consisting of pressing and squeezing techniques performed with the fingers, palm and elbow. Kukui nut, macadamia, or coconut oil may be used. The recipient lies on a mat, or in modern times, a massage table to receive lomi-lomi. Associated methods include baths, bone adjusting techniques, and prayer.

Theory: Lomi-lomi is based in traditional Hawaiian culture, and emphasizes letting go of stress, unconditional love, and opening the heart to harmony, acceptance, and healing.

Reference: *Hawaiian Lomi-Lomi: Big Island Massage* by Nancy S. Kahalewai (Hilo, HI: Island Massage Publishing, 2000).

Web Site: Aunty Margaret Homepage (www.hawaiian.net/~kea/aunty.html)

10. Lymphatic Drainage Massage

Origin: Manual techniques applied to enhance lymphatic system function and treat lymphedema were developed as early as the 1880s. Emil and Astid Vodder developed their Manual Lymph Drainage (MLD), or Vodder Method, in the 1930s in France. In the 1970s, Hungarians Michael and Ethel Foldi combined Vodder's MLD with other modalities to create a treatment for lymphedema called Complete Decongestive Therapy (CDT).

Technique: Lymphatic drainage massage is a specialized form of Western massage consisting of gentle techniques applied to the superficial skin layers to stretch the tissue and open the superficial lymphatic vessels so that lymph fluid can enter the vessels more easily. Classic Vodder techniques include stationary circles, scoop, pump, rotary, and light effleurage applied rhythmically and in specific directions.

Theory: Lymphatic drainage massage is based on Western anatomy and physiology, and knowledge of the lymphatic system. Techniques are applied in such a way to enhance the movement of lymph fluid into superficial vessels and through the system. Lymphatic drainage massage improves immune function, reduces areas of edema, and aids injury healing.

Web Sites: Academy of Lymphatic Studies (www.acols.com)

Dr. Vodder School North America (www.vodderschool.com)

11. Medical Massage

Origin: Massage has been used to treat ailments from time immemorial all over the globe. Historically in Western medicine, it has been called medical rubbing, frictions, massage, massotherapeutics, and physiotherapy. Medical massage is emerging in the 21st century as a specialty within the broader field of therapeutic massage and bodywork. It is sometimes called *clinical massage*.

Technique: Medical massage is a specialty of Western massage in which soft tissue manipulation and related techniques are used in the treatment of pathological conditions. A subspecialty is the treatment of musculoskeletal dysfunction.

Theory: Medical massage is based in Western anatomy, physiology, kinesiology, and pathology. Traditional and contemporary massage techniques are used as appropriate in treatment plans.

References: *Basic Clinical Massage Therapy: Integrating Anatomy and Treatment* by James H. Clay and David M. Pounds (Philadelphia: Lippincott Williams & Wilkins, 2003) (Treating Musculoskeletal Dysfunction).

Clinical Massage Therapy: Understanding, Assessing and Treating over 70 Conditions by Fiona Rattray and Linda Ludwig (Toronto, Canada: Talus Incorporated, 2000).

Massage for Orthopedic Conditions by Thomas Hendrickson (Philadelphia: Lippincott Williams & Wilkins, 2003).

Medical Massage by Ross Turchaninov and Connie Cox (Scottsdale, AZ: Stress Less Publishing, 1998).

12. Myofascial Massage

Origin: Manual techniques that target the myofascial tissues were developed in the 1950s by Ida Rolf (1896–1979) in her system of Rolfing®, and by osteopath Robert Ward as myofascial release technique in the 1960s. Since then several systems of bodywork that treat myofascial tissues have been developed.

Technique: Myofascial massage techniques apply traction to the skin and underlying tissues to slowly and gently push, pull, and stretch fascial tissues and break fascial adhesions. They are applied without oil so that restrictions can be palpated and techniques applied without slipping.

Theory: Myofascial massage is based in Western anatomy and physiology. It focuses on connective or myofascial tissues that surround muscles, nerves, blood vessels, and all organs of the body. Restrictions in fascial tissues can cause a variety of dysfunctions, including limited mobility, postural distortion, poor cellular nutrition, and pain. Myofascial massage produces a softening of tissues and freeing of fascial restrictions.

Reference: *The Myofascial Release Manual*, 3rd edition, by Carol J. Manheim (Thorofare, NJ: Slack, Inc., 2001)

13. Neuromuscular Therapy (NMT)

Origin: A precursor to today's NMT was developed by a natural healer named Stanley Lief in the 1920s. Trigger Point Therapy was brought to public attention through the work of Janet Travell, MD (1901–1997), an expert in myofascial pain, and her treatment of Presidents Kennedy and Johnson in the 1960s. Fitness expert Bonnie Prudden developed a popular system of NMT called Myotherapy® in the 1970s.

Technique: Neuromuscular Therapy is a form of contemporary Western massage in which trigger points, i.e., hyperirritable taut bands in the myofascial tissues, are located and deactivated using ischematic compression. Pressure is applied to trigger points for about 30 seconds using the thumb, fingers, or small hand tool. A stretch of the affected muscle follows application of pressure on trigger points.

Theory: A trigger point is a taut band or irritable spot in myofascial tissue that causes muscle pain at the trigger point and in its referral zones. It also causes muscle shortening, and decreased strength. Under a microscope, trigger points appear to be bands of contracted muscle tissue.

References: Travell, J. G., & Simons, D. G. (1999). *Myofascial pain and dysfunction: The trigger point manual, Volume 1—Upper half of the body*, 2nd editon. Baltimore: Williams & Wilkins.

Travell, J. G., & Simons, D. G. (1992). *Myofascial pain and dysfunction: The trigger point manual, Volume 2—The lower extremities*. Baltimore: Williams & Wilkins.

Web Site: Bonnie Prudden Myotherapy (www.bonnieprudden.com)

14. Polarity Therapy

Origin: Polarity Therapy was developed by Randolph Stone (1890–1981) in the 1930–1950s. Stone combined Western knowledge with theories from Chinese and Ayurvedic medicine, particularly regarding energy balancing. Upon his retirement in 1973, Stone's successors taught Polarity Therapy throughout the United States. The American Polarity Therapy Association was founded in 1984.

Technique: Polarity Therapy is an eclectic form of energy bodywork. Most Polarity Therapy techniques consist of placing the hands in different positions on the body to affect the free flow of energy. Other techniques include pressing, gentle rocking, and brushing.

Theory: Polarity Therapy techniques aim to remove obstructions to the free flow of energy in the body. Stone developed his own esoteric theories of energy flow after studying Chinese and Ayurvedic medicine.

Web Site: American Polarity Therapy Association (www.polaritytherapy.org)

15. Reflexology

Origin: Modern reflexology was developed by Eunice Ingham Stopfel (1889–1974), who combined the theory of Zone Therapy with compression massage of the feet and hands. She mapped the feet for their corresponding zones of reference, and developed pressure techniques for stimulating points on the feet to affect specific organs and structures of the body. She started her work in the 1930s, and taught throughout the United States in the 1950–1960s.

Technique: Reflexology is performed primarily on the feet. Pressure is applied to areas of the feet to stimulate other parts of the body. Reflexology techniques include thumb walking, finger walking, hook and backup, along with Western massage and joint movements applied to the feet.

Theory: Reflexology is based in Zone Therapy, which postulates that 10 longitudinal zones of the body end in the feet and the hands. Pressure to a zone in the feet causes stimulation of the entire zone. Reflexology charts map out which specific organs or body structures will be affected by pressure on specific areas of the feet. Reflexology is thought to normalize function, improve circulation, and promote relaxation. Knowledge of Western anatomy, physiology, and pathology are important in reflexology.

Web Sites: Home of Reflexology (www.reflexology.org)

International Institute of Reflexology (www.reflexology-usa.net)

16. Rolfing® Structural Integration

Origin: Rolfing was developed by Ida P. Rolf (1896–1979), and brought to public recognition during the 1970s within the human potential movement. The Rolf Institute® of Structural Integration was founded in 1971, and provides training and certification for Rolfing practitioners.

Technique: Rolfing is a form of contemporary Western bodywork, also called Structural Integration. It includes soft tissue manipulation and movement education. In Rolfing, myofascial tissues are manipulated so that they lengthen and glide, to balance the body around its vertical axis, achieving proper alignment or posture. In the process of working with deep myofascial tissues, past emotional trauma is also released.

Theory: Rolfing is based in Western anatomy and physiology, especially of fascial tissues, and psychology.

Web Site: The Rolf Institute for Structural Integration (www.rolf.org)

17. Shiatsu—Namikoshi

Origin: Shiatsu evolved from traditional Japanese massage called Amma. Tokujiro Namikoshi (1905–) developed a system of finger pressure to treat various ailments. He founded the first Shiatsu Institute of Therapy on Hokkaido in 1925, and the Japan Shiatsu Institute in Tokyo in 1940. His son, Toru Namikoshi (1931–), popularized Shiatsu in Japan and throughout the world in the 1950–1970s.

Technique: Shiatsu is a form of Asian Bodywork Therapy. Shiatsu literally means finger pressure (shi-atsu) in Japanese. Pressure is applied along energy (ki) meridians and to acupoints with the thumbs, fingers, or elbow. Recipient is either lying on a mat on the floor or on a bodywork table.

Theory: Shiatsu, as developed by Namikoshi, combines traditional Chinese medicine and Western anatomy and physiology. Important acupoints are pressed to elicit desired results.

Web Site: American Organization of Bodywork Therapies of Asia (www.aobta.org)

18. Sports Massage

Origin: Sports massage can be traced to ancient Greece and Rome where massage was given in the gymnasia and public baths. Massage prepared athletes for exercises, and helped in recovery from competition. In the late 19th century, rubbers and athletic masseurs used massage in the training of athletes. Sports massage was revived in the 1970s within the context of Western massage.

Technique: Sports massage is a specialty within Western massage. Western massage techniques are applied to enhance athletic performance, prevent injuries, prepare for and recover from competition, and in rehabilitation of injuries. Modern sports massage given at events emphasizes the technique of compression and other forms of petrissage. Individual practitioners may add other bodywork approaches to achieve the goals of the athlete.

Theory: Sports massage is based in Western anatomy, physiology, kinesiology, pathology, and sports science.

Reference: *Understanding Sports Massage* by Patricia J. Benjamin & Scott Lamp (Champaign, IL: Human Kinetics, 1996).

19. Stone Massage

Origin: Stones have been used in healing practices all over the world, including Asia. Healing or hot stone massage is a treatment that gained popularity in North American spas in the 1990–2000s.

Technique: Stone massage is a form of contemporary bodywork and spa treatment. Stones of various sizes, shapes and textures are used as massage tools, and as a form of thermal therapy. As massage tools, stones are used instead of the hands to apply pressure during techniques such as effleurage. As thermal therapy, stones may be heated and

placed on the body over certain anatomical structures or in patterns over energy centers and meridians; or cooled and used as cryotherapy to reduce swelling and cool tissues.
Theory: Stone massage is practiced as an eclectic form of bodywork incorporating Western anatomy and physiology with traditional Asian medicine. Geological properties of various kinds of stones are considered. Hot stones applied to the body impart weight and heat that promotes relaxation, normal body function, and energy balancing.
References: *Healing Stone Massage*. Video with Carollanne Crichton (Real Bodywork, 2001).
Japanese Hot Stone Massage by Mark Hess and Shogo Mochizuki (Kotobuki Publications, 2002).

20. Swedish Massage

   Origin: Swedish massage and related techniques were developed in Europe in the early 1800s, and brought to North America in the 1860s. It can be traced historically to the work of two men, Pehr Henrick Ling (1776–1839) of Sweden, and Johann Mezger (1838–1909) of Amsterdam. The heyday of Swedish massage in the United States was the 1930–1950s, when it was offered in health clubs, salons, and as part of physiotherapy.
   Technique: Swedish massage is a form of traditional Western massage. The five classic technique categories of Swedish massage soft tissue manipulation are effleurage (stroking, sliding), petrissage (kneading, compression), tapotement (percussion), friction, and vibration. Joint movements and hydrotherapy are also within the scope of Swedish massage.
   Theory: Swedish massage is based in Western anatomy, physiology, and pathology. It is applied to support the normal function of the human body and its systems, as well as enhance its innate healing capacity.
   See Western Massage.

21. Thai Massage

   Origin: Nuad bo-Rarn means "ancient massage" in the language of Thailand. It has been practiced for over 2500 years. At the Temple of the Reclining Buddha in Bangkok, 200 year–old stone engravings illustrate the energy lines and points, and techniques of this ancient practice. Thai massage is passed down in families, and also taught at schools of Traditional Thai Medicine.
   Technique: In Thai massage, the practitioner uses passive movement, yoga-like stretching, and pressure techniques to stimulate energy channels called *sen lines*, and release tension in the body. Application is gentle and rhythmic. Recipients lie on floor mats to receive Thai Massage.
   Theory: Thai massage is based on Ayurvedic (India) and Chinese medicine, and was influenced by yoga, as it evolved in ancient Thailand. Techniques stimulate the free flow of energy through channels.
   Web Site: Institute of Thai Massage (www.thai-massage.org)

22. Therapeutic Touch (TT)

   Origin: Therapeutic Touch was developed by Delores Krieger, a professor of nursing, and her teacher, Dora Kunz in the 1960–1970s. It is a modification of the ancient practice of laying on of the hands.
   Technique: Therapeutic Touch is a system of energy bodywork performed in five steps: (1) centering of the practitioner, (2) assessment of the energy field of the recipient with the palms of the hands, (3) clearing blockages, imbalances or congestion of energy with sweeping hand movements, (4) establishing harmony in the energy field using the mind, (5) smoothing out the energy field by sweeping the hands outward toward the periphery of the field.
   Theory: Therapeutic Touch is based in theories of bioelectricity and electromagnetic energy fields. The sweeping hand movements of TT move energy to create balance and harmony in a person's energy field. Imbalances, blockages, and congestion in the energy field are thought to result in disease and dysfunction. TT is used in the treatment of many different ailments.
   Web Sites: Nurse Healers–Professional Associates International (www.therapeutic touch.org)

23. Trager® Approach

   Origin: Trager Approach, also known as Psychophysical Integration, was developed by Milton Trager, MD (1908–1997). After earning a medical degree after World War II, Trager opened a practice in Hawaii in 1959, and gave a public demonstration of his work in 1973.

   Technique: The Trager Approach is a system of contemporary Western bodywork that combines tissue and joint mobilization, relaxation and movement re-education. The practitioner applies continuous rhythmic movement to different joints in the body with the recipient lying on a table. Recipients recreate the easy, light, free movements of the table work in a system of active exercise called Mentastics.

   Theory: Trager focuses on creating the sensations of lighter, easier, and freer movement through affecting neurological mechanisms of the body. It imparts an experience of deep relaxation, and greater joint mobility.

   Web Site: Trager International (www.trager.com)

24. Tuina

   Origin: The origin of Tuina, or Chinese medical massage, is clouded in the mists of time. It developed from the same roots as acupuncture in Chinese medicine. Tuina is written about in several ancient medical texts, and a Tuina department was set up in the Imperial Health Administration in the Tang Dynasty (618–907 CE). Tuina for infants and children became popular in the Qing Dynasty (1644–1911 CE)

   Technique: Tuina is a form of Chinese medical massage, i.e., Asian Bodywork Therapy. Techniques of Tuina include stroking, pushing, grasping, pressing, palm-rubbing, twisting, pinching, rubbing, rolling, tapping, stretching, kneading, lifting, and holding. Techniques are applied to stimulate acupoints and affect blood circulation. Tuina also includes joint manipulation, herbal remedies, and therapeutic exercise.

   Theory: Tuina is based in theory of Chinese medicine including *qi* or energy, energy channels, and yin-yang. Modern Tuina incorporates knowledge of Western anatomy, physiology, and pathology. Tuina is used to treat ailments recognized by Chinese medicine, as well as Western pathology.

   Reference: *Chinese Tuina Therapy* by Wang Fu (Bejing, China: Foreign Languages Press, 1994).

25. Western Massage

   Origin: Western massage can be traced to health and healing practices of ancient Greece and Rome. Techniques of soft tissue manipulation were further developed through the centuries in Europe and North America. Western massage today is an outgrowth of Swedish massage, massage used in Western medicine, and various contemporary systems of massage and bodywork.

   Description: Western massage techniques include classic Swedish massage techniques, plus various forms of contemporary massage, e.g., neuromuscular therapy, myofascial massage, lymphatic drainage massage, and other forms of massage therapy based in Western anatomy, physiology, and pathology. Western massage practitioners tend to be eclectic, incorporating various techniques, including energy approaches, with classic Swedish massage.

   Theory: Western massage is based in Western anatomy, physiology, and pathology. It aims to enhance the normal functioning of the body and its systems, including the innate healing power in each person.

   Web Sites: American Massage Therapy Association (www.amtamassage.org) Associated Bodywork & Massage Professionals (www.abmp.com)

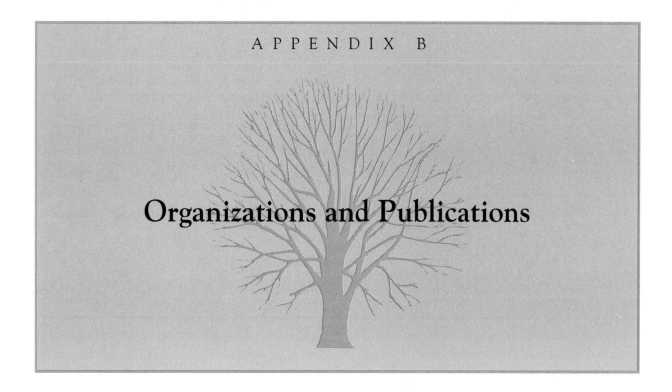

APPENDIX B

Organizations and Publications

ORGANIZATIONS

American Massage Therapy Association (AMTA)
820 Davis Street, Suite 100
Evanston, IL 60201-4444
(847) 864-0123
www.amtamassage.org

AMTA Foundation
820 Davis Street, Suite 100
Evanston, IL 60201-4444
(847) 869-5019
www.amtafoundation.org

American Organization for Bodywork Therapies
    of Asia (AOBTA)
1010 Haddonfield-Berlin Rd., Suite 408
Voorhees, NJ 08043
(856) 782-1616
www.aobta.org

American Polarity Therapy Association (APTA)
P.O. Box 19858
Boulder, CO 80308
(303) 545-2080
www.polaritytherapy.org

Associated Bodywork & Massage Professionals (ABMP)
1271 Sugarbush Drive
Evergreen, CO 80439-7347
(800) 458-2267
www.abmp.com

Canadian Massage Therapist Alliance (CMTA)
344 Lakeshore Road East, Suite B
Oakville (Ontario)
Canada L6J 1J6
(905) 849-8606
www.cmta.ca

Canadian Touch Research Center
760 Saint-Zotique Street East
Montreal (Quebec)
Canada H2S 1M5
(514) 272-5141
www.ccrt-ctrc.org

Commission on Massage Therapy Accreditation (COMTA)
820 Davis Street, Suite 100
Evanston, IL 60201-4444
(847) 869-5039
www.comta.org

Day-Break Geriatric Massage Institute
7434-A King George Drive
Indianapolis, IN 46240
(317) 722-986
www.daybreak-massage.com

Dr. Vodder School of North America
P.O. Box 5701
Victoria (British Columbia)
Canada V8R 6S8
(250) 598-9862
www.vodderschool.com

International Association of Infant Massage Instructors (US)
1891 Goodyear Avenue, Suite 622
Ventura, CA 93003
www.iaim-us.com

International Institute of Reflexology, Inc.
5650 First Avenue North
P.O. Box 12642
St. Petersburg, FL 33733-2642
(727) 343-4811
www.reflexology-usa.net

International Loving Touch Foundation (infant massage)
P.O. Box 16374
Portland, OR 97292
(503) 253-8482
www.lovingtouch.com

International Spa Association (ISPA)
2365 Harrodsburg Road, Suite A325
Lexington, KY 40504
(888) 651-4772
www.experienceispa.com

Jin Shin Do® Foundation for Bodymind Acupressure™
P.O.Box 416
Idyllwild, CA 92549
(909) 659-5707
www.jinshindo.org

National Center of Complementary and Alternative Medicine
National Institutes of Health
Bethesda, Maryland 20892
www.nccam.nih.gov

National Certification Board for Therapeutic Massage and Bodywork (NCBTMB)
8201 Greensboro Drive, Suite 300
McLean, VA 22102
(800) 296-664 or (703) 610-9015
www.ncbtmb.com

National Certification Commission for Acupuncture and Oriental Medicine (NCCAOM)
11 Canal Center Plaza, Suite 300
Alexandria, VA 22314
(703) 548-9004
www.nccaom.org

National Association of Nurse Massage Therapists (NANMT)
P.O. Box 24004
Huber Hts., OH 45424
(800) 262-4017
www.nanmt.org

Nurse Healers–Professional Associates International (Therapeutic Touch)
3760 South Highland Drive Suite 429
Salt Lake City, Utah 84106
(801) 273-3399
www.therapeutic-touch.org

Rolf Institute of Structural Integration®
205 Canyon Blvd.
Boulder, CO 80302
(800) 530-8875 or (303) 449-5903
www.rolf.org

TouchPro Institute
(Professional Chair Massage)
584 Castro Street, #555
San Francisco, CA 94114
(800) 999-5026
www.TouchPro.com

Touch Research Institutes (TRI)
University of Miami School of Medicine
P.O. Box 016820
Miami, FL 33101
(305) 243-6781
www.miami.edu/touch-research

World of Massage Museum (WOMM)
1636 W. First Avenue, Suite 100
Spokane, WA 99204
(800) 872-1282
www.worldofmassagemuseum.com

PUBLICATIONS

Massage Magazine
1636 W. First Avenue, Suite 100
Spokane, WA 99204
(800) 872-1282
www.massagemag.com

Massage & Bodywork Magazine
(Published by Associated Bodywork & Massage
   Professionals)
1271 Sugarbush Drive
Evergreen, CO 80439
(800) 458-2267
www.massageandbodywork.com

Massage Therapy Canada
1088 Fennell Avenue East, 2nd Floor
Hamilton (Ontario)
Canada L8T 1R8
(888) 247-2176
www.massagetherapycanada.com

Massage Therapy Journal
(Published by American Massage Therapy Association)
820 Davis Street, Suite 100
Evanston, IL 60201-4444
(847) 864-0123
www.amtamassage.org

Massage Today
P.O. Box 4139
Huntington Beach, CA 92605
(714)230-3150
www.masssagetoday.com

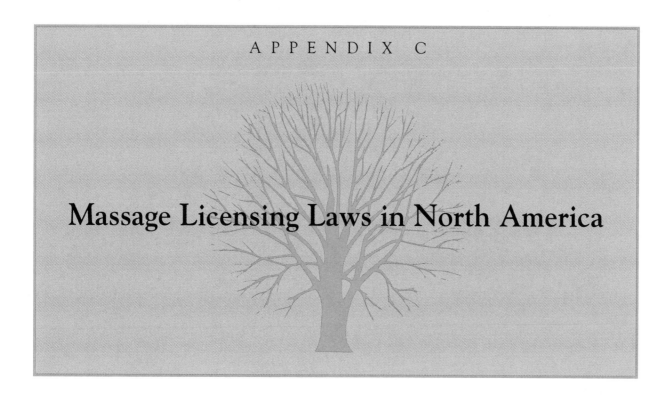

APPENDIX C

Massage Licensing Laws in North America

The following list contains information about state (U.S.) and provincial (Canada) licensing for massage therapists. It is current up to the time of publication of this text.

Please check one of the following Web sites for more current information: [www.amtamassage.org; www.abmp.com; massagemag.com]; or the state agency responsible for licensing.

UNITED STATES

Alabama Massage Therapy Board
610 S. McDonough St.
Montgomery, AL 36104
(334) 269-9990
www.almtbd.state.al.us
Education required: 600 hours*
Exam: NCETMB

Arizona (Effective date: July 2004)
www.massagetherapy.az.gov
Education required: 500 hours*
Exam: NCETMB

Arkansas State Board of Massage Therapy
103 Airways
Hot Springs, AR 71903
(501) 623-0444
www.state.ar.us
Education required: 500 hours*
Exam: NCETMB or state exam

Education required only lists massage therapy education required. States may also require CPR and other education. Most require graduation from a state-approved or accredited massage school or program. Check state law for most complete information.

NCETMB refers to the National Certification Examination for Therapeutic Massage and Bodywork.

Connecticut—Massage Therapy Licensure
Department of Public Health
410 Capitol Avenue—MS#12APP
P.O. Box 340308
Hartford, CT 06134
(860) 509-7573
www.dph.state.ct.us
Education required: 500 hours*
Exam: NCETMB

Delaware Board of Massage and Bodywork
Cannon Building
861 Silver Lake Blvd., #203
Dover, DE 19904
(302) 744-4506
www.professionallicensing.state.de.us/boards/massagebody
  works
Education required: 500 hours*
Exam: NCETMB

District of Columbia Massage Therapy Board
Occupational and Professional Licensing
  Administration
941 N. Capitol St., N.E., 7th Floor
Washington, DC 20002
(202) 727-7185
www.dcra.org/main.htm
Education from approved school required
Exam: State exam

Florida Board of Massage Therapy
Department of Health
2020 Capitol Circle S.E., Bin #C09
Tallahassee, FL 32399
(850) 488-0595
www.doh.state.fl.us/mqa/massage/mahome.html
Education required: 500 hours*
Exam: NCETMB

State of Hawaii
Board of Massage Therapy
P.O. Box 3469
Honolulu, HI 96801
(808) 586-2699
www.state.hi.us/dcca/pvl
Education required: 570 hours*
Exam: State exam

Illinois Department of Professional Regulation
320 West Washington St., 3rd Floor
Springfield, IL 62786
(217) 785-0800
www.ildpr.com
Education required: 500 hours*
Exam: NCETMB
(Effective date: January 2005)

Iowa Department of Health
Board of Massage Therapy Examiners
Lucas State Office Building, 5th Floor
321 E. 12th St.
Des Moines, IA 50319
(515) 281-6959
www.idph.state.ia.us/licensure
Education required: 500 hours*
Exam: NCETMB

Kentucky Board of Licensure for Massage Therapy
P.O. Box 1360
Frankfort, KY 406021
(502) 564-3296
www.state.ky.us/agencies/finance/occupations
Education required: 600 hours*
Exam: NCETMB

Louisiana Board of Massage Therapy
12022 Plank Road
Baton Rouge, LA 70811
(225) 771-4090
www.lsbmt.org
Education required: 500 hours*
Exam: NCETMB

Maine Board of Massage Therapy
Department of Professional and Financial Regulation
35 State House Station
Augusta, ME 04333
(207) 624-8613
www.state.me.us/pfr/led/massage
Education required: 500 hours*
Exam: NCETMB

Maryland Board of Chiropractic Examiners
Massage Therapy Advisory Committee
4201 Patterson Ave., 5th Floor
Baltimore, MD 21215
(410) 764-4738
www.mdmassage.org
Education required: 500 hours massage* + 60 hours college
Exam: NCETMB

Mississippi State Board of Massage Therapy
P.O. Box 12489
Jackson, MS 39236
(601) 856-6127
www.msbmt.state.ms.us
Education required: 700 hours
Exam: NCETMB

Missouri Massage Therapy Board
3605 Missouri Blvd.
P.O. Box 1335
Jefferson City, MO 65102

(573) 522-6277
www.ecodev.state.mo.us/pr
Education required: 500 hours*
Exam: NCETMB or approved exam

Nebraska Massage Therapy Board
Health and Human Services
Credentialing Division
301 Centennial Mall South, 3rd Floor
Lincoln, NE 68509
(402) 471-2115
www.hhs.state.ne.us/crl/massagerules.htm
Education required: 1000 hours*
Exam: NCETMB + practical exam

New Hampshire Office of Program Support
Board of Massage Therapy
Health Facilities Administration
129 Pleasant Street
Concord, NH 03301
(603) 271-5127
www.nhes.state.nh.us/elmi/licertoccs/massa01.htm
Education required: 750 hours*
Exam: NCETMB or state exam

New Jersey Board of Nursing
Massage, Bodywork & Somatic Therapy Examining
  Committee
P.O. Box 45010
Newark, NJ 07101
www.state.nj.us/lps/ca/nursing
Education required: 500 hours or NCETMB
(Effective date: 2003)

New Mexico
Board of Massage Therapy
2055 Pacheco St., #400
Santa Fe, NM 87504
(505) 476-7090
www.rld.state.nm.us/b&c/massage
Education required: 650 hours*
Exam: NCETMB

New York State Board of Massage Therapy
Cultural Education Center, #3041
Albany, NY 12230
(518) 473-1417
www.op.nysed.gov/massage.htm
Education required: 1000 hours*
Exam: State exam

North Carolina Board of Massage
  and Bodywork Therapy
P.O. Box 2539
Raleigh, NC 27602
(919) 546-0050

www.bmbt.org
Education required: 500 hours*
Exam: NCETMB

North Dakota Board of Massage
P.O. Box 218
Beach, ND 58621
(701) 872-4895
www.ndboardofmassage.com
Education required: 750 hours*
Exam: Written and practical state exam

Ohio Massage Therapy Board
77 South High Street, 17th Floor
Columbus, OH 43266
(614) 466-3934
www.state.oh.us/med
Education required: 600 hours*
Exam: State exam

Oregon Board of Massage Technicians
State Office Building
3218 Pringle Road S.E., #250
Salem, OR 97302
(503) 365-8657
www.oregonmassage.org
Education required: 500 hours*
Exam: NCETMB + practical test

Rhode Island Department of Health
Professional Regulation
3 Capitol Hill, Room 104
Providence, RI 02908
(401) 222-2827
www.health.state.ri.us
Education required: 500 hours*
Exam: NCETMB

South Carolina Department of Labor
Licensing and Regulation
P.O. Box 11329
Columbia, SC 29211
(803) 896-4588
www.myscgov.com
Education required: 500 hours*
Exam: NCETMB

Tennessee Massage Licensure Board
Cordell Hull Building, 1st Floor
425 Fifth Ave. N.
Nashville, TN 37247
(615) 532-3202
www.state.tn.us/hh.html
Education required: 500 hours*
Exam: NCETMB

Texas Department of Health
1100 West 49th St.
Austin, TX 78756
(512) 834-6616
www.tdh.state.tx.us/hcqs/plc/massage.html
Education required: 300 hours*
Exam: Written and practical exam

State of Utah Department of Commerce
Board of Massage Therapy
P.O. Box 146741
Salt Lake city, UT 84144
(801) 530-6964
www.commerce.state.ut.us/dopl/wp-app.htm
Education required: 600 hours*
Exam: NCETMB

Virginia Board of Nursing
6606 W. Broadway St., 4th Floor
Richmond, VA 23230
(804) 662-9909
www.vdh.state.va.us
Education required: 500 hours*
Exam: NCETMB

State of Washington Department of Health
1300 S.W. Quince St.
P.O. Box 47867
Olympia, WA 98504
(360) 236-4700
www.don.wa.gov
Education required: 500 hours*
Exam: NCETMB

State of West Virginia
Board of Massage Therapy
200 Davis St., #1
Princeton, WV 24740
(304) 487-1400
www.wvmassage.org
Education required: 500 hours*
Exam: NCETMB

Wisconsin Department of Regulation and Licensing
Massage Therapy Board
1400 E. Washington Ave.
Madison, WI 53703
(608) 266-0145
www.state.wi.us/regulation
Education required: 600 hours*
Exam: State approved exam

CANADA

British Columbia
Registered Massage Therapist
(604) 736-3404
Education required: 3,000 hours*

Newfoundland and Labrador
Registered Massage Therapist
(709) 739-7181
Education required: 2,200 hours*

Ontario
Massage Therapist
(416) 489-2626
Education required: 2–3 year program*

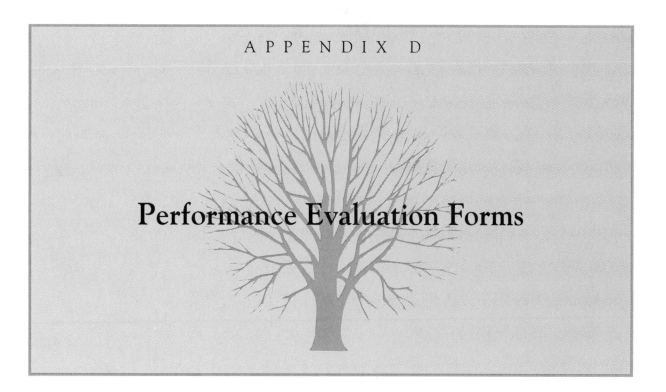

APPENDIX D

Performance Evaluation Forms

The performance evaluation, or practical testing, of massage techniques and their applications is important in the educational setting. Students benefit from receiving feedback about their performance as they are learning how to give safe and effective massage. Teachers need to determine if students have achieved a minimum level of competency.

The following forms are offered as examples of a format that can be used in giving performance evaluations to students of massage. The general format takes into consideration the need for giving a numerical value or grade to what is essentially a subjective evaluation. It also honors the teachers' more intuitive sense of how students are grasping the material to be learned, while encouraging teachers to be specific about what they are seeing.

One of the most important elements in developing an evaluation instrument is determining which items will receive evaluation. These are taken from the learning outcomes for the course of study. The following instruments have been developed for evaluating performance of the Western massage techniques described in Chapter 7; the application of skills in giving a full-body mas-sage session as described in Chapter 9; and the application of skills in giving treatment to a specific part of the body, for a specific medical condition, or to a special population as described throughout the text.

The rating scale used is from 0 to 5. Zero indicates total incompetence; 1 = very poor; 2 = poor; 3 = adequate; 4 = good; 5 = excellent. A simple way for evaluators to use the rating scale is to first determine whether students are adequate (rating = 3) using their experience and judgment in observing performance, and taking into consideration all relevant factors. If students are not at least "adequate," evaluators can identify specific factors that are detracting from the performance and determine if the rating is 2, 1, or 0. If students appear more than adequate, evaluators can identify specific factors that make the performance good or excellent and choose a rating of 4 or 5. Reasons for the rating given and ways to improve performance may be noted in the "comments" section. The more specific evaluators can be about what they are looking for, the more objective and consistent evaluations will be.

The comments section of the form provides a place for evaluators to identify the factors they observed that had an impact on the rating. For example, an observation that the student forgot to put a bolster under the knees of a recipient who was supine might help account for the rating given for "positioning." Students receive specific feedback about their performance from the comments. In this sense, an evaluation is also a learning tool.

In the school setting, translating a rating into a grade is a matter of determining the level of competence desired in students who pass a course or section of a course. In some situations, an average rating of 3 or adequate is considered satisfactory or passing. Other situations may call for more than adequate performance for a passing grade. Traditional schools may want to translate numerical evaluations into A, B, C, D, or F grades. These performance evaluation forms provide a basis for assigning grades, but do not dictate what a passing grade is. The particular school or teacher needs to take that next step in assigning grades.

Performance Evaluation of Individual Massage Techniques: Western Massage

Student's Name: Date of Evaluation:
Evaluator's Name: Class:

0 = incompetent; 1 = very poor; 2 = poor; 3 = adequate; 4 = good; 5 = excellent

Effleurage techniques slide or glide over the skin with a smooth continuous motion.

Technique/Rating	Comments

1. Basic sliding effleurage

    0   1   2   3   4   5

2. Bilateral tree stroking

    0   1   2   3   4   5

3. Three-count stroking of the trapezius

    0   1   2   3   4   5

4. Horizontal stroking

    0   1   2   3   4   5

5. Mennell's superficial stroking

    0   1   2   3   4   5

6. Nerve strokes

    0   1   2   3   4   5

7. Knuckling

    0   1   2   3   4   5

8. Sedating effleurage of the back

    0   1   2   3   4   5

Petrissage techniques lift, wring, or squeeze soft tissues in a kneading motion; or press or roll the tissues under or between the hands.

9. Basic two-handed kneading

    0   1   2   3   4   5

10. One-handed kneading

    0   1   2   3   4   5

11. Alternating one-handed kneading

    0   1   2   3   4   5

12. Circular two-handed petrissage

    0   1   2   3   4   5

13. Alternating fingers-to-thumb petrissage

0   1   2   3   4   5

14. Skin rolling

0   1   2   3   4   5

15. Compression

0   1   2   3   4   5

Friction is performed by rubbing one surface over another repeatedly.

16. Superficial warming friction

0   1   2   3   4   5

17. Sawing friction

0   1   2   3   4   5

18. Superficial friction using knuckles

0   1   2   3   4   5

19. Deep cross-fiber friction

0   1   2   3   4   5

20. Circular deep friction

0   1   2   3   4   5

Tapotement consists of a series of brisk percussive movements following each other in rapid, alternating fashion.

21. Hacking

0   1   2   3   4   5

22. Cupping

0   1   2   3   4   5

23. Clapping

0   1   2   3   4   5

24. Slapping

0   1   2   3   4   5

25. Tapping

0   1   2   3   4   5

26. Pincement

0   1   2   3   4   5

27. Quacking

0   1   2   3   4   5

Vibration may be described as an oscillating, quivering, or trembling motion; or movement back and forth, or up and down, performed quickly and repeatedly.

28. Fine vibration with fingertips

    0   1   2   3   4   5

29. Light effleurage with vibration

    0   1   2   3   4   5

30. Shaking—coarse vibration

    0   1   2   3   4   5

31. Jostling—coarse vibration

    0   1   2   3   4   5

Touch without movement

32. Passive touch

    0   1   2   3   4   5

33. Direct static pressure

    0   1   2   3   4   5

Total Points _____ /33 = _____ **Average Rating**   **Student's Name:**

Performance Evaluation of Full-Body Massage

Student's Name: Date of Evaluation:

Evaluator's Name: Class:

0 = incompetent; 1 = very poor; 2 = poor; 3 = adequate; 4 = good; 5 = excellent

Items   **Comments**

1. Professional demeanor

   0 1 2 3 4 5

2. Environment

   0 1 2 3 4 5

3. Draping

   0 1 2 3 4 5

4. Positioning the receiver

   0 1 2 3 4 5

5. Body mechanics

   0 1 2 3 4 5

6. Use of lubricant

   0 1 2 3 4 5

7. Organization of session

   0 1 2 3 4 5

8. Application of techniques

   0 1 2 3 4 5

9. Pressure

   0 1 2 3 4 5

10. Rhythm and pacing

    0 1 2 3 4 5

11. Safety considerations

    0 1 2 3 4 5

12. Overall effectiveness

    0 1 2 3 4 5

Total points _____/12 = _____ Average Rating   Student's Name:

Performance Evaluation of Massage Treatment

Student's Name: Date of Evaluation:

Evaluator's Name: Class:

Special condition/assessment/diagnosis: _____.

Part of body treated: _____.

Treatment goals: _____.

0 = incompetent; 1 = very poor; 2 = poor; 3 = adequate; 4 = good; 5 = excellent

Items for Evaluation   **Comments**

1. Professional demeanor

   0   1   2   3   4   5

2. Environment

   0   1   2   3   4   5

3. Draping

   0   1   2   3   4   5

4. Positioning the receiver

   0   1   2   3   4   5

5. Body mechanics

   0   1   2   3   4   5

6. Choice of techniques (appropriateness)

   0   1   2   3   4   5

7. Skill in application of techniques

   0   1   2   3   4   5

8. Adjunct modalities used

   0   1   2   3   4   5

9. Organization of session

   0   1   2   3   4   5

10. Safety precautions observed

    0   1   2   3   4   5

11. Effectiveness of treatment

    0   1   2   3   4   5

Total points _____/11 = _____ Average Rating   Student's Name:

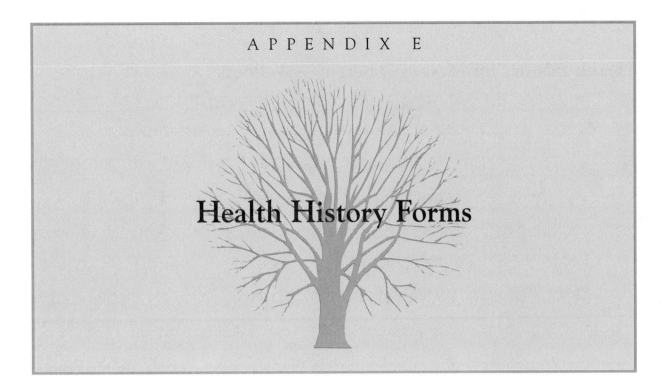

APPENDIX E

Health History Forms

Health history information is essential for planning safe and effective massage sessions. In the wellness model, health information is used to plan massage sessions that help the receiver progress further along the path to high-level wellness. In the treatment model, information about medical conditions, diagnoses from health care providers, and treatment goals help the therapist apply massage to alleviate the condition for which massage is indicated.

An important purpose of health history information is to alert the practitioner to situations for which massage is contraindicated, or for which special cautions apply. The receiver may not be aware that massage can be harmful under certain conditions, and so it is the practitioner's responsibility to gather enough information to make such a judgment. Certain areas of the body may be avoided, certain techniques omitted, or applications modified based on information from health history.

The following two examples of health history forms may serve as models for developing a written form that fits your practice and your potential clients or patients. One form may be used to gather information for a general wellness session, and the other asks for more detailed medical information.

Health History for Massage Therapy—Wellness

Name _____ Date of initial visit _____

Address _____ Phone _____

Occupation _____ Date of birth _____

Sports/physical activities/hobbies _____

The following information will be used to help plan safe and effective massage sessions. Please answer the questions to the best of your knowledge.

1. Have you had professional massage before?   Yes   No

2. Do you have any difficulty lying on your front, back, or side?   Yes   No

   If yes, please explain _____

3. Do you have allergic reactions to oils, lotions, ointments, liniments, or other substances put on your skin?   Yes   No

   If yes, please explain _____

4. Do you wear contact lenses ( ) dentures ( ) a hearing aid ( )?

5. Do you sit for long hours at a workstation, computer, or driving?   Yes   No

   If yes, please describe _____

6. Do you perform any repetitive movement in your work, sports, or hobby?   Yes   No

   If yes, please describe _____

7. Do you experience stress in your work, family, or other aspect of your life?   Yes   No

   If yes, how do you think it has affected your health? muscle tension ( ) anxiety ( ) insomnia ( ) irritability ( ) other _____

8. Is there a particular area of the body where you are experiencing tension, stiffness, or other discomfort?   Yes   No

   If yes, please identify _____

9. Do you have any particular goals in mind for this massage session?   Yes   No

   If yes, please explain _____

In order to plan a massage session that is safe and effective, we need some general information about your medical history.

10. Are you currently under medical supervision?   Yes   No

    If yes, please explain _____

11. Are you currently taking any medication?   Yes   No

    If yes, please list _____

12. Please check any condition listed below that applies to you:

_____ contagious skin condition

_____ open sores or wounds

_____ easy bruising

_____ recent accident or injury

_____ current fever

_____ swollen glands

_____ allergies

_____ heart condition

_____ high or low blood pressure

_____ circulatory disorder

_____ contagious skin condition
      varicose veins
      atherosclerosis
      phlebitis

_____ joint disorder
      rheumatoid arthritis

_____ osteoporosis

_____ epilepsy

_____ headaches

_____ cancer

_____ epilepsy

_____ diabetes

_____ decreased sensation

_____ recent surgery

_____ joint disorder

_____ artificial joint

Comments:

_____

_____

_____

13. For women: Are you pregnant?   Yes   No   If yes, how many months? _____

14. Is there anything else about your health history that you think would be useful for your massage practitioner to know to plan a safe and effective massage session for you?

_____

_____

_____

_____

I understand that these massage sessions are for general wellness purposes and that I should see a doctor or other appropriate health care provider for diagnosis and treatment of any suspected medical problem. Also, that it is my responsibility to keep my massage practitioner informed of any changes in my health, and any medications that I may begin to take in the future.

Signature _____ Date _____

Health History for Massage Therapy Treatment

Name _____ Date of initial visit _____

Address _____ Phone _____

Occupation _____ Date of birth _____

Name of physician _____ Phone _____

Other health care provider _____

Referred by _____

1. Have you had massage therapy before?   Yes   No

2. For women: Are you pregnant?   Yes   No   If yes, how many months? _____

3. Do you have any difficulty lying on your front, back, or side?   Yes   No
    If yes, please explain _____

4. Do you have allergic reactions to oils, lotions, ointments, liniments, or other substances put on your skin?   Yes   No
    If yes, please explain _____

5. Do you wear contact lenses ( ) dentures ( ) a hearing aid ( )?

6. Do you sit for long hours at a workstation, computer, or driving?   Yes   No
    If yes, please describe _____

7. Do you perform any repetitive movement in your work, sports, or hobby?   Yes   No
    If yes, please describe _____

8. Do you experience stress in your work, family, or other aspect of your life?   Yes   No
    How would you describe your stress level?   Low   Medium   High   Very high
    If high, how do you think stress has effected your health? muscle tension ( ) anxiety ( ) insomnia ( ) irritability
    ( ) other _____

9. Is there a particular area of the body where you are experiencing tension, stiffness, or other discomfort?   Yes   No
    If yes, please identify _____

In order to plan a massage session that is safe and effective, we need some general information about your medical history.

10. Are you currently under medical supervision?   Yes   No
    If yes, please explain _____

11. Are you currently taking any medication?   Yes   No
    If yes, please list _____

12. Please check any condition listed below that applies to you:

_____ Skin condition (e.g., acne, rash, skin cancer, allergy, easy bruising, contagious condition)

_____ Allergies

_____ Recent accident, injury, or surgery (e.g., whiplash, sprain, broken bone, deep bruise)

_____ Muscular problems (e.g., tension, cramping, chronic soreness)

_____ Joint problems (e.g., osteoarthritis, rheumatoid arthritis, gout, hypermobile joints, recent dislocation)

_____ Lymphatic condition (e.g., swollen glands, nodes removed, lymphoma, lymphedema)

_____ Circulatory or blood conditions (e.g., atherosclerosis, varicose veins, phlebitis, arrhythmias, high or low blood pressure, heart disease, recent heart attack or stroke, anemia)

_____ Neurologic condition (e.g., numbness or tingling in any area of the body, sciatica, damage from stroke, epilepsy, multiple sclerosis, cerebral palsy)

_____ Digestive conditions (e.g., ulcers)

_____ Immune system conditions (e.g., chronic fatigue, HIV/AIDS)

_____ Skeletal conditions (e.g., osteoporosis, bone cancer, spinal injury)

_____ Headaches (e.g., tension, PMS, migraines)

_____ Cancer

_____ Emotional difficulties (e.g., depression, anxiety, panic attacks, eating disorder, psychotic episodes). Are you currently seeing a psychotherapist for this condition?   Yes   No

_____ Previous surgery, disease, or other medical condition that may be affecting you now (e.g., polio, previous heart attack or stroke, previously broken bones)

Comments:

_____

_____

_____

13. Is there anything else about your health history that you think would be useful for your massage practitioner to know to plan a safe and effective massage session for you?

_____

_____

_____

14. Has your physician or other health care provider recommended massage for any of the conditions listed above?   Yes   No

If yes, please explain _____

15. Do you have any particular goals in mind for this massage session related to any of the conditions mentioned above?   Yes   No

If yes, please explain _____

I understand that I should see a doctor or other appropriate health care provider for diagnosis and treatment of any suspected medical problem. It may be beneficial for my massage practitioner to speak to my doctor about my medical condition to determine how massage may help the healing process, and to avoid worsening the condition. I will be asked for permission to contact my doctor, if the massage practitioner thinks that it might be useful. I also understand that it is my responsibility to keep my massage practitioner informed of any changes in my health, and any medications that I may begin to take in the future.

Signature _____ Date _____

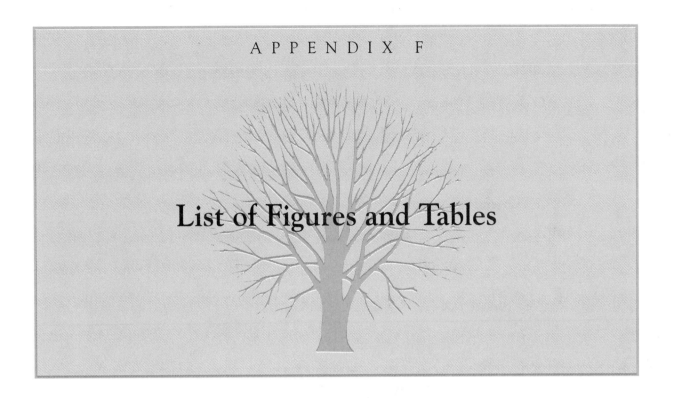

APPENDIX F

List of Figures and Tables

8   Joint Movements
Figure

11   Hydrotherapy / Thermal Therapies

12   Myofascial Massage

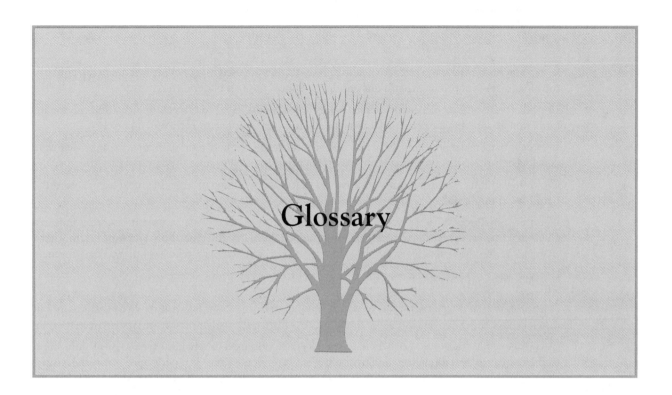

Glossary

Active movements are performed voluntarily by a person with no or some assistance from a practitioner. Types of active movements are free, assistive, and resistive.

Acupressure is a Western term for a form of Asian bodywork therapy based on Chinese meridian theory in which acupuncture points are pressed to stimulate the flow of energy or *chi*.

Alternative therapy refers to methods or systems of healing outside of mainstream medicine.

Amma is a term for traditional Japanese massage.

Asian bodywork therapies (ABT) are forms of massage and bodywork whose theoretical basis is Traditional Asian (Chinese) Medicine.

Assistive movement is a type of active movement in which the recipient initiates the movement, and the practitioner helps perform the movement. Also called **assisted movement.**

Ayurvedic massage is a system of soft tissue manipulation based in traditional theories of health and disease from India, i.e., Ayurvedic medicine.

Benefits are positive outcomes. The benefits of massage are experienced by recipients when the effects of massage support their general health and wellbeing.

Body-centered therapy refers to methods of healing that work primarily through the physical body, but which affect the whole person — body, mind, emotions, and spirit.

Body mechanics refers to the posture and biomechanics of the practitioner when performing massage. Good body mechanics protect the practitioner from injury and maximize the efficiency of technique applications.

Bodywork is a general term for practices involving touch and movement in which the practitioner uses manual techniques to promote health and healing of the recipient. The healing massage techniques described in this text are considered forms of bodywork.

Boundaries refer to practices that clearly delineate and maintain practitioner and client roles within the therapeutic relationship.

CAM is an acronym for Complementary and Alternative Medicine.

Clinical massage therapy describes applications of massage for the treatment of pathologies. Also called **medical massage.**

Complementary therapy   refers to healing methods that are used as secondary treatments to enhance the effectiveness of primary treatments, and that contribute to a patient's recovery.

Confidentiality   is an ethical principle that upholds clients' right to privacy, and prohibits giving information about clients to others without the client's permission. See **HIPAA.**

Contemporary massage and bodywork   is a general category for systems of manual therapy that were developed in the 20th century, e.g., myofascial massage, neuromuscular therapy, polarity therapy.

Contraindications   are conditions or situations that make receiving massage inadvisable because of the harm that it might do.

Counter-transference   is a psychological phenomenon that occurs when a practitioner responds to a client as if they were relating to someone important in their, i.e., the practitioner's, past (e.g., mother), and transferring those positive or negative feelings onto the therapeutic relationship. See **transference.**

Cryotherapy   is the application of cold (e.g., ice) for its therapeutic effects.

Deep friction   is a type of friction in which the practitioner's fingers do not move over the skin, but instead, move the skin over tissues underneath. Cross-fiber and circular friction are types of deep friction.

Deep transverse friction   is a specific type of deep friction used in rehabilitation to break adhesions, facilitate healthy scar formation, and treat muscle and tendon lesions. It is performed across the tissues, causing broadening and separation of fibers. Deep transverse friction was popularized by James Cyriax. Also called **Cyriax friction.**

Direct pressure, or direct static pressure,   is the application of force to compress tissues in a specific spot; it is applied with a thumb, finger, elbow, or knuckle. It can be considered a form of compression without movement and has also been called **static friction.**

Draping   refers to the use of sheets, towels, or other materials to cover recipients of massage to preserve their privacy and modesty, to maintain professional boundaries, and for warmth.

Eclectic practitioners   combine two or more systems of massage and bodywork into their own unique approach to manual therapy.

Effects of massage   refer to the basic physiological and psychological changes that occur to the recipient during a massage session.

Effectiveness   of a massage performance refers to the degree to which intended goals are achieved and to which the recipient is satisfied.

Effleurage   is a Western massage technique category that includes movements that slide or glide over the body with a smooth continuous motion.

Endangerment sites   are areas of the body where delicate body structures are less protected and, therefore, may be more easily damaged when receiving massage.

Environment   for massage includes the room, air quality, lighting, sound, dressing arrangements, equipment, and overall cleanliness and neatness of the space in which a session is given.

Esalen massage   is a genre of bodywork based on a simplified form of Swedish massage, whose main purpose is to enhance nonverbal connection with the inner self and with others. It emphasizes the sensual aspects of massage. It was developed at the Esalen Institute in Big Sur, California in the 1970s as part of the human potential movement.

Evidence-based therapy   is founded on scientific research that provides verifiable evidence of the effectiveness of a specific treatment.

Folk and native massage traditions   are found all over the world among families, tribes, and villages. They are based on tradition and experience and often involve herbal remedies, ritual, and religious beliefs.

Foot reflexology   *See* **reflexology.**

Free active movements or free exercises   are performed entirely by a person with no assistance from a practitioner.

Friction   is a Western massage technique category that includes movements that rub one surface over another repeatedly and includes superficial and deep friction.

Full-body Western massage   refers to a massage session lasting from 30 to 90 minutes, in which traditional Western massage techniques are combined into a routine to address the whole body. These sessions are generally wellness oriented and aim to improve circulation, relax the muscles, improve joint mobility, induce general relaxation, promote healthy skin, and create a general sense of wellbeing.

General contraindications   are conditions or situations that make receiving *any* massage inadvisable because of the harm that it might do.

Healing   means enhancing health and wellbeing. It is the process of regaining health or optimal functioning after an injury, disease, or other debilitating condition. "To heal" means to make healthy, whole, or sound; restore to health; or free from ailment.

HIPAA   is an acronym for the Health Insurance Portability and Accountability Act of 1996.

HIPAA Privacy Rules   specify how medical records must be secured, who may have access to medical records, and under what conditions records may be shared with others. *See* **confidentiality.**

Holistic massage   refers to forms of massage which take into account the wholeness of human beings, i.e., body, mind, emotions, and spirit.

Human potential movement   is an historical social movement in the 1960–1970s United States that advocated exploring the limits of human potential, and spawned many forms of massage and bodywork. *See* **Esalen massage.**

Hydrotherapy   is the use of water in different forms for its therapeutic effects. *See* **thermal therapies.**

Indication   is used in the treatment model to mean that when a specific medical condition is present, a particular modality is indicated or advised to alleviate the condition. Massage is indicated as a treatment for a number of medical conditions.

Infant massage   involves soft tissue manipulation and joint movements designed to enhance the growth and development of newborns and children.

Informed consent   is a procedure used to ask for explicit permission from a client to touch a certain body area, or perform a specific technique.

Integrative health care   is an approach to healing in which mainstream medicine and alternative healing methods are offered as equal options for treating patients.

Intention   is the aim that guides the action, that is, what the practitioner hopes to accomplish.

Intervention model   is a procedure used to clarify a possible misunderstanding of intention by a client (e.g., sexual intent), and to make a decision whether to stop or continue with a massage session.

Jin Shin Do®   is a modern synthesis of traditional Chinese acupressure/acupuncture theory and techniques, breathing exercises, Taoist philosophy, and modern psychology. It was developed by Iona Marsaa Teeguarden in the 1970s in the United States.

Joint manipulations,   sometimes called adjustments or chiropractic adjustments, refer to techniques that take a joint beyond its normal range of motion and that are specific attempts to realign a misaligned joint, usually using a thrusting movement. Joint manipulations are not part of Western massage and are not within the scope of this text.

Joint movements   are techniques that involve motion in the joints of the body, and include mobilizing techniques and stretching.

Local contraindications   are conditions or situations that make receiving massage on a particular part of the body inadvisable because of the harm that it might do. Also called **regional contraindications.**

Lubricants   are topical substances used in some massage sessions to enhance the effects of techniques and to minimize skin friction. Common lubricants include vegetable and mineral oils, jojoba, lotions, and combinations of these substances.

Lymphatic drainage massage (LDM)   is a form of contemporary massage designed to assist the function of the lymphatic system by the application of slow, light, and repetitive strokes that help move lymph fluid through the system of vessels and nodes (also **manual lymph drainage**).

Manual therapy   refers to healing methods applied with the practioner's hands touching or moving the recipient's body.

Massage   is the intentional and systematic manipulation of the soft tissues of the body to enhance health and healing. Joint movements and stretching are commonly performed as part of massage. The primary characteristics of massage are touch and movement.

Massage therapy   is a general term for health and healing practices involving touch and movement, which are based in massage and related manual techniques. It is sometimes used synonymously with the term **bodywork.** The term *massage therapy* has been adopted by some massage practitioners to define their profession, which is a licensed profession in many states.

Medical massage   *See* **clinical massage.**

Mobilizing techniques   Mobilizing techniques are free and loose non-specific joint movements within the normal range of joint motion.

Modality   is a method of treating a medical condition. Massage is considered a modality in the tradition of physiotherapy, along with other modalities such as ice packs, hot packs, ultrasound, or whirlpool baths.

Myofascial massage   is a general term for techniques aimed at restoring mobility in the body's fascia and softening connective tissue that has become rigid. Also called **myofascial release** and **myofascial unwinding.**

Natural healing   refers to a philosophy that shows preference for methods of healing derived from nature, the belief in an innate healing force, and a holistic view of human life.

Natural healing arts   are methods of healing derived from nature, for example, nutritious food, herbs, water therapy, exercise, relaxation, fresh air, sunshine, and massage.

Neuromuscular therapy (NMT)   is a form of contemporary massage focused on deactivating myofascial trigger points. *See* **trigger points.**

Organization of a session   refers to the overall structure of a massage session into beginning, middle, and end; the progression from one section of the body to another; and the ordering of techniques into sequences. Organization includes the use of opening techniques, transitions, and finishing techniques.

Pacing   refers to the speed of performing techniques, which may vary from very slow to very fast for different effects.

Palliative care   refers to methods of reducing symptoms and discomfort associated with certain diseases or their treatment.

Passive movements   are body movements initiated and controlled by the practitioner, while the recipient remains relaxed and receptive.

Passive touch   is simply laying the fingers, one hand, or both hands on the body. Passive touch may impart heat to an area, have a calming influence, or help balance energy.

Person-centered massage   refers to maintaining awareness of the whole person during a session, as opposed to focusing strictly on the pathology, i.e., pathology centered.

Petrissage   is a Western massage technique category that includes movements that lift, wring, or squeeze soft tissues in a kneading motion; or press or roll the soft tissues under or between the hands.

Polarity therapy   is a form of bodywork that uses simple touch and gentle rocking movements with the intention to balance life energy and to encourage relaxation. It was developed by Randolph Stone in the mid-20th century.

Positioning the receiver   refers to placing the recipient of massage in a position (e.g., supine, prone, side-lying, seated) to maximize his or her comfort and safety. Bolsters and other props may be used to support specific body areas.

Practitioner   refers to someone trained in massage techniques and who uses massage in the practice of his or her profession.

Pregnancy massage   refers to massage and bodywork adapted to meet the needs of pregnant women, and relieve some of the discomforts related to the pregnant state.

Pressure   is related to the force used in applying techniques and to the degree of compaction of tissues as techniques are applied. The amount of pressure used in massage will depend on the intended effect and the tolerance or desires of the recipient.

Principle-based massage   utilizes a broad base of knowledge and skills to plan a unique session or treatment strategy, as opposed to relying on a set protocol or formula.

Professional demeanor   refers to the appearance, language, and behavior of practitioners, which meets professional standards and inspires trust and respect.

Professional library   includes the resources a practitioner has accessible within their own office, including some basic sources of information about conditions, pathologies, and special populations commonly encountered in their massage practice.

Reflexology   is a form of bodywork based on the theory of zone therapy, in which specific spots on the feet or hands are pressed to stimulate corresponding areas in other parts of the body.

Research literacy   refers to knowledge and skills needed to understand and use scientific research. It includes an understanding of the scientific method, locating research articles, and reading, analyzing, and evaluating research studies.

Resistive movements   are a type of active movement in which the practitioner offers resistance to the motion, thereby challenging the muscles used. Also called **resisted movements.**

Rhythm   refers to a recurring pattern of movement with a specific cadence, beat, or accent and may be described as smooth, flowing, or uneven.

Seated massage   refers to massage given with the recipient seated in an ordinary or a special massage chair. It is called **on-site massage** when the chair is taken to a public place such as an office or commercial establishment. Also called **chair massage.**

Scope of practice   describes the legally allowed, or professionally defined, methods used by a certain profession, as well as their intention in performing them. Different professions have different scopes of practice as defined by law or by the profession. Massage techniques fall within the scope of practice of several professions.

Session   refers to a period of time in which massage is given to a recipient by a practitioner. Sessions have logical organization, have a wellness or a treatment purpose, and generally vary from 10 minutes to two hours.

Shiatsu   is a general term for Japanese bodywork based on Chinese meridian theory and Western science, in which *tsubo* (i.e., acupoints) are pressed to balance the flow of energy or *ki*.

Sports massage   is the science and art of applying massage and related techniques to ensure the health and wellbeing of the athlete and to enhance athletic performance. The major applications of sports massage are recovery, remedial, rehabilitation, maintenance, and event (i.e., pre-, inter-, and post-event).

Standards of practice   are documents developed by professional associations that outline acceptable ethical professional conduct.

Stretching   is a passive movement performed to the limit of the range of motion of a joint. Stretching increases flexibility in a joint; lengthens the muscles and connective tissues that cross a joint; and helps relax muscles involved.

Superficial friction   is a type of friction in which the hand rubs briskly back and forth over the skin to improve circulation in superficial tissues and to create heat.

Swedish massage   is a genre of bodywork that includes traditional Western massage, Swedish movements, hydrotherapy, heat lamps, and other modalities. Swedish massage is a popular form of massage in health clubs, spas, and resorts.

Swedish Movement Cure   refers to Pehr Ling's system of medical gymnastics that was developed in the early 1800s and which, along with Mezger's massage, is the forerunner of today's Western massage.

Tapotement   is a Western massage technique category consisting of brisk percussive movements that are performed in rapid rhythmic fashion. Forms of tapotement include hacking, rapping, cupping, clapping, slapping, tapping, and pincement.

Technique   refers to the technical aspects of the application of massage, or how the body moves while performing massage. The broader concept of the term technique also includes the intent.

Therapeutic relationship   is a model for understanding the separate and unique roles of the practitioner and the client in the therapeutic setting.

Thermal therapies   involve the application of hot and cold modalities for their therapeutic effects, e.g., hot packs, ice. See **hydrotherapy.**

Touch   means "to come into contact with." Massage practitioners touch their clients or patients in many ways, but primarily with their hands. Touch may happen on a physical or an energetic level.

Touch without movement   is a Western massage technique in which the practitioner comes in contact with the recipient either physically or energetically, but no perceptible movement occurs that fits into the five traditional classic Western massage categories. Two common types of touch without movement are passive touch and direct static pressure.

Traditional Asian Medicine (TAM)   is a system of healing based on Chinese medicine, and includes concepts such as yin/yang, the five elements, energy (Qi), and energy channels.

Transference   is a psychological phenomenon that occurs when clients respond to practitioners as if they were relating to someone important in their past (e.g., father), and transferring those positive or negative feelings onto the therapeutic relationship. See **counter-transference.**

Treatment   refers to interventions aimed at alleviating a specific medical condition.

Treatment model   is a concept that explains the intention of using specific interventions or modalities to alleviate medical conditions.

Trigger points   are small, hyperirritable spots in muscle or related connective tissue that may cause local pain or pain in a distant referral zone. Trigger points may be relieved manually with ischemic compression techniques, deep friction, deep stripping, and stretching. See **neuromuscular therapy (NMT).**

Vibration   is a Western massage technique category that includes oscillating, quivering, or trembling movements; or movement of soft tissues back and forth, or up and down, performed quickly and repeatedly. Vibration may be described as fine or coarse (e.g., shaking, jostling).

Wellness   refers to a condition of optimal physical, emotional, intellectual, spiritual, social, and vocational wellbeing.

Wellness massage   is massage performed with the intention of promoting the receiver's general wellbeing. It goes beyond the treatment of specific conditions to help the receiver achieve high-level wellness.

Wellness Massage Pyramid   is a model for understanding the possible contributions of massage therapy to high-level wellness. Pyramid levels from the base to the top are: treatment, recovery, prevention, neutral zone, health maintenance, personal growth, and life enjoyment.

Wellness model   is a concept that explains good health and wellbeing as aimed at living a healthy, vibrant, and meaningful life. It goes beyond the idea of health as the absence of disease and emphasizes personal responsibility. Also called the **wellness perspective.**

Western massage   is a form of soft tissue manipulation and related techniques developed in Europe and the United States over the past 200 years. The technique categories commonly used to describe Western massage are effleurage, petrissage, tapotement, friction, vibration, touch without movement, and joint movements. See **Swedish massage.**

Zen Shiatsu   is a form of Asian Bodywork Therapy from Japan developed by Shizuto Masunaga.

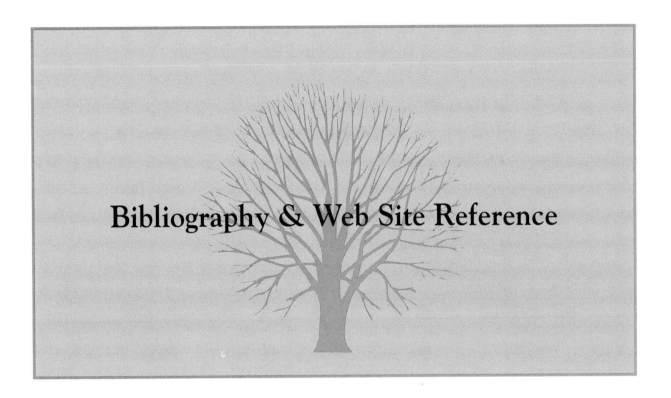

Bibliography & Web Site Reference

BOOKS AND ARTICLES

No Author

_____ *Alternative Medicine: Expanding Medical Horizons: A Report to the National Institutes of Health on Alternative Medicine Systems and Practices in the United States* (1994). Available from the Office of Alternative Medicine, National Institutes of Health, 6120 Executive Blvd., #450, Rockville, MD 20892-9904.

_____ (1996) Massage helps lower stress of working, taking final exams. In *Massage* magazine, 62 (July/August), 148.

A

AMTA (2002) *Demand for massage therapy use and acceptance increasing.* Retreved: March 2003 (*http://amtamassage.org*).

Anderson, K. N., & Anderson, L. E. (1990). *Mosby's pocket dictionary of medicine, nursing, & allied health.* St. Louis: C. V. Mosby.

Andrade, C., and P. Clifford. (2001). *Outcomes-based massage.* Philadelphia: Lippincott Williams & Wilkins.

Andrews, H. (1910). *Massage & training.* London: Health & Strength, Ltd.

Arano, L. C. (1976). *The medieval health handbook: Tacuinum sanitatis.* New York: George Braziller.

Armstrong, D., & Armstrong, E. M. (1991). *The great American medicine show: Being an illustrated history of hucksters, healers, health evangelists, and heroes from Plymouth Rock to the present.* New York: Prentice Hall.

B

Badger, C. (1986). The swollen limb. *Nursing Times* (England, 82(31), pp. 40–41.

Barclay, J. (1994) *In good hands: The history of the chartered society of physiotherapy 1894–1994.* London: Butterworth-Heinemann.

Barnes, J. F. (1987). Myofascial release. *Physical Therapy Forum*, September 16.

Barr, J. S., & N. Taslitz (1970). Influence of back massage on autonomic functions. *Physical Therapy, 50*, pp. 1679–1691.

Bauer, W. C., & Dracup, K. A. (1987). Physiological effects of back massage in patients with acute myocardial infarction. *Focus on Critical Care, 14*(6), pp. 42–46.

Baumgartner, A. J. (1947). *Massage in athletics.* Minneapolis, MN: Burgess.

Beals, K. R. (1978). Clubfoot in the Maori: A genetic study of 50 kindreds. *New Zealand Medical Journal, 88*, pp. 144–146.

Beard, G., & Wood, E. C. (1964). *Massage principles and techniques.* Philadelphia: W. B. Saunders.

Belanger, A.-Y. (2002). *Evidenced-based guide to therapeutic physical agents*. Philadelphia: Lippincott Williams & Wilkins.

Bell, A. J. (1964). Massage and the physiotherapist. *Physiotherapy, 50,* 406–408.

Benjamin, B. E. (1995). Massage and body work with survivors of abuse: Part I. *Massage Therapy Journal, 34*(3), pp. 23–32.

Benjamin, B. E., & Sohnen-Moe, C. (2003). *The ethics of touch*. Tuscon, AZ: SMA Inc.

Benjamin, P. J. (1989a). Eunice Ingham and the development of foot reflexology in the United States. Part one: The early years—to 1946. *Massage Therapy Journal,* Spring, pp. 38–44.

Benjamin, P. J. (1989b). Eunice Ingham and the development of foot reflexology in the United States. Part two: On the road, 1946–1974. *Massage Therapy Journal,* Winter, pp. 49–55.

Benjamin, P. J. (1993). Massage therapy in the 1940's and the College of Swedish Massage in Chicago. *Massage Therapy Journal, 32*(4), pp. 56–62.

Benjamin, P. J. (1994). *On-site therapeutic massage: Investment for a healthy business*. Information brochure. Rockford, IL: Hemingway Publications.

Benjamin, P. J. (1996). The California revival: Massage therapy in the 1970–80's. Presentation at the AMTA National Education Conference in Los Angeles, CA, June 1996.

Benjamin, P. J. (2002). Shampooing—A journey to the East. *Massage Therapy Journal, 41*(2), pp. 140–144.

Benjamin, P. J., & Lamp, S. P. (1996). *Understanding sports massage*. Champaign, IL: Human Kinetics.

Beresford-Cooke, C. (1999). *Shiatsu theory and practice*. Edinburgh: Churchill Livingstone.

Berube, R. (1988). *Evolutionary traditions: Unique approaches to lymphatic drainage & circulatory massage techniques*. Hudson, NH: Robert Berube.

Bilz, F. E. (1898). *The natural method of healing: A new and complete guide to health*. Translated from the latest German edition. Leipiz: F. E. Bilz.

Bohm, M. (1913). *Massage: Its principles and techniques*. Translated by Elizabeth Gould. Philadelphia: Lippincott.

Brown, C. C., ed. (1984). *The many facets of touch*. Johnson & Johnson Baby Products Company.

Beeken, J., et al. (1998) Effectiveness of neuromuscular release massage therapy on chronic obstructive lung disease. *Clinical Nursing Research. 7*(3), pp. 309–325.

Bunce, I. H., Mirolo, B. R., Hennessy, J. M., et al. (1994). Post-mastectomy lymphedema treatment and measurement. *Medical Journal,* Australia, *161,* pp. 125–128.

Byers, D. C. (1997). *Better health with foot reflexology*. Revised. St. Petersburg, FL: Ingham Publishing.

C

Cady, S. H., & G. E. Jones. (1997) Massage therapy as a workplace intervention for reduction of stress. *Perceptual and Motor Skills, 84*(1), pp. 157–158.

Cailliet, R. (1981). *Shoulder pain*, 2nd ed. Philadelphia: F. A. Davis.

Calvert, R. N. (2002). *The history of massage: An illustrated survey from around the world*. Rochester, VT: Healing Arts Press.

Cantu, R. I., & Grodin, A. J. (1992). *Myofascial manipulation: Theory and clinical application*. Gaithersburg, MD: Aspen Publishers.

Capra, F. (1984). *The Tao of physics*. New York: Bantam Books.

Chaitow, L. (1996). *Modern neuromuscular techniques*. London: Churchill Livingston.

Chamness, A. (1996). Breast cancer and massage therapy. *Massage Therapy Journal, 35*(1, Winter) pp. 44–46.

Cheng, X. (1993) *Chinese Acupuncture and Moxibustion,* Beijing, China: Foreign Languages Press.

Cherkin, D. C., Eisenberg, D. et al. (2001). Randomized trial comparing traditonal Chinese medical acupuncture, therapeutic massage, and self-care education for chronic low back pain. *Archives of Internal Medicine 161*(8), pp. 1081–1088.

Chopra, D. (1991). *Perfect health: The complete mind/body guide*. New York: Harmony Books.

Claire, T. (1995). *Bodywork: What type of massage to get, and how to make the most of it*. New York: William Morrow.

Collinge, W. (1996). *The American Holistic Health Association complete guide to alternative medicine*. New York: Warner Books.

Connelly, D. (1979). *Traditional acupuncture: The law of the Five Elements*. Columbia, Maryland: The Center for Traditional Acupuncture.

Corwin, E. J. (1996). *Handbook of pathophysiology*. Philadelphia: Lippincott.

Crosman, L. J., Chateauvert, S. R., & Weisburg, J. (1985). The effects of massage to the hamstring muscle group on range of motion. *Massage Journal,* pp. 59–62.

Croutier, A. L. (1992) *Taking the waters: Spirit, art, sensuality*. New York: Abbeyville Press.

Cunliffe, B. (1978). *The Roman baths: A guide to the baths and Roman museum*. City of Bath: Bath Archeological Trust.

Curties, D. (1999) *Breast massage*. Moncton, New Brunswick, Canada: Curties-Overzet Publications.

Curties, D. (1994). Could massage therapy promote cancer metastasis. *Journal of Soft Tissue Manipulation,* April–May.

Curties, D. (1999) *Massage therapy and cancer*. Toronto, Canada: Curties-Overzet Publications.

Curtis, M. (1994) The use of massage in restoring cardiac rhythm. *Nursing Times* (England), *90*(38), pp. 36–37.

Cyriax, J. H., & Cyriax, P. J. (1993). *Illustrated manual of orthopedic medicine*, 2nd ed. Boston: Butterworth & Heinemann.

D

Deadman, P. (1998). *A manual of acupuncture*. East Sussex, England: Journal of Chinese Medicine Publications.

de Bruijn, R. (1984). Deep transverse friction: Its analgesic effect. *International Journal of Sports Medicine, 5*, pp. 35–36.

DeDomenico, G. & Wood, E. C. (1997). *Beard's massage*. 4th Ed. Philadelphia, W. B. Saunders.

Dieter, J. N. I., & E. K. Emory (2002). "Supplemental tactile and kinesthetic stimulation for preterm infants." Chapter 7 in *Massage therapy: The evidence for practice*. Rich, G. J., Editor. New York: Mosby.

Dixon, Marian W. (2001). *Body mechanics and self-care manual*. Upper Saddle River, NJ: Prentice Hall.

Downing, G. (1972). *The massage book*. New York: Random House.

Drinker, C. K., & Yoffey, J. M. (1941). *Lymphatics, lymph and lymphoid tissue: Their physiological and clinical significance*. Cambridge: Harvard University Press.

Dychtwald, K. (1977). *Body-mind*. New York: Jove Publications.

E

Eisenberg, D. M., Kessler, R. C., Foster, C., Norlock, F. E., Calkins, D. R., & Delblanco, T. L. (1993). Unconventional medicine in the United States. *New England Journal of Medicine, 328*(4), pp. 246–252.

Eisenberg, D. M., Davis, R. B., Ettner, S. L. et al. (1998). Trends in alternative medicine use in the United States, 1990–1997. *Journal of the American Medical Association, 280* (18), pp. 1569–1575.

Elkins, E. C., Herrick, J. F., Grindlay, J. H., et al. (1953). Effects of various procedures on the flow of lymph. *Archives of Physical Medicine, 34*, 31.

Ellis, V., Hill, J. & Campbell, H. (1995) Strengthening the family unity through the healing power of massage. *Journal of Hospice & Palliative Care*, V12, pp. 19–20.

Evans, W., & Rosenberg, E. H. (1991). *Biomarkers*. New York: Simon & Schuster.

F

Fakouri, C., & Jones, P. (1987). Relaxation ℞: Slow stroke back rub. *Journal of Gerontological Nursing, 13*(2), pp. 32–35.

Fanslow, C. (1984). Touch and the elderly. In *The many facets of touch*, edited by C. C. Brown. Skillman, NJ: Johnson & Johnson Baby Products Company.

Fay, H. J. (1916). *Scientific massage for athletes*. London: Ewart, Seymour & Co.

Ferrell-Torry, A. T., & Glick, O. J. (1993). The use of therapeutic massage as a nursing intervention to modify anxiety and the perception of cancer pain. *Cancer Nursing, 16*(2), pp. 93–101.

Field, T. (2000) *Touch therapy*. New York: Churchill Livingston.

Field, T. (2001) *Touch*. Cambridge, MA: The MIT Press.

Field, T., Fox, N., Pickens, J., Ironsong, G., & Scafidi, F. (1993). Job stress survey. Unpublished manuscript. Touch Research Institute, University of Miami School of Medicine. Reported in *Touchpoints: Touch Research Abstracts, 1*(1).

Field, T., Hernandez-Reif, M., Hart, S., Teakston, H. (1999). "Pregnant women benefit from massage therapy." *Journal of Psychosomatic Obstetrics and Gynecology, 20*, pp. 31–38.

Field, T., Hernandez-Reif, M., Taylor, S., Quintino, O., Burman, I. (1997) "Labor pain is reduced by massage therapy." *Journal of Psychosomatic Obstetrics and Gynecology.* 18, pp. 286–291.

Field, T., Morrow, C., Valdeon, C., et al. (1992). Massage reduces anxiety in child and adolescent psychiatric patients. *Journal of the American Academy of Child and Adolescent Psychiatry, 31*(1), pp. 125–131.

Field, T., Schanberg, S. M., Scafidi, F., et al. (1986). Tactile/kinesthetic stimulation effects on preterm neonates. *Pediatrics, 77*(5), pp. 654–658.

Fitzgerald, W. H & Bowers, E. F. (1917) *Zone therapy*. Columbus, OH: I. W. Long.

Ford, C. W. (1989). *Where healing waters meet: Touching mind & emotion through the body*. Barrytown, NY: Station Hill Press.

Ford, C. W. (1993). *Compassionate touch: The role of human touch in healing and recovery*. New York: A Fireside/Parkside book.

Frazer, J., & Kerr, J. R. (1993). Psychophysiological effects of back massage on elderly institutionalized patients. *Journal of Advanced Nursing, 18*, pp. 238–245.

Frierwood, H. T. (1953). The place of the health service in the total YMCA program. *Journal of Physical Education, 21*.

Frye, B. (2000) *Body mechanics for manual therapists: A functional approach to self-care and injury prevention*. Stanwood, WA: Freytag Publishing.

G

Gach, M. R. (1990). *Acupressure's potent points: A guide to self-care for common ailments*. New York: Bantam Books.

Georgii, A. (1880). *Kinetic jottings*. London: Henry Renshaw.

Gordon, R. (1979). *Your healing hands: The polarity experience*. Santa Cruz, CA: Unity Press.

Grafstrom, A. (1904). *A text-book of mechano-therapy (massage and medical gymnastics), prepared for the use of medical students, trained nurses, and medical gymnasts*. Philadelphia: W. B. Saunders.

Graham, D. (1884). *Practical treatise on massage*. New York: Wm. Wood and Co.

Graham, D. (1902). *A treatise on massage, its history, mode of application and effects.* Philadelphia: Lippincott.

Graham, R. L. (1923). *Hydro-hygiene: The science of curing by water.* New York: The Thompson-Barlow Company.

Greene, E. (1996). Study links stress reduction with faster healing. *Massage Therapy Journal, 35*(1), p. 16.

H

Hammer, W. I. (1993) The use of transverse friction massage in the management of chronic bursitis of the hip and shoulder. *Journal of Manipulation and Physical Therapy, 16*(2), pp. 107–111.

Hecox, B., Mehreteab, T.A., Weisberg, J. (1994). *Physical agents: A comprehensive text for physical therapists.* Norwalk, CT: Appleton & Lange.

Heidt, P. (1981). Effect of therapeutic touch on anxiety level of hospitalized patients. *Nursing Research, 30*(1), pp. 32–37.

Henshall, K. (1992). *A Guide to Remembering Japanese Characters.* Rutland, Vermont: Charles E. Tuttle Company.

Hodge, M., Robinson, C., Boehmer, J., & Klein, S. (2002). "Employee outcomes following work-site acupressure and massage." Chapter 9 in *Massage therapy: The evidence for practice.* New York: Mosby.

Hoffa, A. J. (1900). *Technik der massage,* 3rd ed. Verlagsbuchhandlung, Stuttgart: Ferdinand. Enke. As translated by F. M. Tappan and Ruth Friedlander.

Howdyshell, C. (1998). Complementary therapy: Aromatherapy with massage for geriatric and hospice care for a holistic approach. *Hospice Journal,* V.13, pp. 69–75.

Hoffa, A. (1978). *Technik der massage* (13th ed). Stuttgart, Germany: Ferdinand Enke. Translated for Fran Tappan by Ruth Friedlander.

Huitt, W. G. (2002). Maslow's hierarchy of needs. Retrieved: March 2003 (*http://chiron.valdosta.edu/whuitt/col/regsys/maslow.html*).

I

Ingham, E. D. (1938). *Stories the feet can tell: Stepping to better health.* Rochester, NY, author.

Ironson, G., Field, T. et al. (1996). Massage therapy is associated with enhancement of the immune system's cytotoxic capacity. *International Journal of Neuroscience, 84,* pp. 205–217.

J

Jarmey, C. and Mojay, G. (1991). *Shiatsu: The complete guide,* Hammersmith, London: Thorsons.

Jarrett. L. (2000). *Nourishing destiny: The inner tradition of Chinese medicine,* Stockbridge, Massachusetts: Spirit Path Press.

Joachim, G. (1983). The effects of two stress management techniques on feelings of well-being in patients with inflammatory bowel disease. *Nursing Papers, 15*(5), p. 18.

Johari, H. (1996). *Ayurvedic massage: Traditional Indian techniques for balancing body and mind.* Rochester, VT: Healing Arts Press.

Johnson, W. (1866). *The anatriptic art.* London: Simpkin, Marshall & Co.

Joya, M. (1958). *Mock Joya's things Japanese.* Tokyo: Tokyo News Service, Ltd.

Juhan, D. (1987). *Job's body: A handbook for bodywork.* Barrytown, NY: Station Hill Press.

K

Kaard, B., & Tostinbo, O. (1989). Increase of plasma beta endorphins in a connective tissue massage. *General Pharmacology, 20*(4), pp. 487–489.

Karpen, M. (1995). Dolores Kreiger, PhD, RN: Tireless teacher of Therapeutic Touch. *Alternative & Complementary Therapies,* April/May, pp. 142–146.

Kasseroller, R. (1998). *Compendium of Dr. Vodder's Manual Lymph Drainage.* Heidelberg: Karl F. Haug Verlag.

Keller, E., & Bzdek, V. M. (1986). Effects of therapeutic touch on tension headache pain. *Nursing Research, 35*(2), pp. 101–106.

Kellogg, J. H. (1923). *The art of massage.* Battle Creek, MI: Modern Medicine Publishing Co.

Kellogg, J. H. (1929). *The art of massage: A practical manual for the nurse, the student and the practitioner.* Battle Creek, MI: Modern Medicine Publishing Co.

Kelly, D. G. (2002) *A primer on lymphedema.* Upper Saddle River, NJ: Prentice Hall.

King, R. K. (1996). *Myofascial massage therapy: Towards postural balance.* Self-published training manual by Bobkat Productions, Chicago.

Kleen, E. A. (1921). *Massage and medical gymnastics.* New York: William Wood & Company.

Knaster, M. (1996). *Discovering the body's wisdom: A comprehensive guide to more than fifty mind-body practices.* New York: Bantam Books.

Knight, K. L. (1995). *Cryotherapy in sport injury management.* Champaign, IL: Human Kinetics.

Kramer, N. A. (1990). Comparison of therapeutic touch and casual touch in stress reduction of hospitalized children. *Pediatric Nursing, 16*(5), pp. 483–485.

Kresge, C. A. (1983). Massage and sports. In O. Appenzeller & R. Atkinson (eds.) *Sports medicine: Fitness, training, injuries* (pp. 367–380). Baltimore: Urban & Schwarzenberg.

Kunz, K. and Kunz, B. (1991). *The complete guide to foot reflexology.* Revised. Englewood Cliffs, NJ: Prentice Hall Trade.

Kurz, I. (1986). *Introduction to Dr. Vodder's manual lymphatic drainage.* Vol. 2, Therapy 1. Heidelberg: Haug Publishers.

Kurz, I. (1990). *Introduction to Dr. Vodder's manual lymphatic drainage.* Vol. 3, Therapy 2. Heidelberg: Haug Publishers.

Kurz, W., Wittlinger, G., Litmanovitch, Y. I., et al. (1978). Effect of manual lymph drainage massage on urinary excretion of neurohormones and minerals in chronic lyphedema. *Angiology, 29,* pp. 64–72.

L

Leboyer, F. (1982). *Loving hands: The traditional art of baby massage.* New York: Alfred A. Knopf.

Leonard, G. (1988). *Walking on the edge of the world: A memoir of the sixties and beyond.* Boston: Houghton Mifflin.

Ling, P. H. (1840a). The general principles of gymnastics. In *The collected works of P. H. Ling.* (1866). Stockholm, Sweden. Translated by Lars Agren and Patricia J. Benjamin. Unpublished.

Ling, P. H. (1840b). Notations to the general principles. In *The collected works of P. H. Ling.* (1866). Stockholm, Sweden. Translated by Lars Agren and Patricia J. Benjamin and published in *Massage Therapy Journal,* Winter 1987.

Ling P. H. (1840c). The means or vehicle of gymnastics. Translated by R. J. Cyriax. In *American Physical Education Review, 19*(4), April 1914.

Longworth, J. D. (1982). Psychophysiological effects of slow stroke back massage in normotensive females. *Advances in Nursing Science 4,* pp. 44–61.

Lundberg, P. (1992). *The book of shiatsu.* New York: Simon & Schuster.

M

MacDonald, G. (1999). *Medicine hands: Massage therapy for people with cancer.* Tallahassee, FL: Findhorn Press.

MacDonald, G. (1995). Massage for cancer patients: A review of nursing research. *Massage Therapy Journal,* Summer, 53–56.

Maciocia, G. (1998) *The Foundations of Chinese Medicine: A Comprehensive Text for Acupuncturists and Herbalists.* Edinburgh: Churchill Livingstone.

Maciocia, G. (1994). *The Practice of Chinese Medicine: The Treatment of Diseases with Acupuncture and Chinese Herbs.* Edinburgh: Churchill Livingstone.

MacKenzie, J. (1923) *Angina pectoris.* London: Henry Frowde and Hodder and Stoughton.

Manheim, C. (2001) *The myofascial release manual,* 3rd edition. Thorofare, NJ: Slack Inc.

Martini, F. H., & Bartholomew, M. S. (1999). *Structure and function of the human body.* Upper Saddle River, NJ: Prentice-Hall.

Masunaga, S. (1983). *Keiraku to shiatsu.* Yokosuka: Ido-No-Nihonsha.

Masunaga, S. & Ohashi, W. (1977). *Zen shiatsu: How to harmonize Yin and Yang for better health.* Tokyo: Japan Publications.

McIntosh, N. (1999) *The educated heart: Professional guidelines for massage therapists, bodyworkers and movement teachers.* Memphis, TN: Decatur Bainbridge Press.

McKenzie, R. T. (1915). *Exercise in education and medicine,* 2nd ed. Philadelphia: W. B. Saunders.

McMillan, M. (1921). *Massage and therapeutic exercise.* Philadelphia: W. B. Saunders.

McMillan, M. (1925). *Massage and therapeutic exercise,* 2nd ed. Philadelphia: W. B. Saunders.

Menard, M. B. (2003) *Making sense of research: A guide to research literacy for complementary practitioners.* Toronto: Curties-Overzet Publications.

Mennell, J. B. (1945). *Physical treatment,* 5th ed. Philadelphia: Blakiston.

Mense, S. & D. G. Simons. (2001) "Myofascial pain caused by trigger points." Chapter 9 in *Muscle pain: Understanding its nature, diagnosis, and treatment.* Philadelphia: Lippincott, Williams & Wilkins.

Miesler, D. W. (1990). *Geriatric massage techniques: Topics for bodyworkers no. 2.* Guerneville, CA: Day-Break Productions.

Miller, E. T. (1996). *Day Spa Techniques.* Albany, NY: Milady Publications.

Mitchell, J. K. (1894). The effect of massage on the number and haemoglobin value of the red blood cells. *American Journal of Medical Science, 107,* pp. 502–515.

M'Lean, T. (1814). *Picturesque representations of the dress and manners of the Chinese.* London: Howlett and Brimmer.

Monastersky, R. (2002) "Plumbing ancient rituals: Sweatbaths in Maya cities provide a window into lives long ago." *The Chronicle of Higher Education.* 17 May 2002, pp. A22–23.

Monte, T., & the Editors of East West Natural Health (1993). *World medicine: The East West guide to healing your body.* New York: Putnam.

Montague, A. (1978). *Touching: The human significance of the skin,* 2nd ed. New York: Harper & Row.

Mortimer, P. S., Simmonds, R., Rezvani, M., et al. (1990). The measurement of skin lymph flow by isotope clearance: Reliability, reproducibility, injection dynamics, and the effects of massage. *Journal of Investigative Dermatology, 95,* pp. 666–682.

Moyers, B. (1993) "The Mystery of Chi." Volume 1: *Healing and the Mind*. Video series. Ambrose Video.

Murphy, W. (Ed.) (1995). *Healing the generations: A history of physical therapy and the American Physical Therapy Association*. Lyme, CT: Greenwich Publishing Group.

Murrell, W. (1890). *Massotherapeutics or massage as a mode of treatment*. Philadelphia: Blakiston.

N

Namikoshi, Toru. (1969) *Shiatsu: Japanese finger-pressure*. Tokyo: Japan Publications.

Namikoshi, T. (1981). *The complete book of shiatsu therapy*. Tokyo: Japan Publications.

National Certification Board for Therapeutic Massage and Bodywork (2000) *Standards of Practice*. Retrieved March 2003 (*www.ncbtmb.org*).

Nelson, D. (1994). *Compassionate touch: Hands-on caregiving for the elderly, the ill, and the dying*. Barrytown, NY: Station Hill Press.

Nelson, Dawn. (2001). *From the heart through the hands: The power of touch in caregiving*. Forres, Scotland: Findhorn Press.

Ni, M. (1995). *The Yellow Emperor's classic of medicine: A new translation of the Nei Jing Suwen with commentary*. Boston: Shambhala.

Nissen, H. (1889). *A manual of instruction for giving Swedish movement and massage treatment*. Philadelphia: F. A. Davis.

Nissen, H. (1920). *Practical massage and corrective exercises with applied anatomy*. Philadelphia: F. A. Davis.

Norman, L. & Cowan, T. (1988) *Feet first: A guide to foot reflexology*. New York: Fireside.

O

Ohashi, W. (1976). *Do-it-yourself shiatsu*. New York: E. P. Dutton.

Older, J. (1982). *Touching is healing*. New York: Stein & Day.

Omura, Y. (1982). *Acupuncture medicine*. Tokyo: Japan Publications.

Ostrom, K. W. (1905). *Massage and the original Swedish movements*. Philadelphia: Blakiston.

P

Palmer, D. (1995). The death of on-site massage? *Massage Therapy Journal, 34*(3), pp. 119–120.

Palmer, D. (1995). What is Kata? *TouchPro massage manual*. San Francisco: Skilled Touch Institute of Chair Massage.

Pemberton, R. (1939). Physiology of Massage. In *American Medical Association Handbook of Physical Therapy*, 3rd ed. Chicago: Council of Physical Therapy.

Perrone, B., Stockel, H. H., & Krueger, V. (1989). *Medicine women, curanderas, and women doctors*. Norman, OK: University of Oklahoma Press.

Persad, R. (2001). *Massage therapy & medications: General treatment principles*. Toronto: Curties-Overzet Publications.

Premkumar, K. (1999). *Pathology A to Z—A handbook for massage therapists*. Calgary, Canada: VanPub Books.

Pollard, D. W. (1902). Massage in training. An unpublished thesis, International Young Men's Christian Association Training School, Springfield, MA.

Posse, N. (1895). *The special kinesiology of educational gymnastics*. Boston: Lothrop, Lee & Shepard.

Preyde, M. Effectiveness of massage therapy for subacute low-back pain: A randomized controlled trial. *CMAJ, 162*(13), pp. 1815–1820.

Prudden, B. (1980). *Pain erasure: The Bonnie Prudden way*. New York: M. Evans.

Prudden, B. (1984). *Myotherapy: Bonnie Prudden's complete guide to pain-free living*. New York: Ballantine Books.

Puustjarvi, K., Airaksinen, O., and P. J. Pontinen. (1990) The effects of massage in patients with chronic tension headache. *Acupuncture Electrotherapy Research, 15*(2), pp. 159–162.

R

Rattray, F. S. (1994). *Massage therapy: An approach to treatments*. Toronto, Ontario: Massage Therapy Texts and MA Verick Consultants.

Rattray, F., and L. Ludwig. (2000). *Clinical massage therapy: Understanding, assessing and treating over 700 conditions*. Toronto, Canada: Talus Incorporated.

Reihl, S. (2001). "Beginning myofascial release." Instructional video produced by Real Bodywork.

Remington, R. (2002). "Hand massage in the agitated elderly." Chapter 8 in *Massage therapy: The evidence for practice* by G. J. Rich, editor. New York: Mosby.

Rhiner, M., Ferrell, B. R., Ferrell, B. A., & Grant, M. M. (1993). A structured non-drug intervention program for cancer pain. *Cancer Practice, 1*, pp. 137–143.

Rich, G. J. (2002) *Massage therapy: The evidence for practice*. New York: Mosby.

Robbins, G., Powers, D., & Burgess, S. (1994). *A wellness way of life*, 2nd ed. Madison, WI: Brown & Benchmark.

Roth, M. (1851). *The prevention and cure of many chronic diseases by movements.* London: John Churchill.

Ruebottom, A., Lee, C., Dryden, P. J. (1989). Massage for terminally ill AIDS patients. *International Conference on AIDS,* June.

S

Sampson, C. W. (1926). *A practice of physiotherapy.* St. Louis: C. V. Mosby.

Scheumann, D.W. (2002). *The balanced body: A guide to deep tissue and neuromuscular therapy.* 2nd edition. Philadelphia: Lippincott, Williams & Wilkins.

Schneider, Vimala (2000). *Infant massage: A handbook for loving parents.* New York: Bantam Books.

Schultz, R. L., and R. Feitis. (1996). *The endless web: Fascial anatomy and physical reality.* Berkeley, CA: North Atlantic Books.

Seiger, L., Vanderpool, K., & Barnes, D. (1995). *Fitness and wellness strategies.* Madison, WI: Brown & Benchmark.

Serizawa, K. (1972). *Massage, the oriental method.* Tokyo: Japan Publications.

Serizawa, K. (1976). *Effective tsubo therapy.* Tokyo: Japan Publications.

Serizawa, K. (1984). *Tsubo: Vital points for oriental therapy.* Tokyo: Japan Publications.

Siedman, M. (1982). *Like a hollow flute: A guide to polarity therapy.* Santa Cruz, CA: Elan Press.

Siegel, A. (1986). *Live energy: The power that heals.* Bridgeport, Dorset, England: Prism Press/Colin Spooner.

Sills, Franklin. (2002). *The polarity process: Energy as a healing art.* Berkeley, CA: North Atlantic Books.

Sims, S. (1986). Slow stroke back massage for cancer patients. *Nursing Times, 82,* pp. 47–50.

Stillerman, E. (1992). *Mother-massage: A handbook for relieving the discomforts of pregnancy.* New York: Delta/Delcorte.

Stone, Randolph. (1987). *Dr. Randolph Stone's Polarity Therapy: The complete collected works.* Harlan Tarbell, Illustrator. Sebastopol, CA: CRCS Publications.

Stone, Randolph. (1991) *Health building: The conscious art of living well.* Sebastopol, CA: CRCS Publications.

Sunshine, W., Field, T., et al. (1996) Fibromyalgia benefits from massage therapy and transcutaneous electrical stimulation. *Journal of Clinical Rheum. 2*(1), pp. 18–22.

T

Tedeschi, M. (2000). *Essential anatomy for healing and the martial arts.* Tokyo: Weatherwill.

Teeguarden, I. M. (1978). *Acupressure way of health: Jin Shin Do.* New York/Tokyo: Japan Publications (distributed by Putnam).

Teeguarden, I. M. (1985). Acupressure in the classroom. *East West Journal, 15* (August), p. 22.

Teeguarden, I. M. (1981). *Jin Shin Do handbook,* 2nd ed. Felton, CA: Jin Shin Do Foundation.

Teeguarden, I. M. (1987). *Joy of feeling: Bodymind acupressure.* New York/Tokyo: Japan Publications (distributed by Putnam). Harper & Row.

Teeguarden, I. M. (1996). *A complete guide to acupressure.* New York/Tokyo: Japan Publications (distributed by Putnam).

Thomas, C. L. (ed.) (1985). *Taber's cyclopedic medical dictionary.* Philadelphia: F. A. Davis.

Time-Life Books (1987). *The age of god-kings: Timeframe 3000–1500 B.C.* Alexandria, VA: Time-Life Books.

Tope, D. M., Hann, D. M., & Pinkson, B. (1994). Massage therapy: An old intervention comes of age. *Quality of Life—A Nursing Challenge, 3,* pp. 14–18.

Torres, E. (no date). *The folk healer: The Mexican-American tradition of curanderismo.* Kingsville, TX: Nieves Press.

Travell, J. G., & Rinzler, S. H. (1952). The myofascial genesis of pain. *Postgraduate Medicine,* 11, pp. 425–434.

Travell, J. G., & Simons, D. G. (1983). *Myofascial pain and dysfunction: The trigger point manual.* Baltimore: Williams & Wilkins.

Travell, J. G., & Simons, D. G. (1999). *Myofascial pain and dysfunction: The trigger point manual, Volume 1—Upper half of the body.* 2nd ed. Baltimore: Williams & Wilkins.

Travell, J. G., & Simons, D. G. (1992). *Myofascial pain and dysfunction: The trigger point manual, Volume 2—The lower extremities.* Baltimore: Williams & Wilkins.

Travis, J. W., & Ryan, R. S. (2000). *Wellness workbook.* 2nd edition. Berkeley, CA: Ten Speed Press.

W

Wang, J. (1994). *The history of massage in mainland China.* American Organization for Bodywork Therapies of Asia (AOBTA), Video #13, Boston, MA convention.

Wang, J. (1999), "To treat before sick" from *Pulse,* Voorhees, NJ: AOBTA.

Weinrich, S. P., & Weinrich, M. C. (1990). The effect of massage on pain in cancer patients. *Applied Nursing Research, 3,* pp. 140–145.

Werner, R. (2000). *Massage therapists guide to pathology.* 2nd ed. Philadelphia: Lippincott Williams & Wilkins.

Wheeden, A., Scafidi, F., Field, T., et al. (1993). Massage effects on cocaine-exposed preterm neonates. *Developmental and Behavioral Pediatrics*, *14*(5), pp. 318–322.

White House Commission on Complementary and Alternative Medicine Policy (2002). *Final Report*. Department of Health and Human Services (*www.whccamp.hhs.gov*).

Witt, P. L., & MacKinnon, J. (1986). Trager psychosocial integration: a method to improve chest mobility of patients with chronic lung disease. *Physical Therapy*, *66*(2), pp. 214–217.

Wittinger, H., & Wittinger, G. (1986). *Introduction to Dr. Vodder's manual lymphatic drainage*. Vol. 1, 3rd rev. ed. Heidelberg: Haug Publishers.

Wood, E. C., & Becker, P. D. (1981). *Beard's massage*, 3rd ed. Philadelphia: W. B. Saunders.

Y

Yates, J. (1999). *A physician's guide to therapeutic massage: Its physiological effects and treatment applications*. 2nd edition. Vancouver, BC: Massage Therapists' Association of British Columbia.

Yuen, J. (2001) *Light on the essence of Chinese medicine: The Nei Jing Su Wen*, New England School of Acupuncture, Boston, MA.

Z

Zanolla, R., Monzeglio, C., Balzarini, A., & Martino, G. (1984). Evaluation of the results of three different methods of postmastectomy lymphedema treatment. *Journal of Surgical Oncology*, *26*, pp. 210–213.

Zeitlin, D., et al. (2000). Immunological effects of massage therapy during academic stress. *Psychosomatic Medicine*, *62*, pp. 83–87.

Zukav, G. (1979). *The dancing Wu Li masters: An overview of the new physics*. New York: Bantam Books.

Web Sites

Academy of Lymphatic Studies in Sebastian, Florida (www.acols.com)

Aging Research Centre (ARC) (ww.arclab.org)

Alexander Technique (www.alexandertechnique.com)

Alexander Technique International (www.ati-net.com)

American Massage Therapy Association (www.amtamassage.org)

American Organization for Bodywork Therapies of Asia (www.aobta.org)

American Polarity Therapy Association (www.polaritytherapy.org)

American Society for Alexander Technique (www.alexandertech.org)

American Society on Aging (www.asaging.org)

AMTA Foundation—Research Database (www.amtafoundation.org)

Associated Bodywork & Massage Professionals (www.abmp.com)

Bonnie Prudden Myotherapy (www.bonnieprudden.com)

Canadian Massage Therapist Alliance (www.cmta.ca)

Canadian Touch Research Center (ww.ccrt-ctrc.org)

Center to Advance Palliative Care (ww.capc.org)

Commission on Massage Therapy Accreditation (www.comta.org)

Craniosacral Therapy Association of North America (craniosacraltherapy.org)

Day-Break Geriatric Massage Institute (www.daybreak-massage.com)

Dr Vodder School North America in Victoria, BC, Canada (www.vodderschool.com)

Esalen Institute (www.esalen.org)

Feldenkrais Guild of North America (www.feldenkrais.com)

HIPAA Privacy Guidelines (ww.hhs.gov/ocr/hipaa)

Home of Reflexology (ww.reflexology.org)

Institute of Thai Massage (www.thai-massage.org)

International Association of Infant Massage Instructors (www.iaimi.com)

International Feldenkrais Federation (www.feldenkrais-method.org)

International Institute of Infant Massage (www.infantmassageinstitute.com)

International Institute of Reflexology (www.reflexology-usa.net)

International Loving Touch Foundation (www.lovingtouch.com)

International Spa Association (www.experienceispa.com)

Jin Shin Do® Foundation (www.jinshindo.org)

Lymphatic Research Foundation (www.lymphaticresearch.org)

Massage magazine (www.massagemag.com)

Massage & Bodywork Magazine (www.massageandbodywork.com)

Massage Therapy Canada (www.massagetherapycanada.com)

Massage Therapy Journal (www.amtamassage.org)

Massage Today (www.massagetoday.com)

Myofascial Release. Com (www.myofascial-release.com)

National Association for Holistic Aromatherapy (www.naha.org)

National Association of Nurse Massage Therapists (www.nanmt.org)

National Center of Complementary and Alternative Medicine at NIH, Washington D.C. (www.nccam.nih.gov)

National Certification Board for Therapeutic Massage and Bodywork (www.ncbtmb.com)

National Certification Commission for Acupuncture and Oriental Medicine (www.nccaom.org)

National Council on Aging (NCOA) (www.ncoa.org)

National Hospice and Palliative Care Organization (www.nhpco.org)

National Hospice Foundation (www.hospiceinfo.org)

National Institute on Aging at the National Institutes of Health (www.nia.nih.gov)

National Library of Medicine (www.ncbi.nlm.nih.gov/PubMed)

National Lymphedema Network (www.lymphnet.org)

Nurse Healers-Professional Associates International (www.therapeutic-touch.org)

Reflexology Research Project (www.reflexology-reseach.com)

Rolf Institute of Structural Integration (www.rolf.org)

TouchPro Institute (www.touchpro.org)

Touch Research Institute at the University of Miami (www.miami.edu/touch-research)

Trager International (www.trager.com)

Upledger Institute (www.upledger.com)

U.S. Administration on Aging (AoA) (www.aoa.gov)

Wellness Associates (www.thewellspring.com)

White House Commission on CAM Policy Report (www.whccamp.hhs.gov)

World of Massage Museum (www.worldofmassagemuseum.org)

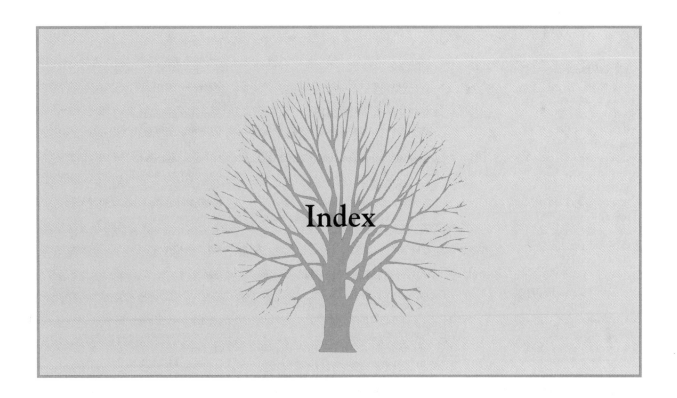

Index

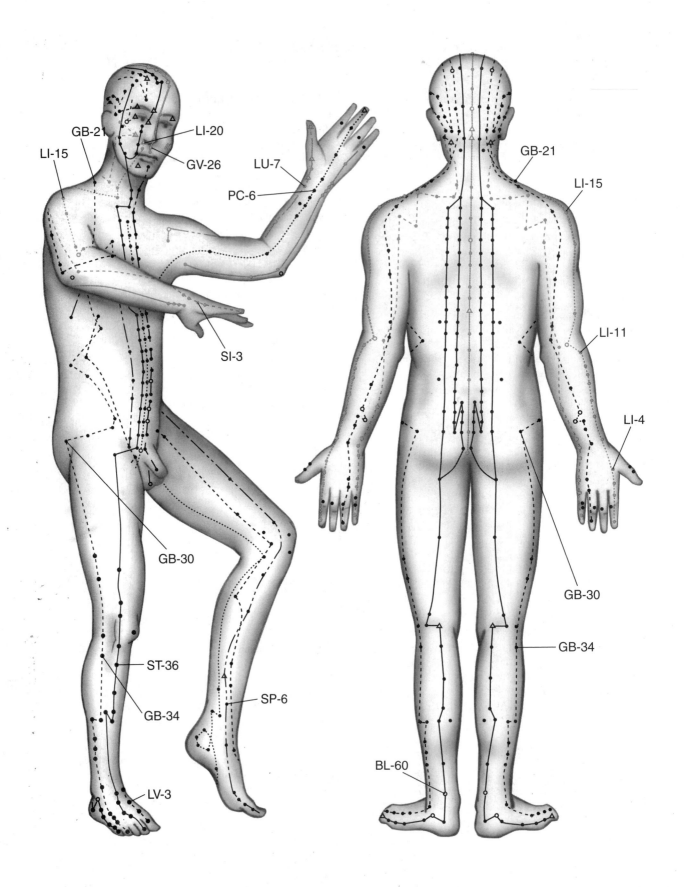